Computer-Aided Drug Discovery and Design: Theory, Methods and Applications

Computer-Aided Drug Discovery and Design: Theory, Methods and Applications

Editor: Holly Lambert

AMERICAN
MEDICAL PUBLISHERS
www.americanmedicalpublishers.com

AMERICAN
MEDICAL PUBLISHERS
www.americanmedicalpublishers.com

Cataloging-in-Publication Data

Computer-aided drug discovery and design : theory, methods and applications / edited by Holly Lambert.
p. cm.
Includes bibliographical references and index.
ISBN 979-8-88740-020-4
1. Drug development--Data processing. 2. Drugs--Computer-aided design. 3. Drugs--Design--Data processing.
4. Pharmaceutical technology. 5. Pharmacology--Data processing. I. Lambert, Holly.
RM301.25 .C663 2023
615.19--dc23

American Medical Publishers,
41 Flatbush Avenue,
1st Floor, New York,
NY 11217, USA

ISBN 979-8-88740-020-4 (Hardback)

Contents

Preface

Modern drug discovery and design programs use computer aided drug discovery (CADD) for identifying and optimizing bioactive compounds used for developing new drugs. It is also known by alternative terms such as in-silico pharmacology and computational therapeutics. CADD approaches are vital in identifying viable drug candidates at a low cost. These approaches are usually divided into two types, namely, structure-based and ligand-based drug design approaches. Both these approaches are used to identify suitable lead molecules. These computational methods are useful for reducing the use of animal models in pharmacological research, assisting in the rational design of novel and safe drug candidates, repositioning marketed drugs, and assisting medicinal chemists and pharmacologists throughout the drug discovery process. This book is a compilation of chapters research papers that discuss the most vital concepts and emerging trends in the usage of computers for drug discovery and design. It will provide comprehensive knowledge to the readers.

After months of intensive research and writing, this book is the end result of all who devoted their time and efforts in the initiation and progress of this book. It will surely be a source of reference in enhancing the required knowledge of the new developments in the area. During the course of developing this book, certain measures such as accuracy, authenticity and research focused analytical studies were given preference in order to produce a comprehensive book in the area of study.

This book would not have been possible without the efforts of the authors and the publisher. I extend my sincere thanks to them. Secondly, I express my gratitude to my family and well-wishers. And most importantly, I thank my students for constantly expressing their willingness and curiosity in enhancing their knowledge in the field, which encourages me to take up further research projects for the advancement of the area.

Editor

1

LigBuilder V3: A Multi-Target *de novo* Drug Design Approach

Yaxia Yuan[1]*, Jianfeng Pei*[2*] *and Luhua Lai*[1,2,3*]

[1] *Beijing National Laboratory for Molecular Sciences, State Key Laboratory for Structural Chemistry of Unstable and Stable Species, College of Chemistry and Molecular Engineering, Peking University, Beijing, China,* [2] *Center for Quantitative Biology, Academy for Advanced Interdisciplinary Studies, Peking University, Beijing, China,* [3] *Center for Life Sciences, Academy for Advanced Interdisciplinary Studies, Peking University, Beijing, China*

***Correspondence:**
Jianfeng Pei
jfpei@pku.edu.cn
Luhua Lai
lhlai@pku.edu.cn

With the rapid development of systems-based pharmacology and poly-pharmacology, method development for rational design of multi-target drugs has becoming urgent. In this paper, we present the first *de novo* multi-target drug design program LigBuilder V3, which can be used to design ligands to target multiple receptors, multiple binding sites of one receptor, or various conformations of one receptor. LigBuilder V3 is generally applicable in *de novo* multi-target drug design and optimization, especially for the design of concise ligands for protein targets with large difference in binding sites. To demonstrate the utility of LigBuilder V3, we have used it to design dual-functional inhibitors targeting HIV protease and HIV reverse transcriptase with three different strategy, including multi-target *de novo* design, multi-target growing, and multi-target linking. The designed compounds were computational validated by MM/GBSA binding free energy estimation as highly potential multi-target inhibitors for both HIV protease and HIV reverse transcriptase. The LigBuilder V3 program can be downloaded at "http://www.pkumdl.cn/ligbuilder3/".

Keywords: *De novo* design, Multi-target drug design (MTDD), multi-target drug optimization, Dual-functional inhibitors, LigBuilder

INTRODUCTION

For most of the twentieth century, drug discovery process was dominated by a reductionist "one disease, one target, one molecule" philosophy (Alcaro et al., 2019). Researchers and pharmaceutical industries around the world have been struggling to develop highly specific regulators against particular targets, which are generally expected to achieve higher potencies while reducing the risk of off-target related side effects (Eaton et al., 1995; Morphy and Rankovic, 2009; Hughes et al., 2011). Although successful drugs have been brought to market with this approach, new drug R&D aiming novel targets was noticeable slowdown and fewer drugs were approved over the last decades (Scannell et al., 2012; Ramsay et al., 2018), which implies the limitation and deficiency of previous single-target drug discovery strategy. Due to the complexity of biological network (Gerstein et al., 2012), disease usually involves multiple factors and biological pathways, so agents that directly interfere individual molecular targets often lack effectiveness at treating complex diseases (Brown and Superti-Furga, 2003; Kamb et al., 2007; Cavalli et al., 2008; He et al., 2016). Moreover, the upstream components of pathways have to be regulated if only one target is aimed at in a multiple pathology related disease, which is more likely to cause unexpected side effects. Consequently, researchers and pharmaceutical industries have been turning their attention to develop therapies that modulate multiple targets simultaneously (Reddy and Zhang, 2013; Zhang et al., 2017; Kumar and Sharma, 2018). Combination therapy and multi-target therapy were proposed to address this problem.

Combination drugs, which is defined as a concerted pharmacological intervention of multiple targets with several compounds, have been used increasingly to treat many types of diseases, such as viral and bacterial infection, cancer, hypertension, and atherosclerosis (Giles et al., 2014; Von Hoff et al., 2014; Blonde et al., 2015; Lu et al., 2018). Although the combination therapy is proposed to set up a new direction for drug discovery, it is not a new concept. In fact, using multi-component mixture extracted from natural products is a historical therapy in traditional medical treatments. Besides, the highly active antiretroviral therapy (HAART) (Lu et al., 2018), which is also known as the "AIDS cocktail," has been the first-line anti-AIDS treatment since the end of last century (Bhatti et al., 2016). Many combination drugs have been launched to market and proved to be effective therapies for complex diseases, however, poor patient compliance has been raised especially in treatment of asymptomatic diseases such as hypertension (Eisen et al., 1990). An alternative way to simplify drug dosing is to mix multiple drug components into single co-formulated tablet, but different PK/PD property of each component may complicate the formulation and raise the risk of drug-drug interaction, and increase the risk and cost of such fix dose combinations strategy (Morphy and Rankovic, 2009).

Multi-target drug, which is defined as single compound that interacts with multiple targets simultaneously, has been paid much attention recently. Multi-target therapy is expected to be new and more effective medications for a variety of complex diseases even with relatively weak activity (Korcsmaros et al., 2007; Zimmermann et al., 2007). The uniform chemical component of multi-target drug will introduce lower risk of drug-drug interaction comparing with multi-components strategy. Moreover, although the discovery process of multi-target drug will be more complicated in the design and optimization stage due to the increased constraints from multiple targets, the risk and costs for the most expensive clinic trial stage are in principle similar with traditional single-target drug development. Consequently, many methods for multi-target ligand discovery were developed (Morphy et al., 2004; Zhan and Liu, 2009; Abdolmaleki et al., 2017; Zhang et al., 2017), such as multi-target QSAR (González-Díaz et al., 2006), fragment linker strategy (Morphy and Rankovic, 2006), framework combination (Morphy and Rankovic, 2006; Chen et al., 2011), and common pharmacophore based virtual screening and cross screening (Wei et al., 2008). Among them, framework combination and cross screening are both widely used approaches for discovering of multi-target lead (Morphy and Rankovic, 2005, 2009, 2010; Wu et al., 2012; Lepailleur et al., 2014; Bottegoni et al., 2016). Framework combination approach is based on the integration of multiple compounds via the fusion of common or similar sub-structure. Although the combined molecule from this approach is usually much smaller than directly linking two distinct structures with flexible chain, the median ligand efficiency is typically lower than general preclinical compounds which may lead to possible poor oral pharmacokinetics (Morphy and Rankovic, 2007). An alternative way is to screen multiple targets with the same compound library and select the consensus hints, namely, cross screening (Geppert et al., 2010). Although reported compounds derived by cross screening are better in ligand efficiency than that of framework combination approach, they are still statistically less efficient than general preclinical compounds. Considering the requirement of interacting with distinct binding sites, we are not surprising in the relative low ligand efficiency of multi-target compounds designed by the above methods (Morphy and Harris, 2012). Therefore, it is critical for multi-target compounds to be "highly integrated" that could make the most of each component group in multiple interactions. Moreover, the optimization of multi-target lead is far more complicated than that of single-target lead, because the "optimization landscape" of multi-target lead is no longer a simple stepwise "group-activity" profile in single-target lead optimization. The requirement of binding affinity balance for multiple binding will significantly reduce the available chemical space of the lead structure, as a result, stepwise optimization in multi-target optimization easily leads to "the blind alley," namely, local minima. The increased dimensions in "optimization landscape" of multi-target lead optimization make the stepwise strategy less efficient, and implies that a more global and extensive structure sampling is necessary in optimization, which may be difficult to be achieved by manual work. It also suggests that a "one-step" design rather than routine "optimizing-bioassay" cycle is more suitable for multi-target drug discovery process. Therefore, the efficient discovery strategy of "highly integrated" ligand for unrelated targets remains challenging and a general strategy of multi-target rational drug design for dissimilar targets needs to be developed.

We developed an innovative multi-target design method, called LigBuilder V3, which enables the *de novo* design and molecular optimization algorithm to handle multiple targets. The chemical space exploration algorithm inherited from LigBuilder V2 (Yuan et al., 2011) has been upgraded to explore more sophisticated structure space of multi-target ligands. As we design the multi-target ligands from scratch with the consideration of multiple interactions of each component group, high ligand efficiency is expected to be achieved with this *de novo* design approach, which is very important for multi-target drugs. Multi-target lead optimization is also implemented in LigBuilder V3, which can help researchers to find possible multi-target optimization solutions. Furthermore, we apply an "ensemble linking" strategy to promote the efficiency of "fragment linking" algorithm and make it available in linking fragments for multi-target design, which is helpful in highly efficient recombination of known ligands and framework combination.

METHOD AND ALGORITHM

Data Structure and Definition

LigBuilder V3 implements the same genetic algorithm (GA) (Fraser, 1957; Bremermann, 1958; Holland, 1975; Whitley, 1994) used in LigBuilder V2. GA is an optimization algorithm inspired by the process of natural selection, and it mimics the evolution of a population under selection pressure. LigBuilder V3 uses the overlapping generation model of GA, that is, new generation of individuals are evolved from previous population and then replace their parents with GA iteration. For a typical overlapping generation model of GA, roulette wheel selection approach

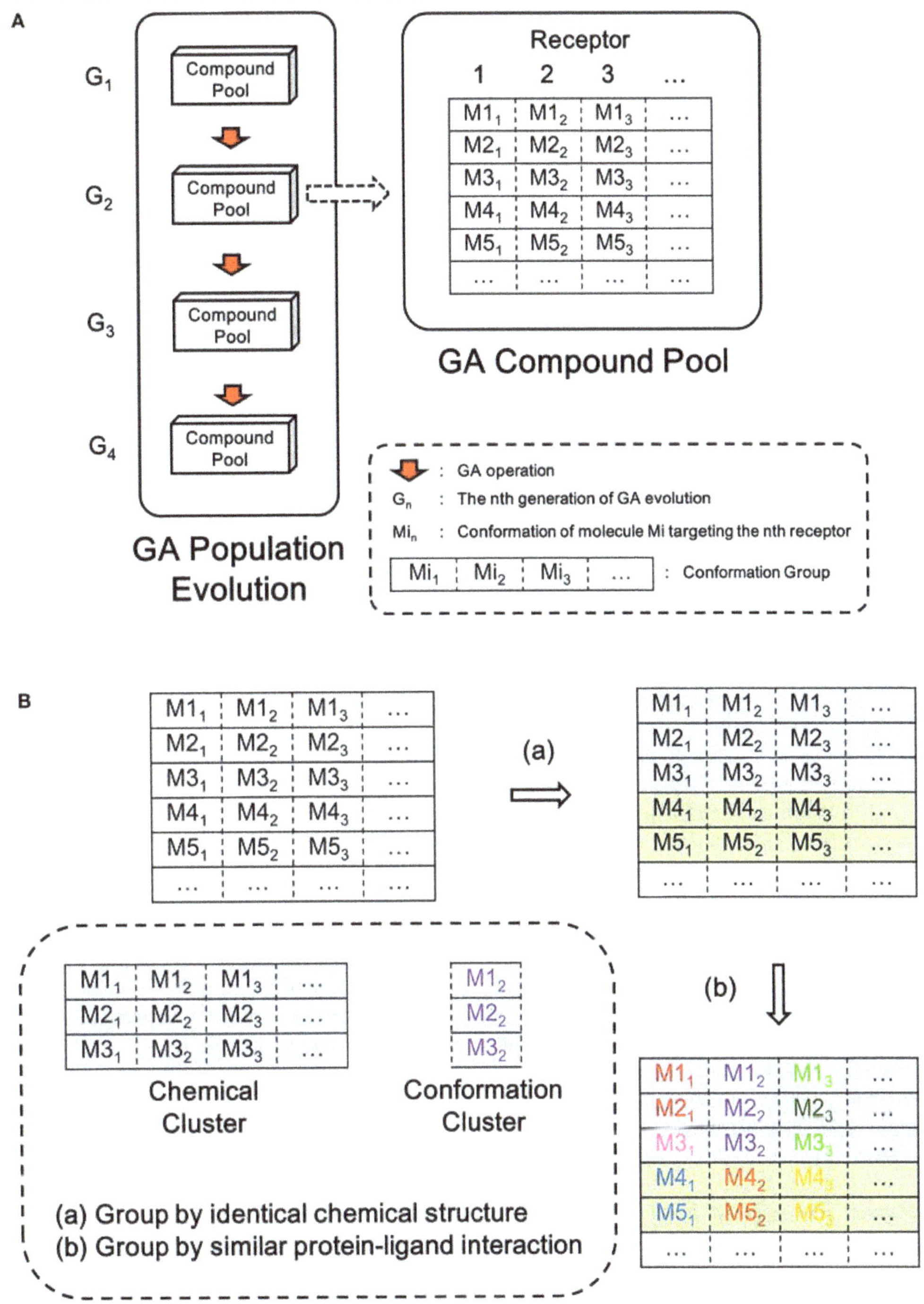

FIGURE 1 | Sketch map of data structure in LigBuilder V3. **(A)** The overview structure of GA evolution and GA compound pool. The GA compound pool includes the ensemble of molecules evolved in GA population. For multi-target design, conformations for each receptor are listed in corresponding column, as a result, each row could represent a solution of multi-target inhibition, and it could be viewed as the basic unit in multi-target GA population, which has similar status as "molecule" in single-target GA population. To avoid confusion, we define each row as a "conformation group" instead of "molecule" or "conformation." **(B)** The definition of chemical cluster and conformation cluster. The compound pool is clustered on two levels: **(a)** all molecules sharing identical chemical structures will be clustered as chemical cluster, which could be synthesized by same route; **(b)** conformations with similar protein-ligand interaction will be clustered as conformation cluster, which represent same interaction mode.

is used to select 10% members from current population as parent for evolving next generation, and all members in current population will be discarded. To balance quality and diversity of population, LigBuilder exempt the top 10% members in current population from elimination, that is, these top members will be directly transferred to next generation. So the quality of member in offspring generation will be better, at least equal to parent generation. We define the GA compound pool as the ensemble of molecules in the newest generation of GA population evolution. The overview of the data structure used in GA evolution is described in **Figure 1A**.

As each molecule produced by multi-target design method involves multiple proteins, we should consider the multiple conformations of the molecule that bind to its corresponding targets. This is different to single target drug design method. To avoid confusion, we use "Conformation Group" instead of "Molecule" and "Conformation" to indicate the multiple binding conformations of multi-target molecule in this manuscript (**Figure 1A**).

We also define the "chemical cluster" and "conformation cluster" to depict the relationship in chemical structure and binding conformation among multi-target molecules (**Figure 1B**). From the perspective of synthesis, molecules with the same chemical structure could be considered as identical. But from the perspective of protein-ligand interaction, the conformations of ligand must be taken into account because the binding of ligand is based on spatial interaction between atoms from ligand and protein. Therefore, we cluster all conformations at two levels: (1) chemical clusters: each conformation of a chemical cluster shares the same two-dimensional (2D) structure, and they could be synthesized via the same reactions estimated by the synthesis-accessibility analysis module inherited from LigBuilder V2; (2) conformation clusters: all the conformations in a conformation cluster also share the same 2D structure, thus the conformation cluster is a subset of chemical cluster. All conformations in a conformation cluster are similar with each other, so they could be consider as sharing same interaction mode. Although all conformations of a conformation cluster are interchangeable from the perspective of interaction mode, we have to keep these "duplicates," because they may provide necessary local perturbation, for example, the members in a conformation cluster may have various orientations of hydrogen atoms. The orientations of hydrogen atoms usually have little effect on protein-ligand binding except being involved in hydrogen bond forming, but it is much sensitive in further evolution of molecules because the hydrogen atom is responsible for growing site for connecting newly added fragments.

Multi-Target Seed Structure Mapping

Seed structure is the starting point structure for lead optimization. The preparation of seed structures for single target lead optimization is straightforward, however, additional steps are needed for preparation of seed structures for multi-target design. As each "multi-target seed structure" indicates a conformation group which is composed by the different binding conformation of the ligand to each target, therefore it is necessary to make one-to-one correspondence between atoms of each member in the conformation group. Because only hydrogen atoms are possible connection site in the whole design process, the seed structure mapping is based on the mapping of hydrogen atoms, namely, hydrogen mapping. Due to the symmetry of molecule, there may be more than one possible solution of hydrogen mapping between two structures.

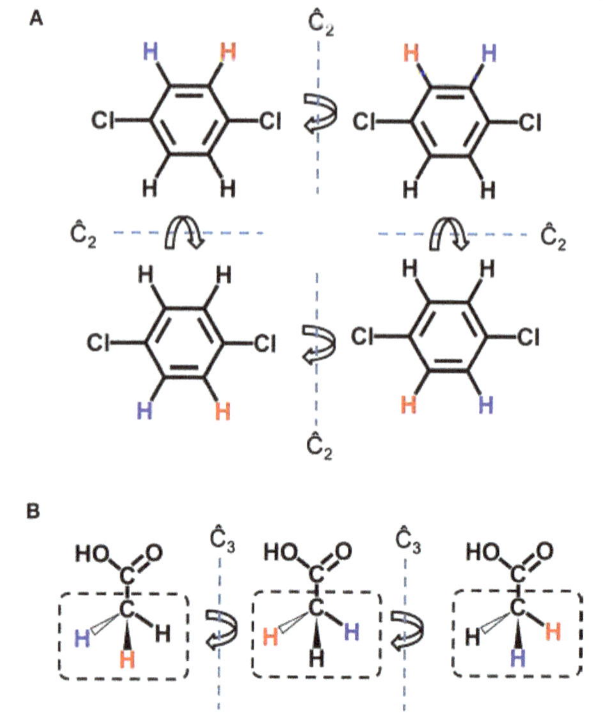

FIGURE 2 | Symmetry in hydrogen mapping. **(A)** Example for the symmetry of structure. 2 C_2 symmetry axis of 1,4-dichlorobenzene conduce to 4 possible hydrogen mappings. **(B)** Example for the symmetry of group. A C_3 symmetry axis of methyl group of acetic acid conduces to three possible hydrogen mappings. The hydrogen atom colored in red and blue indicates the first hydrogen and last hydrogen in hydrogen mapping, respectively.

As depicted in **Figure 2**, two types of symmetry should be taken into account, i.e., the hydrogen symmetry of molecule and the hydrogen symmetry of group. The molecular hydrogen symmetry refers to the rotation symmetry of all hydrogen in the molecule, and the hydrogen symmetry of group refers to the rotation symmetry of multiple hydrogen atoms that connected to one heavy atom. **Figure 2A** shows two C_2 symmetry axises of 1,4-dichlorobenzene, which conduce to 4 possible hydrogen mappings. **Figure 2B** shows a C_3 symmetry axis of the methyl group of acetic acid, which conduces to 3 possible hydrogen mappings. We should note that although some molecules such as the acetic acid are not chiral, the potential chirality is taken into account for the hydrogen mapping in LigBuilder V3, because the further growing operation may bring in chirality to the carbon atom. In other words, both 2D topological and three dimensional (3D) structural information are considered in hydrogen mapping.

Although all the hydrogen atoms in ligand are possible fragment growing site, not every hydrogen atom could serve as growing site because of steric hindrance or user's preference. Thus, LigBuilder V3 only reserves the possible hydrogen mappings with maximal growing sites mapped, named growing site mapping, which increase the possibility of further growing operation to the greatest extent. If there is no possible

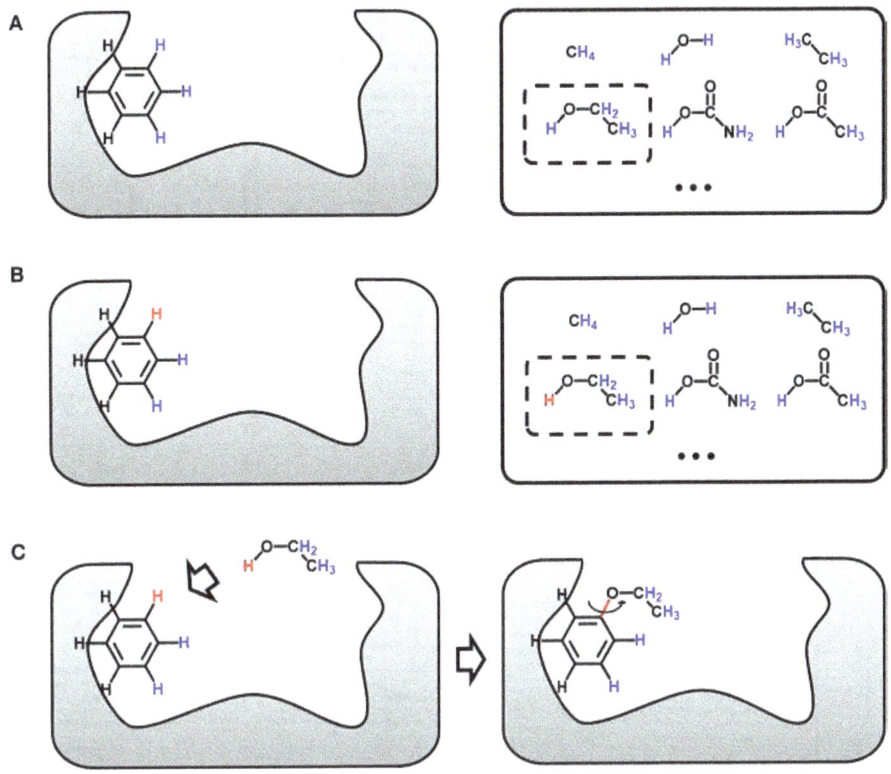

FIGURE 3 | Sketch map of the growing operation. **(A)** The seed structure in the binding site and chosen fragment (dashed box) in the building block library (solid box). All potential growing sites are colored in blue. **(B)** The randomly chosen growing site of seed structure and chosen fragment are colored in red. **(C)** The chosen fragment is moved and then attached to the seed structure. The favorable conformations are determined by uniformly 3 degree-step sampling of the torsion angle along the newly formed bond, which is colored in red.

hydrogen mapping or growing sites mapping, the corresponding conformation group will be ignored. However, if there are more than one solutions of rational hydrogen mappings, LigBuilder V3 will regard them as different seed structures and use them independently in subsequentially design process.

For the case that involves more than two targets, LigBuilder V3 makes hydrogen mapping between the conformation for the first target and each of the remaining targets one by one. As a result, all the rest conformations of the conformation group are mapped to the first conformation, so it is feasible to the find the common growing site mappings of the whole conformation group.

Multi-Target Growing

Lead optimization is the fundamental function of LigBuilder series. Both LigBuilder V1 and V2 provide the "Growing" strategy, which generates derivatives based on the lead structure (i.e., "seed" structure) that has been pre-placed into the binding pocket. In the present study, we extend the "Growing" strategy to multi-target growing (multi-target lead optimization).

Figure 3 is the sketch map of single-target growing operation, which is the basis of multi-target growing operation. The gray area on the left in **Figure 3A** represents the binding site of the target, and the benzene is a representative seed structure. Molecules in the solid box on the right are privileged fragments, which could serve as the building blocks for assembling new structure. Although all hydrogen atoms are feasible for attaching fragments, only a few of them are potential connection site without steric hindrance. Taking **Figure 3A** for example, hydrogen atoms of benzene face to the vacant region of binding site are colored in blue, which indicate the potential growing sites, and the others near to the receptor atoms will be ignored. Meanwhile, all the hydrogen atoms of building blocks will be considered as potential connection site by default. Users can also assign or block certain "growing sites" on seed structures and building blocks to customize the style of molecule. As the seed structure and building block library has been prepared, LigBuilder will randomly choose a fragment from the building block library (the dashed box in **Figure 3A**), and then randomly choose a potential growing site on the seed structure and the chosen building block, respectively (red hydrogen atoms in **Figure 3B**). The building block will be attached to the seed structure along the direction of selected hydrogen atoms (red hydrogen in **Figure 3B**). With uniformly 3 degree-step sampling of the torsion angle along the newly formed bond (red bond in **Figure 3C**), several favorable conformations with local minimal energies will be reserved as candidates in consideration of the flexibility of molecule. GA is applied

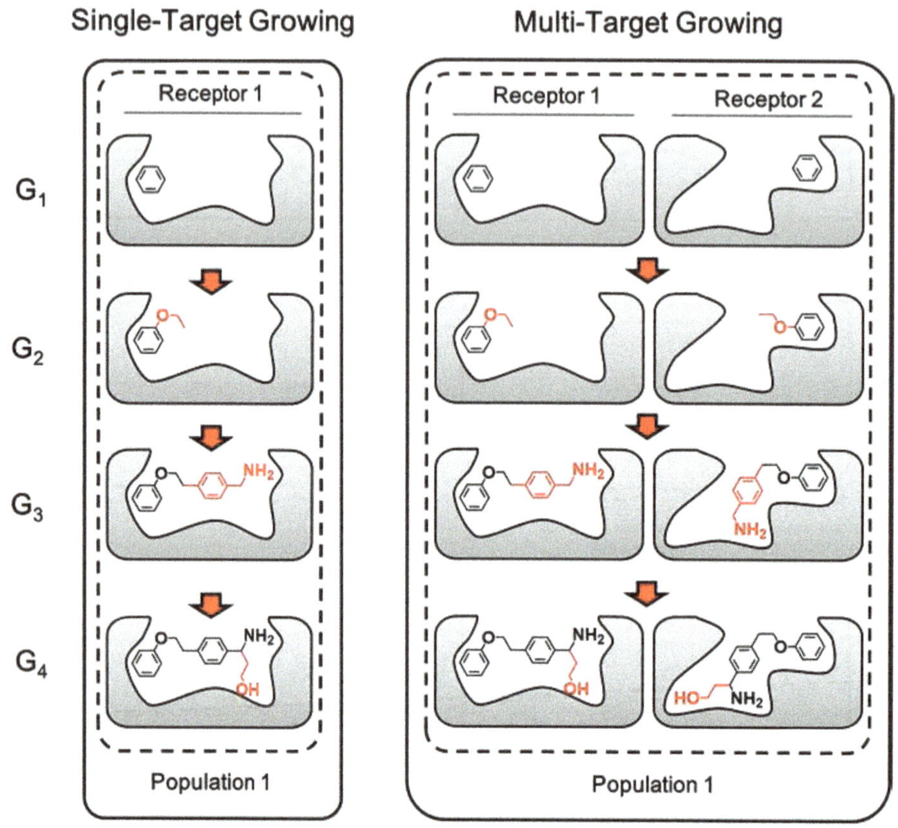

FIGURE 4 | The sketch map of growing process. The multi-target growing operation could be considered as multiple synchronous single-target growing operation. The fragments grown in each step are colored in red (Only one conformation group of each generation are showed here as representatives of the compound pool).

to select elites from these candidates, and these elites will serve as the seed structures for the next growing cycle. This repeated process for each ligand continues until: (1) the ligand is fully designed and there is no available space for adding any new chemical group; (2) the ligand reaches the limitation of molecular weight, which is 480 Da by default; (3) the GA generation number reaches a maximal number, which is 15 by default.

Different from single-target design, the lead structure for multi-target design should be prepared as "seed" conformation group, which is composed by the binding conformation of the lead structure to each target. With a simultaneous operation of growing chemically identical building block on the same site of each member in the conformation group, compounds generated by LigBuilder V3 are expected to be capable of binding to multiple targets. As depicted in **Figure 4**, multi-target growing could be considered as multiple synchronous single-target growing operation. The identical building block and the same growing site in the growing operation will maintain the consistency of 2D structures of the conformation group. Meanwhile, the 3D conformation of ligand is only restrained by its corresponding targets, that is, the conformation in each conformation group is optimized and evaluated independently. Therefore, this strategy could utilize the flexibility of ligand to improve the capability of multi-target binding. Genetic Algorithm (GA) is also applied to manipulate the growing cycle in the same manner as single target growing.

Ensemble Linking

Although assembling several bioactive fragments to generate potent ligand is very promising, the computational method of linking proximal fragments covalently is fraught with challenges. To avoid affecting respective bioactivity, the orientation and position of fragments should be changeless. Therefore, the feasibility of linking is severely limited by the rigid restriction of bond length and bond angle in molecule. Besides, the unfavorable energy of torsion may further reduce the feasibility. Although there may be some solutions existed in huge chemical space, the low efficiency in finding these solutions narrows the application of fragments linking. As a result, there are few successful cases of fragments linking, except using flexible chain as linker. However, although flexible chain could be used to relax the rigid restriction of linking, it may increase the amount of accessible conformation of the structure which brings in unfavorable entropy change during binding process, thus the linked fragments usually do not bind as the same degree as the sum of the individual fragments.

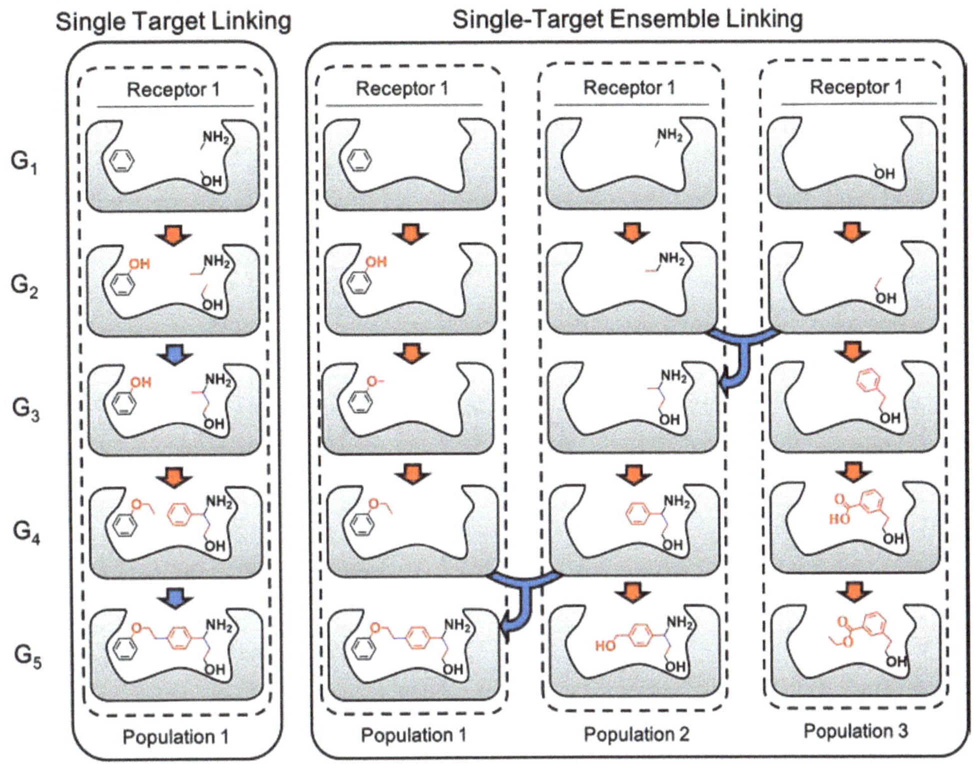

FIGURE 5 | The sketch map of linking and ensemble linking process. The red arrow indicates the growing operation while blue arrow indicates the linking operation. In accordance with the color of arrows, atoms, and bonds formed in growing and linking operation are colored in red and blue, respectively. For previous linking algorithm, the aggregation of certain fragments is regarded as a whole "seed," so the linking process will be constrained by every fragment in the aggregation. Instead, ensemble linking algorithm applies a more flexible linking strategy, which attempts to derive new structures from each of seed fragments independently and then find possible way of linking among these structures. The different populations indicated different independent GA threads.

Moreover, the excessive flexibility of structure may reduce the specificity of ligand.

The ensemble linking algorithm is developed in LigBuilder V3 to improve the efficiency of fragments linking process, which is expected to make this method more practical. To demonstrate the details of the new algorithm, the sketch map of the linking algorithm used in previous versions of LigBuilder series and ensemble linking algorithm used in LigBuilder V3 are compared in **Figure 5**. Previous linking algorithm applies a direct strategy of linking, which aims to linking certain fragments with many building blocks. Instead, ensemble linking algorithm applies a more flexible linking strategy, which attempts to derive new structures from each of seed fragments independently and then find possible way of linking among these structures. Although both algorithms are capable of generating the same final structure in **Figure 5**, ensemble linking strategy is expected to be more efficient. For the general linking algorithm, it is straightforwardly requiring that all the given fragments should be linked, which is usually hard especially for multi-target linking. To overcome this problem, ensemble linking algorithm is based on extra linking fragments, and automatically find the apportioned combination of fragments, which would improve the possibility of finding solution for linking fragments. To be specific, for general linking algorithm, the number of fragments used for linking is limited, for example, user poses 3 fragments into the ligand binding site, and the linking algorithm attempts to find suitable linkers to connect all these 3 specific fragments. For ensemble linking, user could pose several thousands of fragments into the ligand binding site, and the ensemble linking algorithm attempts to find suitable linkers to connect any 3 fragments among all available fragments. Obviously, the ensemble linking algorithm will significantly increase the possibility of finding suitable solution for linking 3 fragments comparing with general linking algorithm. Besides, with dissociation of combined seed fragments in linking algorithm, the whole linking process would be more robust, it would not be dragged by improper derivation or conformation of individual fragment. Moreover, it raises the possibility of comprehensive utilization of more bioactive fragments without exhaustive combination. As a result, LigBuilder V3 could be applied to find possible solutions of linking among hundreds of fragments, which further improves the success rate of linking.

The ensemble linking algorithm will generate many derivative candidates based on the linking fragments to enhance the possibility for finding solution, obviously, although the possibility of linking increases with the number of candidates, the computation cost also will increase by the same rate. So it is important to generate candidates more effective rather than

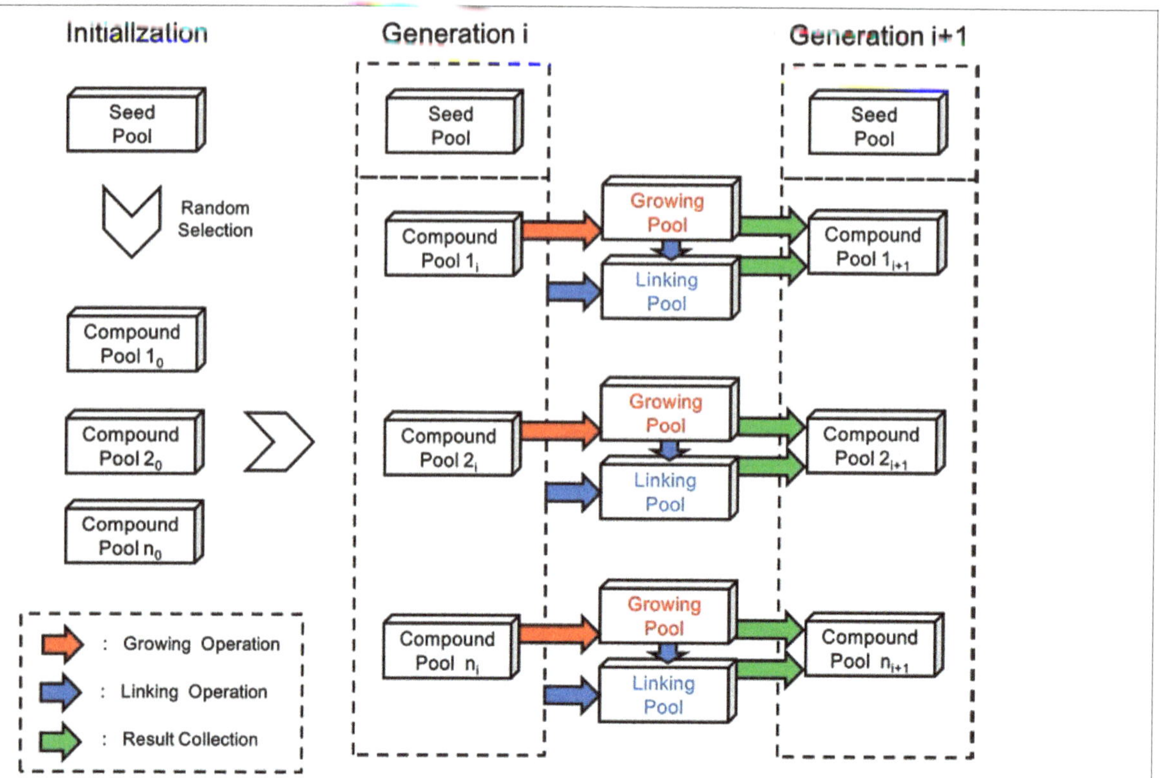

FIGURE 6 | The flow chart of linking process in LigBuilder V3. The structures of initial compound pool are randomly selected from the seed pool in the initialization stage. Then LigBuilder V3 perform the growing and linking operation on each compound pool for producing new generation of compound pools. The growing operation brings in derivation on molecules in previous compound pool and result in a "Growing pool," which is colored in red. Then the linking operation will be performed for finding possible way of linking between these newly formed structures and previous existed structures. The "previous existed structures" in each generation is denoted with the dashed box. As similar with growing operation, the linking results will be collected into a "Linking pool" which is colored in blue. At last, the "Growing pool" and "Linking pool" will be merged into a new generation of compound pool.

increase the number of candidates to improve the efficiency. As all candidates in the GA population have similar molecular weight because they are generated by GA evolution with same number of generations, the linking possibility will reach the peak when candidates in the population occupy about half of the binding site. But it rapidly falls when candidates in the population are too large to be integrated in limited space of binding site. In addition, the linking possibility is also low when the candidates in the population are too small which may make them far away from each other for linking. So we applied a stagger strategy that operating several independent GA threads simultaneously, meanwhile, the starting of each GA threads are staggered so as to make them be in various generation of GA process. That is, ensemble linking algorithm will not only perform "intra-linking" among candidates in a GA process, but also perform "inter-linking" among candidates in different GA threads. With this strategy, the high diversity of molecular weight distribution among all candidates could bring in higher linking possibility and efficiency.

As depicted in **Figure 6**, each generation of ensemble linking can be decomposed into two steps, i.e., the growing step and the linking step. LigBuilder V3 performs the growing operation on all compounds from each compound pool in the growing step, and then finds possible way of linking between the newly formed compounds and all previous existed compounds including seed pool (dashed box in **Figure 6**) in the linking step. Although compounds generated in both steps will be collected together into new generation of compound pools, the compounds generated in the linking step (linking pools in **Figure 6**) will have a certain level of priority in GA process, which make the ensemble linking algorithm trends to link fragments rather than grow for derivation. To be specific, the compounds generated in the linking step indicates a "linking" operation is occurred, on the contrary, compounds generated in the growing step do not link with other fragments in this step. So LigBuilder will elevate the fitness score of compounds from linking step, which encourage the linking behavior. The structures of initial compound pool are randomly selected from the seed pool. After the initialization, LigBuilder V3 will repeat the ensemble linking process for each ligand until: 1) the ligand is fully designed and there is no available space for any new chemical group; 2) the ligand reaches the limitation of molecular weight, which is 480 Da by default; 3) the GA generation number reaches a maximal number, which is 15 by default.

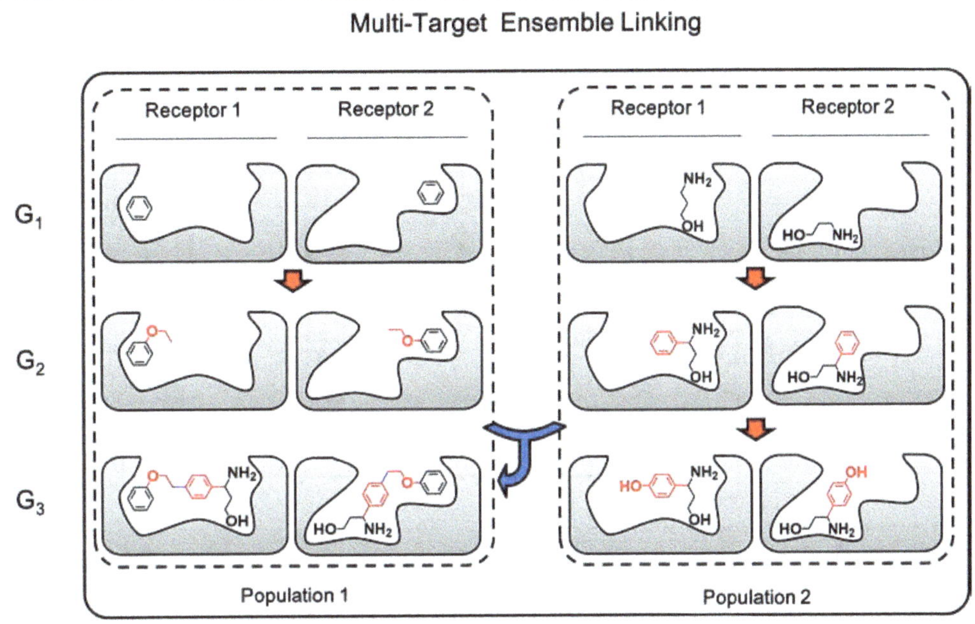

FIGURE 7 | The multi-target ensemble linking operation could be considered as multiple synchronous single-target ensemble linking operation. The red arrow indicates the growing operation while blue arrow indicates the linking operation. In accordance with the color of arrows, atoms, and bonds formed in growing and linking operation are colored in red and blue, respectively.

Multi-Target Linking

A further challenge lies in designing multi-target ligand is linking fragments that interacting with multiple targets. Although many successes occurred in designing single target ligand by fragments linking strategy, few research focus on multi-target linking method. Comparing with lead compound, potential active fragments are much easier to pick by fragment-based approach, such as NMR, DSF, X-ray crystallography, surface plasmon resonance and mass spectrometry (Mashalidis et al., 2013). In addition, computational methods such as fragment docking (Wang et al., 2015) or CrystalDock (Durrant et al., 2011) are also effective ways to identify lead-fragments. Moreover, small fragments are much more likely to interact with multiple targets due to its lower specificity. Therefore, it is feasible and promising to design multi-target ligand by integrating several fragments. So we try to improve our ensemble linking algorithm to handle multi-target fragments linking in LigBuilder V3.

As with the multi-target growing algorithm, the fragments for multi-target linking should also be prepared as "seed" conformation group. Because the ensemble linking algorithm in LigBuilder V3 handle the fragments independently, users no longer have to predetermine which fragments will be linked together in the stage of seed preparation. That is, the procedure of conformation group preparation for linking is same as that for growing. The only difference is that at least 2 conformation groups should be prepared for linking and at least 1 for growing.

Multi-target linking algorithm is based-on the ensemble linking algorithm described in above section, therefore both the growing step and linking step which make up the ensemble linking algorithm will be extended to multiple targets. The growing step of multi-target ensemble linking is exactly the same with multi-target growing, while the linking step applies the same strategy of "multi-target operation" used in multi-target growing. As described above, multi-target growing operation is a simultaneously operation of growing chemical identical building block on the same site of each member in the conformation group. In a similar way, multi-target linking operation in linking step is a simultaneously pairwise operation of linking corresponding members from two conformation groups on the same linking sites (**Figure 7**). That is, the first member of conformation group A will be linked with the first member of conformation group B. Then the second member of both conformation group will be linked together on the same linking sites of the first member. This pairwise process will be repeated until all members have been linked or any failure occurs due to steric hindrance or molecular tension. As a result, these linked structures are expected to be capable of binding to multiple receptor, while they share identical chemical structures.

Multi-Target *de novo* Design

LigBuilder V3 inherits the "Chemical Space Exploring Algorithm" (CSEA) from LigBuilder V2 to create novel scaffolds and structures. In LigBuilder V2, CSEA works in the following way: (1) an sp^3 carbon with 4 hydrogen atoms will be randomly posed in the binding site and serve as the starting point of constructing new molecules with growing operation; (2) newly designed molecules will be split into fragments; (3) fragments with high predicted binding affinity, that is, high contribution fragments will be selected for updating the "seed structure pool," which is used to supply seeds for subsequent design cycles;

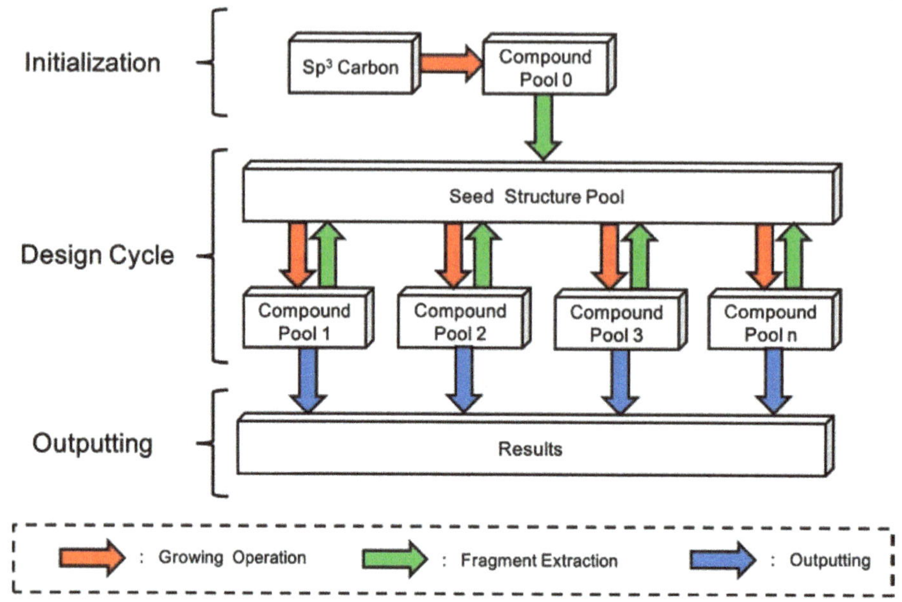

FIGURE 8 | Schema of Chemical Space Exploring Algorithm (CSEA). A randomly positioned sp^3 carbon will be taken as starting point of growing operation for generating the initial compound pool. Then fragments extracted from compound pool will be used to construct a seed structure pool, which contains seed structures that more favorable than the initial sp^3 carbon. As new compound pools could be generated based-on structures in seed structure pool, while fragments extracted from these newly formed compounds will be used to update the seed structure pool, LigBuilder V3 avoids the dependency of initial structure and be promising in exploring larger chemical space.

(4) a structure from "seed structure pool" is randomly select as the starting point of constructing new molecules with growing operation, then the 2–4 steps will be repeated. For LigBuilder V3, CSEA is extended to multi-target design purpose by applying multi-target growing operation instead of single-target growing operation. Meanwhile, the fragment extraction process of single conformation will also be replaced by fragment extraction of "conformation group" (**Figure 8**). With the self-circulation seed generating feature, CSEA can help to avoid the limitations associated with pre-assigned seed structures and explore a broader chemical space, thus greatly improving the novelty and efficiency of design.

As the seed structure pool is used to collect and provide initial fragments of design process, the quality of seed structure pool may significantly affect the design results. Since CSEA could provide a mass of potential seed fragments during the design process, the seed structure pool will be updated to achieve higher binding affinity while maintain diversity of seeds. Then the CSEA will have a higher starting point for generating potent structures, which in turn produce better seed fragments for updating the seed structure pool. Therefore, the seed structure pool will keep evolving during the whole design process, which iteratively optimize the performance of design.

Seed Structure Extraction

The most direct way of extracting component fragments from chemical structure is splitting the molecule by iterating over all single bonds. However, the traversal extraction method would take a lot of computing time when handle millions of compounds, which is a common order of magnitude in CESA process of LigBuilder V3. Therefore, we develop a simplified extraction algorithm for acceleration. To balance the representativeness of fragments and extraction speed, we only focus on the molecular scaffold and key interaction group, which are major determinants of molecular conformation and protein-ligand interaction. As a result, only five categories of fragments are considered in CESA: (1) Single atoms; (2) rigid scaffold (rigid chain and rigid ring system); (3) flexible scaffold (flexible ring system); (4) interaction group (e.g., carboxyl group); (5) scaffold with connected interaction group. If a fragment could be classified into more than one category, it will be put into the category with smallest category number. With this algorithm, LigBuilder V3 is also capable of extracting fragments from known ligands as seed structures, which is convenient for fragments linking or lead optimization.

For multi-target design, as the seed structure is composed of multiple conformations (conformation group) instead of single conformation, seed structures extracted from known ligands of each targets should be paired to construct conformation groups first. LigBuilder V3 extracts fragments from all known ligands in the same way of extracting fragments in single-target design, and then hydrogen mapping algorithm will be implemented among these fragments to find all possible combinations. That is, if a fragment is present in ligand of every targets, it is a common fragment and LigBuilder will mapping this fragment to construct multi-target fragments group as seed structures. However, if this fragment is absent in ligands for any one of the targets, it is not common fragment and the fragment will be discarded.

Multi-Target Ligand Efficiency

Ligand efficiency (LE) is frequently used to prioritize hits from HTS, and it can be regarded as a guide for selecting efficient fragments for further optimization. It is much more important for multi-target design because the ligand efficiency is also the index of "integration degree," which is a more critical index for multi-target drugs. There are various definitions of LE but most widely used approximation is described as the average free energy of binding per heavy atom or average pIC_{50} per heavy atom, which are demonstrated as follows (Hopkins et al., 2004):

$$LE = \frac{-\Delta G}{HAC} \quad or$$
$$LE = \frac{-\log(IC_{50})}{HAC} \qquad (HAC\ is\ heavy\ atom\ count)$$

For multi-target ligand, multi-target ligand efficiency (MLE) could be derived with a similar form of LE. As the multi-target ligand causes multiple binding free energy, MLE could be described as the summation of average free energy of binding per heavy atom or summation of average pIC_{50} per heavy atom, which are demonstrated as follows:

$$MLE_N = \frac{\sum -\Delta G_n}{HAC} \quad or$$
$$MLE_N = \frac{\sum -\log\left(IC_{50_n}\right)}{HAC} \qquad (N\ is\ the\ number\ of\ target)$$

The ligand efficiency is not comparable if the target number is different, so we use the subscript for MLE to indicate the condition of rational comparison and make it distinct from LE of single-target ligands. We should note that the MLE is insufficient for the performance evaluation of multi-target ligand, because the uneven activity of targeting individual binding site may be obscured by summation. However, it is much complicated to evaluate the efficiency of multi-target ligand, because it depends on the specific biological network that it is involved in. So the MLE would be only considered as an index of average efficiency for selecting potential multi-target lead structures.

Other Functional Modules

The other functional modules implemented in LigBuilder V3 are directly inherited from LigBuilder V2, including: (1) drug-like and privileged building blocks; (2) Toxic fragments; (3) Drug-like rules (for example, Lipinski rule); (4) Ligand-binding site detection module; (5) Synthesis analysis modules; (6) Scoring function; (7) LogP module; (8) GA fitness function (composed of scoring function, MLE, toxic fragments filter, and drug-like rules). It should be noted that the binding affinity predicted by scoring function for multi-target ligand is calculated by its average of binding affinity predicted for each target.

Design HIV-PR/HIV-RT Dual-Functional Inhibitor

Structural Preparation

The crystal structures of PR and RT used in this study are downloaded from the RCSB Protein Data Bank (Berman et al., 2003) (PDB code: 3A2O, Hidaka et al., 2009, and 4G1Q, Kuroda et al., 2013, respectively), and both structures are complexes with potent inhibitors solved at high resolution (0.88 and 1.51 Å, respectively). The inhibitor binding sites of PR and RT were defined by binding site detection program Cavity (Yuan et al., 2013; Zhang et al., 2015; Xu et al., 2018), which provides the detailed definition for boundary of "design space." The drug-like and privileged building blocks used in this study were inherited from LigBuilder V2. Then three different design strategies were used to design dual-function inhibitors for PR and RT.

De novo Design Approach

LigBuilder V3 inherited the seed generation and optimization algorithm from LigBuilder V2, that is, LigBuilder V3 could iteratively extract seed structures from designed compounds and use the extract seed structures for design new compounds. The GA parameters were set as follows: GA population size of 1,000, GA parent ratio of 10%, GA generation number of 12. Total 1 million candidate dual-functional compounds were generated by LigBuilder V3 with *de novo* design mode.

Growing Approach

Growing approach is for optimization of prepared seed structures. We collected all protein-ligand binding complex of PR or RT from the RCSB Protein Data Bank (Berman et al., 2003), including 323 PR-ligand complexes and 141 RT-ligand complexes (Listed in **Table S1**). All the PR-ligand complexes were aligned to the PR structure complexed with KNI-1689 (PDB code: 3A2O, Hidaka et al., 2009), and all the RT-ligand complexes were aligned to the RT structure complexed with Rilpivirine (PDB code: 4G1Q, Kuroda et al., 2013) using Pymol (Schrodinger, 2010), which could ensure that all ligands in the complexes are also aligned according to the receptor alignment. With the fragment-extraction function of LigBuilder V3, fragments with no more than 20 heavy atoms were extract from these known PR or RT ligands. As the ligand efficiency is important for the seed structure, fragments with SLE index <0.1 were removed, and a total of 2,386 fragments for PR and 1,442 fragments for RT were obtained at this stage. Then fragments for PR and RT with the same 2D structure were paired with "hydrogen mapping" algorithm mentioned above, and a total of 3,506 paired fragments were prepared. The GA parameters were set as follows: GA population size of 1,000, GA parent ratio of 10%, GA generation number of 12. Total 100 K candidate dual-functional compounds were generated by LigBuilder V3 with growing design mode based on the prepared fragments. As the binding affinity is usually related to the size of molecule, large seed fragments are more competitive than small fragments especially for the genetic algorithm used in LigBuilder. So, each fragment was independently used as the seed structure with multiple runs of LigBuilder to avoid bias to large seed fragments.

Linking Approach

Linking approach is for integrating key fragments into new compounds. The paired fragments used in this approach were prepared in the same way of growing approach. However, all paired fragments were used together in linking approach to maximize the possibility of finding ways for linking fragments.

It would be intuitive that the more fragments provided, the better performance would be expected. The GA parameters were set as follows: GA population size of 10,000, GA parent ratio of 10%, ensemble population number of 10, GA generation number of 12. Total 10 K candidate dual-functional compounds were generated by LigBuilder V3 with linking design mode based on the 3,506 prepared fragments.

Post-processing

As multi-target ligand should bind to different proteins with the same chemical structure, ideally, each moiety of the ligand could contribute to its binding to all targets, so ligand efficiency would be important in evaluating a multi-target ligand. In this study, predicted pKd of all the output compounds are larger than 5.0, so only MSLE index were used to rank and select top 1,000 results with best ligand efficiency from multi-target design procedure for the three approaches. Because LigBuilder V3 only uses a fast empirical scoring function for estimating protein ligand binding affinity, in order to improve the accuracy of calculation, the total 3,000 selected compounds were further subjected to energy minimization and 100 ps short time molecular dynamic (MD) simulation by using the Amber package (Case et al., 2012) for

TABLE 1 | Binding free energy predicted by MM/GBSA method.

	***De novo* design**		**Growing approach**		**Linking approach**		**HIV-PR potent inhibitor**[b]	**HIV-PR weak inhibitor**[c]	**HIV-RT potent inhibitor**[d]	**HIV-RT weak inhibitor**[e]
	Top 10[a]	**Top 1**	**Top 10**	**Top 1**	**Top 10**	**Top 1**				
PR	−28.2	−35	−28.4	−32	−34.9	−35.0	−68.2	−21.9	–	–
RT	−33.6	−34.9	−34.5	−40.3	−38.0	−38.8	–	–	−41.5	−22.6
Ave.	−30.9	−35.0	−31.5	−36.2	**−36.5**	**−36.9**	–	–	–	–

Energy unit is kcal/mol.
[a]Top 10 indicates the average of best 10 compounds; [b]FDA approved drug Darunavir with IC_{50} of 0.15 nM (Shen et al., 2013). Complex structure was from PDB code 4LL3 (Kožíšek et al., 2014). [c]PR weak inhibitor with IC_{50} of 2.3 μM (Jhoti et al., 1994). Complex structure was from PDB code 1HTE (Jhoti et al., 1994). [d]FDA approved drug Efavirenz with IC_{50} of 41 nM (King et al., 2002). Complex structure was from PDB code 1FK9 (Ren et al., 2000). [e]RT weak inhibitor with IC_{50} of 1.2 μM (Chan et al., 2017). Complex structure was from PDB code 5VQS (Chan et al., 2017). Bold values indicate the best average energy among results from three approaches.

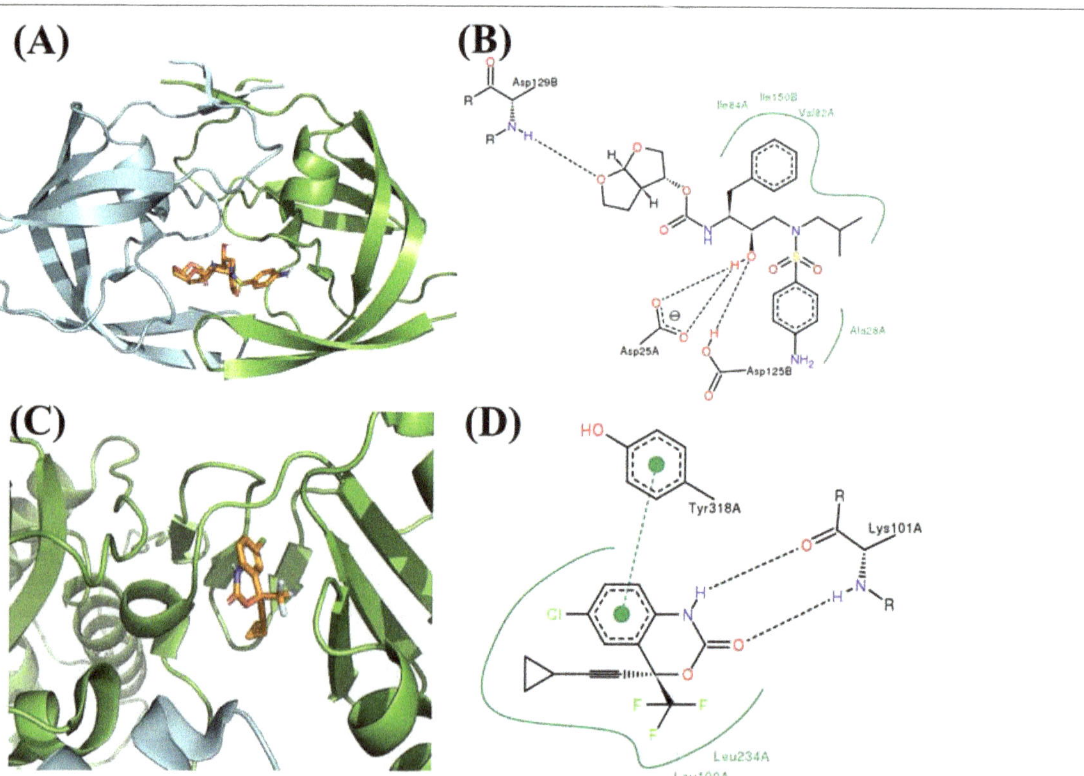

FIGURE 9 | (A) Binding mode of FDA approved PR inhibitor Darunavir. The dimerized PR is showed in green and cyan cartoon style, and the Darunavir is showed in golden stick style (figure generated by Pymol, Schrodinger, 2010). **(B)** The 2D interaction figure for Darunavir binding with PR (figure generated by PoseView, Stierand and Rarey, 2010). **(C)** Binding mode of FDA approved RT inhibitor Efavirenz. **(D)** The 2D interaction figure for Efavirenz binding with RT.

estimating the binding affinity with MM/GBSA method (Rastelli et al., 2010).

Application of LigBuiler V3 in Multi-Target Ligand Design

The concept prototype for growing mode algorithm of LigBuilder V3 has been experimental validated by designing COX2/LTA$_4$H dual-functional inhibitor, which resulted in a single ligand that binding to COX2 and LTA$_4$H with IC$_{50}$ of 7.1 and 7.0 μM, respectively (Shang et al., 2014). Although this work is based on a developing version of LigBuilder V3, and many manual interventions were involved due to immature of the algorithm, the success of this case suggests the feasibility of using LigBuilder V3 to design multi-target ligand. Moreover, LigBuilder V3 were further developed based on the knowledge learned from this case. Besides the improvement of multi-target growing algorithm, both multi-target *de novo* design approach and multi-target linking approach are realized in this version of LigBuilder V3. In this study, we have tested the LigBuilder V3 by designing dual-functional inhibitor targeting two well-characterized virus enzymes, HIV protease (PR) and HIV reverse transcriptase (RT) with all three design modes. As both PR and RT are important drug targets of clinical antiretroviral therapy, the multi-target strategy such as combination of nucleoside reverse transcriptase inhibitors (NRTI) and protease inhibitor (PI) shows significant advantage over each single component and has been broadly used for HIV treatment (Lu et al., 2018). Consequently, researchers have been interesting in developing cocktail drug combinations, and pursue multi-target anti-HIV inhibitors for improving patient compliance. Matsumoto *et al.* have reported the strategy of linking PR and RT inhibitor by spontaneously cleavable linker (Matsumoto et al., 2000). Furthermore, scaffold merging strategy is successfully applied in designing multi-target anti-HIV inhibitors in recent years (Song et al., 2015; Sun et al., 2016). However, both the dependency of known inhibitors and specific requirement of molecular structure limit the practical applications of structure merging strategy. Therefore, we present a more universal solution of multi-target design with the example of designing dual-functional inhibitors for PR and RT by LigBuilder V3. The detailed methods and parameters are described in the Method and Algorithm section.

The top 1,000 compounds from each design modes were selected and subjected to 100 ps short time molecular dynamic simulation, then the binding affinity of each compounds were estimated by MM/GBSA method. The average binding affinity of the top 10 compounds and top 1 compound for each design modes were collected in **Table 1**. Although the designed multi-target compounds could not compare with the super potent PR and RT inhibitors with sub-nanomolar level activity, the designed compounds are predicted to be more potent than micromolar level inhibitor of both PR and RT, that is, these compounds are expected to be dual-functional inhibitor for PR and RT at sub-micromolar level activity for both targets.

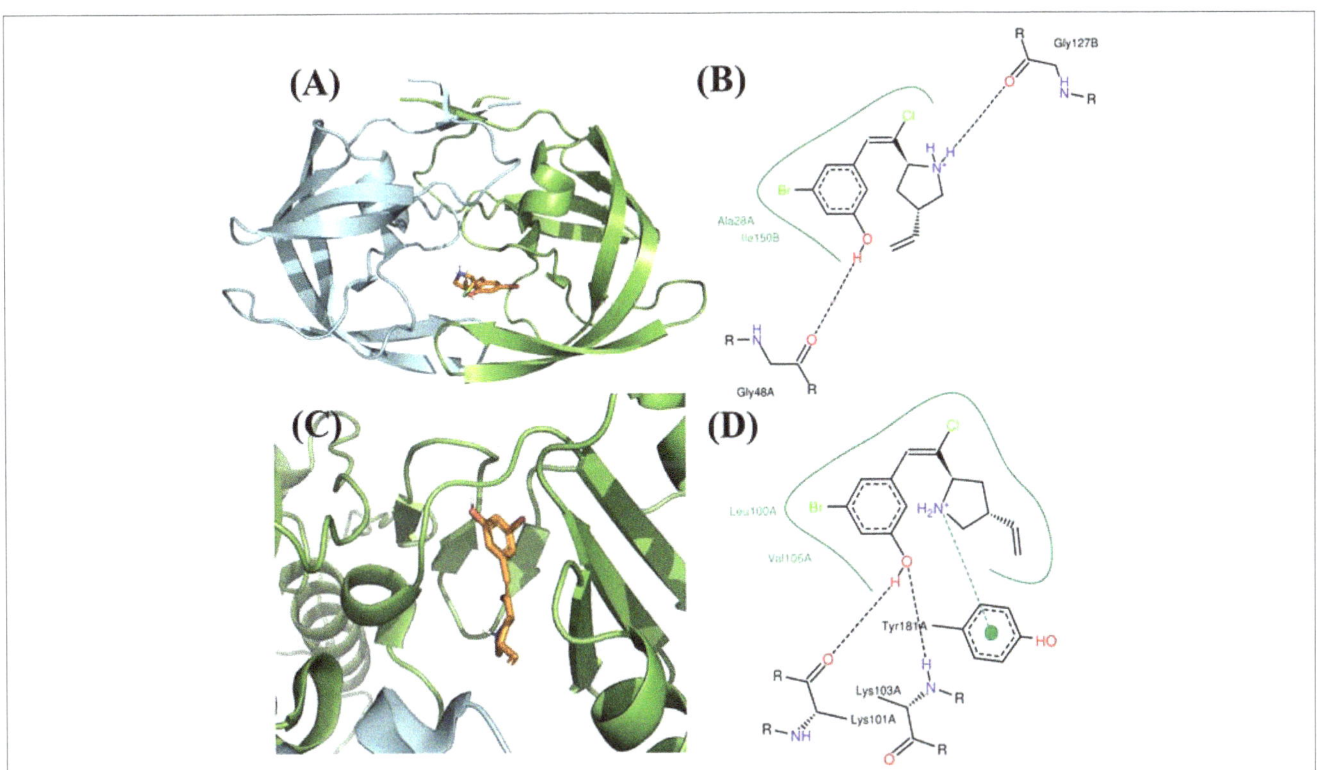

FIGURE 10 | Binding mode of the best compound from *de novo* design approach. **(A)** Binding mode with PR. **(B)** 2D interaction with PR. **(C)** Binding mode with RT. **(D)** 2D interaction with RT.

The binding mode of FDA approved PR inhibitor and RT inhibitor are depicted in **Figure 9**. Obviously, they adopt very distinct protein-ligand interaction modes. The best compound from *de novo* design approach is depicted in **Figure 10**. This compound forms distinct interaction comparing with known PR or RT inhibitors. It is highly compact and fully utilized its polar groups and hydrophobic groups to form interaction with PR and RT in different manner. The best compound from fragments growing approach is depicted in **Figure 11**. This compound is growing from a benzene ring which is one of the most common fragments in PR and RT inhibitors. The best compound from fragments linking approach is depicted in **Figure 12**. This compound is much bigger than compounds from *de novo* approach and growing approach, which indicates its relatively lower ligand efficiency. As linking approach is intensively pursing possible ways for linking provided fragments, the success of linking is more important than ligand efficiency, so the algorithm is preferable to allow generating derivates with much lower ligand efficiency which may enhance the possibility of linking. Overall, all of these compounds are relatively small, and groups in these compounds usually contribute to the binding with different protein in different manner, which is the most need feature for designing highly compact multi-target ligand.

Essentially, the design process of LigBuilder is a kind of "random evolution" process implemented by genetic algorithm. So the quality of design result is expected to be improved along with the total computational time. As the output result could be unlimited, it is not realistic to achieve the maximal quality. For a fair comparison among the results from three strategies, we used different output number to ensure they consumed roughly similar computational time. So we designed 1 million, 100 K, and 10 K compounds for *de novo* approach, growing approach, and linking approach, respectively, which is roughly corresponding to the compound generating efficiency of three approaches in

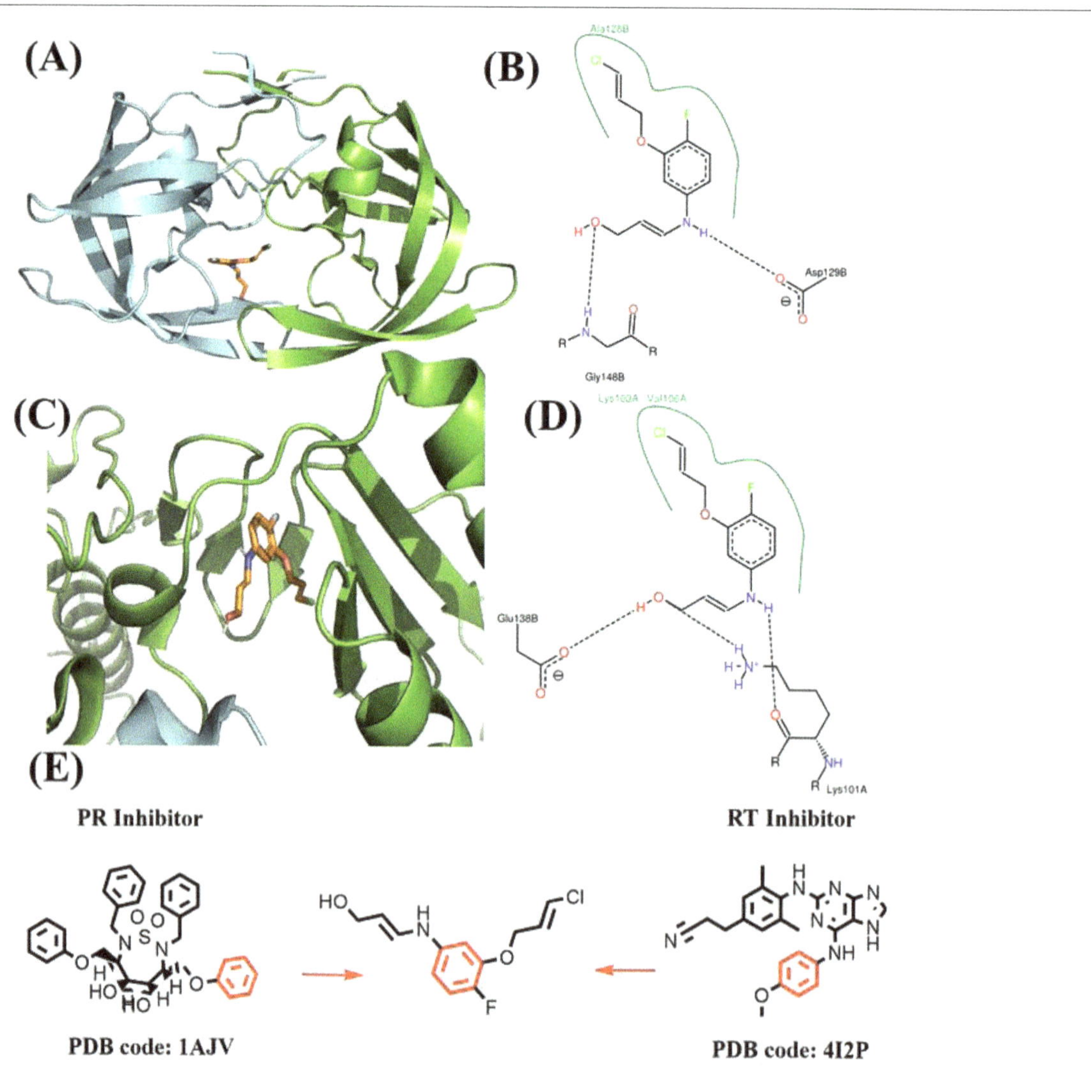

FIGURE 11 | Binding mode of the best compound from growing approach. **(A)** Binding mode with PR. **(B)** 2D interaction with PR. **(C)** Binding mode with RT. **(D)** 2D interaction with RT. **(E)** Source of fragments in PR inhibitor and RT inhibitor for growing are colored in red.

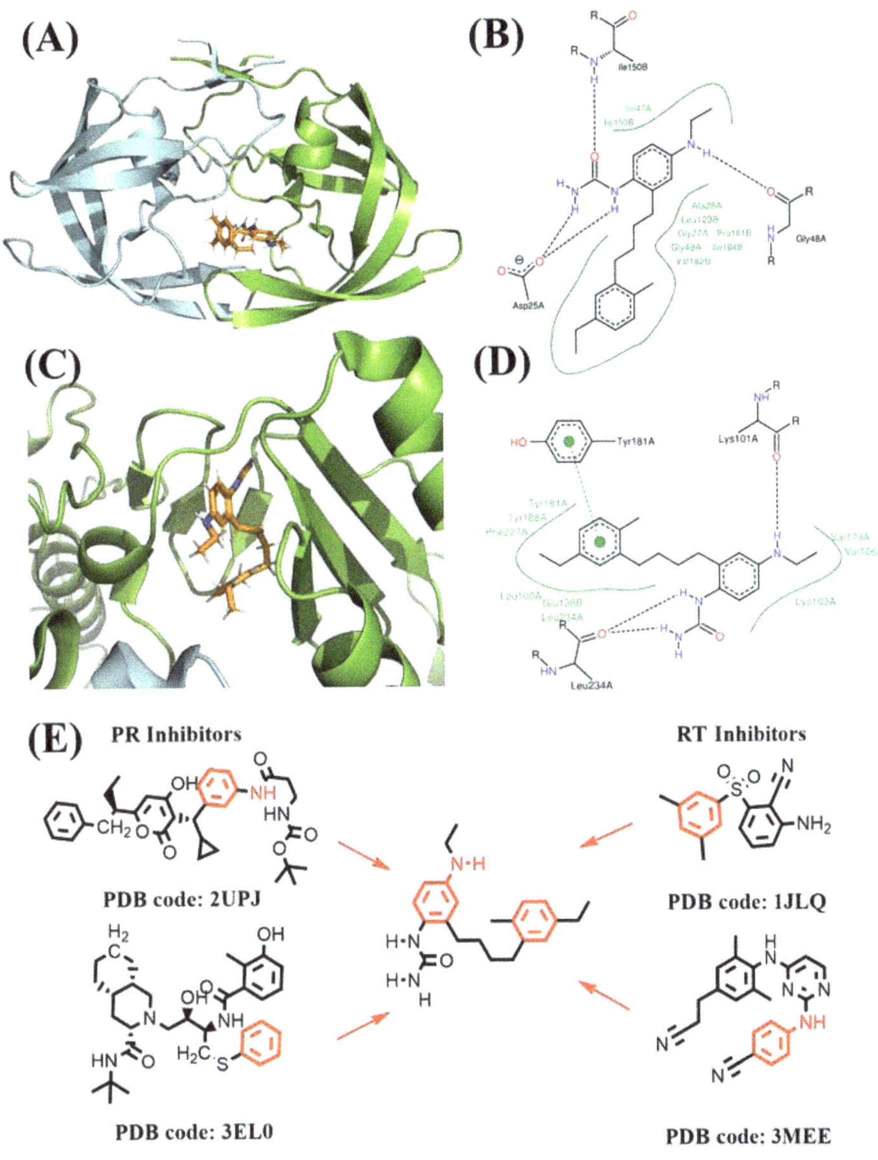

FIGURE 12 | Binding mode of the best compound from linking approach. **(A)** Binding mode with PR. **(B)** 2D interaction with PR. **(C)** Binding mode with RT. **(D)** 2D interaction with RT. **(E)** Source of fragments in PR inhibitor and RT inhibitor for linking are colored in red.

this project. Base on the data in **Table 1**, linking approach is most effective way of design high affinity ligands, and growing approach is also more effective than *de novo* approach. This is not surprising because known fragments would provide good starting points for derivation and significantly reduce searching space. The linking approach uses more known fragments which further improve its efficiency comparing with growing approach using only 1 fragment. However, the results from *de novo* approach demonstrated that this approach could achieve similar design performance to growing approach or linking approach if more computational resource is provided. As the *de novo* approach does not reply on known fragments, it would be very useful for design ligands for new targets or discover novel ligands for known targets. On the other hand, growing approach and linking approach also have their unique advantages comparing with *de novo* approach. Since compounds designed by growing or linking approach contain "validated active fragments," it would reduce the risk of "false positive," which is very common in computer-aided drug discovery. So the three strategies could be complementary in practical drug discovery projects.

CONCLUSION

In this paper, we present the first *de novo* multi-target drug design program LigBuilder V3. In addition, building ligands from scratch, LigBuilder V3 also provides the feasibility of multi-target lead optimization and multi-target fragments linking. This program is generally applicable in rational and elegant multi target drug design and optimization, especially for the design of concise ligands for proteins targets with large difference in binding sites. The developing version of LigBuilder V3 was successfully applied in designing COX2/LTA_4H dual-functional inhibitors with micromolar level activity. In this study, we further demonstrated the three design strategies of LigBuilder V3 with computational evaluation of designing HIV-PR and HIV-RT dual functional inhibitors. We hope the concept and LigBuilder V3 can be validated by applications from the users in the future.

AUTHOR CONTRIBUTIONS

JP and LL conceived the project. YY, JP, and LL designed the experiments, analyzed the results, and wrote the manuscript. YY performed the experiments.

FUNDING

This work was supported in part by the Ministry of Science and Technology of China (2016YFA0502300 and 2015CB910300) and the National Natural Science Foundation of China (21633001 and 21673010).

ACKNOWLEDGMENTS

We thank Dr. Erchang Shang for feedback of experiment data in developing of LigBuilder V3, thank Dr. Daqi Yu, Dr. Yifei Qi, Dr. Changsheng Zhang, Dr. Fangjin Chen, Dr. Weilin Zhang, and Dr. Youjun Xu for providing supports in algorithm.

REFERENCES

Abdolmaleki, A., Ghasemi, J. B., and Ghasemi, F. (2017). Computer aided drug design for multi-target drug design: SAR/QSAR, molecular docking and pharmacophore methods. *Curr. Drug Targets* 18, 556–575. doi: 10.2174/1389450117666160101120822

Alcaro, S., Bolognesi, M. L., García-Sosa, A. T., and Rapposelli, S. (2019). Multi-target-directed ligands (MTDL) as challenging research tools in drug discovery: from design to pharmacological evaluation. *Front. Chem.* 7:71. doi: 10.3389/fchem.2019.00071

Berman, H. M., Bourne, P. E., Westbrook, J., and Zardecki, C. (2003). *The Protein Data Bank in Protein Structure.* Boca Raton, FL: CRC Press. 394–410.

Bhatti, A. B., Usman, M., and Kandi, V. (2016). Current scenario of HIV/AIDS, treatment options, and major challenges with compliance to antiretroviral therapy. *Cureus* 8:e515. doi: 10.7759/cureus.515

Blonde, L., Jendle, J., Gross, J., Woo, V., Jiang, H., Fahrbach, J. L., et al. (2015). Once-weekly dulaglutide versus bedtime insulin glargine, both in combination with prandial insulin lispro, in patients with type 2 diabetes (AWARD-4): a randomised, open-label, phase 3, non-inferiority study. *Lancet* 385, 2057–2066. doi: 10.1016/S0140-6736(15)60936-9

Bottegoni, G., Veronesi, M., Bisignano, P., Kacker, P., Favia, A. D., and Cavalli, A. (2016). Development and application of a virtual screening protocol for the identification of multitarget fragments. *ChemMedChem* 11, 1259–1263. doi: 10.1002/cmdc.201500521

Bremermann, H. J. (1958). *The Evolution of Intelligence: The Nervous System as a Model of its Environment.* Seattle, WA: University of Washington, Department of Mathematics.

Brown, D., and Superti-Furga, G. (2003). Rediscovering the sweet spot in drug discovery. *Drug Discov. Today* 8, 1067–1077. doi: 10.1016/S1359-6446(03)02902-7

Case, D. A., Darden, T. A., Cheatham T. E. III, Simmerling, C. L., Wang, J., Duke, R. E., et al. (2012). *AMBER 12.* San Francisco, CA: University of California.

Cavalli, A., Bolognesi, M. L., Minarini, A., Rosini, M., Tumiatti, V., Recanatini, M., et al. (2008). Multi-target-directed ligands to combat neurodegenerative diseases. *J. Med. Chem.* 51, 347–372. doi: 10.1021/jm7009364

Chan, A. H., Lee, W.-G., Spasov, K. A., Cisneros, J. A., Kudalkar, S. N., Petrova, Z. O., et al. (2017). Covalent inhibitors for eradication of drug-resistant HIV-1 reverse transcriptase: from design to protein crystallography. *Proc. Natl. Acad. Sci. U.S.A.* 114, 9725–9730. doi: 10.1073/pnas.1711463114

Chen, Z., Wu, Y., Liu, Y., Yang, S., Chen, Y., and Lai, L. (2011). Discovery of dual target inhibitors against cyclooxygenases and leukotriene A4 hydrolyase. *J. Med. Chem.* 54, 3650–3660. doi: 10.1021/jm200063s

Durrant, J. D., Friedman, A. J., and Mccammon, J. A. (2011). CrystalDock: a novel approach to fragment-based drug design. *J. Chem. Inf. Model.* 51, 2573–2580. doi: 10.1021/ci200357y

Eaton, B. E., Gold, L., and Zichi, D. A. (1995). Let's get specific: the relationship between specificity and affinity. *Chem. Biol.* 2, 633–638. doi: 10.1016/1074-5521(95)90023-3

Eisen, S. A., Miller, D. K., Woodward, R. S., Spitznagel, E., and Przybeck, T. R. (1990). The effect of prescribed daily dose frequency on patient medication compliance. *Arch. Intern. Med.* 150, 1881–1884. doi: 10.1001/archinte.1990.00390200073014

Fraser, A. S. (1957). Simulation of genetic systems by automatic digital computers ii. Effects of linkage on rates of advance under selection. *Aust. J. Biol. Sci.* 10, 492–500. doi: 10.1071/BI9570492

Geppert, H., Vogt, M., and Bajorath, J. (2010). Current trends in ligand-based virtual screening: molecular representations, data mining methods, new application areas, and performance evaluation. *J. Chem. Inf. Model.* 50, 205–216. doi: 10.1021/ci900419k

Gerstein, M. B., Kundaje, A., Hariharan, M., Landt, S. G., Yan, K.-K., Cheng, C., et al. (2012). Architecture of the human regulatory network derived from ENCODE data. *Nature* 489, 91–100. doi: 10.1038/nature11245

Giles, T. D., Weber, M. A., Basile, J., Gradman, A. H., Bharucha, D. B., Chen, W., et al. (2014). Efficacy and safety of nebivolol and valsartan as fixed-dose combination in hypertension: a randomised, multicentre study. *Lancet* 383, 1889–1898. doi: 10.1016/S0140-6736(14)60614-0

González-Díaz, H., Prado-Prado, F. J., Santana, L., and Uriarte, E. (2006). Unify QSAR approach to antimicrobials. part 1: predicting antifungal activity against different species. *Bioorg Med Chem.* 14, 5973–5980. doi: 10.1016/j.bmc.2006.05.018

He, B., Lu, C., Zheng, G., He, X., Wang, M., Chen, G., et al. (2016). Combination therapeutics in complex diseases. *J. Cell. Mol. Med.* 20, 2231–2240. doi: 10.1111/jcmm.12930

Hidaka, K., Kimura, T., Abdel-Rahman, H. M., Nguyen, J.-T., Mcdaniel, K. F., Kohlbrenner, W. E., et al. (2009). Small-sized human immunodeficiency virus type-1 protease inhibitors containing allophenylnorstatine to explore the S2′ pocket. *J. Med. Chem.* 52, 7604–7617. doi: 10.1021/jm9005115

Holland, J. (1975). *Adaptation in Natural and Artificial Systems.* Ann Arbor, MI: University of Michigan Press.

Hopkins, A. L., Groom, C. R., and Alex, A. (2004). Ligand efficiency: a useful metric for lead selection. *Drug Discov. Today* 9, 430–431. doi: 10.1016/S1359-6446(04)03069-7

Hughes, J. P., Rees, S., Kalindjian, S. B., and Philpott, K. L. (2011). Principles of early drug discovery. *Br. J. Pharmacol.* 162, 1239–1249. doi: 10.1111/j.1476-5381.2010.01127.x

Jhoti, H., Singh, O. M., Weir, M. P., Cooke, R., Murray-Rust, P., and Wonacott, A. (1994). X-ray crystallographic studies of a series of penicillin-derived asymmetric inhibitors of HIV-1 protease. *Biochemistry* 33, 8417–8427. doi: 10.1021/bi00194a005

Kamb, A., Wee, S., and Lengauer, C. (2007). Opinion - why is cancer drug discovery so difficult? *Nat. Rev. Drug Discov.* 6, 115–120. doi: 10.1038/nrd2155

King, R. W., Klabe, R. M., Reid, C. D., and Erickson-Viitanen, S. K. (2002). Potency of nonnucleoside reverse transcriptase inhibitors (NNRTIs) used in combination with other human immunodeficiency virus NNRTIs, NRTIs, or protease inhibitors. *Antimicrob. Agents Chemother.* 46, 1640–1646. doi: 10.1128/AAC.46.6.1640-1646.2002

Korcsmaros, T., Szalay, M. S., Csaba, B., Kovacs, I. A., and Csermely, P. (2007). How to design multi-target drugs: target search options in cellular networks. *Expert Opin. Drug Discov.* 2, 799–808. doi: 10.1517/17460441.2.6.799

KoŽíšek, M., Lepšík, M., Grantz Šašková, K., Brynda, J., Konvalinka, J., and Řezáčová, P. (2014). Thermodynamic and structural analysis of HIV protease resistance to darunavir–analysis of heavily mutated patient-derived HIV-1 proteases. *FEBS J.* 281, 1834–1847. doi: 10.1111/febs.12743

Kumar, A., and Sharma, A. (2018). "Computational modeling of multi-target-directed inhibitors against Alzheimer's disease," in *Computational Modelling Drugs Against Alzheimer's Disease*, ed K. Roy (New York, NY: Springer), 533–571.

Kuroda, D. G., Bauman, J. D., Challa, J. R., Patel, D., Troxler, T., Das, K., et al. (2013). Snapshot of the equilibrium dynamics of a drug bound to HIV-1 reverse transcriptase. *Nat. Chem.* 5:174. doi: 10.1038/nchem.1559

Lepailleur, A., Freret, T., Lemaitre, S., Boulouard, M., Dauphin, F. O., Hinschberger, A., et al. (2014). Dual histamine H3R/serotonin 5-HT4R ligands with antiamnesic properties: pharmacophore-based virtual screening and polypharmacology. *J. Chem. Inf. Model.* 54, 1773–1784. doi: 10.1021/ci500157n

Lu, D.-Y., Wu, H.-Y., Yarla, N. S., Xu, B., Ding, J., and Lu, T.-R. (2018). HAART in HIV/AIDS treatments: future trends. *Infect. Disord. Drug Targets* 18, 15–22. doi: 10.2174/1871526517666170505122800

Mashalidis, E. H., Sled,z, P., Lang, S., and Abell, C. (2013). A three-stage biophysical screening cascade for fragment-based drug discovery. *Nat. Protoc.* 8, 2309–2324. doi: 10.1038/nprot.2013.130

Matsumoto, H., Hamawaki, T., Ota, H., Kimura, T., Goto, T., Sano, K., et al. (2000). 'Double-drugs'—A new class of prodrug form of an HIV protease inhibitor conjugated with a reverse transcriptase inhibitor by a spontaneously cleavable linker. *Bioorg. Med. Chem. Lett.* 10, 1227–1231. doi: 10.1016/S0960-894X(00)00202-X

Morphy, J. R., and Harris, C. J. (2012). Designing multi-target drugs. *R. Soc. Chem.* doi: 10.1039/9781849734912

Morphy, R., Kay, C., and Rankovic, Z. (2004). From magic bullets to designed multiple ligands. *Drug Discov. Today* 9, 641–651. doi: 10.1016/S1359-6446(04)03163-0

Morphy, R., and Rankovic, Z. (2005). Designed multiple ligands. An emerging drug discovery paradigm. *J. Med. Chem.* 48, 6523–6543. doi: 10.1021/jm058225d

Morphy, R., and Rankovic, Z. (2006). The physicochemical challenges of designing multiple ligands. *J. Med. Chem.* 49, 4961–4970. doi: 10.1021/jm0603015

Morphy, R., and Rankovic, Z. (2007). Fragments, network biology and designing multiple ligands. *Drug Discov. Today* 12, 156–160. doi: 10.1016/j.drudis.2006.12.006

Morphy, R., and Rankovic, Z. (2009). Designing multiple ligands-medicinal chemistry strategies and challenges. *Curr. Pharm. Des.* 15, 587–600. doi: 10.2174/138161209787315594

Morphy, R., and Rankovic, Z. (2010). "Design of multitarget ligands," in *Lead Generation Approaches in Drug Discovery*, eds Z. Rankovic and R. Morphy (Hoboken, NJ: John Wiley & Sons), 141–164.

Ramsay, R. R., Popovic-Nikolic, M. R., Nikolic, K., Uliassi, E., and Bolognesi, M. L. (2018). A perspective on multi-target drug discovery and design for complex diseases. *Clin. Transl. Med.* 7:3. doi: 10.1186/s40169-017-0181-2

Rastelli, G., Del Rio, A., Degliesposti, G., and Sgobba, M. (2010). Fast and accurate predictions of binding free energies using MM-PBSA and MM-GBSA. *J. Comput. Chem.* 31, 797–810. doi: 10.1002/jcc.21372

Reddy, A. S., and Zhang, S. (2013). Polypharmacology: drug discovery for the future. *Expert Rev. Clin. Pharmacol.* 6, 41–47. doi: 10.1586/ecp.12.74

Ren, J., Milton, J., Weaver, K. L., Short, S. A., Stuart, D. I., and Stammers, D. K. (2000). Structural basis for the resilience of efavirenz (DMP-266) to drug resistance mutations in HIV-1 reverse transcriptase. *Structure* 8, 1089–1094. doi: 10.1016/S0969-2126(00)00513-X

Scannell, J. W., Blanckley, A., Boldon, H., and Warrington, B. (2012). Diagnosing the decline in pharmaceutical R&D efficiency. *Nat. Rev. Drug Discov.* 11, 191. doi: 10.1038/nrd3681

Schrodinger, Llc, (2010). *The PyMOL Molecular Graphics System*, Version 1.3r1.

Shang, E., Yuan, Y., Chen, X., Liu, Y., Pei, J., and Lai, L. (2014). *De novo* design of multitarget ligands with an iterative fragment-growing strategy. *J. Chem. Inf. Model.* 54, 1235–1241. doi: 10.1021/ci500021v

Shen, Y., Altman, M. D., Ali, A., Nalam, M. N., Cao, H., Rana, T. M., et al. (2013). Testing the substrate-envelope hypothesis with designed pairs of compounds. *ACS Chem. Biol.* 8, 2433–2441. doi: 10.1021/cb400468c

Song, A., Yu, H., Wang, C., Zhu, X., Liu, K., and Ma, X. (2015). Novel dual small-molecule HIV inhibitors: scaffolds and discovery strategies. *Curr. Pharm. Des.* 21, 950–962. doi: 10.2174/1381612820666140929095102

Stierand, K., and Rarey, M. (2010). PoseView–molecular interaction patterns at a glance. *J. Cheminform.* 2:P50. doi: 10.1186/1758-2946-2-S1-P50

Sun, X., Fan, N., Xu, W., Sun, Y., Xie, X., Guo, Y., et al. (2016). Design, synthesis and biological evaluation of caffeoyl benzanilides as dual inhibitors of HIV integrase and CCR5. *MedChemComm* 7, 2028–2032. doi: 10.1039/C6MD00311G

Von Hoff, D. D., Goldstein, D., and Renschler, M. F. (2014). Albumin-bound paclitaxel plus gemcitabine in pancreatic cancer. *N. Engl. J. Med.* 370, 479–480. doi: 10.1056/NEJMc1314761

Wang, T., Wu, M.-B., Chen, Z.-J., Chen, H., Lin, J.-P., and Yang, L.-R. (2015). Fragment-based drug discovery and molecular docking in drug design. *Curr. Pharm. Biotechnol.* 16, 11–25. doi: 10.2174/1389201015666141122204532

Wei, D., Jiang, X., Zhou, L., Chen, J., Chen, Z., He, C., et al. (2008). Discovery of multitarget inhibitors by combining molecular docking with common pharmacophore matching. *J. Med. Chem.* 51, 7882–7888. doi: 10.1021/jm8010096

Whitley, D. (1994). A genetic algorithm tutorial. *Stat. Comput.* 4, 65–85. doi: 10.1007/BF00175354

Wu, Y., He, C., Gao, Y., He, S., Liu, Y., and Lai, L. (2012). Dynamic modeling of human 5-lipoxygenase-inhibitor interactions helps to discover novel inhibitors. *J. Med. Chem.* 55, 2597–2605. doi: 10.1021/jm201497k

Xu, Y., Wang, S., Hu, Q., Gao, S., Ma, X., Zhang, W., et al. (2018). CavityPlus: a web server for protein cavity detection with pharmacophore modelling, allosteric site identification and covalent ligand binding ability prediction. *Nucleic Acids Res.* 46, W374–W379. doi: 10.1093/nar/gky380

Yuan, Y., Pei, J., and Lai, L. (2011). LigBuilder 2: a practical *de novo* drug design approach. *J. Chem. Inf. Model.* 51, 1083–1091. doi: 10.1021/ci100350u

Yuan, Y., Pei, J., and Lai, L. (2013). Binding site detection and druggability prediction of protein targets for structure-based drug design. *Curr. Pharm. Des.* 19, 2326–2333. doi: 10.2174/1381612811319120019

Zhan, P., and Liu, X. Y. (2009). Designed multiple ligands: an emerging Anti-HIV drug discovery paradigm. *Curr. Pharm. Des.* 15, 1893–1917. doi: 10.2174/138161209788453266

Zhang, W., Pei, J., and Lai, L. (2017). Computational multitarget drug design. *J. Chem. Inf. Model.* 57, 403–412. doi: 10.1021/acs.jcim.6b00491

Zhang, W., Yuan, Y., Pei, J., and Lai, L. (2015). "CAVITY: mapping the druggable binding site," in *Part of the Series Methods in Pharmacology and Toxicology*, ed W. Zhang (New York, NY: Humana Press), 111–132.

Zimmermann, G. R., Lehar, J., and Keith, C. T. (2007). Multi-target therapeutics: when the whole is greater than the sum of the parts. *Drug Discov. Today* 12, 34–42. doi: 10.1016/j.drudis.2006.11.008

2

Refinement and Rescoring of Virtual Screening Results

Giulio Rastelli and Luca Pinzi*

Department of Life Sciences, University of Modena and Reggio Emilia, Modena, Italy

***Correspondence:**
Giulio Rastelli
giulio.rastelli@unimore.it

High-throughput docking is an established computational screening approach in drug design. This methodology enables a rapid identification of biologically active hit compounds, providing an efficient and cost-effective complement or alternative to experimental high-throughput screenings. However, limitations inherent to the methodology make docking results inevitably approximate. Two major Achille's heels include the use of approximated scoring functions and the limited sampling of the ligand-target complexes. Therefore, docking results require careful evaluation and further post-docking analyses. In this article, we will overview our approach to post-docking analysis in virtual screenings. BEAR (Binding Estimation After Refinement) was developed as a post-docking processing tool that refines docking poses by means of molecular dynamics (MD) and then rescores the ligands based on more accurate scoring functions (MM-PB(GB)SA). The tool has been validated and used prospectively in drug discovery applications. Future directions regarding refinement and rescoring in virtual screening are discussed.

Keywords: docking, post-docking, virtual screening, molecular dynamics, BEAR, binding free energy

INTRODUCTION

High-throughput screening (HTS) is a widely used method for the discovery of biologically active hits. However, the high costs and the low hit rates characterizing such experiments often make HTS not affordable for academic labs or small companies (Sliwoski et al., 2014). As a consequence, high-throughput docking screenings represent an attractive alternative (Irwin and Shoichet, 2016). Structure-based virtual screenings (SBVSs) require the knowledge of the three-dimensional structure of the target of interest, as well as the access to large libraries of small molecules available in public databases (Kar and Roy, 2013; Rastelli, 2013). Docking programs generate binding poses of compounds in the active site of a target and evaluate the ligand binding strength by means of scoring functions (Lengauer and Rarey, 1996; Kitchen et al., 2004). Several docking software relying on different algorithms have been developed for virtual screening so far (Rarey et al., 1996; Morris et al., 1998; Friesner et al., 2004; Sánchez-Linares et al., 2012). However, although remarkable improvements have been obtained along the years, several drawbacks and limitations still exist (Huang and Zou, 2010; Rastelli, 2013). First of all, sampling the conformational space accessible to ligand-target complexes in an induced-fit context is a difficult and target-dependent task. To help overcoming such limitations, several *in silico* strategies including molecular dynamics or induced fit strategies have been introduced (Sherman et al., 2006; Nabuurs et al., 2007; Caporuscio and Rastelli, 2016). Secondly, docking scores and experimental binding affinities usually do not correlate, because screening large numbers of compounds in a reasonable time requires the use of approximate scoring functions. Together, the two effects imply that a variable number of false-positive and false-negative hits populate the ranked lists, which then require careful evaluation and further post-docking analyses. Hence, it has become general opinion that docking results should be improved by means of more rigorous post-docking processing strategies. Several post-processing strategies have been developed to overcome docking limitations over the past decades. In particular, methods based on binding free energy estimations have demonstrated to provide higher hit rates and to be more suitable for ranking cognate ligands in virtual screening (Hou et al., 2011; Genheden and Ryde, 2015; Pu et al., 2017), the predicted binding free energy usually correlating better with experimental data (Brandsdal et al., 2003). One of the first reported energy-based methods is MM-PB(GB)SA, which was developed to more accurately assess the relative free energy of binding for a given macromolecular system from molecular dynamics simulations (Kollman et al., 2000). This method represented a remarkable step forward to the obtainment of *in silico* predicted binding affinities that are in good agreement with experiments. In fact, it was extensively used to evaluate the free energy of binding for a number of complexes in the last years (Gohlke et al., 2003; Hou and Yu, 2007; Ferri et al., 2009; Yang et al., 2012). For example, it was successfully used for identifying residue *hot-spots* outside the binding interface of the Ras–Raf and Ras–RalGDS protein-protein complexes, discussing also their implications for an allosteric activation of the proteins (Gohlke et al., 2003). More recently, this method was also employed for predicting binding affinities of few inhibitors of HIV-1 protease and to help rationalize drug resistance caused by the mutations on the enzyme binding site (Hou and Yu, 2007). However, it should also be noted that MM-PB(GB)SA results are dependent on the employed parameters and receptor structures used in the calculations (Xu et al., 2013; Sun et al., 2014, 2018; Genheden and Ryde, 2015). More accurate free energy-based methods have also been reported (Brandsdal et al., 2003; Jorgensen and Thomas, 2008; Parenti and Rastelli, 2012; Limongelli et al., 2013; De Vivo et al., 2016). Among them, it is worth mentioning the Free Energy Perturbation (FEP) method, which allows to estimate the free energy of binding of a ligand to a protein by decomposing the system through a series of "alchemical transformations" (Jorgensen and Thomas, 2008; De Vivo et al., 2016). More recently, funnel-metadynamics (FM) methods that use a funnel-shaped potential limiting the sampling space available for a ligand to bind/unbind to a protein have been proposed (Limongelli et al., 2013; De Vivo et al., 2016). However, although these methods demonstrated to accurately estimate ligand binding, they are time-consuming and therefore not suitable for virtual screening rescoring of large databases. With the aim of improving ligand-binding estimations of docking complexes at reasonable computational costs, we developed Binding Estimation After Refinement (BEAR) (Rastelli et al., 2009). BEAR is an automated post-docking tool based on conformational refinement of docking poses with molecular dynamics followed by a more accurate prediction of binding free energies performed with MM-PBSA and MM-GBSA, which take into account desolvation energies (Kuhn et al., 2005; Lyne et al., 2006; Rastelli et al., 2010; Genheden and Ryde, 2015). As it allows accurately rescoring docking poses in reasonable times, BEAR can be considered an efficient tool that could be routinely used for virtual screening. In this article, we will briefly describe the BEAR tool, providing an overview of the validation studies performed so far. Finally, we will describe its prospective applications in drug discovery campaigns and comment on future directions of refinement and rescoring methods.

THE BEAR TOOL

The BEAR workflow (**Figure 1**; Rastelli et al., 2009) consists of an initial pre-processing step in which hydrogen atoms are added to the protein, atomic charges (AM1-BCC) are calculated for the docked molecules, and missing force-field parameters are assigned. Then, topologies for the ligand, the protein, and the ligand-protein complex are built. In particular, ligand atom types are assigned according to the Generalized Amber Force Field (GAFF) (Wang et al., 2004), while, the atom types and charges of amino acids are assigned according to the Amber ff03 force field (Duan et al., 2003). The following iterative three steps procedure is based on molecular mechanics (MM) and molecular dynamics (MD) cycles. In particular, an initial MM energy minimization of the whole protein–ligand complex is performed, followed by a short MD simulation where the ligand is allowed to move, and a final re-minimization of the entire complex. All the minimization tasks are performed through 2000 steps without restraints, and with a distance-dependent dielectric constant $\varepsilon = 4r$ and a cutoff of 12 Å. The MD simulation is performed at 300 K for 100 ps, with the SHAKE parameter turned on and a time-step of 2.0 fs. This protocol allows evaluating the reliability of the predicted docking complex and to establish potential additional ligand-protein interactions resulting from the structural refinement of the complex, thus obtaining more accurate binding energy predictions. After refinement of the complex, the free energy of binding of the ligand is calculated with the MM-PBSA and MM-GBSA methods. These operations are implemented with the use of AMBER modules (Case et al., 2018). Further details about the BEAR tool are described in Rastelli et al. (2009).

BENCHMARKING STUDIES

The post-docking tool BEAR has been extensively validated in various test cases. First of all, the MM/MD protocol described above was investigated on a series of aldose reductase inhibitors with notable chemical diversity. Remarkably, the calculated free energies of binding after refinement of ligand-protein complexes resulted to be highly correlated with experimental affinities. This study demonstrated that different classes of aldose reductase inhibitors could be accurately rescored with our procedure (Ferrari et al., 2007). Extensive validations were also made on *Plasmodium falciparium* dihydrofolate reductase (PfDHFR). These simulations aimed at evaluating the performance of BEAR in virtual screening settings of different size and complexity. Firstly, BEAR performed well in discriminating 14 known inhibitors of PfDHFR from the 1,720 compounds included in the National Cancer Institute diversity database (Rastelli et al., 2009). The achieved performances were clearly superior to those of AutoDock (Morris et al., 1998), demonstrating that rescoring

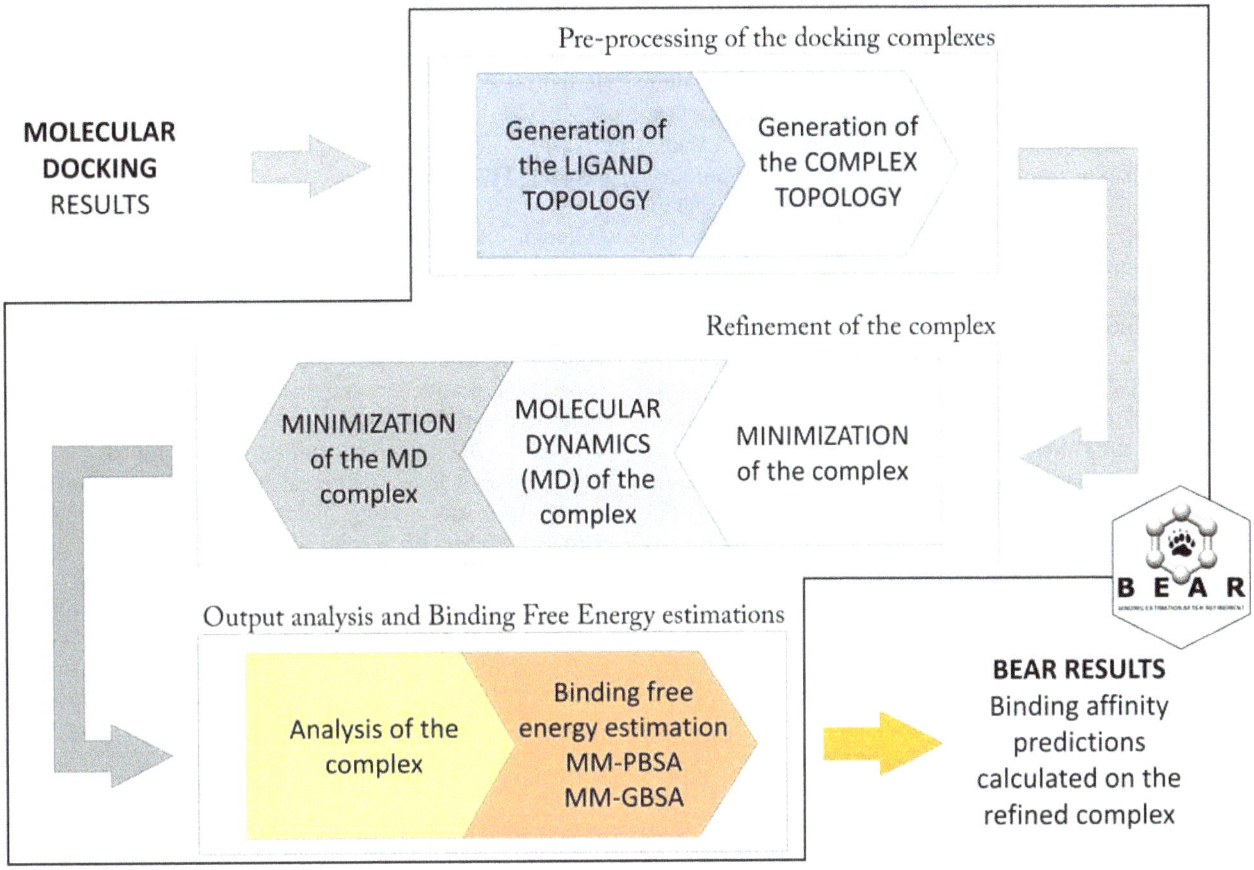

FIGURE 1 | Computational workflow applied in BEAR.

of the predicted docking poses with BEAR heavily improved SBVS results. In a second experiment, enrichment factors (EFs) obtained with BEAR were evaluated by seeding 201 known inhibitors with 7,150 decoys as contained in the DHFR data set of the Directory of Useful Decoys database (Mysinger et al., 2012). Moreover, the same set of ligands was also seeded into the 1.5 million compounds belonging to the lead-like subset of the ZINC database (Irwin et al., 2012), this latter benchmark reflecting a typical virtual screening setting. In both cases, BEAR refinement and rescoring yielded significantly higher EFs compared to docking (Degliesposti et al., 2011). This was also an opportunity for fine-tuning the BEAR parameters, and thus achieving good performances at reasonable computational costs.

The BEAR performance was also assessed on biological targets characterized by flexible binding sites and/or containing water molecules in the binding pocket. Such targets are particularly challenging for SBVS (Elokely and Doerksen, 2013). In fact, certain ligand chemotypes could fit with favorable scores into certain protein conformations but not in others, thus hampering their identification in a virtual screening. To evaluate whether docking into multiple protein conformations (ensemble docking) instead of using a single representative structure would improve BEAR predictions for "difficult" targets (Sgobba et al., 2012), we investigated targets of different families (adenosine deaminase, factor Xa, estrogen receptor, thymidine kinase, aldose reductase, and enoyl ACP reductase). Interestingly, a comparative analysis of the EFs obtained for different proteins and multiple protein conformations revealed that the application of BEAR was able in several cases to yield higher EFs compared to docking. However, in challenging targets such as adenosine deaminase and enoyl ACP reductase, all scoring functions failed in yielding high EFs. This effect was attributed to difficulties in predicting correct ligand binding modes in these two targets. In particular, when the docked pose was completely wrong, for example head-to-tail with respect to the correct binding mode, the MM/MD refinement stage was not enough to turn the binding mode into the correct one. Therefore, the advantage of using MM-PBSA and MM-GBSA in prioritizing active compounds is dependent on the obtainment of correct binding modes, which makes the refinement and rescoring procedures intimately connected.

More recently, BEAR was also applied to screen ligands of G-protein coupled receptors (GPCRs) with known crystal structure, namely β_2-adrenergic (β_2), adenosine A_{2A} (A_{2A}), dopamine D_3 (D_3), and histamine H_1 (H_1) receptors (Anighoro and Rastelli, 2013). Results were analyzed in terms of the ability to recognize known antagonists from decoys, as well as to predict correct binding modes. In all cases except for A_{2A}, significant or dramatic improvements of EFs were obtained after the application of BEAR. A_{2A} was challenging because antagonists participated to an extended water-mediated hydrogen bond network. Interestingly, explicit consideration of a suitable number of these structural waters significantly improved the predictions. This finding is in line with the fact that MM-PB(GB)SA calculations do not explicitly consider water molecules mediating ligand-protein interactions, and binding mode predictions heavily depend on the presence of bridging water molecules participating to hydrogen bond networks. For all GPCRs, a more accurate account of desolvation effects, such as the one performed by MM-PBSA, is important to accurately predict the affinity of the protonated biogenic amines. We also found that five known H_1 and D_3 receptor antagonists were top-scored and ranked well in each of the two target screenings, prospecting for the first time the utility of post-docking tools in multi-target drug design (Anighoro et al., 2014). Indeed, as the free energy of binding calculated by BEAR allows to more accurately predicting the affinity of ligands for their target(s) with a reasonable computer time investment, we envision that *in silico* strategies embedding this tool can be useful to allow the identification of ligands with the desired multi-target profiles.

PROSPECTIVE VALIDATIONS

The BEAR workflow has also been implemented in the computing GRID infrastructure EGEE, as part of the WISDOM (Wide *in silico* DOcking on Malaria) initiative against malaria (Kasam et al., 2009). Then, it was deployed to perform virtual screenings against antimalarial drug targets. One massive data challenge was performed on Plasmepsin II, an aspartic protease involved in the metabolism of *P. falciparum* (Degliesposti et al., 2009). In this work, BEAR was used to refine and rescore the 5,000 top-scoring compounds docked with FlexX (Rarey et al., 1996). Then, the final step of candidates' selection was performed on the top 200 compounds resulting from both MM-PBSA and MM-GBSA ranked lists. Interestingly, an analysis of the BEAR ranked lists, together with an inspection of the protein-ligand complexes and a similarity-based clustering of the ligands allowed selecting 30 compounds belonging to 5 different chemotypes as potential Plasmepsin II inhibitors. Remarkably, 26 of them were active, resulting in an impressive hit rate of 87%, and some of the compounds displayed nanomolar inhibitory activity.

More recently, BEAR was successfully applied in a virtual screening campaign that allowed the identification of the *first-in-class* allosteric inhibitors of CDK2 (Rastelli et al., 2014). In this work, around 600.000 commercially available compounds were screened against a crystal structure of CDK2 with an open type III allosteric pocket, by using AutoDock for docking and BEAR for post-docking analyses. The adopted virtual screening protocol led to the identification of 7 allosteric ligands of CDK2, providing a hit rate of 20%. Interestingly, the most potent compound was able to selectively inhibit CDK2-mediated Retinoblastoma phosphorylation, confirming that its mechanism of action is fully compatible with a selective inhibition of CDK2 phosphorylation in cells. Moreover, some of these ligands inhibited the proliferation of MDA-MB231 and ZR-75-1 breast cancer cells with IC_{50} values in the low micromolar range (Rastelli et al., 2014).

FINAL REMARKS

Although many progresses have been made in molecular docking, limitations deriving from the use of rigid protein conformations and of approximate scoring functions often impair virtual screening results. Therefore, docking results require careful evaluation and further post-docking analyses. BEAR is a post-processing tool that performs binding free energy estimations after MM and MD refinement of docking complexes. Our previous studies demonstrated that BEAR performed well in a number of benchmarking investigations, as well as in discovering biologically active hits in different prospective virtual screening campaigns. Moreover, as it not computationally demanding as other free energy-based methods, it constitutes a reasonable compromise to obtain accurate rescoring of ligands at reasonable computational costs. One might argue that the application of more accurate workflows would require longer computing times with respect to docking. This is especially true considering the recent contributions provided by high performance computing systems to molecular docking, which enable the screening of millions of compounds in a reasonable time (Perez-Sanchez and Wenzel, 2011; Guerrero et al., 2012; Dong et al., 2018). However, future advances in hardware and software will help circumventing such limitation (De Vivo et al., 2016; Wang et al., 2018). Moreover, further advances in our ability to correctly estimate entropies of binding, which are usually not considered in the calculations, will certainly improve post-docking tools, and binding free energy predictions in general. The implementation of enhanced sampling MD protocols in post-docking protocols is another possibility that may enable a more efficient sampling of ligand-protein complexes. Because free energy predictions are heavily dependent on correct binding modes, this may have dramatic consequences on our ability to predict active ligands in virtual screenings. Another interesting question is how to further increase hit rates while enabling post-docking tools to identify significantly vs. moderately active hits. This is an important aspect that would make the subsequent hit-to-lead optimization much easier. Exponential consensus ranking approaches such as the one developed by Palacio-Rodríguez et al. (2019) could be of help, for example to favorably exploit both MM-PBSA and MM-GBSA ranked lists, which generally differ.

AUTHOR CONTRIBUTIONS

GR conceived and wrote the study. LP contributed in writing and editing the manuscript.

REFERENCES

Anighoro, A., Bajorath, J. J., and Rastelli, G. (2014). Polypharmacology: challenges and opportunities in drug discovery. *J. Med. Chem.* 57, 7874–7887. doi: 10.1021/jm5006463

Anighoro, A., and Rastelli, G. (2013). Enrichment factor analyses on G-protein coupled receptors with known crystal structure. *J. Chem. Inf. Model.* 53, 739–743. doi: 10.1021/ci4000745

Brandsdal, B. O., Österberg, F., Almlöf, M., Feierberg, I., Luzhkov, V. B., and Åqvist, J. B. (2003). Free energy calculations and ligand binding in protein simulations. *Adv. Protein Chem.* 66, 123–158. doi: 10.1016/S0065-3233(03)66004-3

Caporuscio, F., and Rastelli, G. (2016). Exploiting computationally derived out-of-the-box protein conformations for drug design. *Future Med. Chem.* 8, 1887–1897. doi: 10.4155/fmc-2016-0098

Case, D. A., Ben-Shalom, I. Y., Brozell, S. R., Cerutti, D. S., Cheatham, T. E. III., Cruzeiro, V. W. D., et al. (2018). *AMBER 2018*. University of California, San Francisco, CA. Available online at: http://www.ambermd.org/ (accessed April 15, 2019).

De Vivo, M., Masetti, M., Bottegoni, G., and Cavalli, A. (2016). Role of molecular dynamics and related methods in drug discovery. *J. Med. Chem.* 59, 4035–4061. doi: 10.1021/acs.jmedchem.5b01684

Degliesposti, G., Kasam, V., Da Costa, A., Kang, H. K., Kim, N., Kim, D. W., et al. (2009). Design and discovery of plasmepsin II inhibitors using an automated workflow on large-scale grids. *ChemMedChem* 4, 1164–1173. doi: 10.1002/cmdc.200900111

Degliesposti, G., Portioli, C., Parenti, M. D., and Rastelli, G. (2011). BEAR, a novel virtual screening methodology for drug discovery. *J. Biomol. Screen.* 16, 129–133. doi: 10.1177/1087057110388276

Dong, D., Xu, Z., Zhong, W., and Peng, S. (2018). Parallelization of molecular docking: a review. *Curr. Top. Med. Chem.* 18, 1015–1028. doi: 10.2174/1568026618666180821145215

Duan, Y., Wu, C., Chowdhury, S., Lee, M. C., Xiong, G., Zhang, W., et al. (2003). A point-charge force field for molecular mechanics simulations of proteins based on condensed-phase quantum mechanical calculations. *J. Comput. Chem.* 24, 1999–2012. doi: 10.1002/jcc.10349

Elokely, K. M., and Doerksen, R. J. (2013). Docking challenge: protein sampling and molecular docking performance. *J. Chem. Inf. Model.* 53, 1934–1945. doi: 10.1021/ci400040d

Ferrari, A. M., Degliesposti, G., Sgobba, M., and Rastelli, G. (2007). Validation of an automated procedure for the prediction of relative free energies of binding on a set of aldose reductase inhibitors. *Bioorg. Med. Chem.* 15, 7865–7877. doi: 10.1016/j.bmc.2007.08.019

Ferri, N., Corsini, A., Bottino, P., Clerici, F., and Contini, A. (2009). Virtual screening approach for the identification of New Rac1 inhibitors. *J. Med. Chem.* 52, 4087–4090. doi: 10.1021/jm8015987

Friesner, R. A., Banks, J. L., Murphy, R. B., Halgren, T. A., Klicic, J. J., Mainz, D. T., et al. (2004). Glide: a new approach for rapid, accurate docking and scoring. 1. Method and assessment of docking accuracy. *J. Med. Chem.* 47, 1739–1749. doi: 10.1021/jm0306430

Genheden, S., and Ryde, U. (2015). The MM/PBSA and MM/GBSA methods to estimate ligand-binding affinities. *Expert Opin. Drug Discov.* 10, 449–461. doi: 10.1517/17460441.2015.1032936

Gohlke, H., Kiel, C., and Case, D. A. (2003). Insights into protein–protein binding by binding free energy calculation and free energy decomposition for the Ras-Raf and Ras-RalGDS complexes. *J. Mol. Biol.* 330, 891–913. doi: 10.1016/S0022-2836(03)00610-7

Guerrero, G. D., Perez-S'nchez, H. E., Cecilia, J. M., and Garcia, J. M. (2012). "Parallelization of virtual screening in drug discovery on massively parallel architectures," in *2012 20th Euromicro International Conference on Parallel, Distributed and Network-based Processing* (Garching), 588–595. doi: 10.1109/PDP.2012.26

Hou, T., Wang, J., Li, Y., and Wang, W. (2011). Assessing the performance of the molecular mechanics/Poisson Boltzmann surface area and molecular mechanics/generalized Born surface area methods. II. The accuracy of ranking poses generated from docking. *J. Comput. Chem.* 32, 866–877. doi: 10.1002/jcc.21666

Hou, T., and Yu, R. (2007). Molecular dynamics and free energy studies on the wild-type and double mutant HIV-1 protease complexed with amprenavir and two amprenavir-related inhibitors: mechanism for binding and drug resistance. *J. Med. Chem.* 50, 1177–1188. doi: 10.1021/jm0609162

Huang, S.-Y., and Zou, X. (2010). Advances and challenges in protein-ligand docking. *Int. J. Mol. Sci.* 11, 3016–3034. doi: 10.3390/ijms11083016

Irwin, J. J., and Shoichet, B. K. (2016). Docking screens for novel ligands conferring new biology. *J. Med. Chem.* 59, 4103–4120. doi: 10.1021/acs.jmedchem.5b02008

Irwin, J. J., Sterling, T., Mysinger, M. M., Bolstad, E. S., and Coleman, R. G. (2012). ZINC: a free tool to discover chemistry for biology. *J. Chem. Inf. Model.* 52, 1757–1768. doi: 10.1021/ci3001277

Jorgensen, W. L., and Thomas, L. L. (2008). Perspective on free-energy perturbation calculations for chemical equilibria. *J. Chem. Theory Comput.* 4, 869–876. doi: 10.1021/ct800011m

Kar, S., and Roy, K. (2013). How far can virtual screening take us in drug discovery? *Expert Opin. Drug Discov.* 8, 245–261. doi: 10.1517/17460441.2013.761204

Kasam, V., Salzemann, J., Botha, M., Dacosta, A., Degliesposti, G., Isea, R., et al. (2009). WISDOM-II: screening against multiple targets implicated in malaria using computational grid infrastructures. *Malar. J.* 8:88. doi: 10.1186/1475-2875-8-88

Kitchen, D. B., Decornez, H., Furr, J. R., and Bajorath, J. (2004). Docking and scoring in virtual screening for drug discovery: methods and applications. *Nat. Rev. Drug Discov.* 3, 935–949. doi: 10.1038/nrd1549

Kollman, P. A., Massova, I., Reyes, C., Kuhn, B., Huo, S., Chong, L., et al. (2000). Calculating structures and free energies of complex molecules: combining molecular mechanics and continuum models. *Acc. Chem. Res.* 33, 889–897. doi: 10.1021/ar000033j

Kuhn, B., Gerber, P., Schulz-Gasch, T., and Stahl, M. (2005). Validation and use of the MM-PBSA approach for drug discovery. *J. Med. Chem.* 48, 4040–4048. doi: 10.1021/jm049081q

Lengauer, T., and Rarey, M. (1996). Computational methods for biomolecular docking. *Curr. Opin. Struct. Biol.* 6, 402–406. doi: 10.1016/S0959-440X(96)80061-3

Limongelli, V., Bonomi, M., and Parrinello, M. (2013). Funnel metadynamics as accurate binding free-energy method. *Proc. Natl. Acad. Sci. U.S.A.* 110, 6358–6363. doi: 10.1073/pnas.1303186110

Lyne, P. D., Lamb, M. L., and Saeh, J. C. (2006). Accurate prediction of the relative potencies of members of a series of kinase inhibitors using molecular docking and MM-GBSA scoring. *J. Med. Chem.* 49, 4805–4808. doi: 10.1021/jm060522a

Morris, G. M., Goodsell, D. S., Halliday, R. S., Huey, R., Hart, W. E., Belew, R. K., et al. (1998). Automated docking using a Lamarckian genetic algorithm and an empirical binding free energy function. *J. Comput. Chem.* 19, 1639–1662.

Mysinger, M. M., Carchia, M., Irwin, J. J., and Shoichet, B. K. (2012). Directory of useful decoys, enhanced (DUD-E): better ligands and decoys for better benchmarking. *J. Med. Chem.* 55, 6582–6594. doi: 10.1021/jm300687e

Nabuurs, S. B., Wagener, M., and de Vlieg, J. (2007). A flexible approach to induced fit docking. *J. Med. Chem.* 50, 6507–6518. doi: 10.1021/jm070593p

Palacio-Rodríguez, K., Lans, I., Cavasotto, C. N., and Cossio, P. (2019). Exponential consensus ranking improves the outcome in docking and receptor ensemble docking. *Sci. Rep.* 9:5142. doi: 10.1038/s41598-019-41594-3

Parenti, M.D., and Rastelli, G. (2012). Advances and applications of binding affinity prediction methods in drug discovery. *Biotechnol. Adv.* 30, 244–250. doi: 10.1016/j.biotechadv.2011.08.003

Perez-Sanchez, H., and Wenzel, W. (2011). Optimization methods for virtual screening on novel computational architectures. *Curr. Comput. Aided. Drug Des.* 7, 44–52. doi: 10.2174/157340911793743565

Pu, C., Yan, G., Shi, J., and Li, R. (2017). Assessing the performance of docking scoring function, FEP, MM-GBSA, and QM/MM-GBSA approaches on a series of PLK1 inhibitors. *Medchemcomm* 8, 1452–1458. doi: 10.1039/c7md00184c

Rarey, M., Kramer, B., Lengauer, T., and Klebe, G. (1996). A fast flexible docking method using an incremental construction algorithm. *J. Mol. Biol.* 261, 470–489. doi: 10.1006/jmbi.1996.0477

Rastelli, G. (2013). Emerging topics in structure-based virtual screening. *Pharm. Res.* 30, 1458–1463. doi: 10.1007/s11095-013-1012-9

Rastelli, G., Anighoro, A., Chripkova, M., Carrassa, L., and Broggini, M. (2014). Structure-based discovery of the first allosteric inhibitors of cyclin-dependent kinase 2. *Cell Cycle* 13, 2296–2305. doi: 10.4161/cc.29295

Rastelli, G., Degliesposti, G., Del Rio, A., and Sgobba, M. (2009). Binding estimation after refinement, a new automated procedure for the refinement and rescoring of docked ligands in virtual screening. *Chem. Biol. Drug Des.* 73, 283–286. doi: 10.1111/j.1747-0285.2009.00780.x

Rastelli, G., Del Rio, A., Degliesposti, G., Sgobba, M., Rio, A., Del Degliesposti, G., et al. (2010). Fast and accurate predictions of binding free energies using MM-PBSA and MM-GBSA. *J. Comput. Chem.* 31, 797–810. doi: 10.1002/jcc.21372

Sánchez-Linares, I., Pérez-Sánchez, H., Cecilia, J. M., and García, J. M. (2012). High-throughput parallel blind virtual screening using BINDSURF. *BMC Bioinformatics* 13:S13. doi: 10.1186/1471-2105-13-S14-S13

Sgobba, M., Caporuscio, F., Anighoro, A., Portioli, C., and Rastelli, G. (2012). Application of a post-docking procedure based on MM-PBSA and MM-GBSA on single and multiple protein conformations. *Eur. J. Med. Chem.* 58, 431–440. doi: 10.1016/j.ejmech.2012.10.024

Sherman, W., Beard, H. S., and Farid, R. (2006). Use of an induced fit receptor structure in virtual screening. *Chem. Biol. Drug Des.* 67, 83–84. doi: 10.1111/j.1747-0285.2005.00327.x

Sliwoski, G., Kothiwale, S., Meiler, J., and Lowe, E. W. (2014). Computational methods in drug discovery. *Pharmacol. Rev.* 66, 334–395. doi: 10.1124/pr.112.007336

Sun, H., Duan, L., Chen, F., Liu, H., Wang, Z., Pan, P., et al. (2018). Assessing the performance of MM/PBSA and MM/GBSA methods. 7. Entropy effects on the performance of end-point binding free energy calculation approaches. *Phys. Chem. Chem. Phys.* 20, 14450–14460. doi: 10.1039/C7CP07623A

Sun, H., Li, Y., Shen, M., Tian, S., Xu, L., Pan, P., et al. (2014). Assessing the performance of MM/PBSA and MM/GBSA methods. 5. Improved docking performance using high solute dielectric constant MM/GBSA and MM/PBSA rescoring *Phys. Chem. Chem. Phys.* 16, 22035–22045. doi: 10.1039/C4CP03179B

Wang, C., Greene, D., Xiao, L., Qi, R., and Luo, R. (2018). Recent developments and applications of the MMPBSA method. *Front. Mol. Biosci.* 4:87. doi: 10.3389/fmolb.2017.00087

Wang, J., Wolf, R. M., Caldwell, J. W., Kollman, P. A., Case, D. A., Wang, J., et al. (2004). Development and testing of a general amber force field. *J. Comput. Chem.* 25, 1157–1174. doi: 10.1002/jcc.20035

Xu, L., Sun, H., Li, Y., Wang, J., and Hou, T. (2013). Assessing the performance of MM/PBSA and MM/GBSA methods. 3. The impact of force fields and ligand charge models. *J. Phys. Chem. B* 117, 8408–8421. doi: 10.1021/jp404160y

Yang, Y., Liu, H., and Yao, X. (2012). Understanding the molecular basis of MK2–p38α signaling complex assembly: insights into protein–protein interaction by molecular dynamics and free energy studies. *Mol. Biosyst.* 8, 2106–2118. doi: 10.1039/C2MB25042J

3

Finding Constellations in Chemical Space Through Core Analysis

J. Jesús Naveja[1,2*] *and José L. Medina-Franco*[2*]

[1] PECEM, School of Medicine, Universidad Nacional Autónoma de México, Mexico City, Mexico, [2] Department of Pharmacy, School of Chemistry, Universidad Nacional Autónoma de México, Mexico City, Mexico

***Correspondence:**
J. Jesús Naveja
naveja@comunidad.unam.mx
José L. Medina-Franco
medinajl@unam.mx

Herein we introduce the constellation plots as a general approach that merges different and complementary molecular representations to enhance the information contained in a visual representation and analysis of chemical space. The method is based on a combination of a sub-structure based representation and classification of compounds with a "classical" coordinate-based representation of chemical space. A distinctive outcome of the method is that organizing the compounds in analog series leads to the formation of groups of molecules, aka "constellations" in chemical space. The novel approach is general and can be used to rapidly identify, for instance, insightful and "bright" Structure-Activity Relationships (StARs) in chemical space that are easy to interpret. This kind of analysis is expected to be especially useful for lead identification in large datasets of unannotated molecules, such as those obtained through high-throughput screening. We demonstrate the application of the method using two datasets of focused inhibitors designed against DNMTs and AKT1.

Keywords: analog series, data visualization, descriptor, scaffold, structure-property relationships

INTRODUCTION

The concept of chemical space is broadly used in drug discovery because of its multiple potential applications; for instance, in library design, compound or dataset classification, compound selection, exploration of structure-activity relationships (SAR), and navigation though structure-property relationships (SPR) in general. However, a precise unique definition of chemical space is not simple. An even more challenging task is the visual representation of this subjective concept.

Chemical space is usually defined as the set of all possible organic compounds (Lipinski and Hopkins, 2004). It is widely recognized that the virtual chemical space is more than astronomically large, as not even all atoms in the universe would suffice to synthesize a single molecule from each of all the 10^{63} possible organic compounds of a size up to 30 atoms (Clayden et al., 2012). Nevertheless, massive efforts have been undertaken to enumerate billions of hypothetical organic compounds, thus allowing large virtual screening campaigns to take place (Reymond, 2015; Lyu et al., 2019).

Along with the increasing size of the mapped chemical space, the interest of applying cartographic methods to visualize the space has expanded (Oprea and Gottfries, 2001). As a result, numerous visualization and conceptualization approaches into chemical space have emerged (Larsson et al., 2007; Osolodkin et al., 2015; Naveja and Medina-Franco, 2017). A cornerstone and key aspect of all proposed methods is the molecular representation and parameters used to define the space where the compounds will reside. Chemical space visualizations have to reduce the dimensionality of the problem of comparing molecular structures, which can be done through algorithms such as principal components analysis and t-distributed stochastic neighbor embedding (see Osolodkin et al., 2015).

In most chemical space approaches, it is desirable that chemical analogs are closer to each other than unrelated and dissimilar molecules since this allows machine learning methods to identify clusters of structurally-related molecules (Medina-Franco et al., 2008; Naveja and Medina-Franco, 2015; Naveja et al., 2016, 2018a). In addition, clustering analog series would allow, at least in principle, to map SAR/SPR into that space. However, due to the vast amplitude of the chemical space and the inevitable loss of information with an initially large space projected into lower dimensions, it is expected that non-analog compounds will end up in the same cluster. Also, when many points in the chemical space are considered at once, visualizations become harder to interpret. To address this issue, approaches such as virtual reality have emerged (Probst and Reymond, 2018).

In parallel to such chemical space approaches based on coordinates, scaffold analysis is a more consistent and chemically-intuitive approach for exploring and identifying collections of analogs (Hu et al., 2011). Ever since the pioneering work by Bemis and Murcko (1996), computational identification of chemical scaffolds has been refined. In this line, Stumpfe et al. (2016) recently introduced the analog series-based scaffold (ASBS), a revolutionary scaffold concept that is more flexible and chemically sound than its predecessors. In fact, the ASBS has proven to yield more biologically meaningful structure-activity/property relationships (SA/PR) than other scaffold definitions (Dimova et al., 2016; Kunimoto et al., 2017; Bajorath, 2018; Dimova and Bajorath, 2018).

Although the chemical space of single analog series can be effectively explored and used, for instance, to guide lead optimization programmes (Vogt et al., 2018), methods for analyzing the relationship among scaffolds of different analog series remain to be explored. Of note, a difficulty in this regard emerges as analog-series based scaffolds tend not to be as consistent as Bemis-Murcko scaffolds, since they result from the retrospective analysis of analog series (Bajorath, 2018). Accordingly, a core framework inspired in the design of the ASBS avoids the shortcoming of inconsistency by allowing molecules to be annotated with more than one putative core (Naveja et al., Submitted). Hence, large libraries containing analogs can be condensed into fewer cores. In this way, SA/PR can be preferentially analyzed for the most explored regions of the chemical space: analog series.

Herein, we present a general methodology for applying the putative core framework to produce more concise and meaningful representations of the chemical space. To our understanding, this is the first method designed for charting multiple analog series into a coordinate-based chemical space, thus combining in a single plot two general and useful approaches of molecular representation and mapping. Of note, since within this framework cores may share analogs (i.e., analog series are allowed to share compounds), such cores can be connected, thus resembling constellations in the chemical space. Therefore, we termed the resulting graphics "constellation plots." As it will be discussed, activity data (or any property of interest) can be mapped into the constellation plot allowing to explore SA/PRs in the space and quickly identify interesting regions in the space. The rest of this methodological paper is organized as follows: first, the concept scheme is presented and the formalism explained through a toy example; thereafter, two case studies using exemplary datasets are presented; finally, we discuss the conclusions and perspectives of this novel approach for combining the scaffold and the chemical space concepts.

METHODS

Datasets Used in the Examples

For illustrating the application of constellation plots in two different context of analysis, we used two benchmark datasets that have been previously explored with other analysis approaches. One set was a group of 827 AKT1 inhibitors extracted and curated from ChEMBL (Gaulton et al., 2017; Naveja et al., 2018b). The second dataset was a collection of 286 compounds tested as inhibitors of DNMT (DNA methyltransferases). This second data set was integrated from multiple sources of information as described in Naveja and Medina-Franco (2018). Since this dataset integrates qualitative (such as those containing crystallographic data) and quantitative databases (such as those containing experimental determination of inhibition curves), for this dataset, we use a categorical classification of activity in "active" or "inactive." The files of the two datasets are included as **Supplementary Information.**

Chemical Space and Analog Series

As mentioned above, constellation plots fuse two ligand-based concepts: chemical space and core analysis. Standard chemical space analysis is carried out by computing descriptors for a collection of molecules (e.g., physicochemical properties and/or structural features) and then applying dimensionality reduction approaches (Rosén et al., 2009; Osolodkin et al., 2015; González-Medina et al., 2016; Prieto-Martínez et al., 2016; Naveja and Medina-Franco, 2017; Borrel et al., 2018). As a result, every data point represents a single molecule (see **Figure 1**). This can render many visualizations hard to read and analyze by the naked eye. Furthermore, the numerous descriptors used are combined, such that every axis in the visualization turns out to have a quite abstract meaning. Herein, for the purpose of charting chemical space, *t*-distributed stochastic neighbor embedding (*t*-SNE) is used. This methodology reduces the number of data points in the center of the map as compared to other approaches and has been used successfully in chemical space charting (Maaten and Hinton, 2008; Lewis et al., 2015). However, other coordinate-based representations of chemical space can be used in this general approach.

In contrast to chemical space, standard scaffold and analog series analysis aims toward a clear and consistent picture of the relationships among compounds. For instance, a scaffold is a substructure shared by all compounds annotated with it. A state-of-the-art approach for defining analog series-based scaffolds was proposed by Stumpfe et al. (2016). They have reasoned that for a scaffold to be relevant in medicinal chemistry, it should not only be a substructure of a molecule, but it also has to comply with three additional criteria: (i) be a major component of the whole molecule, (ii) be derived from the molecule through retrosynthetic rules, and (iii) summarize an

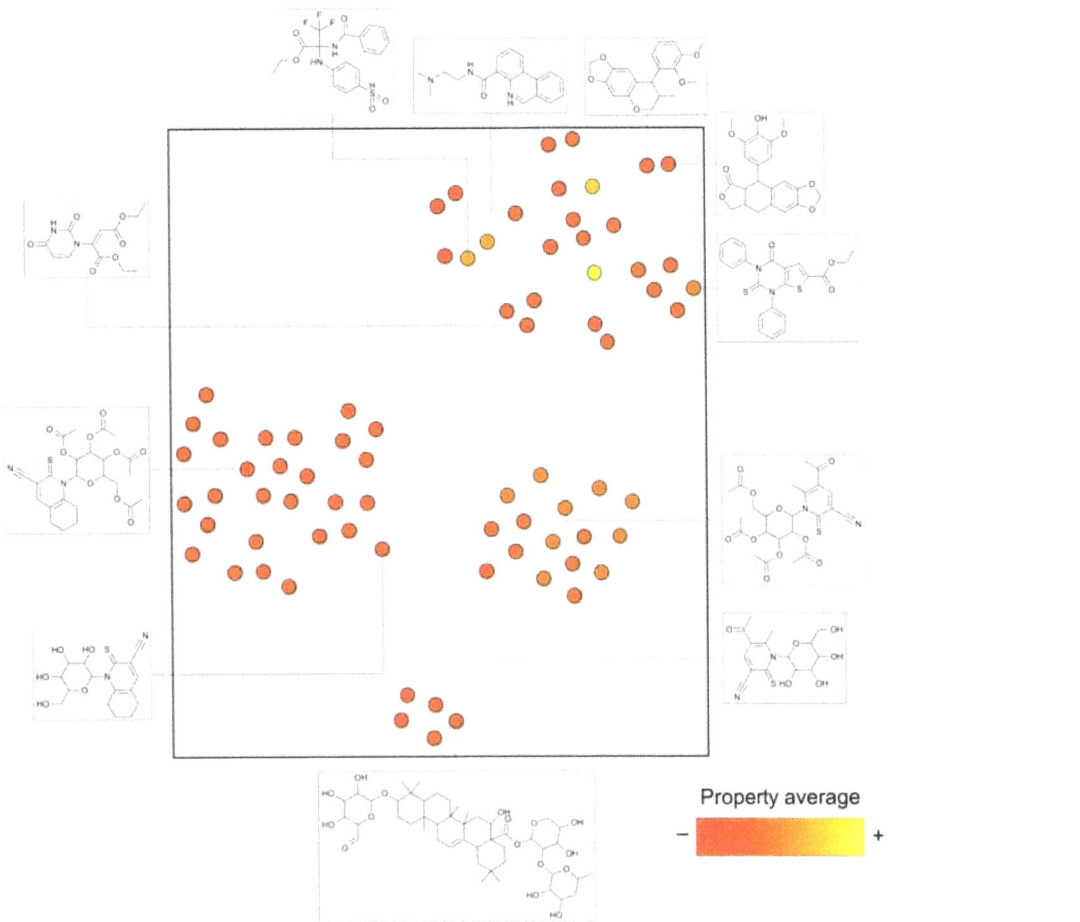

FIGURE 1 | A hypothetical example of a typical chemical space representation based on coordinates. The axes represent the chemical space and have abstract meanings regarding a combination of descriptors. In this case, *t*-SNE using Morgan fingerprints was applied. Every dot represents a single molecule. In activity landscape modeling, color is used to indicate a property (potency in a particular biological endpoint).

analog series in a particular dataset. A number of computational approaches for obtaining ASBS have been proposed (Dimova et al., 2016; Stumpfe et al., 2016; Bajorath, 2018; Naveja et al., 2019). Within these approaches, an analog series is defined as a subnetwork connected by matched molecular pairs (MMPs) (Griffen et al., 2011).

Chemical space analysis of individual analog series has been carried out to measure progression in lead optimization and saturation of analog series (Kunimoto et al., 2018; Vogt et al., 2018; Yonchev et al., 2018). Nevertheless, the fact that assumption (iii) makes analog series inconsistent in as much as the scaffold definition is dependent on the dataset used (Bajorath, 2018) is a limitation for the exploration of chemical space of multiple analog series at once. In a recent study (Naveja et al., Submitted), we discussed that by removing assumption (iii) two effects take place: first, every molecule is allowed to be annotated to more than a single core (equivalent to the term "scaffold"); and second, complete consistency is achieved as no core annotations are ever omitted for any molecule (see **Figure 2**). It is within this general core framework that we propose using constellation plots.

Summarizing Analog Series Information in a Dataset Within the General Core Framework

Since the general core framework can assign multiple cores to single molecules, a useful step prior to mapping cores in the chemical space would be summarizing analog series in the smallest number of cores possible. As illustrated in **Figure 3**, in some instances it is possible to summarize a whole analog series in a single core structure, while in other cases this cannot be done without loss of information. Hence, for avoiding such situations, we did not discard cores unless only one compound mapped to it. Furthermore, if two or more cores mapped to exactly the same compounds, then only the largest core was kept and the others were disregarded from the analysis.

Constellation Plots

After processing a collection of compounds under the general core framework, information is obtained in multiple regards, namely: (a) the chemical structure of every core; (b) the sets of molecules mapping to each core; (c) the molecules annotated to multiple cores; and (d) the analog series to which each compound and core are annotated. We propose a visualization methodology summarizing these four dimensions in a single graphic: the constellation plot that is schematically illustrated in **Figure 4**.

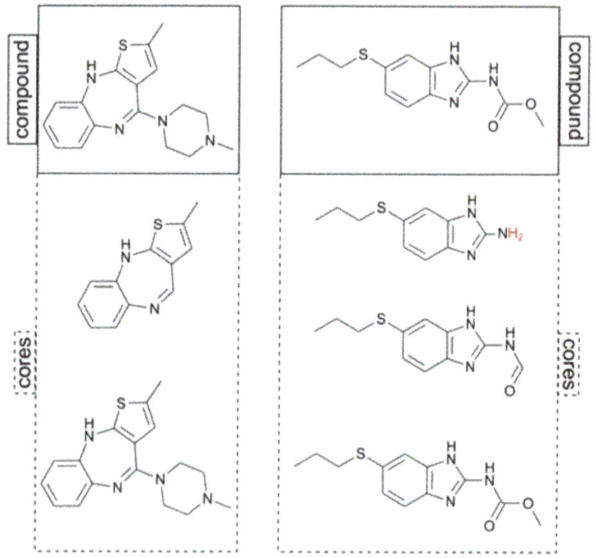

FIGURE 2 | Two examples of putative cores computed for two molecules. Note that in this approach the same chemical structure can be its own core (structures at the bottom). After RECAP fragmentation, hydrogens are added to the core structure to avoid invalid valence (marked in red).

Essentially, in a constellation plot, the chemical structure of representative cores in a database (for example, those annotated with a predefined minimum number of compounds) is used to find descriptors and map them into a chemical space as if they were single molecules. The size of the circles is used to represent the relative number of compounds annotated to each core. Cores sharing compounds are connected by lines forming "constellations" in the chemical space. Every circle is labeled with an identifier for the analog series to which each core belongs. Additionally, a color scale can be used to represent an average of a given property or activity of the compounds annotated with each core, thereby turning constellation plots useful for activity landscape modeling (Waddell and Medina-Franco, 2012). Of note, the activity can be, for instance, measured for a single molecular target. However, the property could also be a representative measure of the selectivity or promiscuity profile of all the compounds sharing a core across multiple biological endpoints (see section Conclusions and Perspectives).

Figure 4, as opposed to **Figure 1**, is able to summarize a larger number of compounds than points depicted and contains information about actual analogs. For instance, analog series I, J, and L form separate clusters, but the cluster top right has multiple chemotypes of distinct analog series. This could not be inferred from clustering algorithms applied to the chemical space information only.

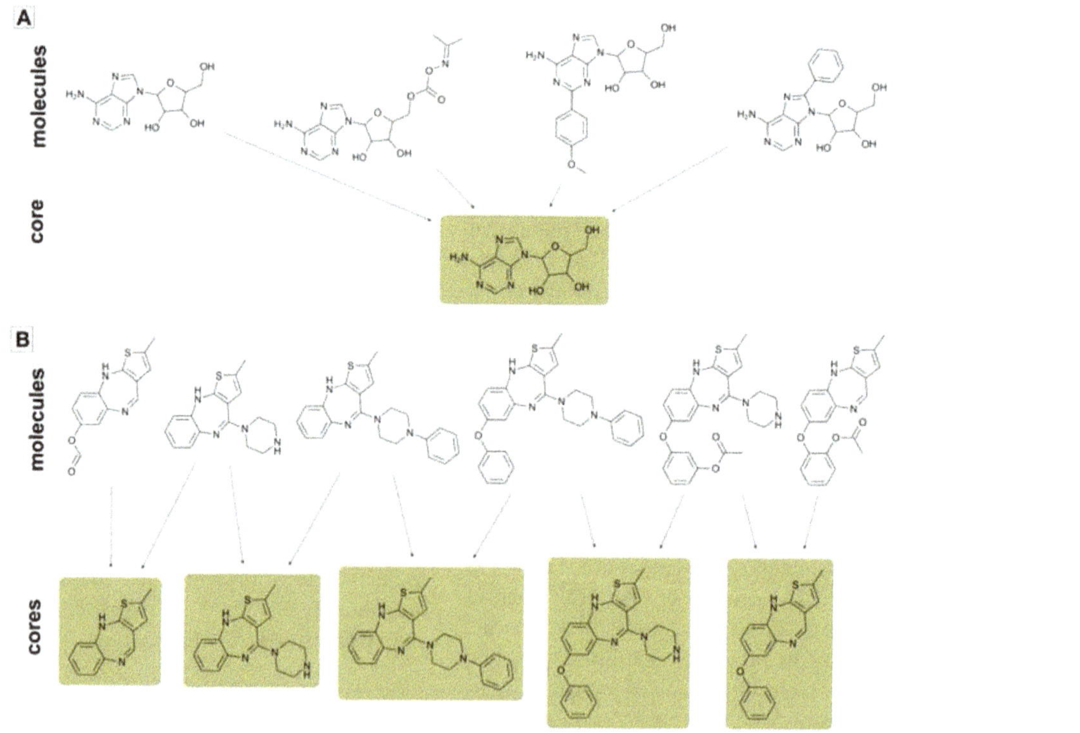

FIGURE 3 | Examples of two analog series with multiple compounds and cores. **(A)** Analog series that can be summarized in a single core; **(B)** Analog series formed by multiple cores. In case **(B)** a single core is not enough for summarizing all information in an analog series.

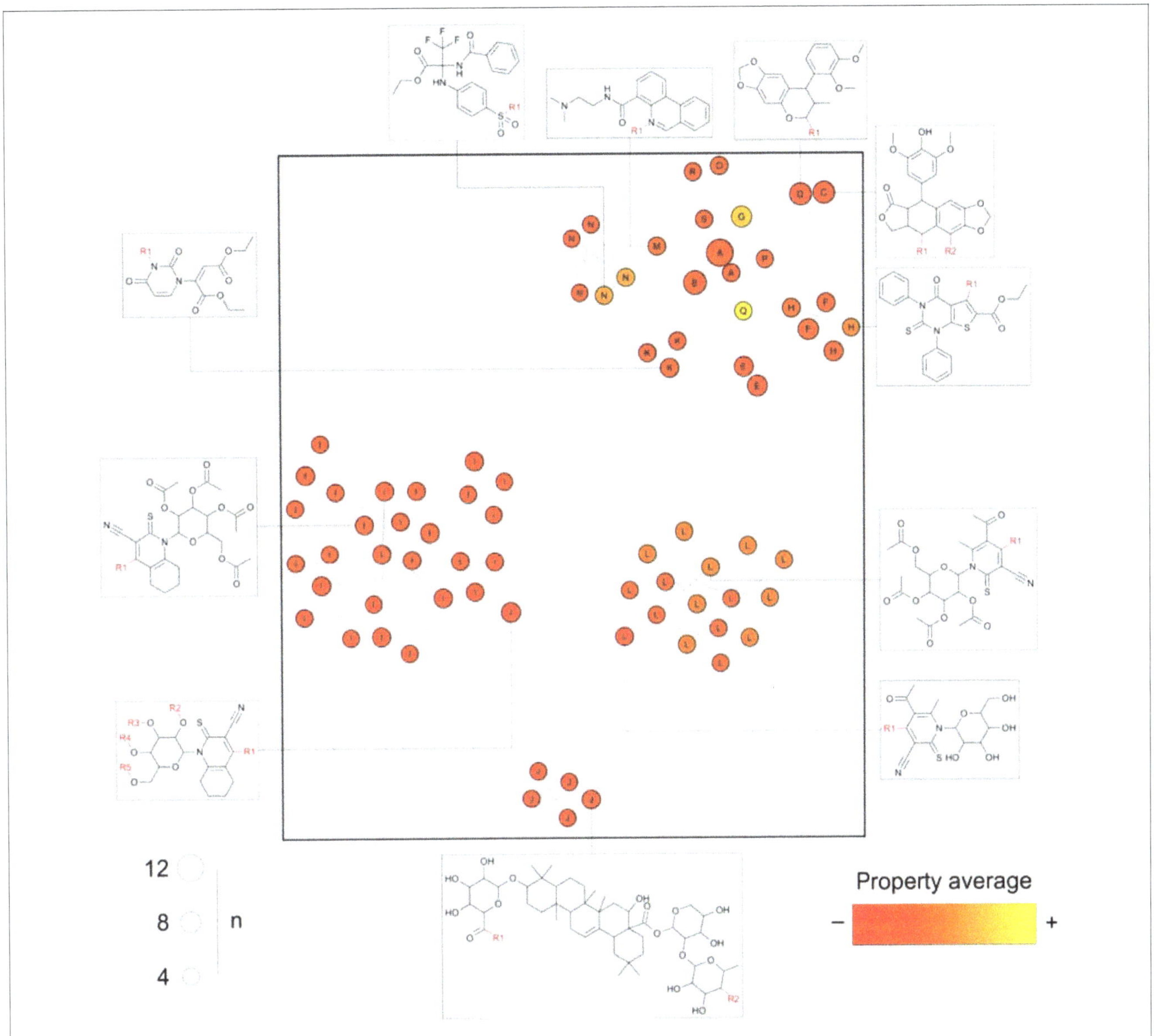

FIGURE 4 | Schematic representation of a general form of a constellation plot. Every circle in the plot represents a core; the axes comprise the coordinates of the chemical structure of the core projected into a 2D representation of the chemical space as computed by any of the standard approaches (e.g., generated using continuous properties or molecular fingerprints and applying *t*-SNE or principal components analysis); the size of the circles indicates the "n" number of compounds annotated to a given core; connected circles are cores sharing compounds; the labels indicate the analog series every point belongs to; the color scale represents the average of a property/activity of the compounds mapping to the core.

Implementation

All scripts required for producing the data herein reported use free Python code and are made freely available in **Supplementary Information**. RDkit was used for computing fingerprints and manipulation of chemical structures (http://www.rdkit.org). Scikit-learn was used for computing *t*-SNE (Pedregosa et al., 2011).

RESULTS AND DISCUSSION

The construction of constellations plots and exemplary applications are illustrated with two case studies of general interest in drug discovery. As mentioned in the section Methods, the first example consists of a dataset of 827 AKT1 inhibitors obtained from ChEMBL (Gaulton et al., 2017) and cheminformatically described in Naveja et al. (2018b). The second example employs a data set of 286 DNA methyltransferase (DNMT) inhibitors obtained from the integration of several databases as described in Naveja and Medina-Franco (2018).

Case Study 1: AKT1 Inhibitors

Analogs in this library could be summarized in 144 cores as discussed in the section Methods. The cores were organized in 79 analog series and contained 440 compounds (about half of the

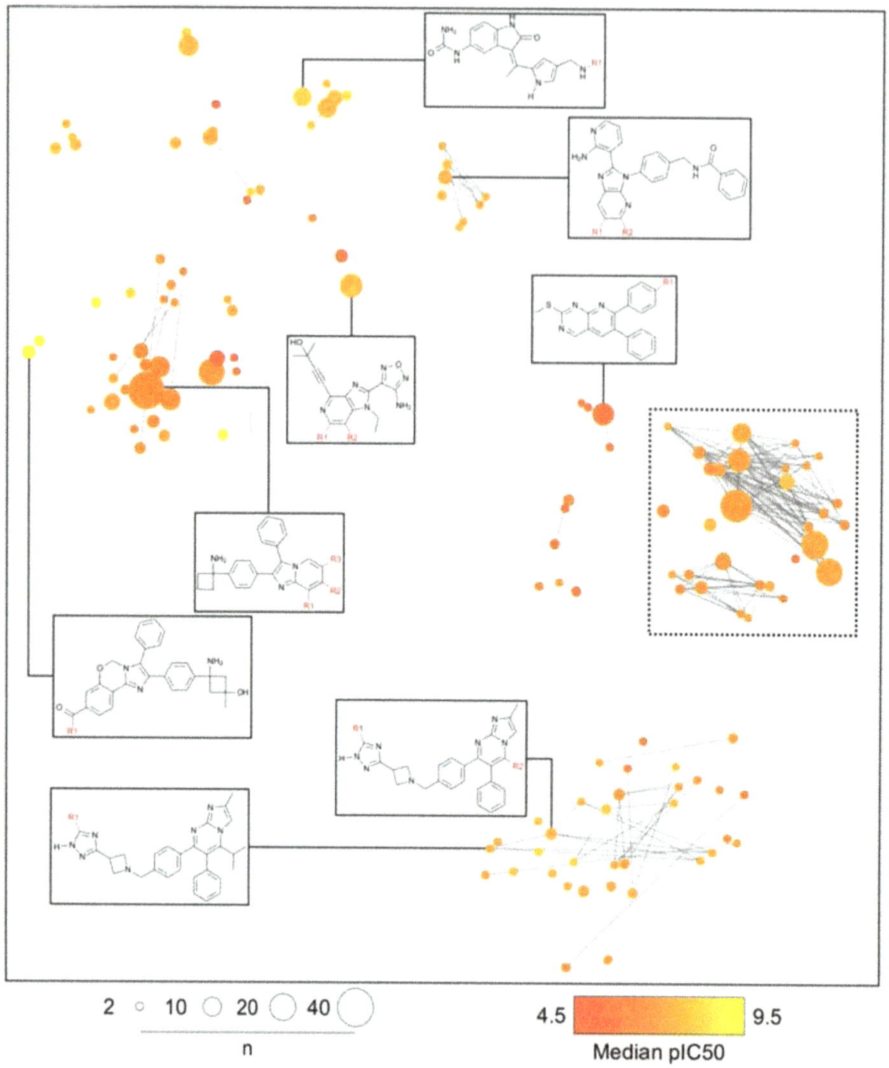

FIGURE 5 | General constellation plot for a dataset of AKT1 inhibitors. It is possible to navigate this map, as observed in **Figure 6**, where the constellation framed within dashed lines is further explored.

initial dataset). **Figure 5** is the constellation plot for these data, where it becomes apparent that chemical space and chemical substructure information play simultaneous roles in describing the SAR. For instance, although some inactive cores are close to active cores in chemical space, they are not usually contained in the same analog series. Therefore, these could be categorized as "scaffold cliffs" rather than simple activity cliffs conceptualized as two small molecules with similar structures and very different activities (Maggiora, 2006). In this case, collections of molecules, rather than single molecules, are being compared.

Figure 6 is a zoomed-in picture into a single "bright" (or predominantly active) constellation comprising five analog series and 55 compounds. As it is readily observed, analog series close in the chemical space have only slight dissimilarities within their scaffolds; in this case, they all share a naphthyridine or naphthyridinone scaffold. Constellation plots allow for a more precise visual SAR analysis and generation of hypotheses. For instance, the core associated to analog series 62 has only a different position for the nitrogens in the rings as well as where substitutions occur. Structural studies could then be conducted to elucidate which are the most relevant features for this kind of scaffolds to be active against AKT1. In this regard, a recent publication co-crystallizing 1,6-naphthyridinone derivatives similar to those in analog series 20 has shown that this scaffold is relevant in forming a π-π stacking interaction with the side chain of Trp80 of the PH-domain (Uhlenbrock et al., 2019). Nonetheless, variation of the position of nitrogen atoms in the scaffold were not considered in the cited study. Indeed, previous SAR studies of these analogs have found the position of the nitrogen atoms in these scaffolds to be critical for the activity against AKT (Zhao et al., 2005; Bilodeau et al., 2008).

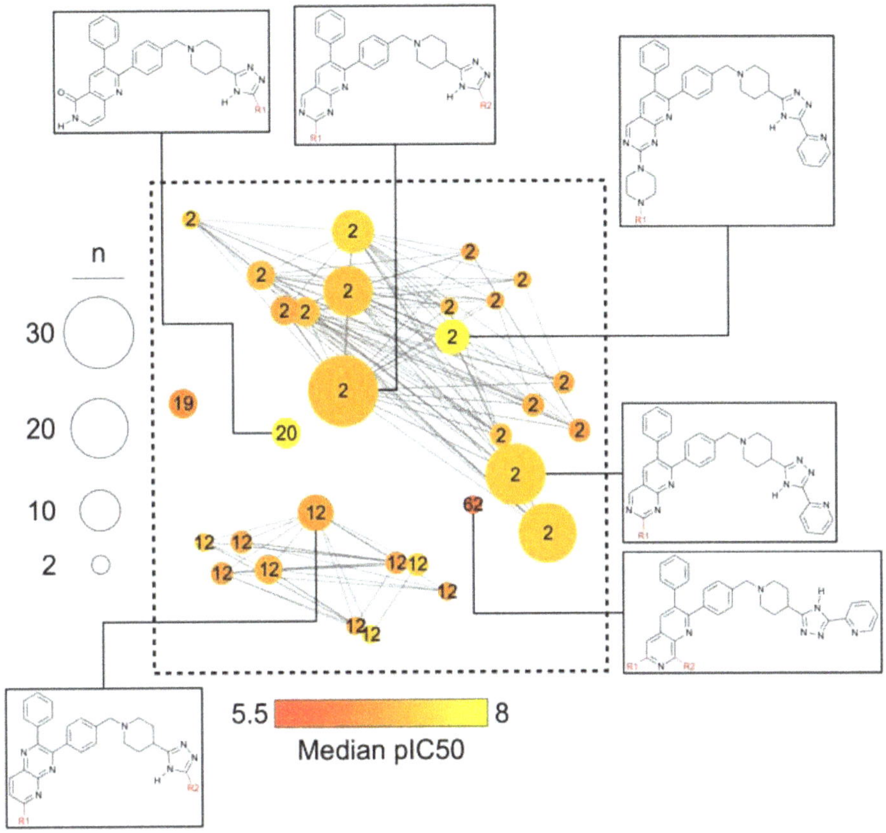

FIGURE 6 | "Zoom-in" into the constellation plot for AKT1 inhibitors selected from **Figure 5**. The core in analog series 62 is not as active as the nearby cores in analog series 2 and 12. Few structural differences can be noted for the compounds in this constellation.

Case Study 2: DNMT Inhibitors

Analogs in this library could be summarized in 23 cores following the procedure discussed in the section Methods. The cores were organized in 13 analog series and contained 46 compounds (about 16% of the initial dataset). Compounds in this library have annotated activity with DNMT1, DNMT3A, and/or DNMT3B. **Figure 7** shows three constellations plots, where chemical space is the same and colors change to represent the activities against each DNMT. As elaborated on the section Methods, each circle in the plot represents a core in which coordinates in the 2D graph is given by similarity measurements computed from Morgan fingerprints using *t*-SNE for dimensionality reduction. Labels indicate the analog series to which cores belong. The color represents the percentage of active compounds sharing that core using a continuous color scale from red (less active cores) to yellow (more active cores). For this example of use of the constellation plots, the definition of "active" was determined from integrating qualitative and quantitative data sources as described in Naveja and Medina-Franco (2018). Circles in gray indicate cores with no reported activity for that particular DNMT. The size of the circle indicates the number of compounds sharing the core. Connected circles are cores sharing compounds. **Figure 7** also shows the chemical structures of representative cores.

The constellation plots for DNMT inhibitors in **Figure 7** allow for rapidly getting several interesting insights of the SAR. For instance, cores at the top left part of the plot from analog series "A" are a bright constellation against DNMT1, i.e., a region in chemical space with active analogs. However, these analogs have not been tested against the other DNMT isoenzymes, which would help determine whether these inhibitors are selective.

Of note, there is a "dark" (or predominantly inactive) constellation in the chemical space of DNMT1 formed by six cores from analog series "D." This dark constellation, however, is more active overall against DNMT3A and appears to be active against DNMT3B. Furthermore, not all cores in this constellation have been tested against DNMT3A and DNMT3B, where they have greater chances of being active.

The plot also reveals a constellation of nucleoside analogs from series "B" at the bottom-right region of the plot that is, overall, selective toward DNMT3B vs. DNMT1. This series has not been tested against DNMT3A yet. Moreover, most of the cores have been tested in DNMT1 only, thus hindering discussions on selectivity. In this regard, analysis of constellation plots is visually helpful in guiding multitarget drug discovery campaigns and in finding opportunities for selectivity.

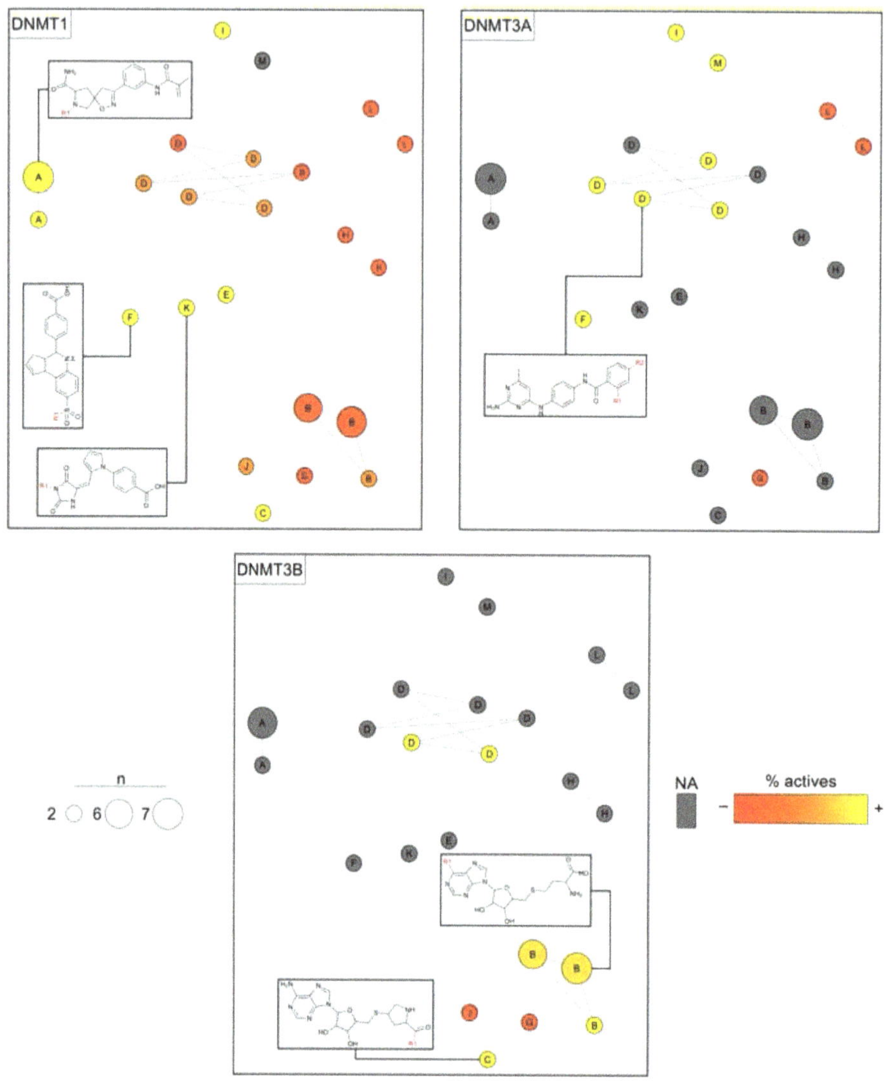

FIGURE 7 | Constellation plots for a dataset of DNA methyltransferase (DNMT) inhibitors tested with DNMT1, DNMT3A, and DNMT3B.

CONCLUSIONS AND PERSPECTIVES

We introduced a novel approach for combining chemical space and analog series methodologies into a single descriptive analysis that can be summarized in a constellation plot. Adding the analog series concept into the chemical space facilitates discussions of regions in the space, as every point summarizes a collection of analogs. A so-called "constellation in chemical space" can be conceptualized as those regions in chemical space formed by core scaffolds with similar structure (as defined by a coordinate-based projection). Mapping activity on the plot readily uncovers active and inactive zones, e.g., bright or dark regions, in chemical space. Of note, constellation plots would be useful for exploring virtually any chemical property, such as biological activity (as demonstrated with two case studies), but also physicochemical properties, complexity or selectivity statistics. In this regard, constellation plots are a flexible approach with multiple potential applications in academia and industry, aiding in the quest of finding potential leads from large collections of screening data (e.g., such as that produced by high-throughput screening campaigns). One of the next steps of this work is the application of the constellations plots to navigate through cell selectivity data of a comprehensive screening dataset. Results will be disclosed in due course.

AUTHOR CONTRIBUTIONS

JN participated in the conceptualization, data gathering, data analysis, and drafted the first version of the manuscript. JM-F participated in the conceptualization, data analysis, and revision of the manuscript.

ACKNOWLEDGMENTS

JN was thankful to CONACyT for the granted scholarship number 622969. We also thank Consejo Nacional de Ciencia y Tecnología (CONACyT) for grant 282785.

REFERENCES

Bajorath, J. (2018). Improving the utility of molecular scaffolds for medicinal and computational chemistry. *Future Med. Chem.* 10, 1645–1648. doi: 10.4155/fmc-2018-0106

Bemis, G. W., and Murcko, M. A. (1996). The properties of known drugs. 1. Molecular frameworks. *J. Med. Chem.* 39, 2887–2893. doi: 10.1021/jm9602928

Bilodeau, M. T., Balitza, A. E., Hoffman, J. M., Manley, P. J., Barnett, S. F., Defeo-Jones, D., et al. (2008). Allosteric inhibitors of Akt1 and Akt2: a naphthyridinone with efficacy in an A2780 tumor xenograft model. *Bioorg. Med. Chem. Lett.* 18, 3178–3182. doi: 10.1016/j.bmcl.2008.04.074

Borrel, A., Kleinstreuer, N. C., and Fourches, D. (2018). Exploring drug space with ChemMaps.com *Bioinformatics* 34, 3773–3775. doi: 10.1093/bioinformatics/bty412

Clayden, J., Greeves, N., and Warren, S. (2012). *Organic Chemistry*. Oxford, UK: Oxford University Press. Available online at: http://global.oup.com/ukhe/product/organic-chemistry-9780199270293?cc=mx&lang=en&

Dimova, D., and Bajorath, J. (2018). Collection of analog series-based scaffolds from public compound sources. *Future Sci. OA* 4:FSO287. doi: 10.4155/fsoa-2017-0135

Dimova, D., Stumpfe, D., Hu, Y., and Bajorath, J. (2016). Analog series-based scaffolds: computational design and exploration of a new type of molecular scaffolds for medicinal chemistry. *Future Sci. OA* 2:FSO149. doi: 10.4155/fsoa-2016-0058

Gaulton, A., Hersey, A., Nowotka, M., Bento, A. P., Chambers, J., Mendez, D., et al. (2017). The ChEMBL database in 2017. *Nucleic Acids Res.* 45, D945–D954. doi: 10.1093/nar/gkw1074

González-Medina, M., Prieto-Martínez, F. D., Naveja, J. J., Méndez-Lucio, O., El-Elimat, T., Pearce, C. J., et al. (2016). Chemoinformatic expedition of the chemical space of fungal products. *Future Med. Chem.* 8, 1399–1412. doi: 10.4155/fmc-2016-0079

Griffen, E., Leach, A. G., Robb, G. R., and Warner, D. J. (2011). Matched molecular pairs as a medicinal chemistry tool. *J. Med. Chem.* 54, 7739–7750. doi: 10.1021/jm200452d

Hu, Y., Stumpfe, D., and Bajorath, J. (2011). Lessons learned from molecular scaffold analysis. *J. Chem. Inf. Model.* 51, 1742–1753. doi: 10.1021/ci200179y

Kunimoto, R., Dimova, D., and Bajorath, J. (2017). Application of a new scaffold concept for computational target deconvolution of chemical cancer cell line screens. *ACS Omega* 2, 1463–1468. doi: 10.1021/acsomega.7b00215

Kunimoto, R., Miyao, T., and Bajorath, J. (2018). Computational method for estimating progression saturation of analog series. *RSC Adv.* 8, 5484–5492. doi: 10.1039/C7RA13748F

Larsson, J., Gottfries, J., Muresan, S., and Backlund, A. (2007). ChemGPS-NP: tuned for navigation in biologically relevant chemical space. *J. Nat. Prod.* 70, 789–794. doi: 10.1021/np070002y

Lewis, R., Guha, R., Korcsmaros, T., and Bender, A. (2015). Synergy maps: exploring compound combinations using network-based visualization. *J. Cheminform.* 7, 36. doi: 10.1186/s13321-015-0090-6

Lipinski, C., and Hopkins, A. (2004). Navigating chemical space for biology and medicine. *Nature* 432, 855–861. doi: 10.1038/nature03193

Lyu, J., Wang, S., Balius, T. E., Singh, I., Levit, A., Moroz, Y. S., et al. (2019). Ultra-large library docking for discovering new chemotypes. *Nature* 566, 224–229. doi: 10.1038/s41586-019-0917-9

Maaten, L., and Hinton, G. (2008). Visualizing data using t-SNE. *J. Mach. Learn. Res.* 9, 2579–2605. Available online at: http://www.jmlr.org/papers/volume9/vandermaaten08a/vandermaaten08a.pdf

Maggiora, G. M. (2006). On outliers and activity cliffs–why QSAR often disappoints. *J. Chem. Inf. Model.* 46, 1535. doi: 10.1021/ci060117s

Medina-Franco, J., Martinez-Mayorga, K., Giulianotti, M., Houghten, R., and Pinilla, C. (2008). Visualization of the chemical space in drug discovery. *CAD* 4, 322–333. doi: 10.2174/157340908786786010

Naveja, J. J., Cortés-Benítez, F., Bratoeff, E., and Medina-Franco, J. L. (2016). Activity landscape analysis of novel 5α-reductase inhibitors. *Mol. Divers.* 20, 771–780. doi: 10.1007/s11030-016-9659-x

Naveja, J. J., and Medina-Franco, J. L. (2015). Activity landscape sweeping: insights into the mechanism of inhibition and optimization of DNMT1 inhibitors. *RSC Adv.* 5, 63882–63895. doi: 10.1039/C5RA12339A

Naveja, J. J., and Medina-Franco, J. L. (2017). ChemMaps: Towards an approach for visualizing the chemical space based on adaptive satellite compounds. *F1000Res.* 6:Chem Inf Sci-1134. doi: 10.12688/f1000research.12095.2

Naveja, J. J., and Medina-Franco, J. L. (2018). Insights from pharmacological similarity of epigenetic targets in epipolypharmacology. *Drug Discov. Today* 23, 141–150. doi: 10.1016/j.drudis.2017.10.006

Naveja, J. J., Norinder, U., Mucs, D., López-López, E., and Medina-Franco, J. L. (2018a). Chemical space, diversity and activity landscape analysis of estrogen receptor binders. *RSC Adv.* 8, 38229–38237. doi: 10.1039/C8RA07604A

Naveja, J. J., Oviedo-Osornio, C. I., Trujillo-Minero, N. N., and Medina-Franco, J. L. (2018b). Chemoinformatics: a perspective from an academic setting in Latin America. *Mol. Divers.* 22, 247–258. doi: 10.1007/s11030-017-9802-3

Naveja, J. J., Vogt, M., Stumpfe, D., Medina-Franco, J. L., and Bajorath, J. (2019). Systematic extraction of analogue series from large compound collections using a new computational compound-core relationship method. *ACS Omega* 4, 1027–1032. doi: 10.1021/acsomega.8b03390

Oprea, T. I., and Gottfries, J. (2001). Chemography: the art of navigating in chemical space. *J. Comb. Chem.* 3, 157–166. doi: 10.1021/cc0000388

Osolodkin, D. I., Radchenko, E. V., Orlov, A. A., Voronkov, A. E., Palyulin, V. A., and Zefirov, N. S. (2015). Progress in visual representations of chemical space. *Expert Opin. Drug Discov.* 10, 959–973. doi: 10.1517/17460441.2015.1060216

Pedregosa, F., Varoquaux, G., Gramfort, A., Michel, V., Thirion, B., Grisel, O., et al. (2011). Scikit-learn: machine learning in Python. *J. Mach. Learn. Res.* 12, 2825–2830. Available online at: http://www.jmlr.org/papers/volume12/pedregosa11a/pedregosa11a.pdf

Prieto-Martínez, F. D., Gortari, E. F., Méndez-Lucio, O., and Medina-Franco, J. L. (2016). A chemical space odyssey of inhibitors of histone deacetylases and bromodomains. *RSC Adv.* 6, 56225–56239. doi: 10.1039/C6RA07224K

Probst, D., and Reymond, J.-L. (2018). Exploring drugbank in virtual reality chemical space. *J. Chem. Inf. Model.* 58, 1731–1735. doi: 10.1021/acs.jcim.8b00402

Reymond, J.-L. (2015). The chemical space project. *Acc. Chem. Res.* 48, 722–730. doi: 10.1021/ar500432k

Rosén, J., Lövgren, A., Kogej, T., Muresan, S., Gottfries, J., and Backlund, A. (2009). ChemGPS-NP(Web): chemical space navigation online. *J. Comput. Aided Mol. Des.* 23, 253–259. doi: 10.1007/s10822-008-9255-y

Stumpfe, D., Dimova, D., and Bajorath, J. (2016). Computational method for the systematic identification of analog series and key compounds representing series and their biological activity profiles. *J. Med. Chem.* 59, 7667–7676. doi: 10.1021/acs.jmedchem.6b00906

Uhlenbrock, N., Smith, S., Weisner, J., Landel, I., Lindemann, M., Le, T. A., et al. (2019). Structural and chemical insights into the covalent-allosteric inhibition of the protein kinase Akt. *Chem. Sci.* 10, 3573–3585. doi: 10.1039/c8sc05212c

Vogt, M., Yonchev, D., and Bajorath, J. (2018). Computational method to evaluate progress in lead optimization. *J. Med. Chem.* 61, 10895–10900. doi: 10.1021/acs.jmedchem.8b01626

Waddell, J., and Medina-Franco, J. L. (2012). Bioactivity landscape modeling: chemoinformatic characterization of structure-activity relationships of compounds tested across multiple targets. *Bioorg. Med. Chem.* 20, 5443–5452. doi: 10.1016/j.bmc.2011.11.051

Yonchev, D., Vogt, M., Stumpfe, D., Kunimoto, R., Miyao, T., and Bajorath, J. (2018). Computational assessment of chemical saturation of analogue series under varying conditions. *ACS Omega* 3, 15799–15808. doi: 10.1021/acsomega.8b02087

Zhao, Z., Leister, W. H., Robinson, R. G., Barnett, S. F., Defeo-Jones, D., Jones, R. E., et al. (2005). Discovery of 2,3,5-trisubstituted pyridine derivatives as potent Akt1 and Akt2 dual inhibitors. *Bioorg. Med. Chem. Lett.* 15, 905–909. doi: 10.1016/j.bmcl.2004.12.062

4

Structural, Thermodynamic and Kinetic Traits of Antiestrogen-Compounds Selectively Targeting the Y537S Mutant Estrogen Receptor α Transcriptional Activity in Breast Cancer Cell Lines

Matic Pavlin[1†], Luca Gelsomino[2†], Ines Barone[2], Angelo Spinello[1], Stefania Catalano[2], Sebastiano Andò[2] and Alessandra Magistrato[1*]*

[1] National Research Council – Institute of Materials (IOM) at International School for Advanced Studies (ISAS), Scuola Internazionale Superiore di Studi Avanzati (SISSA), Trieste, Italy, [2] Department of Pharmacy, Health and Nutrition Sciences, Centro Sanitario, University of Calabria, Rende, Italy

***Correspondence:**
Sebastiano Andò
sebastiano.ando@unical.it
Alessandra Magistrato
alessandra.magistrato@sissa.it

† These authors have contributed equally to this work

The most frequently diagnosed cancers in women are the estrogen receptor (ER)-positive breast cancer subtypes, which are characterized by estrogen dependency for their growth. The mainstay of clinical treatment for this tumor relies on the modulation of ERα action or on the suppression of estrogen biosynthesis via the administration of Selective ERα Modulators/Down-regulators (SERMs/SERDs) or aromatase inhibitors, respectively. Nevertheless, *de novo* and acquired resistance to these therapies frequently occurs and represents a major clinical concern for patient survival. Recently, somatic mutations affecting the hormone-binding domain of ERα (i.e., Y537S, Y537N, D538G) have been associated with endocrine resistance, disease relapse and increased mortality rates. Hence, devising novel therapies against these ERα isoforms represents a daunting challenge. Here, we identified five molecules active on recurrent Y537S ERα polymorphism by employing *in silico* virtual screening on commercial databases of molecules, complemented by ER-transactivation and MTT assays in MCF7 and MDA-MB-231 breast cancer cells expressing wild type or mutated ERα. Among them, one molecule selectively targets Y537S ERα without inducing any cytotoxicity in breast cell lines. Multi-microseconds (4.5 μs) of biased and unbiased molecular dynamics provided an atomic-level picture of the structural, thermodynamics (i.e., binding free energies) and the kinetic (i.e., dissociation free energy barriers) of these active ligands as compared to clinically used SERM/SERDs upon binding to wild type and distinct ERα variants (Y537S, Y537N, D538G). This study contributes to a dissection of the key molecular traits needed by drug-candidates to hamper the agonist (active)-like conformation of ERα, normally selected by those polymorphic variants. This information can be useful to discover mutant specific drug-candidates, enabling to move a step forward toward tailored approaches for breast cancer treatment.

Keywords: estrogen receptor, breast cancer, SERM, SERD, molecular dynamics, Y537S, resistant breast cancers

INTRODUCTION

Breast Cancer (BC) is the most frequent cancer type and the second leading cause of death in women, representing 25% of all cancers. In ~70% of the BC cases detected after the menopause, cellular proliferation is mediated by estrogens (**1**; **Figure 1**) binding to their specific nuclear hormone receptor [Estrogen Receptor α (ERα, *ESR1*)] (Fanning and Greene, 2019).

This latter is a ligand-activated transcription factor, which upon estrogen binding, decreases apoptosis and/or promotes cell proliferation, ultimately playing a pro-oncogenic role. Hence, in the most diffused BC type cell proliferation relies on the expression of ERα, and on the presence of blood circulating estrogens, being hence classified as ER sensitive (ER+). Gold standard endocrine treatments against ER+ BC consist in suppressing estrogen biosynthesis, via the administration of aromatase inhibitors, or in counteracting ERα pro-oncogenic action via the drugging of selective ERα modulators (SERMs) or downregulators (SERDs). Namely, SERMs [tamoxifen and its most abundant metabolite endoxifen (END)] act as antagonists, occupying the estrogen binding site and inducing a conformational change of ERα toward an inactive conformation. SERDs [fulvestrant (FULV)], instead, also foster ERα ubiquitination and degradation (Fanning et al., 2016; Pavlin et al., 2018).

Similarly to other nuclear receptors, ERα presents a puzzling tridimensional structure which atomic-level organization remains controversial (Huang et al., 2018). This is composed out of five distinct functional domains (**Supplementary Figure 1**), among which only the structures of the DNA-binding domain and the ligand-binding domain (LBD) have been characterized. The LBD is active as a homodimer with each monomer hosting a ligand binding cavity (LBC). The LBD crystal structures (**Supplementary Figure 2**) revealed that upon binding of an agonist or an antagonist molecule, helix 12 (H12) can undergo a conformational switch between the active and inactive form, respectively (Joseph et al., 2016). In the agonist (active) state, H12 faces helices H3, H5/6, and H11, closing the LBC (**Supplementary Figure 2A**; Robinson et al., 2013). Conversely, in the antagonist (inactive) form, H12 rearranges, as a consequence of SERM/SERD-binding, moving toward the groove lined by H3 and H5 (**Supplementary Figure 2B**; van Kruchten et al., 2015; Joseph et al., 2016).

In the last decades, SERMs have been proved to be highly beneficial, substantially decreasing the mortality rates of woman affected by BC cancer type by 25–30 %. The most effective ERα antagonists in clinical use are: (i) tamoxifen (**2**; **Figure 1**), a SERM, which in spite of its beneficial action in breast tissues, is plagued by agonistic effects in peripheral ones (endometrium), and is active through its metabolite, endoxifen (**3**; **Figure 1**), and (ii) FULV (**4**; **Figure 1**), a potent SERD (Nilsson and Gustafsson, 2011; van Kruchten et al., 2015) characterized, however, by poor solubility. This makes its administration arduous and therefore probably limiting its efficacy. These adjuvant therapies are administered over extended time frame (5–10 years) to control tumor growth, or, even, to prevent disease in case of BC-prone

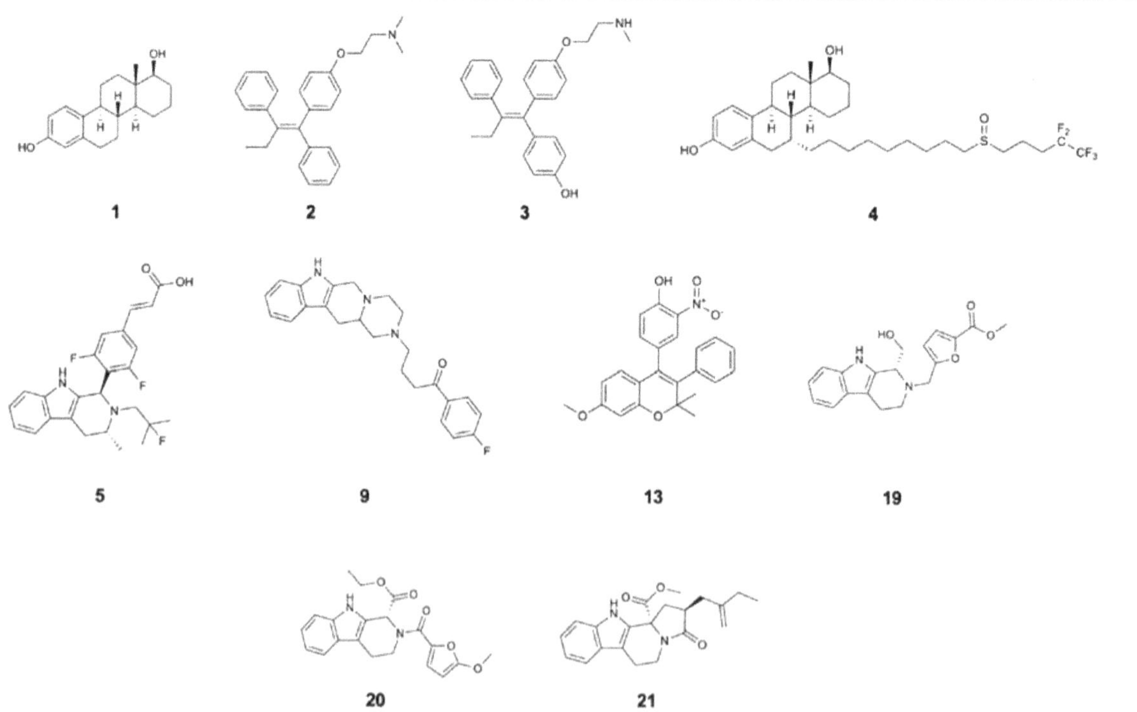

FIGURE 1 | Structures of 17β-estradiol (**1**), tamoxifen (**2**), endoxifen (**3**), fulvestrant (**4**), AZD-9496 (**5**), and compounds **9**, **13**, **19**, **20**, **21** which are the identified drug-candidates active against Y537S ERα.

genetic profiles. Nevertheless, after prolonged exposure to these therapies, tumors evolve by adapting to the pharmacological pressure. Distinct studies highlighted a stunningly complex, composite, and multifactorial genomic landscape as responsible of tumor refractoriness to treatments (Spinello et al., 2019b). This has mostly been associated to an alteration of mitogen activated kinase pathway (MAPK) or of a deregulated estrogen receptor transcriptional activity (Razavi et al., 2018). This latter takes place when ERα acquires new structural traits, eventually leading to resistance and relapse to therapies. Scaringly, almost 50 % of all ER+ BC patients, initially benefiting from first-line therapy, will eventually develop resistance after prolonged treatments (acquired resistance). This ultimately results in a shortening of their survival time.

It is nowadays well-established (Merenbakh-Lamin et al., 2013; Robinson et al., 2013; Toy et al., 2013; Jeselsohn et al., 2014) that distinct ERα polymorphisms (mERαs), located in the vicinity of LBC (i.e., E380Q), between H9 and H10, or in the loop connecting H11 and H12 (i.e., L536Q, L536R, Y537C, Y537N, Y537S, and D538G), are recurrently observed in metastatic BC patients relapsing after extended treatments regimens. The most abundant ERα polymorphisms observed in LBD are D538G (occurrence of 21–36 % of cases (Jeselsohn et al., 2014; Chandarlapaty et al., 2016; Toy et al., 2017), Y537N (5–33 %) (Jeselsohn et al., 2014; Toy et al., 2017), and Y537S (13–22 %) (Jeselsohn et al., 2014; Chandarlapaty et al., 2016; Toy et al., 2017). This latter remains the most aggressive isoform (survival rate of 20 months as compared to 26 of D538G) (Chandarlapaty et al., 2016). Most of these mutations are insensitive to tamoxifen, while still responding to FULV. As such, tumors proliferation still depends on ERα expression, underlying the still unmet oncological need of a complete inhibition/abrogation of its signaling pathway (Busonero et al., 2019).

Targeted therapy counteracting mERα is a current object of intense preclinical and early clinical interest, as also evidenced by the significant number of studies aiming at identifying orally bioavailable SERDs, eventually able to overcome resistance (De Savi et al., 2015; Fanning et al., 2018; Hamilton et al., 2018; Sharma et al., 2018; Kahraman et al., 2019; Scott et al., 2019). Among these GDC-810, AZD9496 (**5**; **Figure 1**) (hereafter AZD, a drug in preclinical use as oral SERD, for which a first clinical study have been recently accomplished) (Weir et al., 2016; Hamilton et al., 2018), and LSZ102 have been identified (Scott et al., 2019).

Aiming at selectively targeting specific and aggressive ERα variants, we have recently meticulously annotated the structural and dynamical alterations induced to ERα structure by each recurrent polymorphism, disclosing that each of them triggers the acquisition of a different agonist-like (intrinsically active) conformation of H12. As a result, tumors bearing these isoforms proliferate irrespectively of estrogen production, with SERMs and aromatase inhibitors' efficacy being lost after their appearance (Spinello et al., 2019b). Since these ER+ BC cells are sensitive to FULV and AZD, we also performed extensive MD simulations typifying the structural features responsible of distinct efficacy of FULV and AZD on mutant (m)ERα, as opposite to END.

Stunningly, our computational assays disclosed that the FULV and AZD's elongated shape, owing to their aliphatic and carboxylic moiety, respectively, was the key structural determinant counteracting the acquisition of an H12 agonist-like conformation (Fanning et al., 2016; Pavlin et al., 2018). Understanding the structural signature needed by drugs able to effectively fight metastatic and refractory BC types was a necessary prerequisite for the rational discovery of mutant-specific SERMs/SERDs. Building on this knowledge, here, we performed virtual screenings on existing database of molecules, and we tested their efficacy on MCF7 and MDA-MB-231 cell lines harboring Wild Type (WT) and Y537S, D538G, and Y537N ERα variants. As a result, we identified five molecules able to counteract the enhanced transcriptional activity of Y537S ERα isoform, with one being non-cytotoxic and preferentially active toward the Y537S variant. The structural and dynamical impact of the five active molecules, as well as their thermodynamic and kinetic properties (of the best molecule) were also explored via biased and unbiased classical Molecular Dynamics (MD) simulations, and compared with those of END, AZD, and FULV in order to dissect the source of their distinct efficacy profiles. These outcomes may lead toward the discovery of isoform-selective drug-candidates, providing a therapeutic option for the specific genomic profile of ER+ BC patients relapsing mainstay therapies.

MATERIALS AND METHODS

In silico Screening

The NCI (https://cactus.nci.nih.gov/download/nci/) library Release 4 Files Series—May 2012 (containing 265,242 structures) was used for virtual screening (VS) studies. Compounds were filtered using the Schrodinger Suite 2017-1 Ligfilter tool (2017). In order to eliminate molecules possessing poor absorption and permeation we applied Lipinski's rule of five (Lipinski et al., 2001). Further, filtering was applied to compounds bearing more than 10 rotatable bonds, since high ligand flexibility implies higher entropic contributions and reduces oral availability (Veber et al., 2002). Next, QikProp (2017) was employed to predict LogP values of the compounds to assess information on their solubility in water.

After ligand preparation *in silico* screening of the library was performed on different mERα structures. Namely, in order to account for receptor's flexibility in the screening we considered five different ERα conformations as target structures (Pavlin et al., 2018). These were selected from the populated cluster extracted from 500 ns-long classical MD simulations trajectories of AZD and FULV in complex with the Y537S, Y537N, and D538G isoforms obtained in our previous study (Pavlin et al., 2018). In this respect, we employed two conformations for Y537S ERα (in complex with AZD and FULV), one for Y537N (in complex with FULV, since conformation of this mutant complex with AZD was similar to that of Y537S), and two structures for D538G (in complex with AZD and FULV). A van der Waals (vdW) radius scaling factor of 0.80 Å for protein and ligands atoms having a partial charge < 0.15 was used to account for protein flexibility. Size of the box for *in silico* screenings was determined by considering the residues interacting with different antagonists placed inside the binding site and those residues pinpointed as critical for antagonizing ERα activation in our previous work (Pavlin et al., 2018).

In order to obtain a set of promising ligands for experimental testing, we followed two protocols of VS. First, a workflow based on three subsequent steps of docking with increasing level of accuracy for each ERα conformation, was adopted by using the Glide program (Friesner et al., 2004). Namely, (i) a fast high-throughput virtual screening (HTVS) was initially performed in order to efficiently select promising ligands among ~220,000 of compounds from the pre-filtered NCI library; (ii) 10 % of the best ranked ligands (~22,000 structures per each ERα conformation) were retained and a single precision (SP) docking calculation was done; (iii) the top 10 % of the resulting compounds (~2,200 structures per each ERα conformation) were screened using the extra precision (XP) protocol. This latter should eliminate false positives by using a more extensive sampling and more accurate scoring functions. END, AZD, and FULV were also docked to assess the quality of our results as reported in **Supplementary Table 1**. The molecules resulting from the screening were sorted according to GlideScore scoring function. The selection criterion for further investigation was that the screened compounds had docking score lower than −8.5 kcal/mol and that displayed favorable interactions with at least one of the five mERαs target structures (i.e., two structures extracted from the MD trajectory of Y537S ERα in complex with AZD and FULV, one for Y537N in complex with FULV, and two structures for D538G in complex with AZD and FULV). This was done in order to find a good compromise between the number of molecules selected for experimental screening and the quality of the docking score. Moreover, our reference molecules FULV and AZD exhibit on the target structure the same range of docking score values.

In the second protocol, we initially performed ligand-based screening using the CANVAS program (Duan et al., 2010; Sastry et al., 2010). Here the searching criteria were based on the scaffold that antagonist should possess. The latter was defined considering the common structural features that an effective SERD should have according to our previous study (Pavlin et al., 2018), more precisely, selected ligand should have scaffold based either on the END scaffold or on the tri-membered ring scaffold of AZD in order to stabilize ligand inside LBC, together with a polar tail that is able to form hydrogen bonds (H-bonds) with the H11-12 loop. The 415 selected ligands were then screened to all five mERαs conformations by using XP protocol. In this second case, the cut-off docking score for selection of ligands was −7.5 kcal/mol, and the ligands were selected only when displaying favorable interactions with at least two distinct mERα structures among the five target structures used and at least one was within the cut-off range. These molecules were available as donation of the National Cancer Institute USA. Other known activities of the five molecules observed to be active on Y537S in this study are reported in **Supplementary Table 7**.

Reagents, Antibodies, and Plasmids

17β-estradiol was purchased from Sigma (St. Louis, MO, USA). Antibodies against ERα and GAPDH were from Santa Cruz Biotechnology (Santa Cruz, CA, USA). Yellow fluorescent protein (YFP)-tagged expression constructs, YFP-WT, YFP-Y537S, YFP-Y537N and YFP-D538G ERα were generated as previously described (Gelsomino et al., 2016, 2018) XETL plasmid, containing an estrogen-responsive element, was provided by Dr. Picard (University of Geneva, Geneva, Switzerland).

Cell Cultures

Human MCF-7 and MDA-MB-231 BC cells were acquired in 2015 from American Type Culture Collection, stored and cultured according to supplier's instructions. Cells were used within six-months after frozen-aliquot resuscitations and regularly tested for Mycoplasma-negativity (MycoAlert, Lonza, Basilea, Switzerland).

Immunoblot Analysis

Equal amounts of proteins were resolved on 10% SDS-PAGE as previously described (Giordano et al., 2016). The antigen-antibody complex was revealed using the ECL System (Bio-rad, Hercules, CA, USA). Images were acquired using Odissey FC from Licor (Lincoln, Nebraska, USA). Blots are representative of three independent experiments.

ERα Transactivation Assay

ERα transactivation assay was performed as previously reported (Barone et al., 2011). Briefly, MCF-7 and MDA-MB-231 cells (50,000/well) were plated in phenol red-free with 5 % charcoal-stripped FBS in 24-well plates. After 24 h, cells were co-transfected with 0.5 μg of reporter plasmid XETL plus 0.1 μg of YFP-tagged expression constructs and 20 ng of TK Renilla luciferase plasmid as an internal control. Transfection was performed using the Lipofectamine 2000 reagent (Life Technologies, Carlsbad, CA, USA) as recommended by the manufacturer. Six hours after transfection, the medium was changed and the cells were treated as indicated for 24 h. Firefly and Renilla luciferase activities were measured using a Dual Luciferase kit (Promega, Madison, WI, USA). The firefly luciferase data for each sample were normalized on the basis of transfection efficiency measured by Renilla luciferase activity (Rizza et al., 2014). Data represent three independent experiments, carried out in triplicate.

MTT Cell Viability Assay

1,000 cells were plated into 96-well plates in phenol red-free medium containing 5 % charcoal-stripped FBS. After 24 h, cells were exposed to the different treatments as indicated. One day later, cell viability was assessed by (3-(4,5-Dimethylthiazol-2-yl)-2,5-Diphenyltetrazolium-Bromide) (MTT, Sigma-Aldrich) as described (Covington et al., 2013). Results are expressed as fold change relative to vehicle-treated cells. Data represent three-independent experiments, performed in triplicate.

Real-Time RT-PCR Assays

Total RNA was extracted from cells using TRIzol reagent (Life Technologies). Purity and integrity of the RNA were confirmed spectroscopically and by gel electrophoresis before use. One microgram of total RNA was reverse transcribed in a final volume of 20 μL using the RETROscript kit (Life Technologies) and cDNA was diluted 1:3 in nuclease-free water. The evaluation of *TFF1*, *CTSD*, *CCND1* and *MYC* mRNA expression was performed by real-time RT-PCR, using SYBR Green Universal PCR Master Mix (Bio-rad). The relative gene expression levels were calculated using the ΔΔCt method as described (Catalano et al., 2015). Primers are listed in **Supplementary Table 2**.

Statistical Analysis of Experimental Data

Data were analyzed for statistical significance using two-tailed student's Test using GraphPad-Prism5 (GraphPad Software, Inc., San Diego, CA). Standard deviations (S. D.) are shown.

Classical MD Simulations

Of the 17 tested molecules (**Figure 1**, **Supplementary Figure 3**) obtained by both protocols of VS (four from the structure-based strategy and the rest by the ligand-based strategy as reported in **Supplementary Table 1**) five resulted to be active in the *in vitro* tests. These latter were also docked to the WT ERα using the XP protocol. All active molecules were subjected to MD simulations in complex with the WT and Y537S ERα variants. Additionally, compound **19**, showing the most promising results in experimental tests, was also docked and simulated in complex with Y537N and D538G ERα.

Physiological protonation states of ERα were already determined previously (Pavlin et al., 2018) using the webserver H++ (Anandakrishnan et al., 2012). Parm99SB AMBER force field (FF) with ILDN modification was employed for the protein (Wickstrom et al., 2009; Lindorff-Larsen et al., 2010), and the general Amber FF (GAFF) (Wang et al., 2004) was used for ligands. ESP charges (Bayly et al., 1993) were calculated by performing geometry optimizations of the ligands at Hartree-Fock level of theory using a 6-31G* basis set with the Gaussian 09 software (Frisch et al., 2016) and were later transformed in RESP charges with the Antechamber module of Ambertools16 (Wang et al., 2006). Since the dockings were performed on monomers, while the LBD in physiological conditions is a dimer, we built each dimer by superimposing the monomer on each of the two dimers of the corresponding mERα conformation from our previous work (Pavlin et al., 2018).

Each system was solvated using TIP3P waters (Jorgensen et al., 1983) in a truncated octahedron box with minimum distance of 12 Å between solute and the edge of the box, leading to a total of ~95,000 atoms. MD simulations were performed with

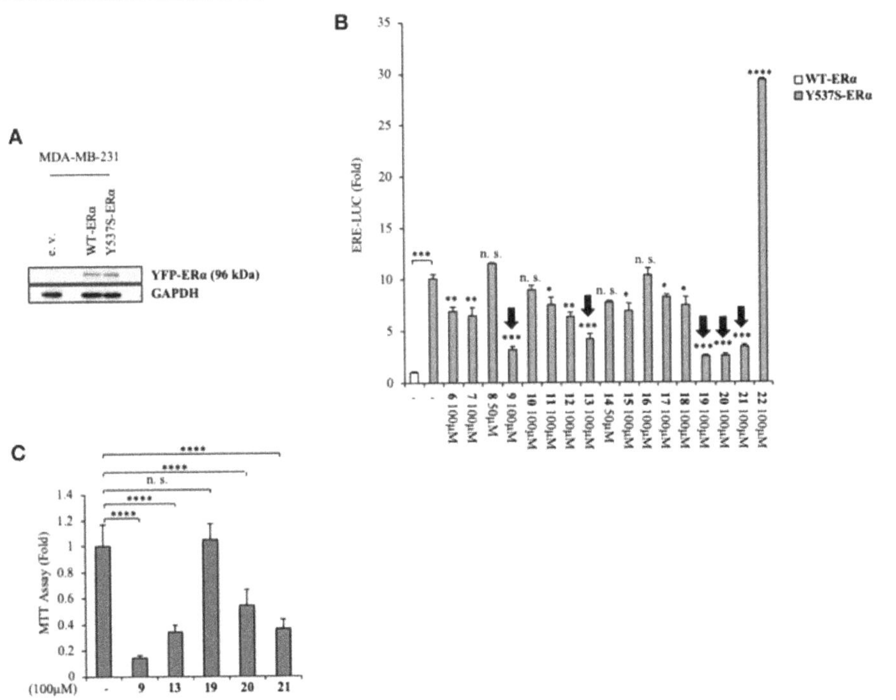

FIGURE 2 | Inhibition of Y537S ERα activation exerted by the compound **19** in MDA-MB-231 breast cancer cells. **(A)** Immunoblotting showing exogenous ERα protein expression in ERα-negative MDA-MB-231 breast cancer cells transiently transfected with an empty vector (e. v.), YFP-WT or YFP-Y537S ERα expression vectors. GAPDH was used as a control for equal loading and transfer. **(B)** ERα-transactivation assay in MDA-MB-231 cells transiently transfected with YFP-WT or YFP-Y537S ERα expressing vectors plus an ERE-luciferase reporter (XETL), and treated with vehicle (-) or the different compounds (**6**-**22**), as indicated. Data are reported as fold change relative to WT-ERα expressing cells. **(C)** MTT cell viability assay in MDA-MB-231 cells treated with vehicle (-) or the different compounds (**9**, **13**, **19**, **20**, **21**, 100 μM), as indicated for 24 h. Results are expressed as fold change relative to vehicle-treated cells. The values represent the mean ± S. D. of three different experiments, each performed in triplicate. n. s., non-significant; $^{*}P < 0.05$; $^{**}P < 0.005$; $^{***}P < 0.0005$; $^{****}P < 0.00005$.

GROMACS 5.0.4 (Abraham et al., 2015). An integration time step of 2 fs was used and all covalent bonds involving hydrogen atoms constrained with the LINCS algorithm (Hess et al., 1997). Particle Mesh Ewald algorithm (Darden et al., 1993) was used in order to account electrostatic interactions. Simulations were performed in the isothermal-isobaric NPT ensemble, at a temperature of 310 K, under control of a velocity-rescaling thermostat (Bussi et al., 2007). Preliminary energy minimization was done with the steepest descend algorithm. Next, all systems were heated to the final temperature of 310 K using 40 steps of simulated annealing (0-90 K in steps of 5 K/25 ps; 90-310 K in steps of 10 K/25 ps). WT ERα models underwent 300 ns long classical MD simulations (last 200 ns were used for analysis), while mERα ones underwent 400 ns long simulations and last 300 ns were used for further analysis.

Metadynamics

In order to further refine the binding poses and better dissect the impact of the kinetic properties on efficacy and selectivity, we performed FF-based Metadynamics (MTD) simulations of AZD and **19**. In particular, MTD runs of 60–130 ns were done to refine the binding pose and study ligand dissociation with GROMACS 5.0.4 using the PLUMED 2.0 plugin (Tribello et al., 2014). Two collective variables (CVs) were used: the first CV (CV1) describes the number of either hydrogen bonds (AZD) or hydrophobic contacts (**19**) between the ligands and the LBC, computed as a coordination number; the second CV (CV2) corresponds to the distance between the center of masses (COM) of the protein and the ligand. Gaussian hills having a height of 0.6 kJ/mol in all systems, while the widths of 0.06 and 0.015 (AZD), 0.40 and 0.025 (**19**), were added, respectively, for CV1 and CV2 every 4 ps of MD. A harmonic wall was used to restrain the exploration of the FES on CV2 at the value of 3.5 nm. Three replicas of the MTD simulations were performed, starting from different frames as extracted from the equilibrated MD trajectory and the uncertainty of the dissociation free energy barriers ($\Delta G^{\#}_{b}$) were estimated from the standard deviation of the barriers obtained out of the three replicas, following a protocol adopted in previous studies (Bisha et al., 2013; Sgrignani and Magistrato, 2015; Spinello et al., 2018, 2019a).

Simulation Analysis

Cluster analysis and root mean square deviation (RMSD) of the MD trajectories were done with the g_cluster tool, based on the Daura et al algorithm (Daura et al., 1999), and g_rms, as implemented in the GROMACS 5.0.4 program (Abraham

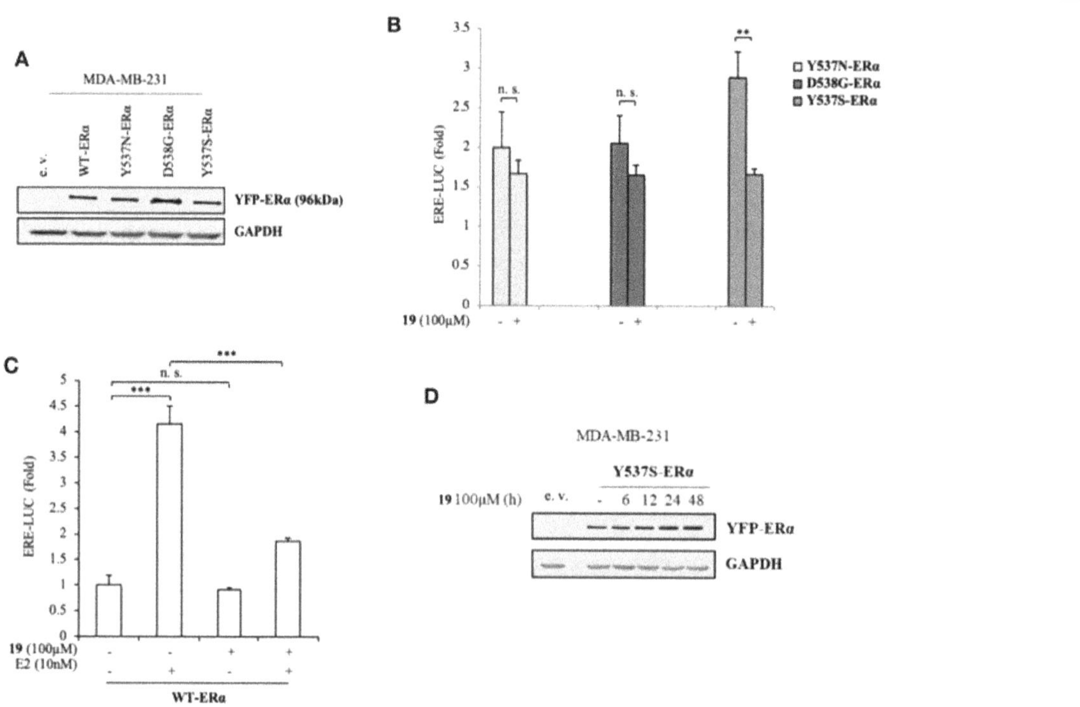

FIGURE 3 | Impact of compound **19** on activation of WT, Y537N, and D538G ERα in MDA-MB-231 breast cancer cells. **(A)** Immunoblotting showing exogenous ERα protein expression in ERα-negative MDA-MB-231 breast cancer cells transiently transfected with an empty vector (e. v.), YFP-WT, YFP-Y537N, YFP-Y537S, or YFP-D538G ERα expressing vectors. GAPDH was used as a control for equal loading and transfer. **(B)** ERα-transactivation assay in MDA-MB-231 cells transiently transfected with YFP-Y537N, YFP-Y537S, or YFP-D538G ERα expressing vectors plus an ERE-luciferase reporter (XETL), and treated with vehicle (-) or the compound **19** at 100 μM. Data are reported as fold change relative to WT-ERα expressing cells. **(C)** ERα-transactivation assay in MDA-MB-231 cells transiently transfected with YFP-WT plus XETL plasmid, and treated with vehicle (-) or the compound **19** (100 μM) in the presence or not of 17β-estradiol (E2, 10 nM). Data are reported as fold change relative to vehicle (-)-treated cells. The values represent the mean ± S. D. of three different experiments, each performed in triplicate. n. s., non-significant; $^{**}P < 0.005$; $^{***}P < 0.0005$. **(D)** Immunoblotting showing ERα protein expression in MDA-MB-231 breast cancer cells transiently transfected with YFP-Y537S ERα expressing vector and treated with the compound **19** (100 μM) at the indicated time. GAPDH was used as a control for equal loading and transfer.

et al., 2015). Molecular Mechanics Generalized Born Surface Area (MM-GBSA) free energy calculation were performed with the MM_PBSA.py tool of Amber 18 program, following a procedure successfully applied in previous studies (Spinello et al., 2019a,c). Visualization of the MD trajectories was done with the VMD program (Humphrey et al., 1996), while the images were prepared using UCSF Chimera1.12 visualization tool (Pettersen et al., 2004).

Correlation Analysis

The covariance matrices were constructed from the atoms position vectors upon an RMS-fit to the starting configuration of the MD run as to remove the rotational and translational motions. Each element in the covariance matrix is the covariance between atoms i and j, defining the i, j position of the matrix. The covariance C_{ij} is defined as

$$C_{ij}=\langle(\vec{r}_i-\langle\vec{r}_i\rangle)(\vec{r}_j-\langle\vec{r}_j\rangle)\rangle, \quad (1)$$

where $\vec{r}_i$ and $\vec{r}_j$ are the position vectors of atoms i and j, and the brackets denote an average over the sampled time period. The diagonalization of the covariance matrix leads to a set of orthogonal collective eigenvectors, each associated to a corresponding eigenvalue. The eigenvalues denote how much each eigenvector is representative of the system dynamics.

The cross-correlation matrices (or normalized covariance matrices) based on the Pearson's correlation coefficients (CC_{ij}) were calculated with the *cpptraj* module of Ambertools 18 from the calculated covariance matrices. Each element of the cross-correlation matrix in the i,j position corresponds to a Pearson's CC_{ij}, i.e., the normalized covariance between atoms i and j calculated with the formula:

$$C_{ij}=\frac{\langle(\vec{r}_i-\langle\vec{r}_i\rangle)(\vec{r}_j-\langle\vec{r}_j\rangle)\rangle}{\left[\left(\langle\vec{r}_i^{\,2}\rangle-\langle\vec{r}_i\rangle^2\right)\left(\langle\vec{r}_j^{\,2}\rangle-\langle\vec{r}_j\rangle^2\right)\right]}, \quad (2)$$

here the normalization factor is the product between the standard deviations of the two position vectors. As a result, CC_{ij} range from a value of -1, for a totally negatively correlated motion between two atoms, and a value of $+1$, which instead means a positively correlated lockstep motion. Here we have also calculated the correlation scores (CSs) between each LBD helix and all the others, dividing each as depicted

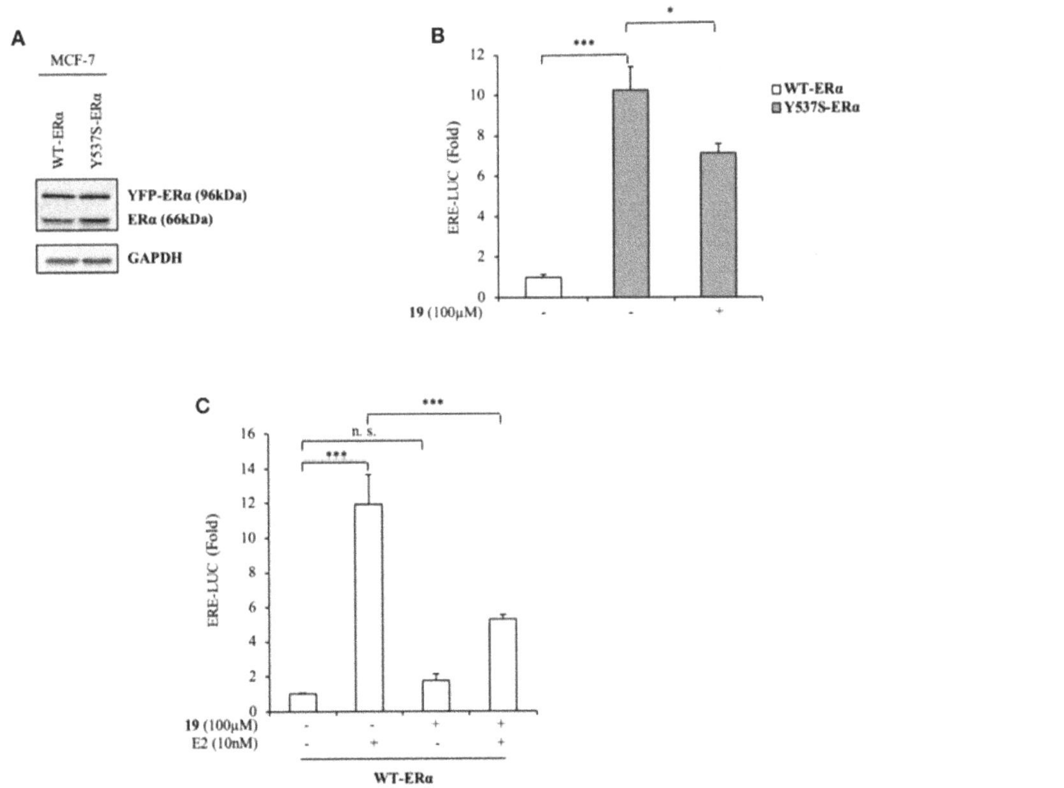

FIGURE 4 | Effects of compound **19** on WT and Y537S ERα activation in MCF-7 breast cancer cells. **(A)** Immunoblotting showing exogenous and endogenous ERα protein expression in ERα-positive MCF-7 breast cancer cells transiently transfected with YFP-WT or YFP-Y537S ERα expressing vectors. GAPDH was used as a control for equal loading and transfer. **(B)** ERα-transactivation assay in MCF-7 cells transiently transfected with YFP-WT or YFP-Y537S ERα expressing vectors plus an ERE-luciferase reporter (XETL), and treated with vehicle (-) or the compound **19** at 100 μM, as indicated. Data are reported as fold change relative to WT-ERα expressing cells. **(C)** ERα-transactivation assay in MCF-7 cells transiently transfected with YFP-WT plus XETL plasmid, and treated with vehicle (-) or the compound **19** (100 μM) in the presence or not of 17β-estradiol (E2, 10 nM). Data are reported as fold change relative to vehicle (-)-treated cells. The values represent the mean ± S. D. of three different experiments, each performed in triplicate. n. s., non-significant; $^{*}P < 0.05$; $^{***}P < 0.0005$.

in **Supplementary Figure 2** (Pavlin et al., 2018). Then, we calculated the sum of CC_{ij} between the residues i belonging to the helix I and the residues j belonging to the helix J. Importantly, the values $-0.6 < CC_{ij} < +0.6$ were discarded in order to eliminate the noise due to uncorrelated motions (Palermo et al., 2016; Casalino et al., 2018) and the sum of the cross-correlation score was divided by the product of the number of residues contributing to the score as a correlation density.

RESULTS

In silico Screening and *in vitro* Studies

Building on our previous classification of structural traits of drugs effectively targeting mERα (Pavlin et al., 2018), we performed *in silico* screening on the structures obtained from MD simulations of Y357S, Y537N, and D538G mutants hosting AZD and FULV in the LBC. A detailed list of the molecules tested as well as their docking score on each specific target structure is reported in **Supplementary Figure 3** and **Supplementary Table 1**, respectively. Remarkably our newly developed VS strategy allows not only to account for the distinct conformations that the receptor can adopt at finite temperature, as in the ensemble docking, but it also encompasses the induced fit effects exerted by the binding of efficacious drugs to distinct ERα isoforms (Spinello et al., 2019a). The best-ranked 17 compounds (**6**-**22**), that were binding to more than one ERα isoform in VS, were then experimentally tested.

Namely, their effect on the transcriptional activity of the mutant Y537S ERα was investigated in cell-based assays, using a standard genomic transcriptional output method (i.e., the estrogen response element (ERE) - luciferase-based gene transactivation system) for assessing their ability to bind ERα and, subsequently, transactivate an ERE-mediated transcription, allowing an assessment of the transcriptional responses of each receptor separately. Thus, human ERα-negative MDA-MB-231 BC cells were cotransfected with either YFP-WT or YFP-Y537S ERα expression vectors along with an ERE-luciferase reporter plasmid (XETL) and treated with the vehicle or the selected compounds (**6**-**22**). As shown in **Figure 2A**, cells expressed similar levels of the 96 kDa protein representing the exogenously added WT or Y537S mutant receptor tagged with YFP. In line with previous results (Toy et al., 2013), reporter gene transactivation assays showed that control basal activity of Y537S ERα was more elevated than that of WT (**Figure 2B**). Importantly, the tested compounds exerted different effects on Y537S ERα transcriptional activity, with **9**, **13**, **19**, **20**, and **21** showing the highest efficacy in reducing the activity of the Y537S mutant (76–57 % decrease) when used at 100 μM concentration. Hence, these were chosen to evaluate their potential toxicity in MDA-MB-231 cells by using MTT cell survival assay (**Figure 2C**). As a result, compounds **9**, **13**, **20**, and **21** markedly reduced cell viability even in MDA-MB-231 cells, whereas the compound **19** did not provoke any significant effects at the dose tested. Thus, among these compounds, **19** represents the best-candidate for further studies. Among these compounds, **9**, **19**, **20**, and **21** share the same chemo-type of the parent compounds AZD.

MDA-MB-231 BC cells transfected with Y537S-ERα vectors and treated with compound **19** at increasing doses (from 1 nM to 100 μM) displayed a dose-dependent decrease of Y537S-ERα transactivation, with the highest inhibition registered at 100 μM concentration (65 ± 10 % inhibition as compared to vehicle) (**Supplementary Figure 4**).

To better clarify the activity of compound **19**, we also evaluated its ability to affect ERα transactivation in cells expressing other two frequently-occurring mutations: YFP-Y537N and YFP-D538G ERα mutations (**Figure 3A**). Surprisingly, **19** has a smaller effect in hampering the transactivation of these mutants (**Figure 3B**), stunningly pinpointing its selectivity in antagonizing preferentially the transcriptional activity of the Y537S ERα isoform.

Next, we inspected its effects on YFP-WT ERα expressing cells in the presence/absence of 17β-estradiol (E2), the endogenous ERα ligand (**Figure 3C**). As expected, E2 treatment was able to trigger luciferase expression through the ERE interaction. Notably its treatment with compound **19**, while not significantly altering WT-ERα transactivation, was associated with a drastic reduction in E2-mediated effects. This suggests that ligand **19** may compete with E2 for the LBC. Interestingly, treatment with **19** was not associated with a down-regulation of Y537S ERα levels (**Figure 3D**).

To expand our investigation, the potency of the compound **19** in affecting Y537S ERα activity was also tested in ER+ MCF-7 BC cells bearing the YFP-WT and YFP-Y537S receptor. These expressed a 66 kDa endogenous ERα, along with a 96 kDa receptor represent the exogenously added WT and mERα tagged with YFP (**Figure 4A**). As previously shown for MDA-MB-231 BC cells, we found a significant increase of YFP-Y537S receptor transcriptional activity as compared to that of YFP-WT ERα and this induction was reduced upon exposure to compound **19** (**Figure 4B**). In addition, **19** antagonized

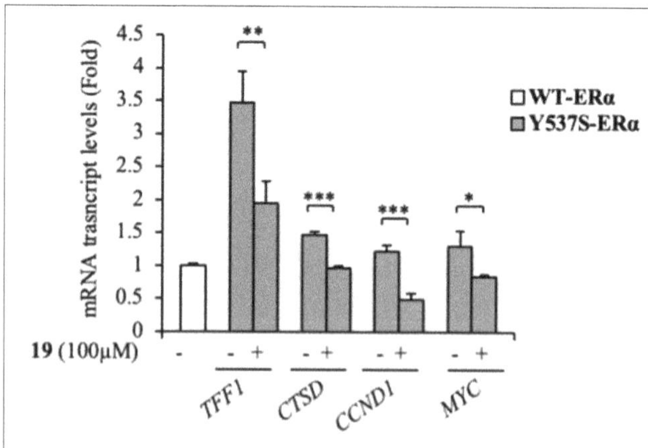

FIGURE 5 | Effects of compound **19** on ERα target genes in YFP-Y537S ERα expressing MDA-MB-231 breast cancer cells. Real time RT-PCR assay for Trefoil Factor 1 (*TTF1*), cathepsin D (*CTSD*), cyclin D1 (*CCND1*) and c-Myc (*MYC*) mRNA expression. The values represent the mean ± S. D. of three different experiments, each performed in triplicate. n. s., non-significant; $^*P < 0.05$; $^{**}P < 0.005$; $^{***}P < 0.0005$.

E2-mediated effects also in YFP-WT ERα MCF-7 expressing cells, without exerting any action on basal WT ERα activity (**Figure 4C**).

At a molecular level, ERα activation and association with the ERE result in an enhanced expression profiles of a number of downstream target genes, including those for trefoil factor 1/pS2, cathepsin D, cyclin D1, and c-Myc (Barone et al., 2010). The biological correlation of the inhibition of Y537S ERα transactivation induced by **19** is the down-regulation of the classical estrogen-regulated genes in MDA-MB-231 cells (**Figure 5**), confirming the binding of this antagonist to ERα, well-fitting with *in silico* predictions.

Atomic-Level Understanding of Drugs Efficacy

In order to identify the structural and dynamics features responsible of the efficacy and the selectivity of compound **19** toward Y537S ERα, while being inefficacious and/or displaying limited efficacy on WT, D538G and Y357N, we performed extensive MD simulations of the five active molecules in complex with the WT and Y537S ERα isoforms, starting from binding poses obtained from docking simulations.

MD simulations revealed two important and common structural traits among the inspected compounds, also shared by AZD and FULV. All molecules occupy the binding cavity

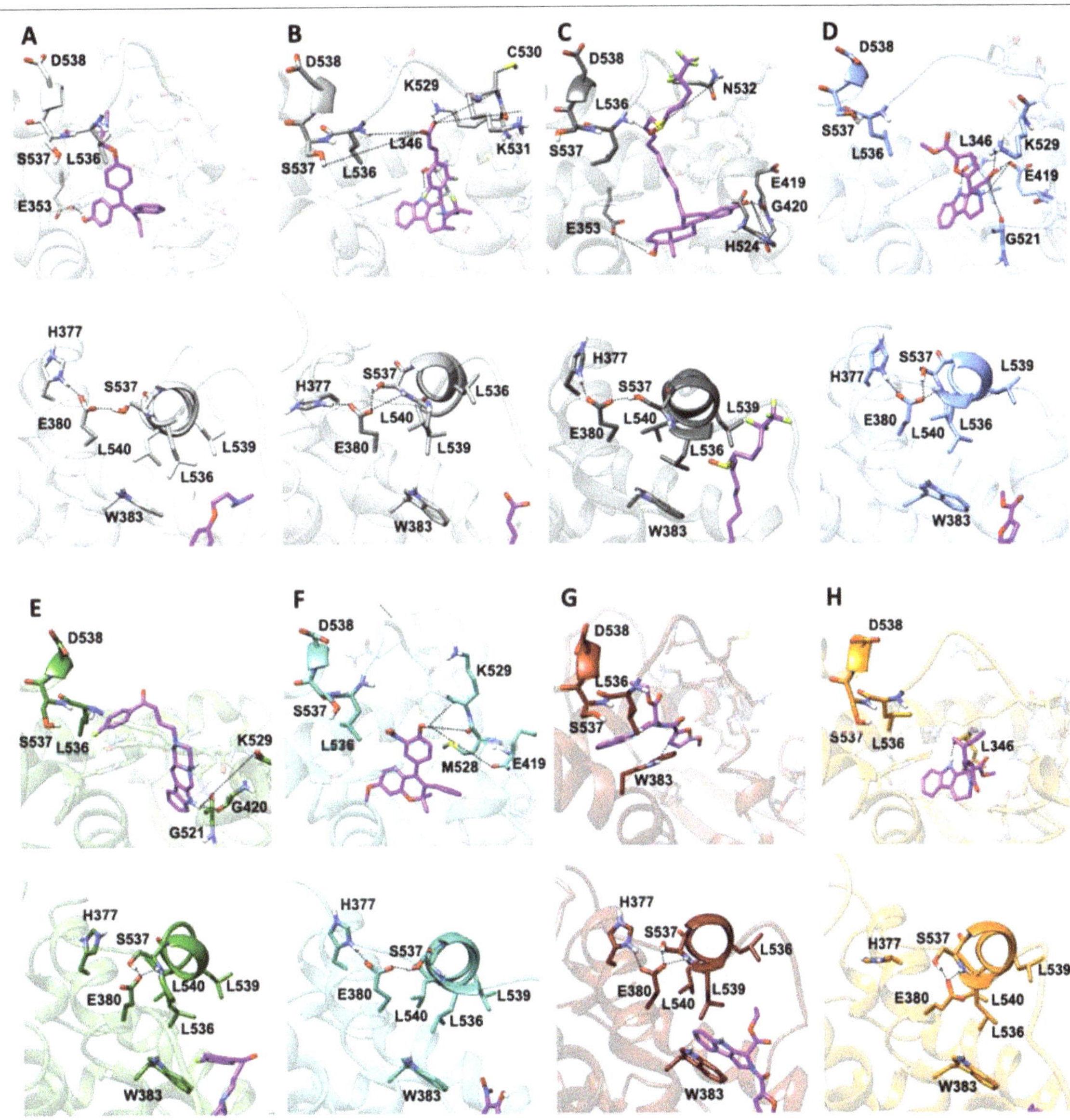

FIGURE 6 | Binding of the five active molecules to Y537S ERα as compared with END, AZD, and FULV. **(A)** END; **(B)** AZD; **(C)** FULV; **(D)** compound **19**; **(E) 9**; **(F) 13**; **(G) 20**; **(H) 21**. Top panels show their placement in the ligand binding cavity, while bottom panels display a close view of E380 H-bond network induced by each ligand. Inhibitors are shown in licorice with carbon atoms in purple color, while oxygen and nitrogen are shown in red and blue, respectively. Protein is depicted in gray new cartoons for END, AZD, FULV, and blue, green, light green purple orange new cartoons for **19**, **9**, **13**, **20**, **21**, respectively.

protruding toward the H11-12 loop, which hosts the Y537S variant (**Figure 6**). Three of them (**9, 19, 20**) establish π-π interactions with W386 in WT (**Supplementary Figure 5**). Due to their different shapes, each ligand engages distinct H-bonds patterns (**Supplementary Table 3**). This network in compounds **13** and **20** involves residues G521, M528, and C530, while **9** and **21** persistently H-bond either to L346, similarly to AZD, or to E419 and G420 (**Supplementary Table 3**). These results show that the selected compounds can either bind in LBC (**9** and **21**) or interact with H11-12 loop (**13** and **20**).

Conversely, **19** is the only ligand firmly anchored to E419 and L346 (**Supplementary Table 3**), at tract H bonding to K529, similarly to AZD in complex with to Y537S (**Figure 6**). This H-bonding motif in our previous paper was indicated as an essential signature of drug-efficacy. Nevertheless, **19** forms a set of low-persistent H-bonds, underlying its high mobility and the need for further optimization in order to improve its efficacy. Surprisingly, compound **19** establishes a well-defined and stable H-bond network only in one LBCs of WT ERα (**Supplementary Table 3**).

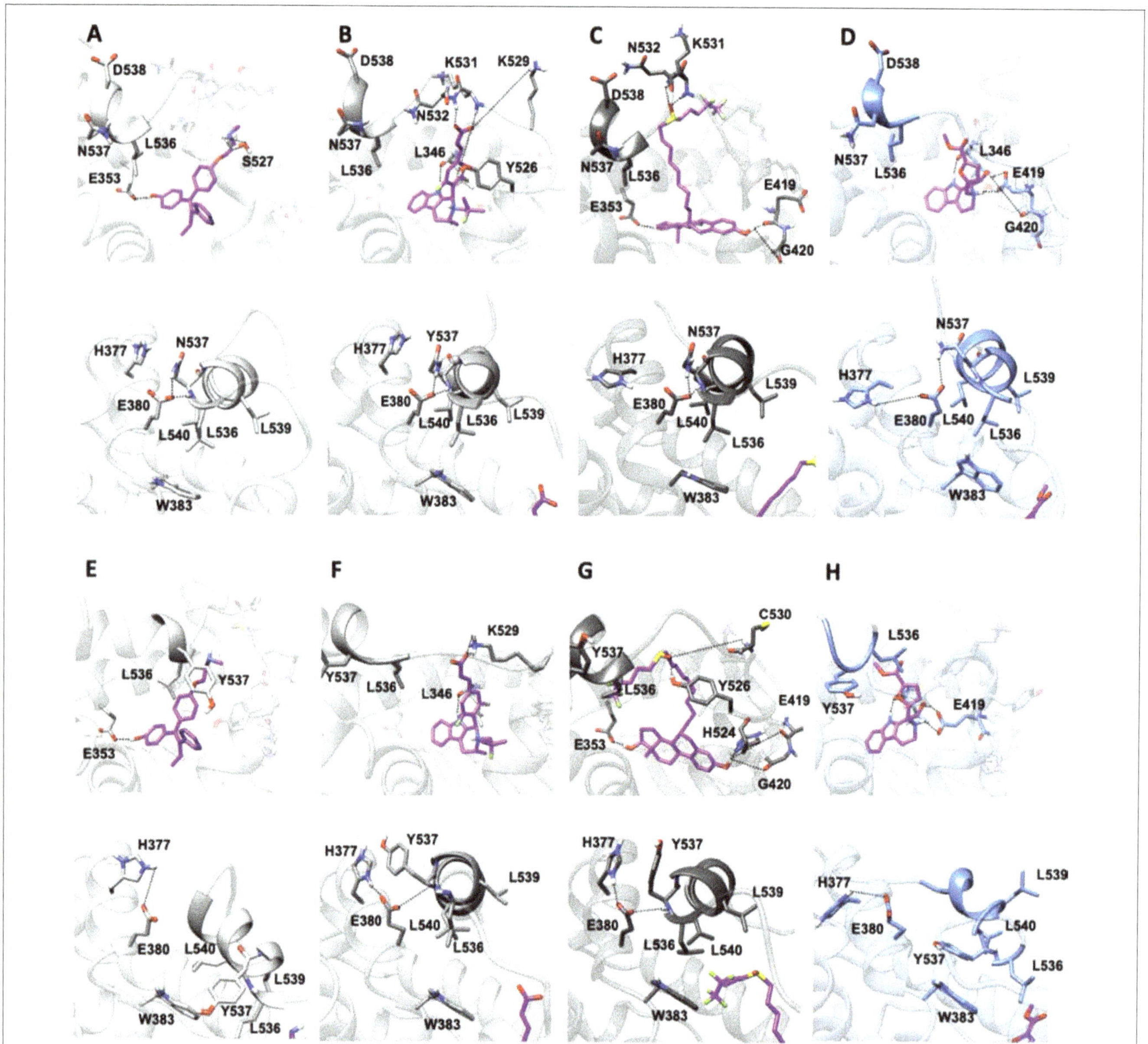

FIGURE 7 | Binding of compound **19** to Y537N and D538G ERα as compared with END, AZD and FULV. Binding to Y537N: **(A)** END; **(B)** AZD; **(C)** FULV; **(D)** Compound **19**. Binding to D538G: **(E)** END; **(F)** AZD; **(G)** FULV; **(H)** Compound **19**. Top panels show their placement in the ligand binding cavity, while bottom panels display a close view of E380 H-bond network induced by each ligand. Inhibitors are shown in licorice with carbon atoms in purple color, while oxygen and nitrogen in red and blue, respectively. Protein is shown in gray new cartoons for END, AZD, FULV, and in blue new cartoons for **19**, respectively.

Next, we inspected how the active drugs counteract the H-bond network responsible of the ERα agonist-like conformation induced by mERα (**Supplementary Table 4**, **Figure 6**). A decrease of the E380-Y537S interaction, previously indicated as structural signature of an intrinsic ERα activation, occurs with all ligands, even if this is less effective than upon FULV or AZD binding. What is more, E380, which strongly H-bonds to S537 in the aggressive Y537S ERα variant, upon binding of **9**, **19**, and **21**, rearranges and engages persistent H-bond to L536. Additionally, in the presence of **19**, there is significant change in the H-bond network of L536 backbone. While this latter strongly interacts with backbone of L539 in the presence of all other compounds, **19** weakens it and, as a result, L536 H-bonds to the backbone of L540 (**Supplementary Table 4**). Remarkably, **19** triggers formation of these H-bonds only in Y537S, but not in WT ERα.

In both Y537N and D538G variants **19** establishes a H-bond network in the binding cavity and in the H11-12 loop region similarly to Y537S (**Supplementary Tables 3**, **4**, and **Figure 7**). Hence, **19** exclusively H-bonds to E419 in all mutants, while only in Y537S can establish week H-bond to K529, similarly to AZD.

We have also calculated the binding free energy (ΔG_b) (**Table 1**) of the five active compounds to WT, Y537S and, for compound **19,** also to the Y537N, D538G variants. Stunningly, **19** dissociates from one monomer of WT ERα due to the lack of H-bonds, rationalizing its preference toward the pathogenic variants. Instead, its ΔG_b is similar in all tested mutants. All other active ligands, but **20**, display a slightly higher affinity for WT ERα, and their ΔG_b is slightly larger than that of **19** toward Y537S, most probably because of their larger size. Nonetheless, the tested ligands do not strongly bind to the LBC, as shown by a comparison of the calculated ΔG_b compared to that AZD. Thus, even small differences in the position of their H-bonding moieties may result in the different binding poses observed for **20** and **13**. To monitor the impact of the distinct ligands size on ΔG_b, we also computed the ligand efficiency (LE, **Supplementary Table 5**), calculated as ΔG_b divided by the number of non-hydrogen atoms. LE differences among ligands are smaller than that of ΔG_bs. **19** presents comparable LE for all mutants tested. Interestingly, compounds **9**, **20**, **21** have a slightly larger LE for Y537S than **19**, suggesting that other features, besides LE or ΔG_b, may be important for ligand selectivity toward the distinct ERα isoforms.

Structural Signatures of (m)ERα Activation/Inactivation

The cross-correlation matrix calculated on the basis of the Pearson correlation coefficients (CC_{ij}) was computed to qualitatively identify the linearly coupled motions between couples of residues along the MD trajectory. A simplified version of this matrix, based on the sum of the of correlation scores (CSs) between each structural elements of (m)ERα (**Supplementary Figure 2**), has been calculated to decrypt the correlation pattern in complex systems (Casalino et al., 2018), among which ERα (Pavlin et al., 2018). In this analysis, a positive/negative score corresponds to a positively (correlated) / negatively (anti-correlated) motion.

In our previous study, the presence of a positive correlation score between H12 and H3-H5 was taken as a structural signature of Y537S ERα intrinsic activation. This was persistent upon END binding, while only FULV and, partially, AZD were able to remove it, in line with the proved activity of these SERDs on the Y537S mutant (Fanning et al., 2016). Hence, we also inspected if the ligands differently affect the internal cross-correlation map. All compounds binding to Y537S remove the contacts between H12 and H3, reducing, in most cases, the cross-correlation score in both monomers

TABLE 1 | Binding free energies (ΔG_b, kcal/mol) of the ligands **9**, **13**, **19**, **20**, and **21**.

	WT		Y537S		Y537N		D538G	
	A	B	A	B	A	B	A	B
Endoxifen	−51.7 ± 3.6	−46.9 ± 3.3	−45.6 ± 3.5	−45.2 ± 3.5	−43.8 ± 3.3	−49.9 ± 4.3	−47.1 ± 3.4	−50.5 ± 3.6
AZD−9496	−45.2 ± 3.6	−43.9 ± 3.7	−42.9 ± 3.7	−53.7 ± 7.7	−45.1 ± 4.1	−42.9 ± 3.9	−45.1 ± 4.0	−43.7 ± 4.3
Fulvestrant	−69.0 ± 6.4	−66.9 ± 6.2	−65.1 ± 5.1	−76.0 ± 5.6	−68.2 ± 6.1	−66.6 ± 5.7	−63.5 ± 6.0	−69.7 ± 6.0
9	−42.7 ± 4.2	−36.7 ± 4.4	−36.9 ± 5.7	−37.3 ± 4.6	/	/	/	/
13	−44.8 ± 4.3	−42.6 ± 3.3	−41.4 ± 3.2	−45.2 ± 4.6	/	/	/	/
19	−21.3 ± 7.2*	−40.9 ± 8.1	−32.3 ± 5.8	−32.3 ± 6.2	−32.9 ± 3.6	−43.0 ± 6.7	−30.8 ± 5.7	−46.8 ± 6.0
20	−38.6 ± 3.3	−35.1 ± 2.6	−40.0 ± 2.9	−38.9 ± 5.0	/	/	/	/
21	−45.4 ± 3.3	−42.5 ± 3.8	−43.6 ± 3.2	−39.2 ± 3.0	/	/	/	/

Absolute values of molecular mechanics Generalized bond surface are (MM-GBSA).‡

‡*Number of atoms/heavy atoms in each ligand:*

Endoxifen – 55/28.

AZD-9496 – 57/32.

Fulvestrant – 88/41.

***9** – 56/29.*

***13** – 51/30.*

***19** – 46/25.*

***20** – 47/27.*

***21** – 50/26.*

**Ligand exits from the binding pocket.*

(**Supplementary Figure 6**). Moreover, compound **19** decreases these contacts also when binding to Y537N and, to a minor extent, to D538G (**Supplementary Figures 7, 8**). Conversely, in WT ERα a smaller positive correlation among H5 and H12 can be observed only for (**20** and **21**; **Supplementary Figure 9**).

In order to capture more quantitatively the relative differences among the activity exerted by these ligands we also analyzed how H12 correlates with all other ERα structural elements in the presence of the distinct active compounds. This analysis clearly shows that ligands **9** and **20** present a cross-correlation

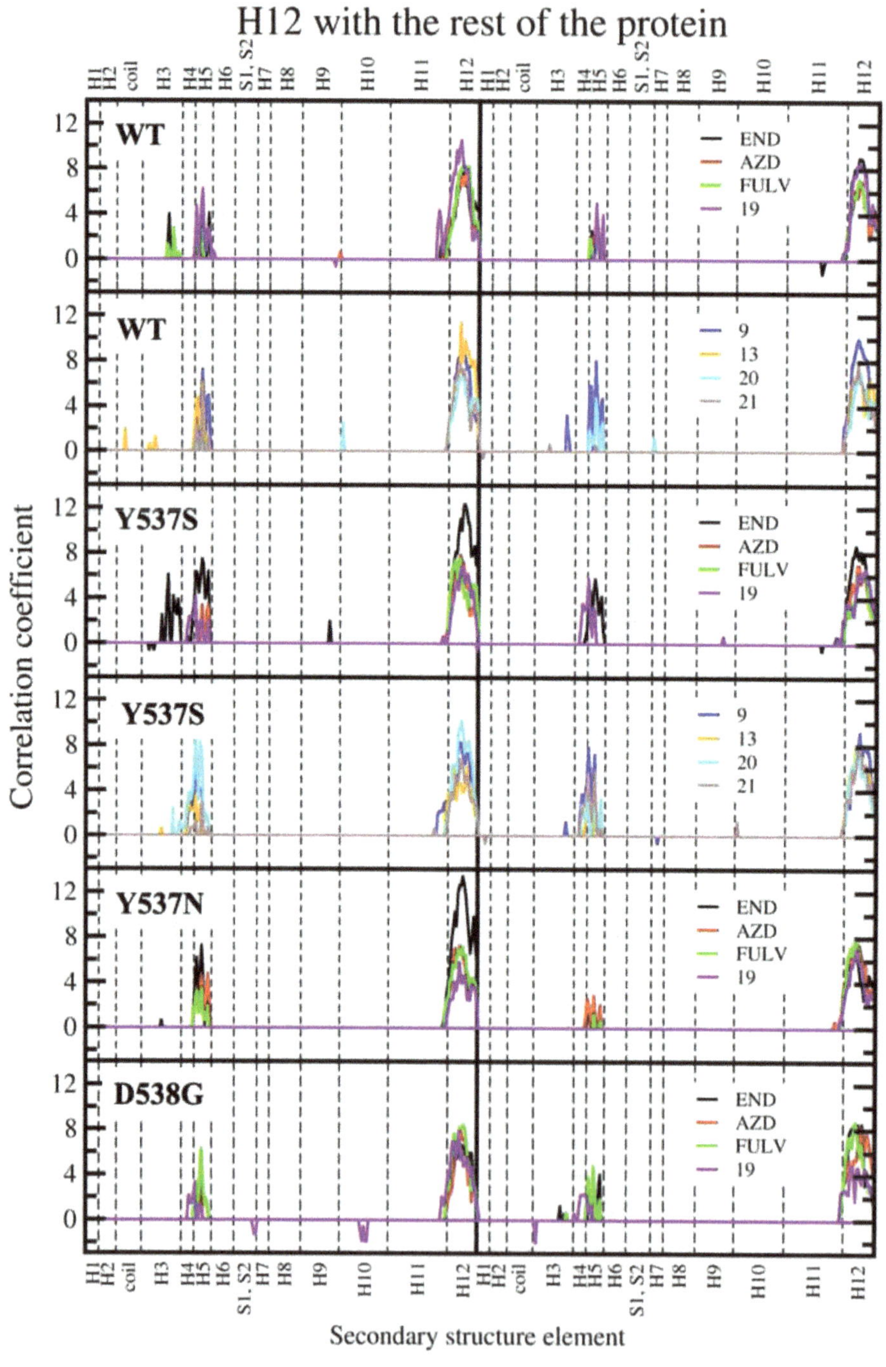

FIGURE 8 | Sum of per-residue cross-correlation coefficients. Left and right columns refer to monomers A and B, respectively. From top to bottom: WT (in complex with END, AZD, FULV, and **19**), WT (with **9**, **13**, **20**, and **21**), Y537S (with END, AZD, FULV, and **19**), Y537S (with **9**, **13**, **20**, and **21**), Y537N, and D538G (in complex with END, AZD, FULV, and **19**). END, AZD, FULV, and compounds **9**, **13**, **19**, **20**, **21** are shown as black, red, green, blue, orange, purple, cyan, and brown lines, respectively.

coupling between H12 and H4-H5 higher or similar to END at least in one Y537S ERα monomer, while **19** effectively reduces this positive correlation in both monomers. This correlation coupling is completely abolished in Y537N and reduced even in D538G (**Figure 8**), pointing to an activity of **19** also against these mutants, even if to a minor extent.

As a result, **19** appears to reduce the transcriptional activity of Y537S cells thanks to its capability of binding in the LBC of both LBD monomers only in the mERαs, where it establishes H-bonds with E415, L346 and K529, similarly to AZD.

Kinetic Characterization of Active Compounds

Since increasing evidences pinpoint the dissociation free energy barriers ($\Delta G_d^{\#}$) of a ligand from its binding cavity to be strongly entwined with the residence time and, thus, with drugs' efficacy (Magistrato et al., 2017), the observed preferential activity of **19** toward Y537S ERα fostered the investigations of its kinetic properties as compared to those of AZD.

The free energy surface (FES) obtained from MTD simulations inducing the dissociation of AZD from the LBC of Y537S ERα shows a wide minimum at Center of Mass (COM) distance between ligand and protein at ~1.2 nm, which, instead, spans the coordination number (CN) 0.2-0.4. A second, narrower, minimum appears at CN around 0 and COM distance ≥ 2.5 nm. By inspecting two-dimensional FES plots of both CVs one can estimate a $\Delta G_d^{\#}$ of 14.1 ± 2.0 kcal/mol for AZD dissociation (**Figure 9A**, **Supplementary Figures 10**, **11**, and **Supplementary Table 6**). The main barrier observed for AZD dissociation is due to the breaking of its H-bond interactions between the carboxylic group of AZD with K529 and C530. These, therefore, appear as pivotal residues for increasing the residence time of this drug in the LBC and possibly its efficacy.

On the other hand, FES for the dissociation of **19** reveals a rather wide minimum at CN = 0.2–0.4, lying at higher distance (COM) between ligand and the LBC as compared to AZD (1.5–1.7 nm) (**Figure 9B**). The second minimum is located in a similar position to that of AZD. In this case, however, the $\Delta G_d^{\#}$ is rather small (3.7 ± 1.9 kcal/mol) (**Supplementary Figures 10**, **11** and **Supplementary Table 6**) and it is associated to the breaking of the H-bond between the hydroxyl group of the ligand and the E418 residue. This latter, therefore, appears to be a distinctive feature of this ligand.

These simulations pinpoint the most important substituents of the ligand that may contribute to improve the kinetic properties of the drugs, and the residues of the LBC that must be engaged in specific interactions for the discovery of mutant-specific anti-estrogen compounds.

DISCUSSION

Breast cancer remains the most diagnosed (1 over 8) and the second leading cause of cancer induced mortality in women. The majority (70 %) of BC is hormone dependent and its proliferation relies on the presence of ERα, which has a pro-oncogenic effect in the presence of estrogens. The gold standard treatment in this type of BC is the hormone adjuvant therapy, which either suppresses estrogen production (aromatase inhibitors) or modulates/degrades the ERα (SERMs/SERDs). The prolonged exposure to these therapies, usually administered consecutively for 5-10 years' time-frame, leads to resistance in half of all luminal BCs after 5 years, in spite of the ERα expression (Toy et al., 2017; Fanning et al., 2018; Busonero et al., 2019; Spinello et al., 2019b).

While the genomic profile of inherited and somatic alterations characterizing each type of BC is well-established, the evolution of the BC's genomic landscape under the evolutionary pressure of systemic therapies is not clearly understood. As well as how this landscape impacts on the clinical outcome of endocrine therapies remains poorly characterized and is currently object of intense research efforts. Resistance onset is, in fact, responsible of refractory BCs and of an increased mortality rate. In this worrisome scenario, the therapeutic options to intervene with personalized treatments based on the patients' evolution of the genomic profiles remains a daunting challenge. This has spurred substantial efforts to characterize the phenotype responsible of drug resistance and propose innovative therapeutic options.

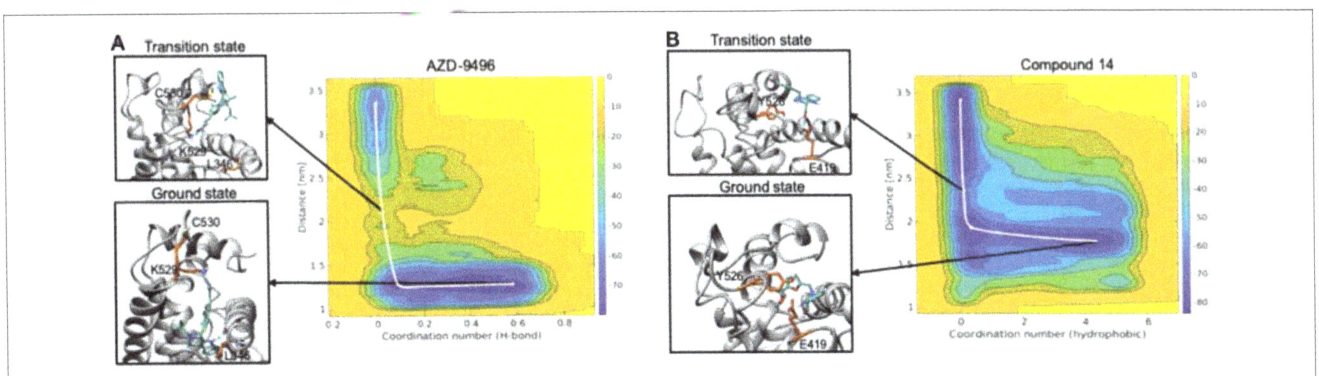

FIGURE 9 | Free energy surface maps from metadynamics simulations for the dissociation of AZD **(A)** and compound **19 (B)** from the ligand binding cavity. On x axis is coordination number (H-bond for AZD and hydrophobic interactions for **19**) and on y axis is COM distance between ligand and receptor. Color scale represents free energy values in kJ/mol. In black squares are encircled structures corresponding to the ligand bound state (ground state), the transition state.

Distinct studies indicated that frequent mutations present in the loop connecting H11 and H12 of the LBD trigger the acquisition of an intrinsically active (agonist-like) ERα conformation, even in the absence of E2. This conformation remains even in the presence of SERMs (Fanning et al., 2016; Pavlin et al., 2018). Our recent computational attempt to identify the key common structural traits that drugs should possess in order to effectively fight resistant BCs was the grounding knowledge for the present study. Indeed, here we carried out *in silico* screening on the structural scaffolds of the Y537S, Y537N, and D538G mutants adapted to known mERα degraders (AZD and FULV), seeking for the structural elements able to protrude toward loop connecting H11-H12. This should allow the ligand to counteract the intrinsic and mutant dependent ERα activation (Pavlin et al., 2018).

From a consensus docking study, we selected 17 molecules (**Supplementary Figure 3**) effectively binding in at least two mutants, among which five resulted to be active on BC cell lines. Some of them were known to be active also on other targets and diseases (**Supplementary Table 7**). Among these compounds, **19** was selective exclusively toward those expressing Y537S (and to a minor extent to Y537N, D538G) ERα (**Figures 2–4**). In spite of its ability to block the transcriptional activity of the receptor only in the high μM range, thus requiring further optimization, the structural scaffold of compound **19** encompasses all the motifs required by an active and mutant-specific drug-candidate. Namely, **19** forms number of H-bonds in the ligand binding cavity (L346 and E419) and with K529. Conversely, E380, a key residue involved in the structural transition toward an agonist-like state of the receptor, persistently H-bonds to H377. This is a previously annotated structural feature able to impede the pro-oncogenic effect of resistant phenotypes. Indeed, compound **19**, to the best of our knowledge, is the only mutant specific modulator of ERα transcriptional activity identified so far. However, its ΔG_b and $\Delta G_d^{\#}$ are remarkably smaller than the parent AZD compound. A detailed comparison among the residues, which optimize these thermodynamics and kinetic properties of the **19** with respect to those of AZD is informative for future knowledge-based drug-design efforts aimed at discovering drug-candidates with superior efficacy.

Since ESR1 mutations are potential clinical biomarkers to guide therapeutic decisions, identification of small molecules able to block proliferation of metastatic tumors expressing one prevalent mERα resistant phenotypes may result in counteracting, preventing and/or delaying their occurrence in early disease stage. In this scenario, our study contributes to move a step forward toward precision and personalized medicine tailored against metastatic and resistant ER+ BCs.

AUTHOR CONTRIBUTIONS

LG and IB performed experiments. MP and AS performed simulations and analysis. IB, SA, SC, and AM designed research and wrote the manuscript.

FUNDING

This work was supported by My First AIRC Grant (MFAG) #16899 to IB, MFAG Grant #17134 to AM, AIRC Investigator Grant (IG) #21414 to SC, AIRC IG #18602 to SA.

ACKNOWLEDGMENTS

The authors thank AIRC for financial support.

REFERENCES

Abraham, M. J., Murtola, T., Schulz, R., Páll, S., Smith, J. C., Hess, B., et al. (2015). GROMACS: High performance molecular simulations through multi-level parallelism from laptops to supercomputers. *SoftwareX* 1–2, 19–25. doi: 10.1016/j.softx.2015.06.001

Anandakrishnan, R., Aguilar, B., and Onufriev, A. V. (2012). H++ 3.0: automating pK prediction and the preparation of biomolecular structures for atomistic molecular modeling and simulations. *Nucl Acids Res.* 40, W537–41. doi: 10.1093/nar/gks375

Barone, I., Brusco, L., and Fuqua, S. A. (2010). Estrogen receptor mutations and changes in downstream gene expression and signaling. *Clin. Cancer Res.* 16, 2702–2708. doi: 10.1158/1078-0432.CCR-09-1753

Barone, I., Brusco, L., Gu, G., Selever, J., Beyer, A., Covington, K. R., et al. (2011). Loss of Rho GDIalpha and resistance to tamoxifen via effects on estrogen receptor alpha. *J. Natl. Cancer Inst.* 103, 538–552. doi: 10.1093/jnci/djr058

Bayly, C. I., Cieplak, P., Cornell, W. D., and Kollman, P. A. (1993). A well-behaved electrostatic potential based method using charge restraints for deriving atomic charges - the RESP model. *J. Phys. Chem.* 97, 10269–10280. doi: 10.1021/J100142a004

Bisha, I., Laio, A., Magistrato, A., Giorgetti, A., and Sgrignani, J. (2013). A candidate ion-retaining state in the inward-facing conformation of sodium/galactose symporter: clues from atomistic simulations. *J. Chem. Theory Comput.* 9, 1240–1246. doi: 10.1021/ct3008233

Busonero, C., Leone, S., Bartoloni, S., and Acconcia, F. (2019). Strategies to degrade estrogen receptor alpha in primary and ESR1 mutant-expressing metastatic breast cancer. *Mol. Cell. Endocrinol.* 480, 107–121. doi: 10.1016/j.mce.2018.10.020

Bussi, G., Donadio, D., and Parrinello, M. (2007). Canonical sampling through velocity rescaling. *J. Chem. Phys.* 126:014101. doi: 10.1063/1.2408420

Casalino, L., Palermo, G., Spinello, A., Rothlisberger, U., and Magistrato, A. (2018). All-atom simulations disentangle the functional dynamics underlying gene maturation in the intron lariat spliceosome. *Proc. Natl. Acad. Sci. U.S.A.* 115, 6584–6589. doi: 10.1073/pnas.1802963115

Catalano, S., Leggio, A., Barone, I., De Marco, R., Gelsomino, L., Campana, A., et al. (2015). A novel leptin antagonist peptide inhibits breast cancer growth *in vitro* and *in vivo*. *J. Cell. Mol. Med.* 19, 1122–1132. doi: 10.1111/jcmm.12517

Chandarlapaty, S., Chen, D., He, W., Sung, P., Samoila, A., You, D., et al. (2016). Prevalence of ESR1 Mutations in cell-free DNA and outcomes in metastatic breast cancer: a secondary analysis of the BOLERO-2 clinical trial. *JAMA Oncol.* 2, 1310–1315. doi: 10.1001/jamaoncol.2016.1279

Covington, K. R., Brusco, L., Barone, I., Tsimelzon, A., Selever, J., Corona-Rodriguez, A., et al. (2013). Metastasis tumor-associated protein 2 enhances metastatic behavior and is associated with poor outcomes in estrogen receptor-negative breast cancer. *Breast Cancer Res. Treat.* 141, 375–384. doi: 10.1007/s10549-013-2709-5

Darden, T., York, D., and Pedersen, L. (1993). Particle mesh ewald: An N.log(N) method for Ewald sums in large systems. *J. Chem. Phys.* 98, 10089–10092. doi: 10.1063/1.464397

Daura, X., Gademann, K., Jaun, B., Seebach, D., van Gunsteren, W. F., and Mark, A. E. (1999). Peptide folding: when simulation meets experiment. *Angew. Chem. Int. Ed.* 38, 236–240.

De Savi, C., Bradbury, R. H., Rabow, A. A., Norman, R. A., de Almeida, C., Andrews, D. M., et al. (2015). Optimization of a novel binding motif to (E)-3-(3,5-difluoro-4-((1R,3R)-2-(2-fluoro-2-methylpropyl)-3-methyl-2,3,4,9-tetrahydro-1H-pyrido[3,4-b]indol-1-yl)phenyl)acrylic Acid (AZD9496), a potent and orally bioavailable selective estrogen receptor downregulator and antagonist. *J. Med. Chem.* 58, 8128–8140. doi: 10.1021/acs.jmedchem.5b00984

Duan, J., Dixon, S. L., Lowrie, J. F., and Sherman, W. (2010). Analysis and comparison of 2D fingerprints: insights into database screening performance using eight fingerprint methods. *J. Mol. Graph. Model.* 29, 157–170. doi: 10.1016/j.jmgm.2010.05.008

Fanning, S. W., and Greene, G. L. (2019). Next-generation ERalpha inhibitors for endocrine-resistant ER+ breast cancer. *Endocrinology* 160, 759–769. doi: 10.1210/en.2018-01095

Fanning, S. W., Hodges-Gallagher, L., Myles, D. C., Sun, R., Fowler, C. E., Plant, I. N., et al. (2018). Specific stereochemistry of OP-1074 disrupts estrogen receptor alpha helix 12 and confers pure antiestrogenic activity. *Nat. Commun.* 9:2368. doi: 10.1038/s41467-018-04413-3

Fanning, S. W., Mayne, C. G., Dharmarajan, V., Carlson, K. E., Martin, T. A., Novick, S. J., et al. (2016). Estrogen receptor alpha somatic mutations Y537S and D538G confer breast cancer endocrine resistance by stabilizing the activating function-2 binding conformation. *eLife* 5:e12792. doi: 10.7554/eLife.12792

Friesner, R. A., Banks, J. L., Murphy, R. B., Halgren, T. A., Klicic, J. J., Mainz, D. T., et al. (2004). Glide: a new approach for rapid, accurate docking and scoring. 1. Method and assessment of docking accuracy. *J. Med. Chem.* 47, 1739–1749. doi: 10.1021/jm0306430

Frisch, M. J., Trucks, G. W., Schlegel, H. B., Scuseria, G. E., Robb, M. A., Cheeseman, J. R., et al. (2016). *Gaussian 09, Revision A.02.* Wallingford CT: Gaussian, Inc.

Gelsomino, L., Gu, G., Rechoum, Y., Beyer, A. R., Pejerrey, S. M., Tsimelzon, A., et al. (2016). ESR1 mutations affect anti-proliferative responses to tamoxifen through enhanced cross-talk with IGF signaling. *Breast Cancer Res. Treat.* 157, 253–265. doi: 10.1007/s10549-016-3829-5

Gelsomino, L., Panza, S., Giordano, C., Barone, I., Gu, G., Spina, E., et al. (2018). Mutations in the estrogen receptor alpha hormone binding domain promote stem cell phenotype through notch activation in breast cancer cell lines. *Cancer Lett.* 428, 12–20. doi: 10.1016/j.canlet.2018.04.023

Giordano, C., Chemi, F., Panza, S., Barone, I., Bonofiglio, D., Lanzino, M., et al. (2016). Leptin as a mediator of tumor-stromal interactions promotes breast cancer stem cell activity. *Oncotarget* 7, 1262–1275. doi: 10.18632/oncotarget.6014

Hamilton, E. P., Patel, M. R., Armstrong, A. C., Baird, R. D., Jhaveri, K., Hoch, M., et al. (2018). A first-in-human study of the new oral selective estrogen receptor degrader AZD9496 for ER(+)/HER2(-) advanced breast cancer. *Clin. Cancer. Res.* 24, 3510–3518. doi: 10.1158/1078-0432.CCR-17-3102

Hess, B., Bekker, H., Berendsen, H. J. C., and Fraaije, J. G. E. M. (1997). LINCS: a linear constraint solver for molecular simulations. *J. Comput. Chem.* 18, 1463–1472.

Huang, W., Peng, Y., Kiselar, J., Zhao, X., Albaqami, A., Mendez, D., et al. (2018). Multidomain architecture of estrogen receptor reveals interfacial cross-talk between its DNA-binding and ligand-binding domains. *Nat. Commun.* 9:3520. doi: 10.1038/s41467-018-06034-2

Humphrey, W., Dalke, A., and Schulten, K. (1996). VMD: Visual molecular dynamics. *J. Mol. Graph.* 14, 33–38, 27–38.

Jeselsohn, R., Yelensky, R., Buchwalter, G., Frampton, G., Meric-Bernstam, F., Gonzalez-Angulo, A. M., et al. (2014). Emergence of constitutively active estrogen receptor-alpha mutations in pretreated advanced estrogen receptor-positive breast cancer. *Clin. Cancer Res.* 20, 1757–1767. doi: 10.1158/1078-0432.CCR-13-2332

Jorgensen, W. L., Chandrasekhar, J., Madura, J. D., Impey, R. W., and Klein, M. L. (1983). Comparison of simple potential functions for simulating liquid water. *J. Chem. Phys.* 79, 926–935. doi: 10.1063/1.445869

Joseph, J. D., Darimont, B., Zhou, W., Arrazate, A., Young, A., Ingalla, E., et al. (2016). The selective estrogen receptor downregulator GDC-0810 is efficacious in diverse models of ER+ breast cancer. *eLife* 5:e15828. doi: 10.7554/eLife.15828

Kahraman, M., Govek, S. P., Nagasawa, J. Y., Lai, A., Bonnefous, C., Douglas, K., et al. (2019). Maximizing ER-alpha degradation maximizes activity in a Tamoxifen-resistant breast cancer model: Identification of GDC-0927. *ACS Med. Chem. Lett.* 10, 50–55. doi: 10.1021/acsmedchemlett.8b00414

Lindorff-Larsen, K., Piana, S., Palmo, K., Maragakis, P., Klepeis, J. L., Dror, R. O., et al. (2010). Improved side-chain torsion potentials for the Amber ff99SB protein force field. *Proteins* 78, 1950–1958. doi: 10.1002/prot.22711

Lipinski, C. A., Lombardo, F., Dominy, B. W., and Feeney, P. J. (2001). Experimental and computational approaches to estimate solubility and permeability in drug discovery and development settings. *Adv. Drug. Deliv. Rev.* 46, 3–26. doi: 10.1016/S0169-409X(00)00129-0

Magistrato, A., Sgrignani, J., Krause, R., and Cavalli, A. (2017). Single or multiple access channels to the CYP450s active site? an answer from free energy simulations of the human aromatase enzyme. *J. Phys. Chem. Lett.* 8, 2036–2042. doi: 10.1021/acs.jpclett.7b00697

Merenbakh-Lamin, K., Ben-Baruch, N., Yeheskel, A., Dvir, A., Soussan-Gutman, L., Jeselsohn, R., et al. (2013). D538G mutation in estrogen receptor-alpha: A novel mechanism for acquired endocrine resistance in breast cancer. *Cancer Res.* 73, 6856–6864. doi: 10.1158/0008-5472.CAN-13-1197

Nilsson, S., and Gustafsson, J. A. (2011). Estrogen receptors: Therapies targeted to receptor subtypes. *Clinical Pharmacol. Ther.* 89, 44–55. doi: 10.1038/clpt.2010.226

Palermo, G., Miao, Y., Walker, R. C., Jinek, M., and McCammon, J. A. (2016). Striking plasticity of CRISPR-Cas9 and key role of non-target DNA, as revealed by molecular simulations. *ACS Cent. Sci.* 2, 756–763. doi: 10.1021/acscentsci.6b00218

Pavlin, M., Spinello, A., Pennati, M., Zaffaroni, N., Gobbi, S., Bisi, A., et al. (2018). A Computational assay of estrogen receptor alpha antagonists reveals the key common structural traits of drugs effectively fighting refractory breast cancers. *Sci. Rep.* 8, 649. doi: 10.1038/s41598-017-17364-4

Pettersen, E. F., Goddard, T. D., Huang, C. C., Couch, G. S., Greenblatt, D. M., Meng, E. C., et al. (2004). UCSF Chimera–a visualization system for exploratory research and analysis. *J. Comput. Chem.* 25, 1605–1612. doi: 10.1002/jcc.20084

Razavi, P., Chang, M. T., Xu, G., Bandlamudi, C., Ross, D. S., Vasan, N., et al. (2018). The genomic landscape of endocrine-resistant advanced breast cancers. *Cancer Cell* 34, 427–438 e426. doi: 10.1016/j.ccell.2018.08.008

Rizza, P., Barone, I., Zito, D., Giordano, F., Lanzino, M., De Amicis, F., et al. (2014). Estrogen receptor beta as a novel target of androgen receptor action in breast cancer cell lines. *Br Cancer Res.* 16:R21. doi: 10.1186/bcr3619

Robinson, D. R., Wu, Y. M., Vats, P., Su, F., Lonigro, R. J., Cao, X., et al. (2013). Activating ESR1 mutations in hormone-resistant metastatic breast cancer. *Nat. Genet.* 45, 1446–1451. doi: 10.1038/ng.2823

Sastry, M., Lowrie, J. F., Dixon, S. L., and Sherman, W. (2010). Large-scale systematic analysis of 2D fingerprint methods and parameters to improve virtual screening enrichments. *J. Chem. Inf. Model.* 50, 771–784. doi: 10.1021/ci100062n

Schrödinger Release 2017-1 (2017). *Small-Molecule Drug Discovery Suite 2017-1.* New York, NY: Schrodinger, LLC.

Scott, J. S., Bailey, A., Buttar, D., Carbajo, R. J., Curwen, J., Davey, P. R. J., et al. (2019). Tricyclic indazoles-a novel class of selective estrogen receptor degrader antagonists. *J. Med. Chem.* 62, 1593–1608. doi: 10.1021/acs.jmedchem.8b01837

Sgrignani, J., and Magistrato, A. (2015). QM/MM MD simulations on the enzymatic pathway of the human flap endonuclease (hFEN1) elucidating common cleavage pathways to RNase H enzymes. *ACS Catal.* 5, 3864–3875. doi: 10.1021/acscatal.5b00178

Sharma, A., Toy, W., Guillen, V. S., Sharma, N., Min, J., Carlson, K. E., et al. (2018). Antagonists for constitutively active mutant estrogen eeceptors: insights into the roles of antiestrogen-core and side-chain. *ACS Chem. Biol.* 13, 3374–3384. doi: 10.1021/acschembio.8b00877

Spinello, A., Martini, S., Berti, F., Pennati, M., Pavlin, M., Sgrignani, J., et al. (2019a). Rational design of allosteric modulators of the aromatase enzyme: an unprecedented therapeutic strategy to fight breast cancer. *Eur. J. Med. Chem.* 168, 253–262. doi: 10.1016/j.ejmech.2019.02.045

Spinello, A., Pavlin, M., Casalino, L., and Magistrato, A. (2018). A dehydrogenase dual hydrogen abstraction mechanism promotes estrogen biosynthesis: can we expand the functional annotation of the aromatase enzyme? *Chem.-Eur. J.* 24, 10840–10849. doi: 10.1002/chem.201802025

Spinello, A., Ritacco, I., and Magistrato, A. (2019b). Recent advances in computational design of potent aromatase inhibitors: open-eye on endocrine-resistant breast cancers. *Expert. Opin. Drug. Discov.* 245:1–12. doi: 10.1080/17460441.2019.1646245

Spinello, A., Vecile, E., Abbate, A., Dobrina, A., and Magistrato, A. (2019c). How can interleukin-1 receptor antagonist modulate distinct cell death pathways? *J. Chem. Inf. Model.* 59, 351–359. doi: 10.1021/acs.jcim.8b00565

Toy, W., Shen, Y., Won, H., Green, B., Sakr, R. A., Will, M., et al. (2013). ESR1 ligand-binding domain mutations in hormone-resistant breast cancer. *Nat. Genet.* 45, 1439–1445. doi: 10.1038/ng.2822

Toy, W., Weir, H., Razavi, P., Lawson, M., Goeppert, A. U., Mazzola, A. M., et al. (2017). Activating ESR1 mutations differentially affect the efficacy of ER antagonists. *Cancer Discov.* 7, 277–287. doi: 10.1158/2159-8290.CD-15-1523

Tribello, G., Bonomi, M., Branduardi, D., Camilloni, C., and Bussi, G. (2014). PLUMED2: New feathers for an old bird. *Comp. Phys. Comm.* 185:606–613. doi: 10.1016/j.cpc.2013.09.018

van Kruchten, M., de Vries, E. G., Glaudemans, A. W., van Lanschot, M. C., van Faassen, M., Kema, I. P., et al. (2015). Measuring residual estrogen receptor availability during fulvestrant therapy in patients with metastatic breast cancer. *Cancer Discov.* 5, 72–81. doi: 10.1158/2159-8290.CD-14-0697

Veber, D. F., Johnson, S. R., Cheng, H. Y., Smith, B. R., Ward, K. W., and Kopple, K. D. (2002). Molecular properties that influence the oral bioavailability of drug candidates. *J. Med. Chem.* 45, 2615–2623. doi: 10.1021/jm020017n

Wang, J., Wang, W., Kollman, P. A., and Case, D. A. (2006). Automatic atom type and bond type perception in molecular mechanical calculations. *J. Mol. Graph. Model.* 25, 247–260. doi: 10.1016/j.jmgm.2005.12.005

Wang, J., Wolf, R. M., Caldwell, J. W., Kollman, P. A., and Case, D. A. (2004). Development and testing of a general amber force field. *J. Comput. Chem.* 25, 1157–1174. doi: 10.1002/jcc.20035

Weir, H. M., Bradbury, R. H., Lawson, M., Rabow, A. A., Buttar, D., Callis, R. J., et al. (2016). AZD9496: an oral estrogen receptor inhibitor that blocks the growth of ER-positive and ESR1-mutant breast tumors in preclinical models. *Cancer Res.* 76, 3307–3318. doi: 10.1158/0008-5472.CAN-15-2357

Wickstrom, L., Okur, A., and Simmerling, C. (2009). Evaluating the performance of the ff99SB force field based on NMR scalar coupling data. *Biophys. J.* 97, 853–856. doi: 10.1016/j.bpj.2009.04.063

5

An Innovative Sequence-to-Structure-Based Approach to Drug Resistance Interpretation and Prediction: The Use of Molecular Interaction Fields to Detect HIV-1 Protease Binding-Site Dissimilarities

Nuno G. Alves [1†], *Ana I. Mata* [1†], *João P. Luís* [1†], *Rui M. M. Brito* [1,2] *and Carlos J. V. Simões* [1,2*]

[1] *Department of Chemistry, Coimbra Chemistry Centre, University of Coimbra, Coimbra, Portugal,* [2] *BSIM Therapeutics, Instituto Pedro Nunes, Coimbra, Portugal*

Correspondence:
Carlos J. V. Simões
carlos.simoes@bsimtx.com

† *These authors have contributed equally to this work*

In silico methodologies have opened new avenues of research to understanding and predicting drug resistance, a pressing health issue that keeps rising at alarming pace. Sequence-based interpretation systems are routinely applied in clinical context in an attempt to predict mutation-based drug resistance and thus aid the choice of the most adequate antibiotic and antiviral therapy. An important limitation of approaches based on genotypic data exclusively is that mutations are not considered in the context of the three-dimensional (3D) structure of the target. Structure-based *in silico* methodologies are inherently more suitable to interpreting and predicting the impact of mutations on target-drug interactions, at the cost of higher computational and time demands when compared with sequence-based approaches. Herein, we present a fast, computationally inexpensive, *sequence-to-structure*-based approach to drug resistance prediction, which makes use of 3D protein structures encoded by input target sequences to draw binding-site comparisons with susceptible templates. Rather than performing atom-by-atom comparisons between input target and template structures, our workflow generates and compares Molecular Interaction Fields (MIFs) that map the areas of energetically favorable interactions between several chemical probe types and the target binding site. Quantitative, pairwise dissimilarity measurements between the target and the template binding sites are thus produced. The method is particularly suited to understanding changes to the 3D structure and the physicochemical environment introduced by mutations into the target binding site. Furthermore, the workflow relies exclusively on freeware, making it accessible to anyone. Using four datasets of known HIV-1 protease sequences as a case-study, we show that our approach is capable of correctly classifying resistant and susceptible sequences given as input. Guided by ROC curve analyses, we fined-tuned a dissimilarity threshold of classification that results in remarkable discriminatory performance (accuracy $\approx$ ROC AUC $\approx$ 0.99), illustrating the high potential of *sequence-to-structure-*, MIF-based approaches in the context of drug resistance prediction. We discuss the complementarity of the proposed methodology to existing prediction algorithms based on genotypic data. The present work represents a new step toward a more comprehensive and structurally-informed interpretation of the impact of genetic variability on the response to HIV-1 therapies.

Keywords: drug resistance prediction, Molecular Interaction Fields, *sequence-to-structure* algorithm, binding-site dissimilarities, HIV-1 protease

INTRODUCTION

Drug resistance is one of the greatest threats of the twenty first century. Fundamentally, the problem resides in the development and spread of resistance-conferring mechanisms among infectious pathogens such as viruses and other microbial targets (McKeegan et al., 2002). Importantly, the selection of random mutations stands out as one of the main mechanisms of acquiring resistance, particularly relevant in viruses which mutate at high frequencies. RNA viruses, for instance, have a mutation rate estimated at 10^{-4} per nucleotide per replication, while DNA viruses have a rate of 10^{-8} per nucleotide per replication (Vere Hodge and Field, 2011; Mason et al., 2018). The extreme variability and rapid mutational spectrum of viral genomes, ongoing viral replication, and prolonged drug exposure linked with the selection and widespread of new drug-resistant strains is still a matter of great concern and importance, particularly in immunocompromised populations (Strasfeld and Chou, 2010; Mason et al., 2018). While a limited number of antiviral drug classes are getting approved for human use, an increasing resistance to some of the most effective available antivirals for HIV/AIDS, herpes, influenza and hepatitis, is being observed. Furthermore, the unpredictability of viral evolution and drug resistance means that antiviral treatments remain costly to the health care systems and are still associated with a significant risk of mortality, particularly in low- and middle-income countries (Irwin et al., 2016). Hence, *a priori* understanding and prediction of resistance against drug targets is of paramount importance toward developing more effective and longer lasting treatment options and regimens.

Antiviral drug resistance has been extensively studied in the rapidly mutating human immunodeficiency virus (HIV). HIV-1, in particular, is one of the most studied virus and the increasingly affordable and accessible genotypic data from clinical HIV-1 strains, together with corresponding data on strain susceptibility or resistance toward several drugs, have sparked the development of several genotypic interpretation systems for prediction of phenotypic drug resistance and therapy response based on genotype (Bonet, 2015). Said systems include (a) rule-based algorithms, including the *Agence Nationale de Recherche sur le Sida* (ANRS) (Brun-Vézinet et al., 2003), the Stanford HIV Drug Resistance Database interface (HIVdb) (Tang et al., 2012), Rega (Van Laethem et al., 2002), and HIV-GRADE (Obermeier et al., 2012a), which heavily rely on the periodic update of mutation-resistance profile lists, and on the knowledge of expert panels; and (b) machine learning-based algorithms trained on large sets of genotype–phenotype pairs to predict the *in vitro* resistance to a specific drug, with renowned examples such as *geno2pheno* (Beerenwinkel et al., 2003) and SHIVA (Riemenschneider et al., 2016). These sequence-based methods are relatively fast and low cost, justifying their routine use to support medical decision in HIV pharmacotherapy (Vercauteren and Vandamme, 2006).

The most relevant computational predictors of antiviral drug resistance currently available share the shortcoming of being purely based on genotypic sequence data. By disregarding the three-dimensional structural context and enzymatic function of the mutated amino acid residues, these systems fail to capture the links between genetic viral mutations and the corresponding mutation-induced structural changes to the effector protein viral machinery (Cao et al., 2005; Weber and Harrison, 2016; Khalid and Sezerman, 2018). This means that such methods are limited in their predictive power and interpretability toward novel mutations and combinations of mutations that go beyond the information accessible for training, such as mutation patterns that are encountered in only a small number of patients.

In contrast, structure-based methods hold potential to help understanding and eventually predicting resistance mechanisms for previously unknown data, shedding light on the elusive link between novel mutations and drug resistance. This may be justified by the fact that such methods can take advantage of available structural information on protein-ligand complexes and structural modeling of point mutations in the protein structure (Hao et al., 2012). Reported examples of the use of structure-based methods include the application of molecular docking to predict resistance or susceptibility of HIV1-PR to different inhibitors (Jenwitheesuk and Samudrala, 2005; Toor et al., 2011), the use of molecular dynamics simulations to study the impact of mutations on enzyme dynamics, stability and binding affinity (Hou and Yu, 2007; Agniswamy et al., 2016; Sheik Amamuddy et al., 2018), and the use of computational mutation scanning protocols to extract insights on free energy and binding affinity changes resulting from active site and non-active site mutations (Hao et al., 2010). Even though these methods are constantly adding new pieces to the puzzle and opening opportunities in the understanding of drug resistance, they suffer from various drawbacks, such as being time-consuming and offering limited predictive accuracy. As a result of such limitations, the primary challenge facing structure-based drug resistance prediction is to achieve an acceptable balance between prediction accuracy and computational efficiency to become both reliable and fast tools to be used in clinic context (Hao et al., 2012). In fact, some of the most recent reports describe the use of machine learning strategies merging both sequence and structural data in attempt to achieve such balance (Masso and Vaisman, 2013; Yu et al., 2014; Khalid and Sezerman, 2018).

In this contribution, we describe a fast, computationally inexpensive, *sequence-to-structure*-based approach to the prediction of drug resistance. The proposed workflow makes use of an archetypal GRID-based method (Goodford, 1985) involving the generation and comparison of Molecular Interaction Fields (MIFs). MIFs may be defined as the spatial variation of interaction energies between a molecular target structure and selected types of chemical probes laid out on a three-dimensional (3D) grid (Cruciani, 2005). The broad range of applications of MIFs extends from ligand-based methodologies, e.g., 3D Quantitative Structure-Activity Relationships (3D-QSAR) models, drug metabolism and pharmacokinetics (DMPK) predictions and pharmacophore elucidation, all the way to structure-based drug design, including binding site detection and molecular docking (Artese et al., 2013). Within the context of viral drug resistance, MIFs hold potential in capturing subtle, mutation-induced, chemical perturbations within the binding site of resistant or susceptible viral structures, thus representing a promising approach to anticipating the impact of mutations on the response to antiviral drugs with atomistic detail.

HIV-1 protease (HIV1-PR) is one of the most characterized viral enzymes, with extensive structural, inhibitor, and mutation data available (Weber and Agniswamy, 2009). As of late 2019, the RCSB Protein Data Bank (RCSB PDB, 2000) ranks HIV-1 as the virus holding the highest number of available structures (2,586), majorly obtained through X-ray crystallography. Of these, the PDB returns 662 entities with at least 90% identity to the HIV1-PR subtype B *consensus* sequence from a BLAST sequence search (Stanford University, 1998a). The search by *consensus* sequences of other HIV-1 subtype B enzymes (Stanford University, 1998a) returns 586 structures for reverse transcriptase and 190 for integrase. With such amount of structural information available, we have built the framework of the present work using HIV1-PR as our first case-study. Commercially available HIV-1 protease inhibitors (PIs) are competitive peptidomimetics with a core structural scaffold that mimics the tetrahedral transition state of HIV1-PR substrate. Although these drugs are chemically distinct, their active conformations are superimposable, and generally establish the same pharmacophoric interactions with their target (Wlodawer and Erickson, 1993; King et al., 2004; Qiu and Liu, 2011; Nayak et al., 2019). Many mutations in HIV1-PR translate into changes in the structure and binding site physicochemical environment, thus affecting the affinity of PIs and representing a hurdle to achieving long-term viral suppression (Irwin et al., 2016; Pawar et al., 2019; Wensing et al., 2019). A quantitative analysis of HIV1-PR drug-resistant mutation frequency, with particular focus on the binding site, was performed using public sequence datasets to support the potential of a MIF-based approach to capturing mutation-induced active site dissimilarities. From this perspective, the workflow proposed here encompasses the use of a conservative structural modeling step for the generation of a HIV1-PR structure from its respective amino acid sequence, and a MIF-based structural alignment and chemical dissimilarity detection step comparing the input *sequence-structure* pair with a carefully selected naïve, susceptible template *sequence-structure* pair. We demonstrate that the quantification of such dissimilarity, depicting the extent of structural, physicochemical and pharmacophoric alterations introduced by mutations, allows for an accurate prediction of HIV1-PR's resistance to PIs.

Compared with previous approaches reported in the literature, and to the best of our knowledge, this work stands out as a first implementation of a fast, *sequence-to-structure*-based algorithm capable of discriminating susceptible and resistant HIV1-PR sequences. Considering that the problem of mutation-induced resistance cuts across virtually all infectious diseases, we believe the approach reported herein may be extended to a wide range of microbial targets besides HIV-1, thus helping rationalize and personalize the therapeutic decision-making process.

MATERIALS AND METHODS

The availability of a public and curated database such as HIVDB (Stanford University, 1998c; Rhee et al., 2003) allows access to HIV1-PR sequences with known levels of resistance, and thus to establish datasets for the development of new methodologies to predict HIV1-PR resistance to protease inhibitors (PIs). This section describes the materials and methods employed in (1) the preparation of sequence datasets with various levels of resistance to PIs; (2) frequency analysis of *major* and *minor* mutations in the sequence datasets in (1); (3) the structural modeling of the reference structure used as template for subsequent modeling of HIV1-PR structures corresponding to each sequence in the datasets; (4) the core components of the proposed algorithm, including the calculation and comparison of pairwise Molecular Interaction Field points between the resulting structural models and the selected naïve template structure; and (5) the performance metrics used to test and evaluate the predictive power of the developed structure-based drug-resistance classification algorithm. A general workflow illustrating (4) and (5) is sketched (draw.io, 2005) in **Figure 1** and the complete script *HIV1predict.sh* for running the sequences is available at GitHub (Alves et al., 2019b). Calculations were run on a 64-bit CentOS 6 Linux server with an Intel Xeon CPU (E5620) at 2.40 GHz (further information as **Supplementary Table S1**).

Datasets of Resistant and Susceptible Sequences

A set of genotype-phenotype correlated HIV1-PR sequences was retrieved from HIVDB, version 8.7 (Stanford University, 1998b,c), and filtered by drug class for PIs. The considered PIs include darunavir, fosamprenavir, atazanavir, indinavir, lopinavir, nelfinavir, saquinavir, and tipranavir. Analyzing the subtype B HIV1-PR sequence of each isolate, i.e., a viral sample obtained from an infected individual, and considering positions with a mixture of amino acids, all possible mutation patterns were written to the FASTA format using a script written in-house (Alves et al., 2018f).

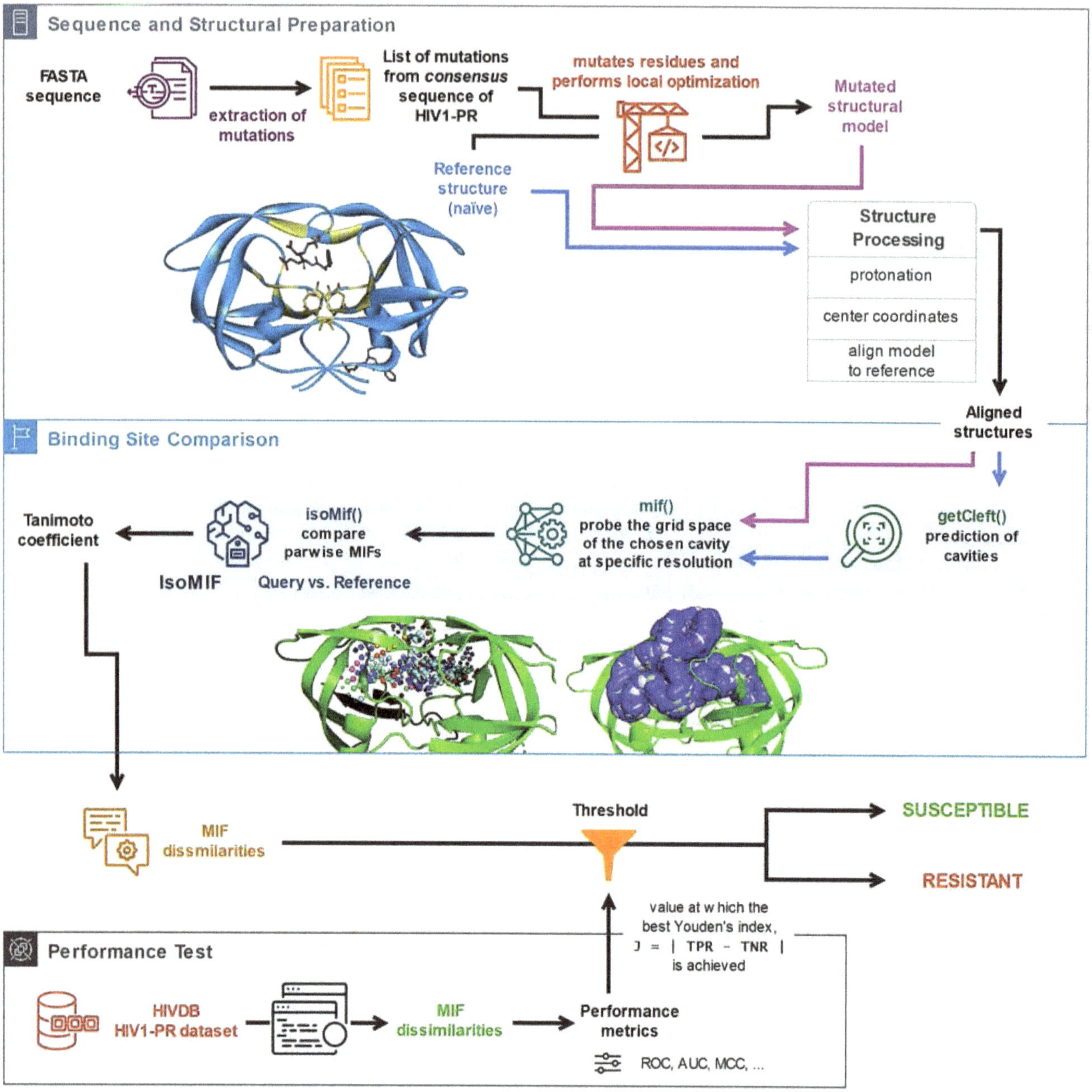

FIGURE 1 | General description of the workflow underlying the proposed *sequence-to-structure*-based drug resistance classifier, holding platform applications to multiple microbial targets. The depicted algorithm starts off with the sequential reading of an amino acid sequence in FASTA format, followed by identification of the present mutations by comparison with the consensus sequence, insertion of the identified mutations in the naïve template, and processing of the structural models for alignment and comparison. Upon structural alignment of the target or database (predicted) structure with the naïve template structure, six types of MIF probe points are computed for the former structure and superimposed with pre-calculated MIF probe points of the latter structure. Calculation of MIF dissimilarities by means of a Tanimoto coefficient proceeds. The bottom panel represents the process of performance evaluation of the proposed classifier based on its application to a large dataset of *sequence-structure* pairs generated for HIV1-PR sequences retrieved from HIVDB. Included are performance metrics such as accuracy, Matthews Correlation Coefficient (MCC), and the area under the receiver-operating-characteristic curve (ROC AUC).

The genotype-phenotype correlation results from the *in vitro* PhenoSense assay (Zhang et al., 2005), which measures the levels of resistance to a PI compared to the wild-type sequence. Following the categorization of susceptibility to PIs described by Rhee et al. (2006), the collected sequences were classified as follows:

- *Susceptible.* Sequences holding <3.0-fold resistance to all PIs in the dataset were considered susceptible (N = 7,768) [Susceptible].
- *Resistant.* Sequences holding more than 20.0-, or 15.0-, or 10.0-fold resistance to all PIs, resulting in three resistant subgroups of increasing degree of resistance: respectively, [Res_{20}] (N =

60) [Res20], [Res_{15}] ($N = 83$) [Res15], which encompasses [Res_{20}] plus 23 sequences holding between 15- and 20-fold resistance, and [Res_{15}] ($N = 873$) [Res10], which encompasses [Res_{20}] and [Res_{15}] plus 790 additional sequences holding between 15- and 10-fold resistance.

Counting of Mutations in HIV1-PR

The quantification of *major* and *minor* mutations (Weber and Agniswamy, 2009) in all datasets was carried out using scripts written in-house (Alves et al., 2018a,b, 2019a) that sequentially read the listing of mutations for each sequence, extract either the *major* or *minor* mutations, and count them for each sequence. Said script was applied to quantify *major* and *minor* mutations in the HIV1-PR binding site.

Preparation of HIV1-PR Structures

Using PDB's BLAST utility (Altschul et al., 1990) to guide the choice of a template for homology modeling, a sequence search, with a 10.0 E-value cut-off and at least 50% identity to the HIV1-PR subtype B *consensus* (Stanford University, 1998a), resulted in 784 entities available. With a more refined query of at least 95% identity to the HIV1-PR subtype B *consensus*, there were still 376 structures available to work with.

Out of these 376 structures, PDB entry 1NH0 for HIV1-PR was chosen as template structure for homology modeling by using PDB's BLAST utility (Altschul et al., 1990). It returned an E-value of 7.20281E-51, but since the intended work was heavily based on structure, our choice was also based on having the best resolution possible. The structure of 1NH0 holds 99% sequence identity (98/99) with the *consensus* B amino acid sequence of protease, HXB2 (henceforth referred to as *consensus sequence*), with one single mutation at position 37 (S37N), has 100% coverage of the sequence, and has been determined at 1.03 Å X-ray resolution. Importantly, this HIV1-PR sequence is known to be susceptible to all PIs.

In this work, Modeler version 9.19 (Šali and Blundell, 1993; Šali, 2019a) was used for predictive modeling of all HIV1-PR structures from their respective sequences. The listing of mutations present in each sequence was automated by scripting (Alves et al., 2018c) and followed by sequentially running the *mutate_model.py* script provided with Modeler (Šali, 2019b) to obtain the correct pattern of mutations and outputting the respective structural model. The procedure implemented in *mutate_model.py* performs local optimization of the mutated residues region and ensures that the obtained structural models are comparable to the template structure. The PDB structure itself (1NH0) was subjected to *mutate_model.py* in order to reverse the mutation present in the template with 99% identity (Asn37, on the outside of the protease) and keep on the *consensus sequence*, remove *HETATM* entries and *alt-locs*—thus yielding the reference template structure. This reference structure was used as template for the generation of the respective structural model of each input FASTA sequence present in the datasets.

All generated structural models were protonated using *Reduce*, version 3.23 (Word et al., 1999). The reference structure was centered to the origin of the axes of the cartesian coordinate system using *VMD*, version 1.9.3 (Humphrey et al., 1996). Structural alignment of all query models onto the centered reference structure was performed with *LovoAlign*, version 16.342 (Martínez et al., 2007).

Workflow for Detection and Scoring of Molecular Interaction Field Dissimilarities

The MIF module of the software package IsoMIF, version dated March 2015 (Chartier and Najmanovich, 2015), was used to generate Molecular Interaction Fields (MIFs) within the HIV1-PR binding sites. MIF-based alignment and calculation of pairwise MIF dissimilarities between reference and dataset binding sites proceeded using the IsoMIF module of the same package. The IsoMIF setup comprises three sequential modules: GetCleft, MIF, and IsoMIF.

Cavity Detection (GetCleft Module)

GetCleft (Gaudreault et al., 2015) was employed to predict cavities in the structure of the reference HIV1-PR (Alves et al., 2018e). This geometry-based method detects cavities by insertion of spheres of radius r between the non-hydrogen protein atoms, reducing such radius if they intersect with any neighboring atoms (clefts defined by the union of overlapping spheres). First, the top five largest cavities were searched at the same time, with a minimum and maximum sphere radius of 1.5 and 4.0 Å, respectively. The largest predicted cavity was visually confirmed to be completely enclosed within the HIV1-PR binding site, using *VMD*, version 1.9.3 (Humphrey et al., 1996). Next, such cavity volume represented by spheres was used to define the location of MIF interaction vectors to be calculated for the reference and all 3D HIV1-PR structural models.

Generation of Molecular Interaction Field (MIF) Probe Points (MIF Module)

The MIF module of IsoMIF was used to compute molecular interaction fields (MIFs) for six different chemical probe types (**Figure 2**): hydrophobic, aromatic, H-bond donor, H-bond acceptor, positive charge and negative charge. The pharmacophoric features shared by PIs (Wlodawer and Erickson, 1993; Nayak et al., 2019) highlight the importance of a conserved physicochemical environment in the binding site. Alterations of this environment are detected with the MIF probes (circled in **Figures 2A,B**) which allow for a quantification of changes caused by the presence of mutations. In this work, a grid resolution of 1.5 Å was defined to calculate the MIFs on the cleft covering the volume of the binding site. Such resolution was selected upon testing to achieve an adequate balance between speed and accuracy of IsoMIF pairwise field dissimilarity calculations.

Alignment of MIF Probe Points and Calculation of Dissimilarities (IsoMIF Module)

Field similarities were computed using the IsoMIF module, which employs a clique-based graph matching approach based on the Bron-Kerbosch algorithm (Bron and Kerbosch, 1973) to perform functional alignments between the probe points under comparison. A grid spacing of 1.5 Å, a geometric distance threshold of 1.0 Å and a maximum of 100 cliques were used as parameters for the calculation of similarities between the

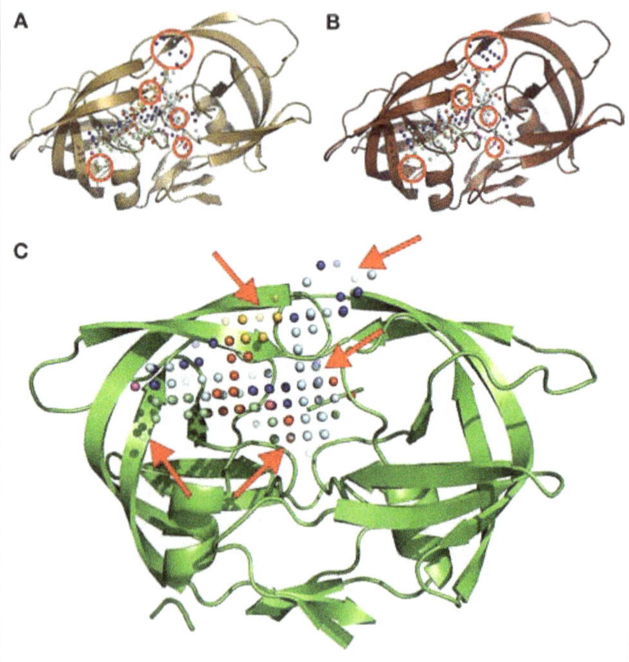

FIGURE 2 | A three-dimensional ribbon depiction of the quaternary structure HIV1-PR dimeric unit, including the six different types of MIF probe points calculated on the enzyme's binding site. (A) Structure and probe points of the reference naïve template. (B) Illustration of the structure and probe points of a mutated model resulting from a sequence holding over 20-fold resistance for PIs. (C) An exemplary output of IsoMIF, highlighting a MIF-based alignment and comparison of both structures: (A,B). The red circles in (A,B) denote areas where the difference in probe points is most visible. The arrows in (C) point to semi-transparent probes, representing the probes which are not shared between the two structures. Legend for the six (6) probe types legend: hydrophobic in light blue, aromatic in orange, H-bond donor in dark blue and acceptor in red, positive in green and negative charge in purple.

binding site of reference and structural models of HIV1-PR. Such similarities were then quantified by the Tanimoto coefficient (T_c), calculated as in Equation 1:

$$T_c = \frac{N_C}{N_R+N_Q-N_C} \quad (1)$$

where N_c is the number of common probe points to the two MIF maps under comparison; N_r and N_q represent the number of probe points present in the reference and query structure, respectively (**Figure 2C**) (Chartier and Najmanovich, 2015). The measurement of dissimilarity (Equation 2) between binding sites is justified by the fact that the focus of this work is set on the discrimination of resistant structures, when compared with a susceptible reference. Therefore, the chosen metric was dissimilarity rather than similarity:

$$\textit{dissimilarity coefficient} = 1.0 - T_c \quad (2)$$

Analysis of Mutation Patterns Across Thousands of HIV1-PR Sequences

Analyses of the number and position of mutations were performed on HIV1-PR sequences in order to obtain information supporting and justifying the development of a *sequence-to-structure-*, MIF-based approach to antiviral resistance classification and prediction.

R version 3.4.3 (R Core Team, 2018) was used to conduct the analysis and generating the associated graphical representations. The R packages used in this work were ggplot2 (Wickham, 2009), *gplots* (Warnes et al., 2019), and ROCit (Khan and Brandenburger, 2019).

"Outlier" Detection on Binding-Site MIF Dissimilarities

Tukey's method (Tukey, 1949; Hoaglin, 2003), also referred to as Tukey's fences method, was used to detect outliers in the binding-site MIF dissimilarities results. Tukey's method is a statistical approach used to determine whether a value should be considered an outlier or not: the method relies on the interquartile range (IQR) measurement, which is calculated by the difference between the first quartile (Q1) and the third quartile (Q3) (see Equation 3). Q1 stands for the value in the dataset that holds 25% of the values below it and Q3 is the value in the dataset that holds 25% of the values above it.

$$IQR = Q3 - Q1 \quad (3)$$

According to Tukey's method, a value is considered an outlier if it is observed in the range described in Equation 4:

$$\begin{gathered} outlier < Q1 - k \times IQR \vee outlier > Q3 + k \times IQR \\ outlier < LowerBound \vee outlier > UpperBound \end{gathered} \quad (4)$$

where $k = 1.5$ indicates an outlier and $k = 3$ indicates an extreme outlier. For the purpose of the present work, only extreme outliers were discarded.

Evaluation of the Algorithm's Predictive Performance

The performance of our method at discriminating resistant from susceptible models was assessed by calculation of several metrics typically employed in the fields of predictive modeling and machine learning, particularly in cases where binary classification occurs. These included the Receiver Operating Characteristic (ROC) and the respective Area Under the Curve (ROC AUC). The ROC curve is a graphical representation of the True Positive Rate (TPR) as a function of the True Negative Rate (TNR), i.e., at various cut-off settings. The TPR is also known as Sensitivity (Equation 5), which measures the proportion of positive cases. On the other hand, the TNR is also calculated as 1—Specificity (Equation 6) and measures the proportion of true negative cases.

$$Sensitivity = \frac{TP}{TP+FN} \quad (5)$$

$$Specificity = \frac{TN}{TN+FP} \quad (6)$$

where *TP* represents the number of correctly identified resistant structures (true positives), *TN*, the number of correctly identified susceptible structures (true negatives), *FP*, the number of susceptible incorrectly predicted as resistant (false positives), and

FN the number of resistant incorrectly predicted as susceptible (false negatives).

Additional performance metrics included Accuracy (Equation 7) and Matthews Correlation Coefficient (MCC; see Equation 8) (Matthews, 1975; Florkowski, 2008; Powers, 2011).

$$Accuracy = \frac{TP+TN}{TP+FP+TN+FN} \quad (7)$$

$$MCC = \frac{TP \times TN - FP \times FN}{\sqrt{(TP+FP)(TP+FN)(TN+FP)(TN+FN)}} \quad (8)$$

The dissimilarity threshold used for classification in resistant or susceptible *sequence-structure* pairs was derived from ROC curves, corresponding to the highest Youden's index (Youden, 1950), J, calculated as in Equation 9:

$$J = Sensitivity + Specificity - 1 \quad (9)$$

This index defines the maximum potential effectiveness of a classifier. It can be determined for all points of an ROC curve, although its maximum value represents the classifier optimal differentiating ability cut-point when equal weight is given to Sensitivity and Specificity (Ruopp et al., 2008).

RESULTS AND DISCUSSION

In this work, we describe a *sequence-to-structure*-, MIF-based method to assess binding-site dissimilarities across *sequence-structure* pairs, with the aim of predicting antiviral resistance—and using HIV1-PR as a case-study. It is generally accepted that the majority of resistance-conferring mutations occur in the binding site regions of viral enzymes (Weber and Agniswamy, 2009; Weber and Harrison, 2016). In order to further support the *rationale* and underlying assumptions of the proposed approach, we performed analysis of *major* and *minor* mutations of HIV1-PR binding site residues focusing on sequences known to be fully resistant and fully susceptible. For the sake of comparison, the quantification of mutations was also extended to *major* and *minor* mutations occurring in the remainder residues, i.e., residues not comprising the binding site region of HIV1-PR.

Counting of PI-Resistant Mutations in HIV1-PR Sequences

Resistance to PIs develops upon accumulation of mutations that increasingly impact the structure of HIV1-PR, resulting in highly-resistant variants of HIV-1. As mentioned by Weber and Agniswamy (2009), PI resistance is linked to the occurrence of primary (*major*) mutations, commonly associated with the active site where HIV PIs typically bind, resulting from structural changes that disrupt the van der Waals contacts and/or hydrogen bonding patterns in the inhibitor-protein interaction and promote direct steric hindrance, by altering the pocket volume or its physicochemical environment. Secondary (*minor*) mutations occur in addition to *major* mutations, acting like accessory mutations that compensate the flaws produced by *major* mutations and enhancing the resistance level (synergistic effect). Being less obvious, they seem to affect HIV1-PR catalysis, dimer stability, inhibitor binding kinetics, and/or active site re-shaping through long-range structural perturbations (Weber and Agniswamy, 2009; Weber and Harrison, 2016).

Our workflow follows a *sequence-to-structure* approach in attempt to capture changes to the structural and physicochemical determinants of HIV1-PR's binding site upon mutation, based on the assumption that these changes represent the main driver of antiviral resistance. To support this assumption, quantification of mutations known to contribute to PI resistance was carried out across the retrieved datasets. The version 8.7 HIVDB (Stanford University, 1998b,c,d) listed the following PI-resistant mutations for HIV1-PR:

- *Major* mutations: D30N, V32I, L33F, M46IL, I47VA, G48VM, I50VL, I54VTALM, L76V, V82AFTSL, I84V, N88SD, and L90M;
- *Minor* mutations: L10FIVRY, V11IL, K20RIMTV, L23I, L24IFM, M36I, K43T, M46V, G48ASTQL, F53LY, I54ST, Q58E, A71VTIL, G73STCADV, T74PS, V82MC, N83DS, I84AC, I85V, N88TG, and L89VT.

Even though not all sequences exhibit the same degree of resistance to each PI, we selected these two groups of *major* and *minor* PI-resistant mutations and quantitatively characterized their presence in our subsets. Since all HIV1-PR sequences in our dataset were retrieved from the same unique source, HIVDB (Stanford University, 1998c; Rhee et al., 2003), the percentage of sequences holding PI-resistant mutations distributed across the entire HIV1-PR sequence, as well as the percentage of PI-resistant mutations manifesting in residues comprising the binding site of HIV1-PR, were determined and compared among all four subsets: [Susceptible], [Res_{10}], [Res_{20}], and [Resistant*]–as represented in **Figure 3**.

Figures 3A,B shows that, as expected, all HIV1-PR sequences belonging to the *Susceptible* subset hold much less PIs-resistant mutations than those belonging to the *Resistant* subsets. The majority (98.24%) of susceptible HIV1-PR sequences does not hold any *major* mutations, while 1.74% contain one *major* mutation, and only one sequence (0.01%) comprises three *major* mutations. The presence of *major* mutations across drug-resistant sequences is higher, ranging from three to seven *major* mutations, implying that among these subsets the *major* mutations appear in the shape of mutation patterns rather than individual mutations. The presence of *minor* mutations (**Figure 3B**) follows a similar trend to that witnessed for *major* mutations, with susceptible sequences denoting a lower number when compared to their resistant counterparts. Approximately 98.25% of the susceptible sequences present two or less *minor* mutations, with about half of susceptible HIV1-PR sequences (53.3 %) displaying no *minor* mutations.

When comparing susceptible vs. drug-resistant sequences, it can be observed that resistance against PIs is linked to the presence of *major* mutations, as implied above (Weber and Harrison, 2016). However, within the subsets of drug-resistant sequences, a direct relation between the number of *major* mutations and the increase of resistance is not observed. Drug-resistant sequences show a higher frequency of *minor*

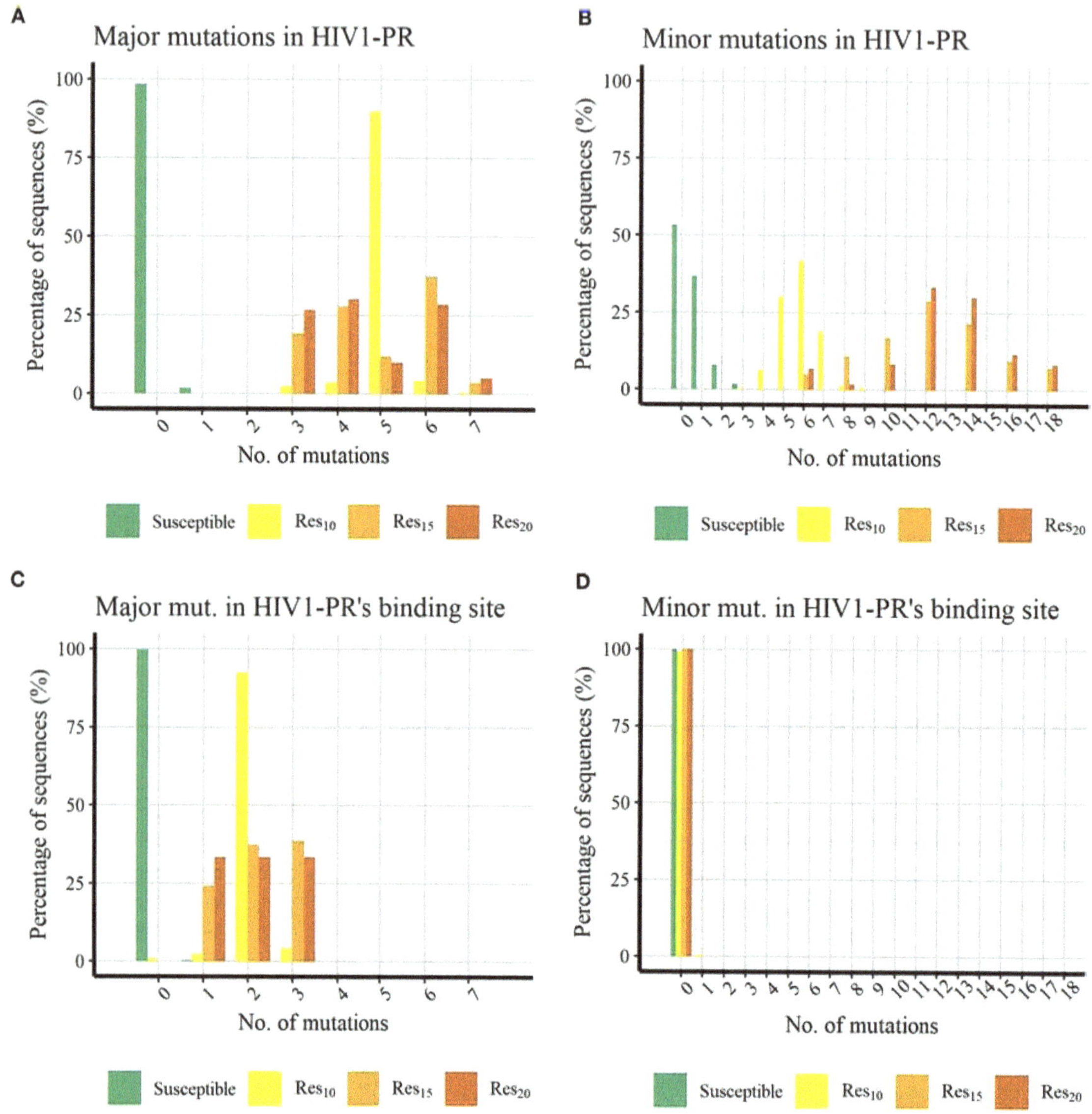

FIGURE 3 | Histograms representing the percentage of PI-resistant mutations in the datasets showing increasing number of PI-resistant mutations in the datasets retrieved from HIVDB. (A) Percentage of major mutations in the whole HIV1-PR. (B) Percentage of minor mutations in the whole HIV1-PR. (C) Percentage of major mutations in the HIV1-PR binding site. (D) Percentage of minor mutations in the HIV1-PR binding site. Represented datasets: [Susceptible] (green); [Res_{10}] (yellow); [Res_{15}] (orange); [Res_{20}] (dark orange).

mutations, ranging from three to 18, with a visual apparent difference between sequences with lower resistance ([Res_{10}]) and the more resistant sequences ([Res_{15}] and [Res_{20}]). In [Res_{10}], 98.2% of the sequences have up to seven *minor* mutations, while 78.3% in [Res_{15}] and 93.3% [Res_{20}] have more than eight *minor* mutations. This trend in the profile of mutation distribution among the resistant sequences is in line with *minor* mutations acting as accessory mutations, appearing as patterns and not as individual mutations, and showing a similar trait as the one observed for the distribution of *major* mutations.

Analysis of *major* mutations located in HIV1-PR's binding site residues (**Figure 3C**), corresponding to sequence positions 30, 32, 47, 48, 50, 82, and 84, shows that 99.78% of the susceptible sequences do not display *major* mutations, while the remainder show only one *major* mutation. In contrast, less than 1% of resistant sequences lack *major* mutations in the drug binding site. Interestingly, the eight sequences representing this small fraction (0.91%) belong to the lower (10-fold) resistance subset ([Res_{10}]). All remaining drug-resistant sequences hold from one to three *major* mutations in the enzyme's binding site.

Counting of mutations in binding site residues of HIV1-PR exposes a systematic presence of *major* mutations in resistant HIV1-PR sequences, while also highlighting the absence of such mutations on 99.78% of their susceptible counterparts. This contrasting trait observed between the binding site region of susceptible and resistant HIV1-PR supports the development of a structure-based drug-resistance classifier focusing on the detection and quantification of binding site dissimilarities.

Regarding the distribution of *minor* mutations across binding site residues, as represented in **Figure 3D**, mutations localized in sequence positions 23, 48, 82, and 84 were quantified among both HIV1-PR susceptible and drug-resistant sequences, revealing that the great majority does not present *minor* mutations in their respective binding sites. Only a small percentage of susceptible (0.01%) and resistant sequences (0.91%) show *minor* mutations in this region. It should be noted that the small subset of resistant sequences holding a *minor* mutation in their binding site region correspond to sequences that do not display *major* mutations in the active site.

These results show that the binding site *minor* mutations are uncommon on the datasets of HIV1-PR sequences—be they resistant or susceptible. Although such mutations appear to be important to increase the enzyme resistance's by stabilizing the mutated protein structure, they seem to produce limited direct effect on the enzyme's binding site, where they are mostly absent. Thus, these results seem to be in agreement with our motivation to explore a quantitative detection of binding-site dissimilarities to predict HIV1-PR resistance to PIs, as the *major* mutations play the main role on altering the binding site conformation, volume and/or physicochemical environment.

The quantification of mutations in the datasets retrieved from HIVDB yielded distinct results between the susceptible and drug-resistant sequences. Most of the resistant sequences show a higher frequency of *major* mutations when compared to the susceptible set. All resistant sequences present at least one mutation in the binding site region, contrasting with 98% of susceptible sequences that do not present any *major* mutations in that site. It is worth noticing that half of the *major* mutations are found in the binding site of resistant sequences. However, when considering the total number of mutations, the increase in the number of mutations per sequence seems to hold a reflection on the increase in the resistance of the observed sequence. Furthermore, binding site *major* mutations are more likely to cause changes on the HIV1-PR binding cleft physicochemical environment when compared with susceptible enzymes which do not have such type of mutations.

A Fast, *Sequence-to-Structure-*, MIF-Based Antiviral Drug Resistance Classifier

The quantification of resistance-conferring mutations in HIV1-PR sequences, using the datasets retrieved from HIVDB, prompted us to further develop a discriminative resistance-classifier approach focused on analysis and comparison of binding-site MIFs. In practice, the proposed workflow involves performing structural modeling of input HIV1-PR sequences using the same template (i.e., 1NH0) and a script (Alves et al., 2018d) that calls *mutate_model.py* (Šali, 2019b) to conduct local energy minimization around the mutated residues of the HIV1-PR structure. Once the generation of structure models is concluded, the modules belonging to the IsoMIF package are deployed for cavity detection (GetCleft module), calculation of MIFs within the selected cavity volume (MIF module), field alignment and quantification of dissimilarities between MIF points computed for the dataset HIV1-PR structural models and those computed for a high quality [Susceptible] reference HIV1-PR structure (1NH0) and, finally, scoring by means of a Tanimoto coefficient (IsoMIF module). The average running time of the workflow is $\approx$ 77 s per sequence (**Supplementary Figure S1** and **Supplementary Datasheet S1**), considering that this value varies with the amount of mutations present in the HIV1-PR.

TABLE 1 | Tukey's method results to determine outliers.

	Susceptible	*Res₁₀*	*Res₁₅*	*Res₂₀*
Q1	0.0057	0.1075	0.1173	0.0649
Q3	0.0225	0.2041	0.2041	0.2171
IQR	0.0168	0.0966	0.0868	0.1522
Lower Bound	−0.0447*	−0.1823*	−0.1431*	−0.3917*
Upper Bound	0.0729	0.4939	0.4645	0.6737

*Quartile 1 (Q1), Quartile 3 (Q3), Inter Quartile Range (IQR), Upper Bound and Lower Bound values for susceptible sequences dissimilarity coefficient distribution. Upper and Lower Bound were calculated as described in Equation 4, with k = 3. Values above the upper bound and below the lower bound were considered outliers. *Negative values are not realistic lower bounds; the minimum value must be 0.*

Analysis of MIF Dissimilarities in HIV1-PR Binding Site

Figure 4 discloses the frequency of HIV1-PR *sequence-structure* pairs scattered across a spectrum of Tanimoto coefficient (Tc) values (varying from 0.00 to 1.00), in turn reflecting binding-site MIF dissimilarities in the subset of susceptible sequences (containing 7,768 *sequence-structure* pairs) against the selected naïve, template structure. Analyzing this profile of binding site dissimilarities, we observe that there are substantially more susceptible sequences concentrated on lower end of the dissimilarity spectrum. However, a small number of sequences ($N = 81$) present higher values, more visibly around the Tc value of 0.35. Since susceptible HIV1-PR *sequence-structure* pairs display a lower frequency of mutations in the binding site residues, we assume that Tc values deviating from the normal trend may highlight inconsistent data, errors and/or any form of outliers worthy of further investigation.

In order to verify if the higher Tc values could reflect true outliers, Tukey's outlier detection method was used (Tukey, 1949; Hoaglin, 2003). **Table 1** shows the result of applying the statistical Tukey method to the MIF dissimilarity Tc values obtained for the dataset of susceptible *sequence-structure* pairs, and to the [Res_{10}], [Res_{15}], and [Res_{20}] subsets. For each of the four groups, **Figure 5** shows boxplots summarizing the distribution of the MIF dissimilarity Tc values. On the susceptible subset, the higher Tc values were identified as significantly different from the central tendency (values were below the determined lower bound; see Equation 4 in Methods). Looking at the dataset of resistant *sequence-structure* pairs, *extreme* outliers (as described in the Methods section) were only found in the [Res_{10}] subset. These outliers were found to be associated with a software limitation wherein the same reference grid

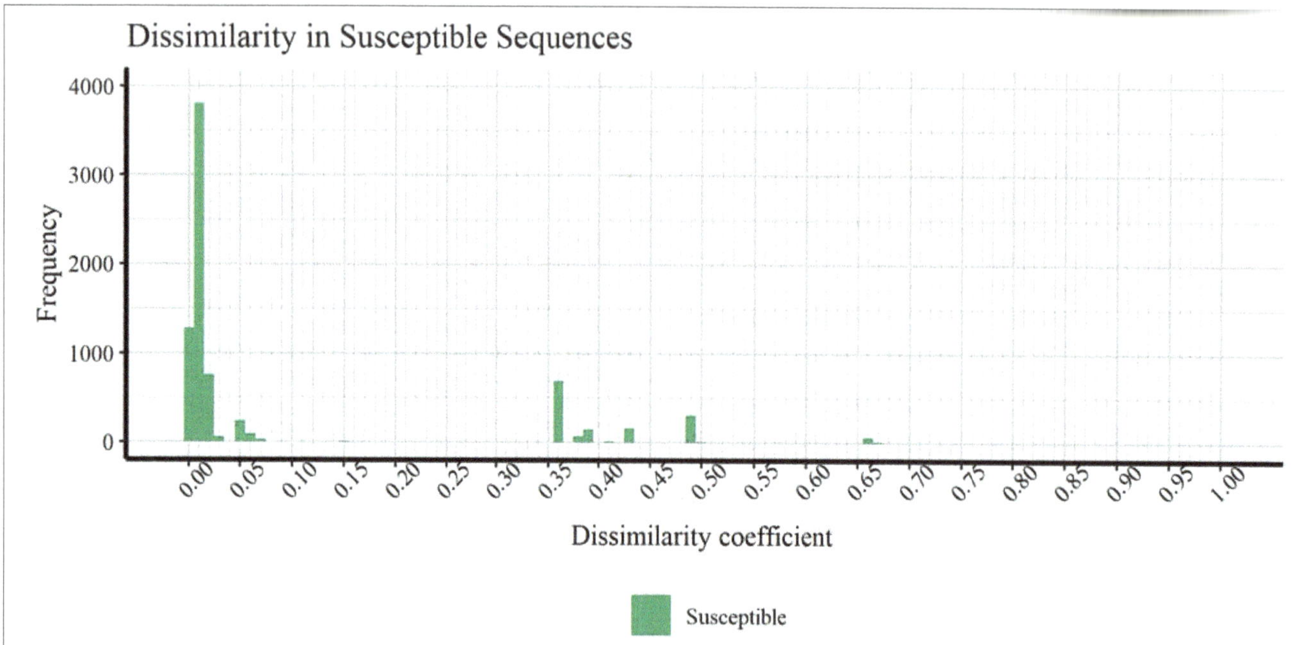

FIGURE 4 | Frequency of susceptible sequences distributed across a range of HIV1-PR binding site 3D dissimilarity coefficients. The maximum value reported is ~0.667.

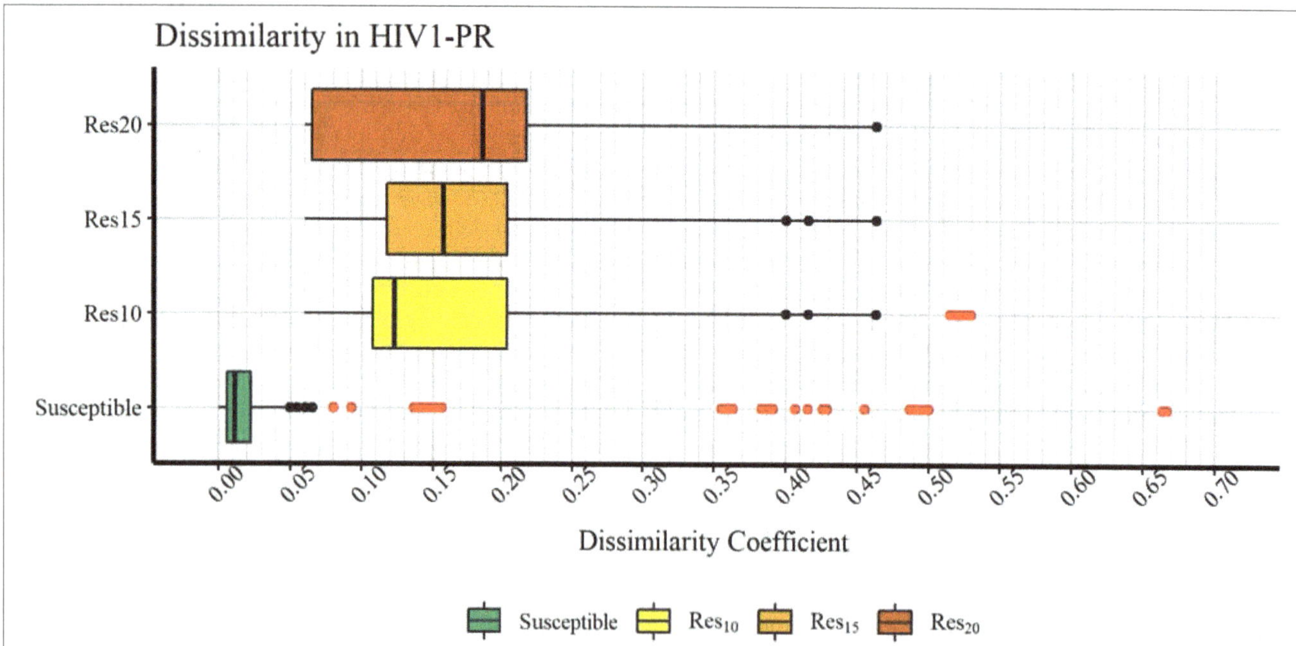

FIGURE 5 | Boxplot representation of dissimilarity coefficients obtained for the HIVDB datasets. The maximum value reported is ~0.667. Outliers are marked in red. Represented datasets: [Susceptible] (green); [Res_{10}] (yellow); [Res_{15}] (orange); [Res_{20}] (dark orange).

(generated by GetCleft), covering the entire binding site volume, was not homogeneous across all HIV1-PR structure models. In fact, a wider grid was calculated for some structures when compared to the reference HIV1-PR structure, which resulted on a different number of grid points, consequently leading to an increase of dissimilarities. Thus, these *sequence-structure* pairs were not considered relevant for performance evaluations, as they could introduce performance bias. The Tukey's boxplot analysis thus allowed the identification and removal of *extreme* outliers in the [Susceptible] and [Res_{10}] subsets, resulting in 6269 and 680 HIV1-PR structural models, respectively. The [Res_{15}] and [Res_{20}] subsets remained unchanged with 83 and 60

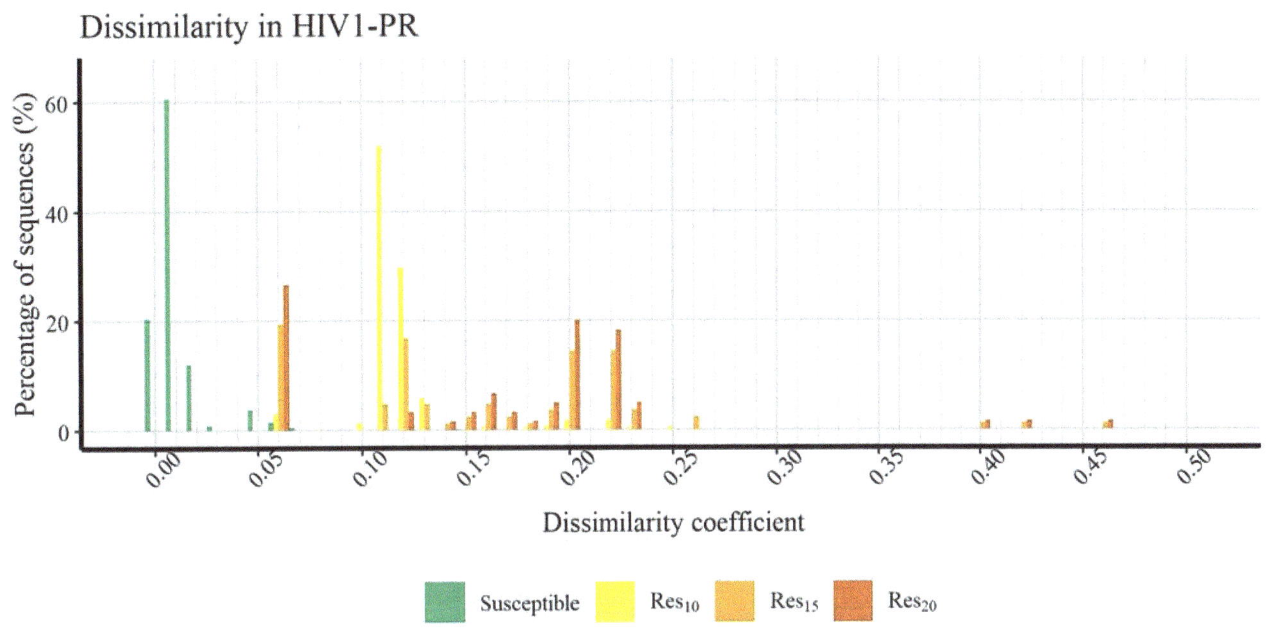

FIGURE 6 | Percentage of sequences distributed across a range of HIV1-PR binding site 3D dissimilarity coefficients. Maximum value reported is ~0.463. Represented datasets: [Susceptible] (green); [Res_{10}] (yellow); [Res_{15}] (orange); [Res_{20}] (dark orange).

HIV1-PR structural models, respectively. The resulting dataset has been used for further statistical analysis and as *test set* for performance calculations.

Figure 6 shows a profile of the HIV1-PR binding-site MIF dissimilarities across the susceptible dataset withdrawn of extreme outliers ([Susceptible*]) and the stratified resistant data set (encompassing [Res_{10}], [Res_{15}], and [Res_{20}]) also withdrawn of extreme outliers ([Susceptible*]). As seen, susceptible HIV1-PR structures tend to present very low to null binding-site MIF dissimilarities compared to the ([Susceptible]) structure modeled from the *consensus* sequence. In fact, 93.91% of the *sequence-structure* pairs in the susceptible group show dissimilarities lower than 0.02, indicating a considerable degree of conservation within the binding site. Overall, these results show a segregation between susceptible and resistant *sequence-structure* pairs, when analyzing their binding-site MIF dissimilarities against a susceptible reference sequence-structure pair, suggesting that our method is able to quantitatively capture differences among susceptible and resistant HIV1-PR structures.

Evaluation of the Classification Performance of Our Drug Resistance Classifier

At the current stage of development, the proposed workflow only performs binary classification, meaning that each input sequence gets classified as either susceptible or resistant. Sequence data are used exclusively for the generation of the structural models on which dissimilarities are analyzed, but not to aid the classification itself. It is worth highlighting that our workflow relies on the detection of structural and chemical changes in viral enzymes that dictate susceptibility or resistance to drugs—rather than on the training of predictive models using sequences with known phenotypic response to drugs. Therefore, instead of using performance evaluation methods, such as cross-validation, that assess the impact of hiding a portion of training data (observations) on the accuracy of the resulting predictions, we resorted to the calculation of metrics of overall performance of our binary classifier.

The Receiver Operating Characteristic (ROC) curve was used to assess the overall discriminatory performance of our method. The score assigned to each dataset entry (here used for testing), corresponding to binding-site dissimilarities between each input *sequence-structure* pair and the template *consensus sequence*-structure, were thus plotted as a ROC curve. ROC curves are conceptually simple plots that depicts a binary classifier's discriminative capability as its discrimination threshold is varied. Such graphical plots are created by plotting the method's true positive rate (sensitivity) against its false positive rate (1-specificity), at varying thresholds. The area under the ROC curve (ROC AUC) value is a single scalar value varying between 0 and 1, providing a measure of the overall discriminatory power of the method. A ROC AUC value of 1 (or 100%) entails a *perfect* discrimination, a value of 0.5 represents random classification, while values above 0.8 are commonly accepted as indicators of an acceptable discriminatory performance (Fawcett, 2006; Pines and Everett, 2008; Powers, 2011; Tape). Furthermore, several performance measures, such as the Sensitivity (Equation 5), Specificity (Equation 6), Accuracy (Equation 7), and MCC (Equation 8) were also determined.

Figure 7 represents the obtained ROC curves and their respective ROC AUC values for the susceptible and resistant HIV1-PR binding-site MIF dissimilarities. ROC AUC values for [Res_{10}], [Res_{15}], and [Res_{20}] subsets were

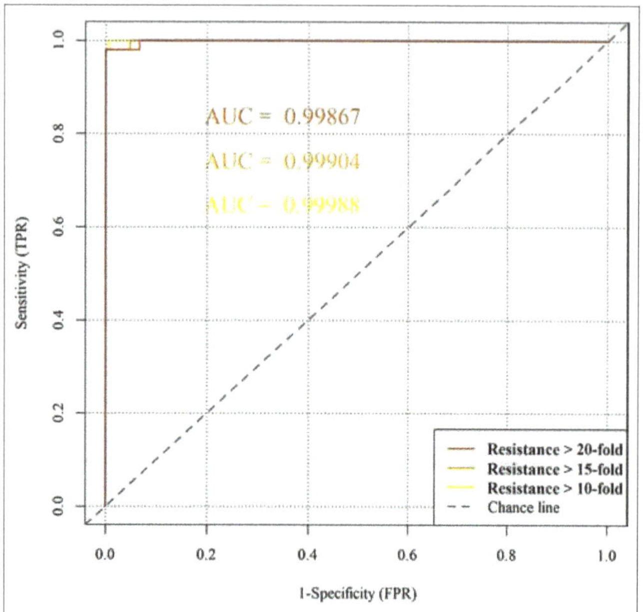

FIGURE 7 | Predictive performance of the binary classification (resistant vs. susceptible) produced by the algorithm/workflow presented herein, quantified by means of Receiver Operating Characteristic (ROC) curves and their respective Area Under the Curve (ROC AUC). The colors represent the ROC curves as follows: yellow for HIV1-PR sequences associated with 10-fold resistance; orange for HIV1-PR sequences associated with 15-fold resistance; and dark orange for HIV1-PR sequences associated with 20-fold resistance.

found to be similarly very high-—0.9999, 0.9990, and 0.9987, respectively – suggesting that the method holds significant discriminatory power to distinguishing susceptible from fully resistant HIV1-PR *sequence-structure* pairs—based on their binding-site MIF dissimilarities to the [Susceptible] reference *sequence-structure* pair.

We have also used ROC curve analysis to guide the definition of an *optimal* discrimination threshold based on Youden's index (Equation 9) (Youden, 1950). The optimal threshold observed corresponded to a 0.06 dissimilarity Tc for all [Res_{10}], [Res_{15}], and [Res_{20}] subsets. **Table 2** presents the values of each performance metric obtained for each subset, when applying a classification threshold of 0.06. At this classification cut-off, the specificities and sensitivities were found to be 0.997 and 0.994 for the [Res_{10}] subset, 0.997 and 0.952 for the [Res_{15}] subset and 0.997 and 0.933 for the [Res_{20}] subset, respectively. In all cases, there is strong discriminative performance toward susceptibility or resistance—as it can be appreciated by the high accuracy values highlighted in **Table 2**. Nevertheless, the best results are found for the [Res_{10}] subset, with an accuracy of about 0.997. On the other hand, the subsets with increasing degree of resistance, [Res_{15}] and [Res_{20}], show only slightly worst results concerning Sensitivity determined at a threshold of 0.06.

The overall predictive performance of our method was also evaluated by the Matthews correlation coefficient (MCC) on the three resistant subsets, which summarizes the sensitivity and the specificity of a classification method within a unique value, also varying between 0 and 1. A higher value of MCC indicates that

TABLE 2 | Performance metrics obtained using a dissimilarity threshold of 0.0603.

Dissimilarity Threshold = 0.0603	Res_{10}	Res_{15}	Res_{20}
ROC AUC	0.99988	0.99904	0.99867
Sensitivity	0.994118	0. 951807	0. 933333
Specificity	0.992184	0. 992184	0. 992184
Accuracy	0.99669	0.996379	0.996366
MCC	0.98151	0.874199	0.833085

the method has a better discriminatory performance. For the [Res_{10}], [Res_{15}], and [Res_{20}] groups, MCC values of 0.982, 0.874, and 0.833 were, respectively, obtained. Still, such performance metrics seems to highlight the clear potential of our MIF-based method to predict drug resistance, especially within the most populated [Res_{10}] group (MCC value close to 1).

Positioning and Differentiation vs. Sequence-Based, PI-Resistance Prediction Tools

More than a decade ago, Lengauer and Sing pointed out the lack of commonly agreed benchmark (or test) datasets to assess and compare the performance of different prediction methods (Lengauer and Sing, 2006). The amount of available information on matched HIV genotype–resistance phenotype has increased significantly over recent years, with HIVDB embodying an important role as a centralized data repository (Rhee et al., 2003). As expected, sequence-based methods can make use of as much information as available to train their predictions, resulting in that they become proficient at "predicting" the phenotypic response for the sequences they have been trained on. Only in a few cases do we witness a concern in drawing prospective validation on unseen sequence sets and in making those test sets available to the community (Tarasova et al., 2018). This hinders the design of fair comparisons with methods that do not make direct use of sequence data for training, such as the one we propose here. On the other hand, over the past years genotypic-based methods have reached a level of sophistication that allows them to perform resistance predictions to specific drugs, exclusively based on sequence data matched to phenotypic response, while, at its current stage of development, our MIF-based method can only perform binary classification (susceptible or resistant) of input sequences.

Taken together, these aspects render the comparison of our algorithm with existing, sequence-trained, multi-classification predictors *non-trivial* to say the least. Further developments of our methodology, aiming at a more exhaustive exploration of specific MIF areas around the mutated binding sites, may enable stratification of classification into multiple drug classes by detecting the determinants of resistance to specific PIs. For the time being, we center the analysis of differentiation of our method on the answer to a recurrent question in the mind virologists or physicians who prescribe HIV-1 medications: *would it be possible to accurately predict whether a new, unknown HIV-1 strain will be susceptible to known PIs?*

TABLE 3 | Performance metrics for exemplary sequence-based prediction tools tested against the datasets compiled in this work.

PI-resistance predictor	$Sensitivity_{(A)}$	$Sensitivity_{(B)}$	Specificity	$FN_{(A)}$‡	$FN_{(B)}$‡	FP‡
HIV-GRADE 07/2019	1.0000	0.1471	0.9809	0	580 *12*	120 *8*
ANRS 29_11/2018	1.0000	0.1868	0.8493	0	553 *14*	945 *61*
HIVdb 8.9.1	1.0000	1.0000	0.8818	0	0	741 *21*
Rega 10.0.0	1.0000	0.0838	0.9804	0	623 *7*	123 *10*
MIF-based Drug Resistance Classifier†	0.9941	0.9941	0.9922	4 *1*	4 *1*	49 *11*

†The proposed MIF-based drug resistance classifier is shown in the last row for comparison purposes.
‡False negatives (FN) corresponds to the number of sequences belonging to the Resistant dataset (withdrawn of extreme outliers) that were predicted susceptible to all PIs. False positives (FP) corresponds to the number of sequences belonging to the Susceptible* dataset (withdrawn of extreme outliers) that were predicted resistant to at least one PI. In italics are indicated the number of viral isolates to which the sequences misclassified as FP belong. Rules for sensitivity analysis in (1) benchmark A [$Sensitivity_{(A)}$]: resistance to one or more PIs is considered a correct prediction; and (2) benchmark B [$Sensitivity_{(B)}$]: resistance to all PIs is considered a correct prediction.*

In order to answer to this question, we first converted our *test set* containing susceptible and resistant HIV1-PR sequences withdrawn of *extreme* outliers ($N = 6{,}269$ [[Susceptible*]] and $N = 680$ [[Resistant*]], respectively) into codon code, using the EMBOSS Backtranseq online tool (Madeira et al., 2019a,b), and then submitted it to the HIV-GRADE web server (Obermeier et al., 2012a,b) for comparison with the sequence-based algorithms ANRS-rules (Brun-Vézinet et al., 2003), HIVdb (Rhee et al., 2003; Tang et al., 2012) and Rega (Van Laethem et al., 2002; Camacho et al., 2017). Unexpectedly, we were not able to obtain predictions from *geno2pheno* via HIV Grade due to a technical issue of the web platform. To eschew this problem, we tried to submit the *test set* directly through *geno2pheno*'s web server, but the interface is limited to an unpractical maximum of 20 sequences per run.

Because the existing sequence-based interpretation systems try to predict phenotypical susceptibility or resistance to the individual drugs for a given genotype, whereas our approach only performs binary classification (susceptibility or resistance to all PIs), in order to draw comparison between the methods we tried to "level the playing field" by converting the predictions made by *sequence-based* algorithms into simpler binary classifications. In a first benchmark (benchmark A), the prediction outputs were converted into (i) susceptibility to all PIs ([Susceptible]) or (ii) resistance to any PI (*Resistant*). In a second, more challenging benchmark (benchmark B), the outputs were encoded as either (i) susceptible to all PIs (*Susceptible*) or (ii) resistant to all PIs (*Resistant*). The full list of criteria applied to the conversion of multiple classifiers into binary classification is given in **Supplementary Table S2**. The full raw output of HIV-GRADE is available in **Supplementary Datasheet S2**.

The ability to accurately predict the susceptibility of the input sequences to all PIs was assessed by determining the rate of correct predictions, with reflection into the calculated methods' Sensitivity (Equation 5) and Specificity (Equation 6). **Table 3** lists calculated performance metrics for the *sequence-based* algorithms on both benchmarks A and B, contrasted with the performance of our *sequence-to-structure-*, MIF-based algorithm. $Sensitivity_{(A)}$ and the number of detected false negatives $FN_{(A)}$ translate the methods' ability to classifying a HIV1-PR sequence known to be resistant to all PIs as *Resistant to at least one PI.* In contrast, $Sensitivity_{(B)}$ and $FN_{(B)}$ translate the methods' ability to correctly predict the same sequences (known to be resistant to all PIs) as *resistant to all PIs.* From the methods' sensitivity viewpoint, the assessment of the results of both benchmarks A and B has been important to counterbalance the crudeness of the conversion of a multiple classifier of resistance toward specific PIs into a binary classification. Benchmark A clearly biases sensitivity in favor of a multi-classifier by considering any resistance prediction (in number or kind of PI) for sequences known to be resistant to all PIs as *correct*, whereas benchmark B offers a more stringent evaluation of sensitivity wherein only *resistant-to-all-PIs* predictions for the same set of fully resistant sequences are considered as *correct.*

As expected the discriminatory power of the methods in benchmark A is in stark contrast with that calculated for benchmark B. $Sensitivity_{(A)}$ suggests that *sequence-based* methods slightly outperform our *sequence-to-structure-*, MIF-based classifier, with 100% correct predictions of *Resistant* sequences vs. a $Sensitivity_{(A)}$ value of 0.994 obtained by our method. By contrast, benchmark B shows a considerable drop in performance by *sequence-based* methods at correctly predicting HIV1-PR sequences resistant to all PIs—aside HIVdb, which retains a Sensitivity of 1.000.

The results in **Table 3** indicate that our workflow outperforms all other algorithms at identifying sequences susceptible to all PIs, with a Specificity of approximately 0.992, while its sequence-based counterparts display Specificities ranging from approximately 0.849 to 0.981. Still, it is worth noting that the large number of FP from the other *sequence-based* methods mostly come from the same isolates, similarly as mentioned above for $FN_{(B)}$. This fact highlights the advantage of accounting for structural information besides genotypic data. While MIFs allow searching for differences in the structural and physicochemical environment of proteins, which might not be significantly affected by mutations for similar amino acids, *sequence-based* approaches will consistently search for mutations at positions of interest and consistently assign them the same classification. At an early-stage of development, our workflow's performance is quite satisfactory, considering that the ability of correctly classifying a sequence as susceptible to all PIs is a highly relevant step at the beginning of antiretroviral therapy—where a false positive weights more on the flexibility of first-line therapy regimens and, consequently, quality of life of the patient.

CONCLUSION AND FUTURE PERSPECTIVES

In recent years, the availability of data in the form of matched HIV genotype–resistance phenotype has expanded greatly, enabling further training of statistical learning methods relating genotype to different levels of phenotypic resistance and against specific drugs. However, in spite of the increased access to and routine sequencing of HIV's genome in many countries, as well as the constant evolution of machine learning (ML)-based techniques, HIV's high mutation rate (estimated in 3×10^{-5} per nucleotide per replication) will continue to pose significant challenges: not only in terms of the constant demand for curation of genotypic and phenotypic data to be fed into ML algorithms, but also from the viewpoint of the interpretability and translation of said data into knowledge to assist the design of novel anti-microbial agents. Therefore, the exploration of innovative structure-based *in silico* approaches to the prediction of drug resistance, focusing at the molecular interface that bridges to drug design, holds clear interest and appeal as alternative or complement to some of the most developed sequence-based statistical methods.

In this contribution, we propose a novel approach to drug resistance prediction, which captures structural and physicochemical modifications induced by mutations in the binding site of an extensively studied viral target, HIV1-PR. We demonstrate that, even at an early, proof-of-principle stage of development, our methodology can identify HIV1-PR *sequence-structure* pairs belonging to three levels of increasing resistance—with impressively high accuracy—thus anticipating, on a purely structural basis, whether a given HIV1-PR sequence will translate into phenotypic resistance or susceptibility to PIs. Since our *sequence-to-structure*-based classifier does not rely on *training* from genotypic data and only uses an individual input sequence to derive the corresponding viral enzyme structure and yield a prediction, its potential real-world value in supporting clinical decision is clearly relevant. Due to the fact that the proposed workflow produced predictions of complete drug susceptibility to the HIV1-PR datasets with high predictive accuracy, said results highlight this methodology as a potential valuable resource on clinical practice. Being able to use the clinical isolate sequence data to accurately predict susceptibility to known PIs, before starting a therapeutic regimen, is of paramount importance to allow the initiation of PI-based therapy with the less expensive 1st generation PIs, resulting in an economic benefit to the healthcare systems. Importantly, even though the method performs analysis on thousands of structural data points (atomic coordinates and MIF points), classification into *susceptible* or *resistant* takes place in a *couple-of-minutes* time scale.

It is worth emphasizing, nevertheless, that there is obvious room for methodological improvement and expansion. The upgrade to multi-classification functionality, where target structures known to be susceptible to specific inhibitors and drugs are used as template for structural modeling, is a critical milestone that will pave the way to predicting resistance to those specific anti-microbial agents. The growing amount of three-dimensional structural data on microbial target-inhibitor complexes, coupled with more elaborate use of sequence data, fuels our belief in that an improved *sequence-to-structure* -, MIF-based drug resistance classifier, will be able to combine the strengths and overcome the shortcomings of current approaches.

Claims of greatness must be backed by adequate validation designs. While the current version of our workflow does not allow drawing comprehensive and direct comparisons with more advanced sequence-based predictors of resistance to specific HIV1-PR inhibitors, further developments to our method will also be accompanied by the assembly and sharing of stratified benchmark sets of susceptible and resistant microbial target sequences—enabling fairer comparisons to be made both by ourselves and the scientific community.

As implied in our concluding words, a clear expectation around this work involves extending the application of our method to other targets, other than HIV1-PR, with inherent and multiple patterns of genetic variation. We realize, however, that this expectation may only be fulfilled if workable amounts of data are shared among the scientific community. Undoubtedly, one of the most critical aspects facing drug resistance prediction is the development of community-wide efforts to prepare and share useful datasets and tools to facilitate improvement and performance evaluation of existing and novel methodologies—which should be a clear priority for researchers working in the field. By basing its development on the use of freeware, our method is freely-available for non-commercial use.

To conclude, we see the results presented here as a promising example of the potential application of combined sequence- and structure-based *in silico* methods to achieve a more detailed interpretation and prediction of the impact of mutations in drug resistance. The ever-increasing emergence and widespread of drug-resistance calls in for the development of more efficient strategies to combat microbial threats in several fronts—be that in the drug discovery research setting or the clinical and medical therapeutic decision realm.

AUTHOR CONTRIBUTIONS

CS and RB developed the idea for the present work and provided critical revisions. NA, AM, and JL contributed equally to its conception, literature search, and manuscript writing. All authors contributed to manuscript revision, read, and approved the submitted version.

ACKNOWLEDGMENTS

NA, AM, JL, CS, and RB thank Daniela Vaz, João Vaz, and Vítor Duque for the informative discussions on the HIV1 drug resistance topic, which lead to devising and developing of the present work. NA, AM, JL, CS, and RB also thank the Coimbra Chemistry Centre (CQC) supported by the Portuguese Agency for Scientific Research, Foundation for Science and Technology (FCT), through Project UID/QUI/00313/2019. NA, AM, and JL acknowledge the MedChemTrain Ph.D. programme (PD/00147/2013) in Medicinal Chemistry—Ministry of Science, Technology, and Higher Education (MCTES), Portugal—for Ph.D. fellowships PD/BD/135287/2017, PD/BD/135289/2017 and PD/BD/135292/2017, respectively.

REFERENCES

Agniswamy, J., Louis, J. M., Roche, J., Harrison, R. W., and Weber, I. T. (2016). Structural studies of a rationally selected multi-drug resistant HIV-1 protease reveal synergistic effect of distal mutations on flap dynamics. *PLoS ONE* 11:e0168616. doi: 10.1371/journal.pone.0168616

Altschul, S. F., Gish, W., Miller, W., Myers, E. W., and Lipman, D. J. (1990). Basic local alignment search tool. *J. Mol. Biol.* 215, 403–410. doi: 10.1016/S0022-2836(05)80360-2

Alves, N. G., Mata, A. I., and Luís, J. P. (2018a). *GitHub: FilterMajor.sh*. Available online at: https://github.com/subject-am/PI-resistance_Prediction/blob/fasta-processing/filterMajor.sh (accessed October 27, 2019).

Alves, N. G., Mata, A. I., and Luís, J. P. (2018b). *GitHub: FilterMinor.sh*. Available online at: https://github.com/subject-am/PI-resistance_Prediction/blob/fasta-processing/filterMinor.sh (accessed October 27, 2019).

Alves, N. G., Mata, A. I., and Luís, J. P. (2018c). *GitHub: MutModels.sh*. Available online at: https://github.com/subject-am/PI-resistance_Prediction/blob/model-structures/MutModels.sh (accessed October 27, 2019).

Alves, N. G., Mata, A. I., and Luís, J. P. (2018d). *GitHub: Pattern_HIVp.sh*. Available online at: https://github.com/subject-am/PI-resistance_Prediction/blob/model-structures/pattern-HIVp.sh (accessed October 27, 2019).

Alves, N. G., Mata, A. I., and Luís, J. P. (2018e). *GitHub: Ref_process.sh*. Available online at: https://github.com/subject-am/PI-resistance_Prediction/blob/isomif_run/ref_process.sh (accessed October 27, 2019).

Alves, N. G., Mata, A. I., and Luís, J. P. (2018f). *GitHub: Separate_sets.sh*. Available online at: https://github.com/subject-am/PI-resistance_Prediction/blob/Dataset-processing/Separate_sets.sh (accessed October 27, 2019).

Alves, N. G., Mata, A. I., and Luís, J. P. (2019a). *GitHub: Count_mut.sh*. Available online at: https://github.com/subject-am/PI-resistance_Prediction/blob/fasta-processing/count_mut.sh (accessed October 27, 2019).

Alves, N. G., Mata, A. I., and Luís, J. P. (2019b). *GitHub: HIV1predict.sh*. Available online at: https://github.com/subject-am/PI-resistance_Prediction/blob/master/bin/HIV1predict.sh (accessed November 30, 2019).

Artese, A., Cross, S., Costa, G., Distinto, S., Parrotta, L., Alcaro, S., et al. (2013). Molecular interaction fields in drug discovery: recent advances and future perspectives. *Wiley Interdiscip. Rev. Comput. Mol. Sci.* 3, 594–613. doi: 10.1002/wcms.1150

Beerenwinkel, N., Däumer, M., Oette, M., Korn, K., Hoffmann, D., Kaiser, R., et al. (2003). Geno2pheno: estimating phenotypic drug resistance from HIV-1 genotypes. *Nucleic Acids Res.* 31, 3850–3855. doi: 10.1093/nar/gkg575

Bonet, I. (2015). Machine learning for prediction of HIV drug resistance: a review. *Curr. Bioinform.* 10, 579–585. doi: 10.2174/1574893610666151008011731

Bron, C., and Kerbosch, J. (1973). Algorithm 457: finding all cliques of an undirected graph. *Commun. ACM* 16, 575–577. doi: 10.1145/362342.362367

Brun-Vézinet, F., Descamps, D., Ruffault, A., Masquelier, B., Calvez, V., Peytavin, G., et al. (2003). Clinically relevant interpretation of genotype for resistance to abacavir. *AIDS* 17, 1795–1802. doi: 10.1097/00002030-200308150-00008

Camacho, R., Laethem, K., Van Geretti, A. M., Verheyen, J., Paredes, R., and Vandamme, A.-M. (2017). *Algorithm for the Use of Genotypic HIV-1 Resistance Data (Version Rega v10.0.0)*. Available online at: https://rega.kuleuven.be/cev/avd/software/rega-hiv1-rules-v10.pdf

Cao, Z. W., Han, L. Y., Zheng, C. J., Ji, Z. L., Chen, X., Lin, H. H., et al. (2005). Computer prediction of drug resistance mutations in proteins. *Drug Discov. Today* 10, 521–529. doi: 10.1016/S1359-6446(05)03377-5

Chartier, M., and Najmanovich, R. (2015). Detection of binding site molecular interaction field similarities. *J. Chem. Inf. Model* 55, 1600–1615. doi: 10.1021/acs.jcim.5b00333

Cruciani, G. (2005). *Molecular Interaction Fields*. Weinheim: FRG, Wiley-VCH Verlag GmbH and Co. KGaA.

draw.io. (2005). *Flowchart Maker & Online Diagram Software*. Available online at: https://www.draw.io/ (accessed October 25, 2019).

Fawcett, T. (2006). An introduction to ROC analysis. *Pattern Recognit. Lett.* 27, 861–874. doi: 10.1016/j.patrec.2005.10.010

Florkowski, C. M. (2008). Sensitivity, specificity, receiver-operating characteristic (ROC) curves and likelihood ratios: communicating the performance of diagnostic tests. *Clin. Biochem. Rev.* 29(Suppl 1), S83–S87.

Gaudreault, F., Morency, L.-P., and Najmanovich, R. J. (2015). NRGsuite: a PyMOL plugin to perform docking simulations in real time using FlexAID. *Bioinformatics* 31, 3856–3858. doi: 10.1093/bioinformatics/btv458

Goodford, P. J. (1985). A computational procedure for determining energetically favorable binding sites on biologically important macromolecules. *J. Med. Chem.* 28, 849–857. doi: 10.1021/jm00145a002

Hao, G., Yang, G., and Zhan, C. (2010). Computational mutation scanning and drug resistance mechanisms of HIV-1 protease inhibitors. *J. Phys. Chem. B* 114, 9663–9676. doi: 10.1021/jp102546s

Hao, G.-F., Guang-Fu, Y., and Zhan, C.-G. (2012). Structure-based methods for predicting target mutation-induced drug resistance and rational drug design to overcome the problem. *Drug Discov. Today* 17, 1121–1126. doi: 10.1016/j.drudis.2012.06.018

Hoaglin, D. C. (2003). John W. Tukey and data analysis. *Stat. Sci.* 18, 311–18. doi: 10.1214/ss/1076102418

Hou, T., and Yu, R. (2007). Molecular dynamics and free energy studies on the wild-type and double mutant HIV-1 protease complexed with amprenavir and two amprenavir-related inhibitors: mechanism for binding and drug resistance. *J. Med. Chem.* 50, 1177–1188. doi: 10.1021/jm0609162

Humphrey, W., Dalke, A., and Schulten, K. (1996). VMD: visual molecular dynamics. *J. Mol. Graph.* 14, 33–38. doi: 10.1016/0263-7855(96)00018-5

Irwin, K. K., Renzette, N., Kowalik, T. F., and Jensen, J. D. (2016). Antiviral drug resistance as an adaptive process. *Virus Evol.* 2:vew014. doi: 10.1093/ve/vew014

Jenwitheesuk, E., and Samudrala, R. (2005). Prediction of HIV-1 protease inhibitor resistance using a protein-inhibitor flexible docking approach. *Antivir. Ther.* 10, 157–166.

Khalid, Z., and Sezerman, O. U. (2018). Prediction of HIV drug resistance by combining sequence and structural properties. *IEEE/ACM Trans. Comput. Biol. Bioinformatics* 15, 966–973. doi: 10.1109/TCBB.2016.2638821

Khan, R. A., and Brandenburger, T. (2019). *ROCit. Performance Assessment of Binary Classifier with Visualization*. Available online at: https://cran.r-project.org/package=ROCit

King, N. M., Prabu-Jeyabalan, M., Nalivaika, E. A., Wigerinck, P., de Bethune, M.-P., and Schiffer, C. A. (2004). Structural and thermodynamic basis for the binding of TMC114, a next-generation human immunodeficiency virus type 1 protease inhibitor. *J. Virol.* 78, 12012–12021. doi: 10.1128/JVI.78.21.12012-12021.2004

Lengauer, T., and Sing, T. (2006). Bioinformatics-assisted anti-HIV therapy. *Nat. Rev. Microbiol.* 4, 790–797. doi: 10.1038/nrmicro1477

Madeira, F., Mi Park, Y., Lee, J., Buso, N., Gur, T., Madhusoodanan, N., et al. (2019a). EMBOSS Backtranseq. *Nucleic Acids Res.* 47, W636–W641. doi: 10.1093/nar/gkz26

Madeira, F., Mi Park, Y., Lee, J., Buso, N., Gur, T., Madhusoodanan, N., et al. (2019b). The EMBL-EBI search and sequence analysis tools APIs in 2019. *Nucleic Acids Res.* 47, W636–W641. doi: 10.1093/nar/gkz268

Martínez, L., Andreani, R., and Martínez, J. M. (2007). Convergent algorithms for protein structural alignment. *BMC Bioinformatics* 8:306. doi: 10.1186/1471-2105-8-306

Mason, S., Devincenzo, J. P., Toovey, S., Wu, J. Z., and Whitley, R. J. (2018). Comparison of antiviral resistance across acute and chronic viral infections. *Antiviral Res.* 158, 103–112. doi: 10.1016/j.antiviral.2018.07.020

Masso, M., and Vaisman, I. I. (2013). Sequence and structure based models of HIV-1 protease and reverse transcriptase drug resistance. *BMC Genomics* 14:S3. doi: 10.1186/1471-2164-14-S4-S3

Matthews, B. W. (1975). Comparison of the predicted and observed secondary structure of T4 phage lysozyme. *Biochim. Biophys. Acta Protein Struct.* 405, 442–451. doi: 10.1016/0005-2795(75)90109-9

McKeegan, K. S., Borges-Walmsley, M. I., and Walmsley, A. R. (2002). Microbial and viral drug resistance mechanisms. *Trends Microbiol.* 10, 8–14. doi: 10.1016/S0966-842X(02)02429-0

Nayak, C., Chandra, I., and Singh, S. K. (2019). An *in silico* pharmacological approach toward the discovery of potent inhibitors to combat drug resistance HIV-1 protease variants. *J. Cell. Biochem.* 120, 9063–9081. doi: 10.1002/jcb.28181

Obermeier, M., Pironti, A., Berg, T., Braun, P., Däumer, M., Eberle, J., et al. (2012a). HIV-GRADE: a publicly available, rules-based drug resistance interpretation algorithm integrating bioinformatic knowledge. *Intervirology* 55, 102–107. doi: 10.1159/000331999

Obermeier, M., Pironti, A., Berg, T., Braun, P., Däumer, M., Eberle, J., et al. (2012b). HIV-GRADE: HIV-1 Tool. *Intervirology* 55, 102–107.

Pawar, S., Wang, Y.-F., Wong-Sam, A., Agniswamy, J., Ghosh, A. K., Harrison, R. W., et al. (2019). Structural studies of antiviral inhibitor with HIV-1 protease bearing drug resistant substitutions of V32I, I47V and V82I. *Biochem. Biophys. Res. Commun.* 514, 974–978. doi: 10.1016/j.bbrc.2019.05.064

Pines, J. M., and Everett, W. W. (2008). *Evidence-Based Emergency Care*, 2nd Edn, eds J. M. Pines, C. R. Carpentee, A. S. Raja, and J. D. Schuur. Oxford: Blackwell Publishing Ltd.

Powers, D. M. W. (2011). Evaluation: from precision, recall and F-factor to ROC, informedness, markedness and correlation. *J. Mach. Learn. Technol.* 2, 37–63. Available online at: http://bioinfopublication.org/viewhtml.php?artid=BIA0001114

Qiu, X., and Liu, Z.-P. (2011). Recent developments of peptidomimetic HIV-1 protease inhibitors. *Curr. Med. Chem.* 18, 4513–4537. doi: 10.2174/092986711797287566

R Core Team (2018). *R: A Language and Environment for Statistical Computing*. R Found. Stat. Comput. Available online at: https://www.r-project.org/

RCSB PDB (2000). *RCSB PDB*. Available at: https://www.rcsb.org/ (accessed September 7, 2019).

[Res_{10}] Alves, Nuno G., Ana Isabel Mata, and João Pedro Luís. (2019) HIV-1 protease isolates from HIVdb Stanford University with more than 10-fold resistance to all inhibitors. GitHub. 20181102. https://github.com/subject-am/PI-resistance_Prediction/blob/Dataset-processing/PI_dataset-res10

[Res_{15}] Alves, Nuno G., Ana Isabel Mata, and João Pedro Luís. (2019) HIV-1 protease isolates from HIVdb Stanford University with more than 15-fold resistance to all inhibitors. GitHub. 20181102. https://github.com/subject-am/PI-resistance_Prediction/blob/Dataset-processing/PI_dataset-res15

[Res_{20}] Alves, Nuno G., Ana Isabel Mata, and João Pedro Luís. (2019) HIV-1 protease isolates from HIVdb Stanford University with more than 20-fold resistance to all inhibitors. GitHub. 20181102. https://github.com/subject-am/PI-resistance_Prediction/blob/Dataset-processing/PI_dataset-res20

[Resistant*] Alves, Nuno G., Ana Isabel Mata, and João Pedro Luís. (2019) HIV-1 protease isolates from HIVdb Stanford University with more than 10-fold resistance to all inhibitors, without extreme outliers. GitHub. 20181102. https://github.com/subject-am/PI-resistance_Prediction/blob/Dataset-processing/Resistant_noOut

Rhee, S.-Y., Gonzales, M. J., Kantor, R., Betts, B. J., Ravela, J., and Shafer, R. W. (2003). Human immunodeficiency virus reverse transcriptase and protease sequence database. *Nucleic Acids Res.* 31, 298–303. doi: 10.1093/nar/gkg100

Rhee, S.-Y., Taylor, J., Wadhera, G., Ben-Hur, A., Brutlag, D. L., and Shafer, R. W. (2006). Genotypic predictors of human immunodeficiency virus type 1 drug resistance. *Proc. Natl. Acad. Sci. U. S. A.* 103, 17355–17360. doi: 10.1073/pnas.0607274103

Riemenschneider, M., Hummel, T., and Heider, D. (2016). SHIVA - a web application for drug resistance and tropism testing in HIV. *BMC Bioinformatics* 17:314. doi: 10.1186/s12859-016-1179-2

Ruopp, M. D., Perkins, N. J., Whitcomb, B. W., and Schisterman, E. F. (2008). Youden index and optimal cut-point estimated from observations affected by a lower limit of detection. *Biometrical J.* 50, 419–430. doi: 10.1002/bimj.200710415

Šali, A. (2019a). *Modeller*. Available at: https://salilab.org/modeller/ (accessed August 20, 2019).

Šali, A. (2019b). *Modeller Wiki*. Available online at: https://salilab.org/modeller/wiki/Mutate model (accessed September 30, 2019).

Šali, A., and Blundell, T. L. (1993). Comparative protein modelling by satisfaction of spatial restraints. *J. Mol. Biol.* 234, 779–815. doi: 10.1006/jmbi.1993.1626

Sheik Amamuddy, O., Bishop, N. T., and Tastan Bishop, Ö. (2018). Characterizing early drug resistance-related events using geometric ensembles from HIV protease dynamics. *Sci. Rep.* 8:17938. doi: 10.1038/s41598-018-36041-8

Stanford University (1998a). *HIVDB: Consensus B Amino Acid Sequences*. Available online at: https://hivdb.stanford.edu/pages/documentPage/consensus_amino_acid_sequences.html (accessed November 2, 2019).

Stanford University (1998b). *HIVDB: Genotype-Phenotype Datasets*. Available online at: https://hivdb.stanford.edu/pages/genopheno.dataset.html (accessed November 2, 2018).

Stanford University (1998c). *HIVDB: HIV Drug Resistance Database*. Available online at: https://hivdb.stanford.edu/ (accessed October 23, 2019).

Stanford University (1998d). *HIVDB: PI Resistance Notes*. Available online at: https://hivdb.stanford.edu/dr-summary/resistance-notes/PI/ (accessed October 23, 2019).

Strasfeld, L., and Chou, S. (2010). Antiviral drug resistance: mechanisms and clinical implications. *Infect. Dis. Clin. North Am.* 24, 413–437. doi: 10.1016/j.idc.2010.01.001

[Susceptible] Alves, Nuno G., Ana Isabel Mata and João Pedro Luís. (2019) HIV-1 protease isolates from HIVdb Stanford University susceptible to all inhibitors. GitHub. 20181102. https://github.com/subject-am/PI-resistance_Prediction/blob/Dataset-processing/PI_dataset-susceptible

[Susceptible*] Alves, Nuno G., Ana Isabel Mata, and João Pedro Luís. (2019) HIV-1 protease isolates from HIVdb Stanford University susceptible to all inhibitors, without *extreme* outliers. GitHub. 20181102. https://github.com/subject-am/PI-resistance_Prediction/blob/Dataset-processing/Susceptible_noOut

Tang, M. W., Liu, T. F., and Shafer, R. W. (2012). The HIVdb system for HIV-1 genotypic resistance interpretation. *Intervirology* 55, 98–101. doi: 10.1159/000331998

Tape, T. G. (1990). *Interpreting Diagnostic Tests*. University of Nebraska Medical Center. Available online at: http://gim.unmc.edu/dxtests/ (accessed October 24, 2019).

Tarasova, O., Biziukova, N., Filimonov, D., and Poroikov, V. (2018). A computational approach for the prediction of HIV resistance based on amino acid and nucleotide descriptors. *Molecules* 23:2751. doi: 10.3390/molecules23112751

Toor, J. S., Sharma, A., Kumar, R., Gupta, P., Garg, P., and Arora, S. K. (2011). Prediction of drug-resistance in HIV-1 subtype C based on protease sequences from ART naive and first-line treatment failures in North India using genotypic and docking analysis. *Antiviral Res.* 92, 213–218. doi: 10.1016/j.antiviral.2011.08.005

Tukey, J. W. (1949). Comparing individual means in the analysis of variance. *Biometrics* 5:99. doi: 10.2307/3001913

Van Laethem, K., De Luca, A., Antinori, A., Cingolani, A., Perna, C. F., and Vandamme, A.-M. (2002). A genotypic drug resistance interpretation algorithm that significantly predicts therapy response in HIV-1-infected patients. *Antivir. Ther.* 7, 123–9.

Vercauteren, J., and Vandamme, A.-M. (2006). Algorithms for the interpretation of HIV-1 genotypic drug resistance information. *Antiviral Res.* 71, 335–342. doi: 10.1016/j.antiviral.2006.05.003

Vere Hodge, A., and Field, H. J. (2011). "General mechanisms of antiviral resistance," in *Genetics and Evolution of Infectious Disease*, ed M. Tibayrenc (Amsterdam: Elsevier), 339–362.

Warnes, G. R., Bolker, B., Bonebakker, L., Gentleman, R., Liaw, W. H. A., Lumley, T., et al. (2019). *gplots: Various R Programming Tools for Plotting Data.* Available online at: https://cran.r-project.org/package=gplots

Weber, I. T., and Agniswamy, J. (2009). HIV-1 protease: structural perspectives on drug resistance. *Viruses* 1, 1110–1136. doi: 10.3390/v1031110

Weber, I. T., and Harrison, R. W. (2016). Tackling the problem of HIV drug resistance. *Postepy Biochem.* 62, 273–279.

Wensing, A. M., Calvez, V., Ceccherini-Silberstein, F., Charpentier, C., Günthard, H. F., Paredes, R., et al. (2019). 2019 update of the drug resistance mutations in HIV-1. *Top. Antivir. Med.* 27, 111–121. Available at: http://www.ncbi.nlm.nih.gov/pubmed/31634862

Wickham, H. (2009). *ggplot2: Elegant Graphics for Data Analysis.* New York, NY: Springer-Verlag. Available online at: https://ggplot2-book.org/. doi: 10.1007/978-0-387-98141-3

Wlodawer, A., and Erickson, J. W. (1993). Structure-based inhibitors of HIV-1 protease. *Annu. Rev. Biochem.* 62, 543–585. doi: 10.1146/annurev.bi.62.070193.002551

Word, J. M., Lovell, S. C., Richardson, J. S., and Richardson, D. C. (1999). Asparagine and glutamine: using hydrogen atom contacts in the choice of side-chain amide orientation. *J. Mol. Biol.* 285, 1735–1747. doi: 10.1006/jmbi.1998.2401

Youden, W. J. (1950). Index for rating diagnostic tests. *Cancer* 3, 32–35.

Yu, X., Weber, I. T., and Harrison, R. W. (2014). Prediction of HIV drug resistance from genotype with encoded three-dimensional protein structure. *BMC Genomics* 15:S1. doi: 10.1186/1471-2164-15-S5-S1

Zhang, J., Rhee, S.-Y., Taylor, J., and Shafer, R. W. (2005). Comparison of the precision and sensitivity of the antivirogram and phenosense HIV drug susceptibility assays. *J. Acquir. Immune Defic. Syndr.* 38, 439–444. doi: 10.1097/01.qai.0000147526.64863.53

6

Fast Screening of Inhibitor Binding/Unbinding Using Novel Software Tool CaverDock

Gaspar P. Pinto [1,2†], Ondrej Vavra [1,2†], Jiri Filipovic [3], Jan Stourac [1,2], David Bednar [1,2] and Jiri Damborsky [1,2*]*

[1] Loschmidt Laboratories, Department of Experimental Biology and RECETOX, Faculty of Science, Masaryk University, Brno, Czechia, [2] International Centre for Clinical Research, St. Anne's University Hospital Brno, Brno, Czechia, [3] Institute of Computer Science, Masaryk University, Brno, Czechia

***Correspondence:**
David Bednar
222755@mail.muni.cz
Jiri Damborsky
jiri@chemi.muni.cz

† These authors have contributed equally to this work

Protein tunnels and channels are attractive targets for drug design. Drug molecules that block the access of substrates or release of products can be efficient modulators of biological activity. Here, we demonstrate the applicability of a newly developed software tool CaverDock for screening databases of drugs against pharmacologically relevant targets. First, we evaluated the effect of rigid and flexible side chains on sets of substrates and inhibitors of seven different proteins. In order to assess the accuracy of our software, we compared the results obtained from CaverDock calculation with experimental data previously collected with heat shock protein 90α. Finally, we tested the virtual screening capabilities of CaverDock with a set of oncological and anti-inflammatory FDA-approved drugs with two molecular targets—cytochrome P450 17A1 and leukotriene A4 hydrolase/aminopeptidase. Calculation of rigid trajectories using four processors took on average 53 min per molecule with 90% successfully calculated cases. The screening identified functional tunnels based on the profile of potential energies of binding and unbinding trajectories. We concluded that CaverDock is a sufficiently fast, robust, and accurate tool for screening binding/unbinding processes of pharmacologically important targets with buried functional sites. The standalone version of CaverDock is available freely at https://loschmidt.chemi.muni.cz/caverdock/ and the web version at https://loschmidt.chemi.muni.cz/caverweb/.

Keywords: binding, docking, channel, unbinding, virtual screening, inhibitors, substrates, tunnel

INTRODUCTION

Until the beginning of the new millennium, drug design mostly relied on experimental high-throughput screening (Kansy et al., 1998; Zhang et al., 1999; Bleicher et al., 2003). These techniques evolved rapidly up to the beginning of the nineties. However, although at that time they seemed promising and the best techniques for drug design and discovery, they were expensive in both time and labor (Bajorath, 2002; Bielska et al., 2014). More cost-effective methods emerged with the introduction of docking algorithms and thorough analysis of protein-ligand interactions. This boom in docking approaches led to the development of over 60 software tools for docking (Sousa et al., 2010; Pagadala et al., 2017). At the beginning of the new millennium, a new technique for drug design called "virtual screening" started to gain recognition (Clark, 2008; Ripphausen et al., 2010).

Virtual screening is now a well-established technique for drug design (Bottegoni et al., 2016), both in academic research and the pharmaceutical industry (Mangoni et al., 1999; Clark, 2008; Huang et al., 2008; Totrov and Abagyan, 2008; Cheng et al., 2012; Kaczor et al., 2016). Many docking programs are available for virtual screening and several comparisons and benchmarks have been published (Cummings et al., 2005; Cross et al., 2009; Lavecchia and Di Giovanni, 2013; Bielska et al., 2014; Chaput et al., 2016; Kim et al., 2016). These programs help in the first step of the drug design process and follow a general protocol of screening a large database of small compounds on a chosen target (receptor). After selecting a target, a library of ligands is chosen. The ligands can be taken from many publically available or commercial libraries. Of these, ZINC (http://zinc15.docking.org/) (Sterling and Irwin, 2015), ChEMBL (https://www.ebi.ac.uk/chembl/) and PubChem (https://pubchem.ncbi.nlm.nih.gov/) are among the most widely used and largest ligand libraries. However, other databases with fewer compounds may be useful when searching for compounds with specific characteristics. An example is Drugbank (https://www.drugbank.ca/) (Law et al., 2014), which is a database of drugs approved by the FDA and Canadian Agency for Drugs and Technologies in Health. It also enables selection of experimental, investigational and illicit drugs.

The success of virtual screening boosted the development of techniques used for drug design and in recent years, binding kinetics has gained increased momentum in the drug design community. A research program supported by the European Innovative Medicine Initiative has, for the last 6 years, focused on understanding target binding kinetics (Laverty et al., 2012; Goldman et al., 2013; Kush and Goldman, 2014). Although there has been a steep rise in the development of methods for drug design, there is still space for further improvements.

The binding of a substrate and release of the products of an enzymatic reaction have been studied using different computational approaches (Straatsma and McCammon, 1992; Kollman, 1993; Lamb and Jorgensen, 1997). Classical and accelerated molecular dynamics simulations have been used to calculate ligand binding affinities. These methods use the free energy perturbation approach to calculate the relative binding free energy between a receptor and two ligands based on the thermodynamic cycle (Kruse et al., 2012; Tomić et al., 2015). However, such methods are computationally demanding and not suitable for screening large libraries. Development of new approaches for analysis of ligand binding and unbinding is clearly needed.

Several computational tools have been developed for searching the best binding positions in the active site pocket of a target molecule and then binding positions with increasing distance from the active site. PELE is a web server that incorporates a wide range of different types of calculation, including protein local motions (Lucas and Guallar, 2012). PELE also enables ligand binding refinement, binding site searches and ligand migration. The latter three scripts yield multiple-pose docking results through all protein free space, which cannot be achieved with simple docking algorithms (Guallar et al., 2009; Hernández-Ortega et al., 2011; Espona-Fiedler et al., 2012; Madadkar-Sobhani and Guallar, 2013). MOMA-LigPath (Devaurs et al., 2013) has a robotics algorithm for space search, not only in the active site pocket but also along an unbinding trajectory. However, as the tool does not output information on the energy of conformations, it is not possible to prioritize individual pathways. SLITHER (Lee et al., 2009) is a web server built to generate conformations of substrates while traveling through membrane channels. It is based on both the AUTODOCK (Morris et al., 2009) and MEDock (Chang et al., 2005) docking algorithms. Energetic information is available from these calculations. However, docking trajectories are often sparse.

We have developed a fast method based on analysis of protein tunnels (Marques et al., 2017) combined with molecular docking in a single implementation—called CaverDock—and used it to address important biochemical problems. Protein tunnels are structural features connecting the buried active site cavities with the protein surface. First, tunnels in proteins are identified using the specialized software Caver (Chovancova et al., 2012). Then, an extensively optimised version of AutoDock Vina (Trott and Olson, 2010) is used to dock a ligand along the tunnel to produce a continuous trajectory. Algorithms implemented in CaverDock (Filipovic et al., 2019; Vavra et al., 2019) can be used to run a virtual screening protocol for binding a library of ligands into and from the active site. This procedure identifies energetically favorable binding sites located outside the active site, providing a profile of potential energies. The goal of CaverDock, in current implementation, is not the calculation of the free energy of binding. Instead of obtaining several trajectories to calculate the free energy (Jarzynski, 1997; Fernández, 2014), CaverDock calculates the binding energy along the several, predetermined, points along the tunnel.

We have utilized the new CaverDock tool in three applications. The first examined differences between substrates and inhibitors and selection of flexible side chains along tunnels bottlenecks, which serve as potential hot spots for mutagenesis. The datasets used for testing of the flexible simulations consisted of seven proteins with six tunnels and one channel: (i) cytochrome P450 17A1, (ii) leukotriene A4 hydrolase/aminopeptidase, (iii) acetylcholinesterase (AChE), (iv) human plasma cholesteryl ester transfer protein (CETP), (v) inducible nitric oxide synthase (iNOS), (vi) UDP-3-O-N-acetylglucosamine deacetylase (LpxC), and (vii) matrix metalloproteinase-13 (MMP-13). Trajectories were calculated for both the natural substrates and inhibitors. The second application was the study of human N-terminal domain of heat shock protein 90α (N-HSP90), an important pharmaceutical cancer target, with a diverse set of inhibitors. The dataset was obtained from previously published study (Kokh et al., 2018). We compared the resulting conformations from CaverDock with positions of inhibitor molecules found in the crystal structures. Furthermore, we analyzed the correlations between CaverDock energies and measured experimental values (Kokh et al., 2018). The third application was the screening of potential inhibitors and identification of the access pathways through simulation of binding processes. The applicability of CaverDock for virtual screening pharmaceutically important molecules was validated with cytochrome P450 17A1 and a dataset of oncological drugs from the NIH.gov website and with leukotriene A4 hydrolase/aminopeptidase and a dataset of anti-inflammatory drugs from the drugbank.ca website. The presented results demonstrate that CaverDock is a ready-to-use tool that should be of broad interest to biochemists, protein engineers, and medicinal chemists.

METHODS

Protein Targets

Cytochrome P450 17A1 and leukotriene A4 hydrolase/aminopeptidase were selected for flexibility testing as well as the model systems to validate the applicability of CaverDock for the virtual screening of ligand libraries. Seven protein targets were considered, as described below. The description of the structure and function of Acetylcholinesterase (AChE), Cholesteryl ester transfer protein (CETP), Nitric oxide synthase (iNOS), Metal-dependent deacetylase (LpxC), and Matrix metalloproteinase-13 (MMP-13) is provided in the **Supplementary Information**.

Cytochrome P450 17A1 functions as a drug-processing enzyme and was selected as the target protein for both application studies. The starting structure for this work was the crystal structure taken from the Protein Data Bank (Berman et al., 2000) with PDB-ID 3RUK (DeVore and Scott, 2012). The structure comprised an agglomerate of 4 cytochromes P450 17A1, from which we only used chain A. The structure also contained the inhibitor Abiraterone, which blocked access to the active site and was deleted prior to CaverDock screening.

Leukotriene A4 hydrolase/aminopeptidase, with crystal structure PDB-ID 4L2L (Stsiapanava et al., 2014), was selected as the second target for both application studies. Leukotrienes are a family of lipid mediators that play important roles in a variety of allergic and inflammatory reactions (Haeggström et al., 1990; Funk, 2001; Haeggström, 2004; Szul et al., 2016). Leukotriene A4 hydrolase/aminopeptidase (EC 3.3.2.6) is a bifunctional zinc metalloenzyme that catalyzes formation of the chemotactic agent LTB4, a key lipid mediator in the immune response. This enzyme, had an inhibitor, 4-(4-benzylphenyl) thiazol-2-amine, bound to the crystal structure, which had to be removed prior to screening. LTA4H possesses two known activities, both of which are exerted via distinct but overlapping active sites and depend on a catalytic zinc atom. The catalytic zinc atom is bound to the signature HEXXH, known also for other M1 metallopeptidases (Gomis-Rüth et al., 2012; Zhang et al., 2015).

Heat shock protein 90α (HSP90) is a chaperone protein that assists the folding of client proteins. The HSP90 consists of three domains. The highly conserved N-terminal domain with ATP-binding cleft which is responsible for the catalytic activity. The middle domain contains a large hydrophobic surface needed for the folding of client proteins. The C-terminal domain is involved in the dimerization of HSP90 (Li et al., 2012). The function of HSP90 is linked to hydrolysis of ATP and the dimerization. A number of the HSP90 client proteins are part of cancer cell-associated signaling pathways, therefore the HSP90 is an important target in drug design. The function of HSP90 can be blocked by small molecules. This inhibition leads to degradation of the client proteins and impacts tumor growth (Kabakov et al., 2010). In this study, we analyzed the bound (HOLO) crystal structures with several small inhibitors inside the ATP-binding pocket. Furthermore, we conducted CaverDock simulations with a larger set of inhibitors using the unbound (APO) crystal structure of N-HSP90 (Kokh et al., 2018).

Structural Analysis of N-HSP90 HOLO Complexes

We studied the ability of CaverDock to find protein-ligand conformations similar to the crystal structures using the set of previously published complexes (Kokh et al., 2018). We analyzed the 34 crystal complexes of the N-HSP90 with different co-crystallized inhibitors. The list of the PDB IDs is in **Supplementary Table S1**. The crystal structures were aligned by DeepAlign (Wang et al., 2013) to simplify the following analyses. The tunnels for CaverDock runs were calculated by Caver 3.02 (Chovancova et al., 2012) in each inhibitor-free structure starting from the catalytic residues 93 and 138 with the probe radius, shell radius and shell depth set to 1.5, 20, and 20 Å, respectively. The tunnel leading through the main opening of the ATP-binding cleft to the active site was selected, discretized with 0.3 Å steps and extended by 20 Å to ensure complete unbinding of the tested inhibitor molecules. The receptor and ligand PDBQT files for CaverDock were prepared by MGLtools (Morris et al., 2009).

Energy Analysis of N-HSP90 HOLO and APO Complexes

Based on the previously published kinetic data (Kokh et al., 2018), we prepared two datasets. The first dataset consists of a subset of 32 inhibitors and HOLO structures from the HOLO structure analysis dataset described above. The kinetic data for two inhibitors (compound_01 and compound_04) was not complete in the original publication. The second dataset was created to check the findings from the HOLO dataset. It consists of 68 inhibitors. In this case, we ran the CaverDock calculations with the APO structure of N-HSP90 (PDB ID 3T0H). The CaverDock calculations were carried out in the same manner as described above for the structural analysis.

Libraries of Small Ligands

Several approaches can be used to choose libraries for virtual screening. For instance, screening as many ligands as possible from a broad dataset of molecules, such as the ZINC database. Another approach is to screen for drug-like compounds with specific biological activities. Virtual screening may also be performed using cognate ligands belonging to a group of compounds that the enzyme naturally binds and/or catalyzes. In the present study, we conducted a virtual screening campaign on a group of drug-like molecules possessing predefined biological activities. The chosen ligands were converted to the AutoDock Vina-compatible PDBQT format using MGLTools v1-5-7rc1 (Morris et al., 2009). We used the inhibitors complexed in the structures for validation of flexible side chains (inhibitor dataset). We built the substrates in Avogadro and minimized them with the UFF forcefield (Hanwell et al., 2012) for the natural substrates (substrate dataset).

A dataset of *133 cancer drugs* was downloaded from the NIH.gov website for the cytochrome P450 17A1. The drugs were all FDA-approved and have been used against different types of cancer. Of the 133 drugs, 105 were used for the screening and 28 were excluded due to being salts or having unconventional atoms that could not be properly handled by AutoDock Vina. Among the 28 excluded drugs, 22 had two ligand molecules in the same file. The other six drugs had some atoms (one with arsenic, three with platinum and two with boron) for which there were no parameters available in the force field of AutoDock Vina. A dataset of *56 anti-inflammatory drugs* was downloaded from the drugbank.ca website for leukotriene A4 hydrolase/aminopeptidase. Out of these 56 drugs, 54 were used and 2 were excluded from the screening. One excluded drug contained a gold atom, for which AutoDock Vina had no defined parameters. The other drug was a silicate mineral with two molecules in the same file.

CaverDock Calculation

The software tool CaverDock is available free of charge at the website https://loschmidt.chemi.muni.cz/caverdock/. The CaverDock protocol (**Figure 1**) starts with finding the tunnels by using Caver (Chovancova et al., 2012). Caver can be used as a standalone program or as a Pymol plugin. The active site is selected as a starting point for the Caver calculation. For all seven proteins, the location of ligand binding in the active site was known (Gerber et al., 1997; Funk, 2001; Thunnissen et al., 2001; Epps and Vosters, 2002; Rudberg et al., 2002; Haeggström et al., 2007; Gattis et al., 2010; Singh and Konwar, 2012; Clayton et al., 2013; Khatri et al., 2014; Yoshimoto and Auchus, 2015). All the other settings were fixed at default values. This step of the protocol yields several tunnels for each protein. The numbering of the tunnels is given by a parameter called priority, which is the ratio between (i) bottleneck radius, (ii) tunnel length and (iii) curvature of the tunnel. The tunnels were represented as a series of sequential spheres.

We only used tunnels with priority 1 for the flexible simulations. These tunnels had the inhibitor already inside, although we removed it before the Caver calculation since we did not relax the protein in any way. Hence, there was an implicit bias for these tunnels. The flexibility in CaverDock arises from the already implemented flexibility capabilities of Autodock Vina. Flexibility on side chains was introduced in three iterations. In the default mode, CaverDock adds flexibility to two residues in each iteration, up to three iterations. These values may be changed by the user to better fit their needs. For each tunnel in the substrate and inhibitor datasets, two flexible bottleneck residues were added in each iteration. These flexible residues were not necessarily the same for the substrate and inhibitor simulations. Since substrates and inhibitors may differ in length and volume, the bottlenecks that they encounter along a tunnel may also differ.

For cytochrome P450 17A1, we used three tunnels for our virtual screening study. The first two tunnels found by Caver were also described in the literature, whereas the third tunnel was ranked as #5 by Caver. By individually inspecting every tunnel, we noted that tunnels ranked #3 and #4 by Caver were too long and narrow to be feasible as a ligand access pathway. For leukotriene A4 hydrolase/aminopeptidase, we used two tunnels ranked #1 and #2 by Caver. The results obtained were consistent

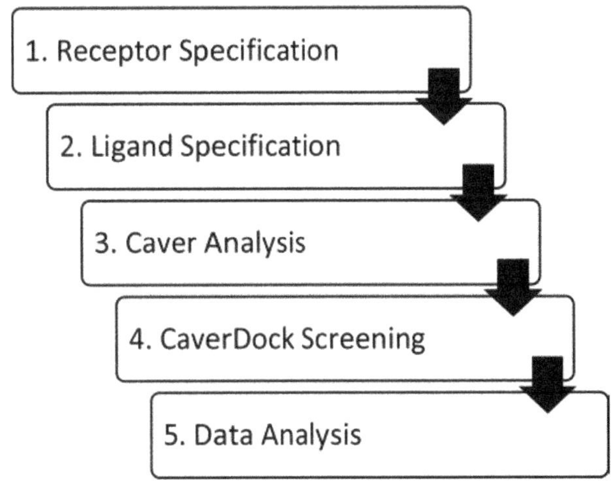

FIGURE 1 | Workflow of virtual screening using CaverDock. (1) Receptor and (2) ligand specification follow established protocols of the software tool AutoDock (Morris et al., 2009). (3) Identification of protein tunnels using Caver (Chovancova et al., 2012). (4) Tunnel discretization and sequential ligand binding study using CaverDock (Filipovic et al., 2019; Vavra et al., 2019). (5) Analysis of docking trajectories and energy profiles, extraction of energy barriers and protein-ligand complexes possessing the lowest energies.

with the literature (Cui et al., 2015), confirming that these two tunnels were used by the protein to transport ligands/drugs in and products out. Since the active site in leukotriene A4 hydrolase/aminopeptidase is inserted deeper into the protein and the protein itself is packed closer together than in cytochrome P450 17A1, only six tunnels were described for this protein vs. 15 tunnels described for cytochrome P450 17A1. A literature search showed that the tunnels ranked highest by Caver were indeed tunnels used by the natural substrate and inhibitors (Yu et al., 2013; Stsiapanava et al., 2014).

After selecting the tunnels to study, the next step in a CaverDock protocol is to discretize the tunnels. Tunnel discretization divides each tunnel into a set of discs. The ligand is *glued* to a disc by one of its atoms and as the disc moves through the tunnel, the software defines a ligand path coordinate. After discretization, we extended the tunnels by two Ångströms. This step ensured that the tunnels were long enough to enable identification of the local binding minima at the tunnel mouth. Having prepared the tunnels, we used MGL tools to set the AutoDock atom types and Gasteiger charges for the receptor and ligands. MGL tools provide scripts that convert pdb and mol2 files into pdbqt file format. Having prepared the receptors and ligands, we next prepared a CaverDock file to run the docking step. This file was equivalent to the one used by AutoDock Vina but with the path to the file containing tunnel information instead of the receptor (Trott and Olson, 2010). We then added information about the studied tunnel from Caver to the configuration file. This new information allowed the "docking" conformation to be searched along the tunnel on each disc. One configuration file needs to be created for each ligand. **Figure 2** shows a representation of a ligand bound along a tunnel taken from several snapshots of a CaverDock calculation.

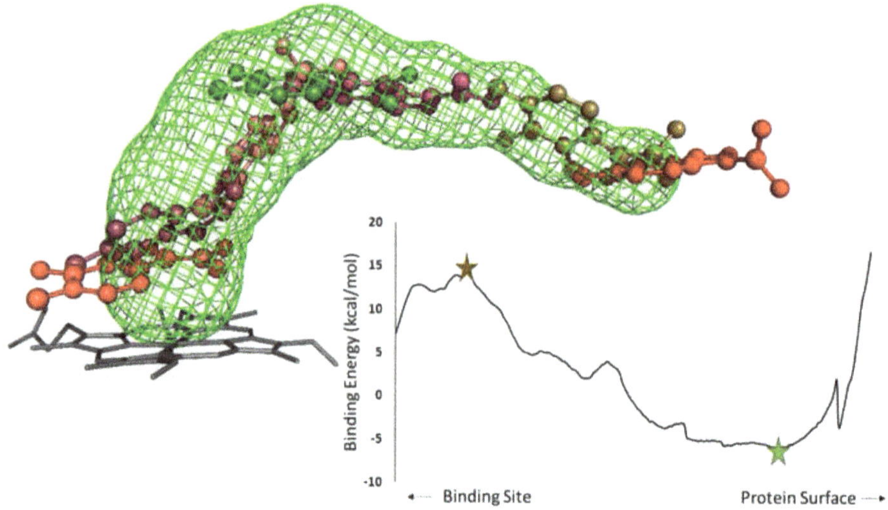

FIGURE 2 | Analysis of an inhibitor passing through a tunnel using CaverDock. Left: structure of cytochrome P450 17A1 and tunnel #3 with seven (7/254) snapshots of a ligand bound along the tunnel. The minimum binding energy conformation is shown in green, whereas the maximum binding energy is shown in brown, in a ball-and-stick representation. Right: energy profile obtained from the CaverDock calculation for cytochrome P450 17A1 and its tunnel #3 with the ligand.

An AutoDock Vina virtual screening was also performed with the same targets as the CaverDock virtual screening. To ensure that AutoDock Vina yielded the best result possible within a reasonable time, we used an exhaustiveness setting of 30. The center of the matrix grid was the same as that used for the CaverDock calculation and the box was 27 Å on each side.

RESULTS

Simulations With Flexible Side Chains

CaverDock allows flexibility of residue side chains along a tunnel. We tested the intrinsic flexibility of AutoDock Vina implemented in CaverDock with the substrate and inhibitor datasets. We introduced flexibility in three iterations by adding two flexible bottleneck residues in each iteration. Thus, iteration 1, 2, and 3 had two, four and six flexible side chains, respectively. The energetic barrier for the substrate and inhibitor to travel from the inside to outside of cytochrome P450 17A1 or leukotriene A4 hydrolase/aminopeptidase was lowered when we added flexible side chains (**Figure 3**). For cytochrome P450 17A1, the binding energy was lowered with each iteration for both the inhibitor and substrate. In the case of the substrate of leukotriene A4 hydrolase/aminopeptidase, the energetic barrier was stabilized with only two flexible side chains and addition of further flexible side chains gave no apparent change in the energetic barrier along the trajectory of the substrate. On the other hand, the inhibitor of leukotriene A4 hydrolase/aminopeptidase had a lower energetic barrier with each iteration. As expected, the inhibitor had a similar or more stable binding energy when compared to the substrate.

We showed that the flexible simulations were able to open parts of the tunnel with high barriers with the substrate and inhibitor datasets (electronic SI). Significant energetic barriers were lost in the iteration with six flexible residues. In this scenario, the ligand was able to leave without any spatial or energetic hindrance. The flexible side chains moved out of the way to let the ligand escape, but the new conformations of side chains were close to the rest of the protein structure. Adding flexible residues did not affect the energetic barrier in iNOS, which showed a similar profile through all iterations in the ligand simulations (electronic SI). In these cases, the tunnel radius was already large enough for unrestricted ligand exchange with no obvious bottleneck.

The usage of the intrinsic AutoDock Vina flexibility in CaverDock is still under development and new algorithms are being tested for obtaining better results. With the current version, users are advised to use both rigid and flexible simulations with four or less flexible side chains. We can get more information about the tunnel with the flexible side chains, e.g., to identify which residues need to be flexible to open the tunnel for ligand passage since these residues are natural hot-spots for potential mutagenesis. However, there is an obvious computational price to pay when using flexible simulations, as shown in **Table 1**. In particular, adding flexible residues leads to longer simulation times. We advise running CaverDock simulations with lower bound trajectories only when running in a rigid mode because rigid trajectories may yield unrealistic high barriers when running upper bound simulations (discussed below).

Comparison of Calculated and Experimental Results

Structural Analysis of HOLO Structures

We calculated the RMSD between the positions of bound inhibitors and the lower-bound CaverDock snapshots. We report the lowest RMSDs and the RMSDs for the lowest energy conformations in **Supplementary Table S1**. Validation of CaverDock in terms of reproducibility of experimental structures of enzyme-inhibitor complexes revealed that the tool identified

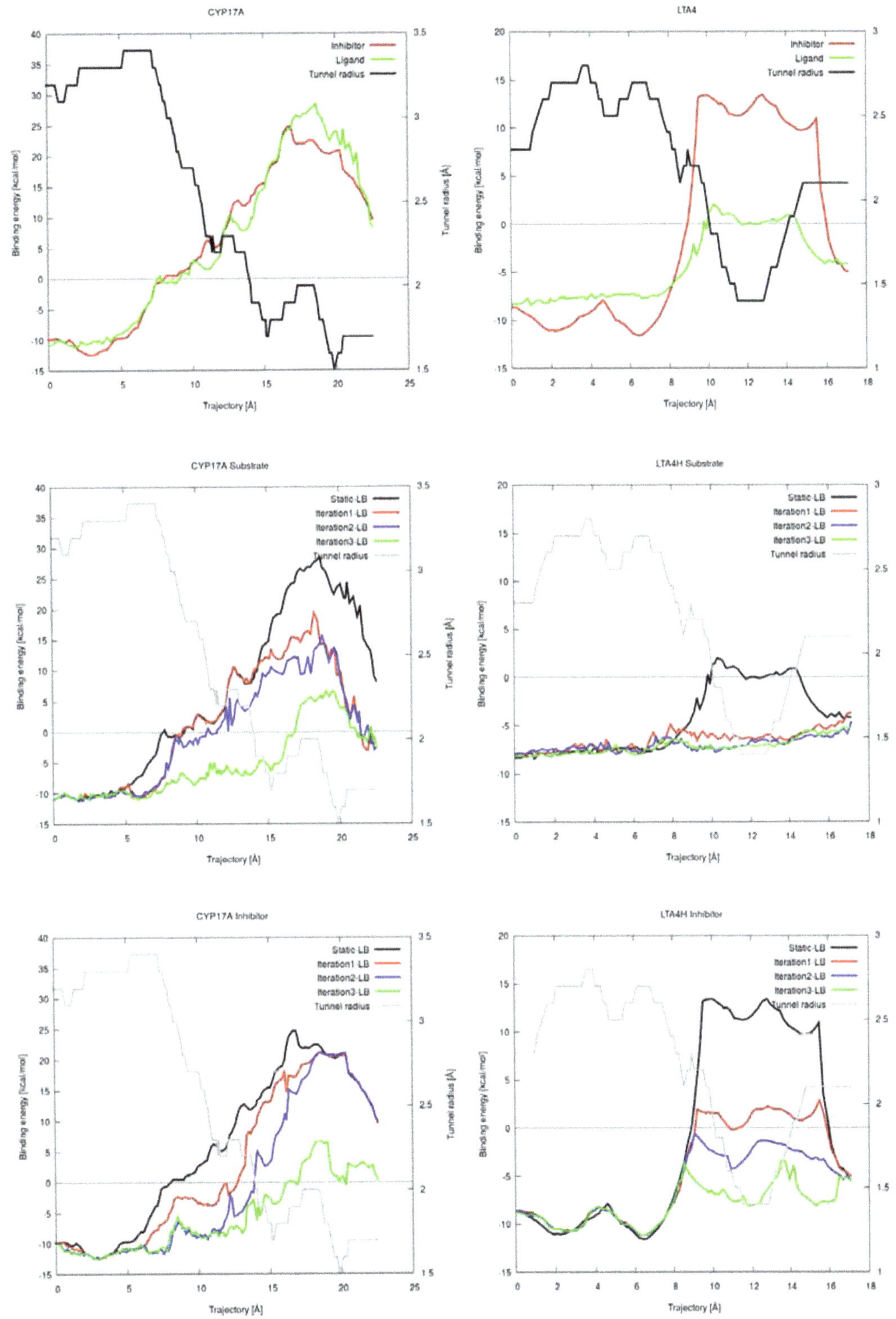

FIGURE 3 | Plots of the binding energies of cytochrome P450 17A1 (left) and leukotriene A4 hydrolase/aminopeptidase (right) obtained from CaverDock with and without flexibility. Binding energies between substrate and inhibitor with tunnel radius present (top). Binding energies from substrate simulations with flexibility, rigid simulation, and tunnel radius on the background (middle). Binding energies from all inhibitor simulations with flexibility, rigid simulation and tunnel radius on the background (bottom).

TABLE 1 | Summary of calculation times for lower bound calculations with rigid and flexible simulations and indication of the flexible residues added on each iteration.

		Cytochrome P450 17A1		Leukotriene A4 hydrolase/aminopeptidase	
		Inhibitors	**Substrates**	**Inhibitors**	**Substrates**
Rigid	Time	47 min 48 s	48 min 13 s	205 min 32 s	24 min 39 s
1st Iteration	Time	110 min 35 s	66 min 18 s	338 min 41 s	50 min 32 s
	Flexible Residues	Ile205, Tyr201	Ile205, Ile246	Val381, Val367	Val367, Phe362
2nd Iteration	Time	252 min 28 s	168 min 3 s	854 min 20 s	112 min 56 s
	Flexible Residues	Arg239, His235	Tyr201, His235	Lys364, Phe362	His360, Lys364
3rd Iteration	Time	436 min 20 s	332 min 22 s	1,994 min 1 s	156 min 11 s
	Flexible Residues	Ile198, Leu242	Leu243, Arg239	His360, Lys385	Gln136, Ile372

Residues are chosen automatically to lower potential energy at bottlenecks.

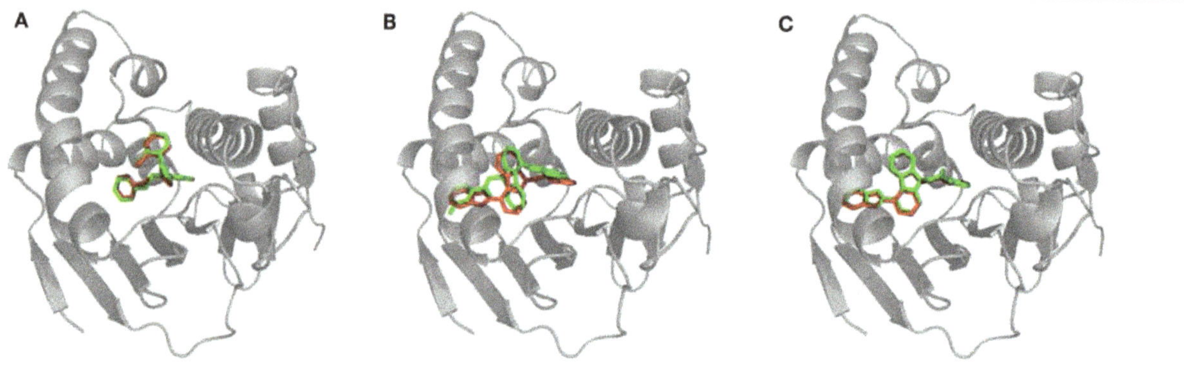

FIGURE 4 | Structural comparison of CaverDock binding poses and X-ray structures. **(A)** Compound_14 correctly predicted by CaverDock (green) with low RMSD compared to the original crystal structure (red). **(B)** Compound_70 wrongly fitted in the pocket by CaverDock (green) with the original size of the tunnel. The overall position is similar, but orientation of the compound is incorrect. **(C)** Compound_70 correctly fitted in the pocket with the increased size of the tunnel. CaverDock (green) predicted a pose in equivalent position to the original crystal structure (red).

proper location and configuration in a vast majority (29 out of 34) cases. We show the example of correct fit in **Figure 4A**. In the case of compound_11, compound_19, compound_38, and compound_70 the correct pose was found by CaverDock but was not correctly identified. A different pose with the lowest energy was picked. In the case of the compound_18, CaverDock failed to find the correct conformation both for the closest and the lowest energy case. The high RMSDs may be caused by incorrect orientation of the ligand and also by the location of the inhibitor. The conformations of inhibitors which are deeper in the protein structure and are out of the tunnel may become unreachable for CaverDock since the ligand is always spatially constrained to the disks.

We experimented with the settings of CaverDock and recalculated the trajectories for the five problematic cases. We found out that by extending the radius of discretized tunnel discs by 10 Å, CaverDock is able to explore deeper parts of the cavity since the ligand has more freedom for movement. The resulting changes of RMSD are shown in **Supplementary Table S2**. The RMSDs were lowered and the binding poses were improved tremendously in case of compound_18, compound_19, and compound_70. This improvement in geometry for the compound_70 is shown in **Figures 4B,C**. The lowest energy pose for the compound_38 was still not identified correctly. Based on these findings, we decided to implement the tunnel extension for our future CaverDock calculations since the improvements were substantially beneficial.

Energy Analysis of N-HSP90 HOLO and APO Forms

CaverDock was used to analyze the unbinding of inhibitors from corresponding HOLO structures. We studied 32 cases with available kinetic data (Kokh et al., 2018). Selected energy values were extracted from the energy profiles: the energy minimum close to the start of the trajectory corresponding with the ligand-bound in the active site (E_{Bound}) and the energy at the tunnel mouth—the last disk of the original tunnel—related with the surface-bound ligand ($E_{Surface}$). In this specific case, there were no visible barriers as shown in the energy profiles **Supplementary Figure S1**. Therefore, we had to use the difference between bound and surface state, the ΔE_{BS} as possible energy barrier which needs to be overcome during the process of unbinding. We calculated the correlation between ΔE_{BS} and the experimentally measured values for k_{on}, K_D, and k_{off}. We found a significant correlation of 0.53 for ΔE_{BS} with $\log(k_{off})$. Comparison of our results with

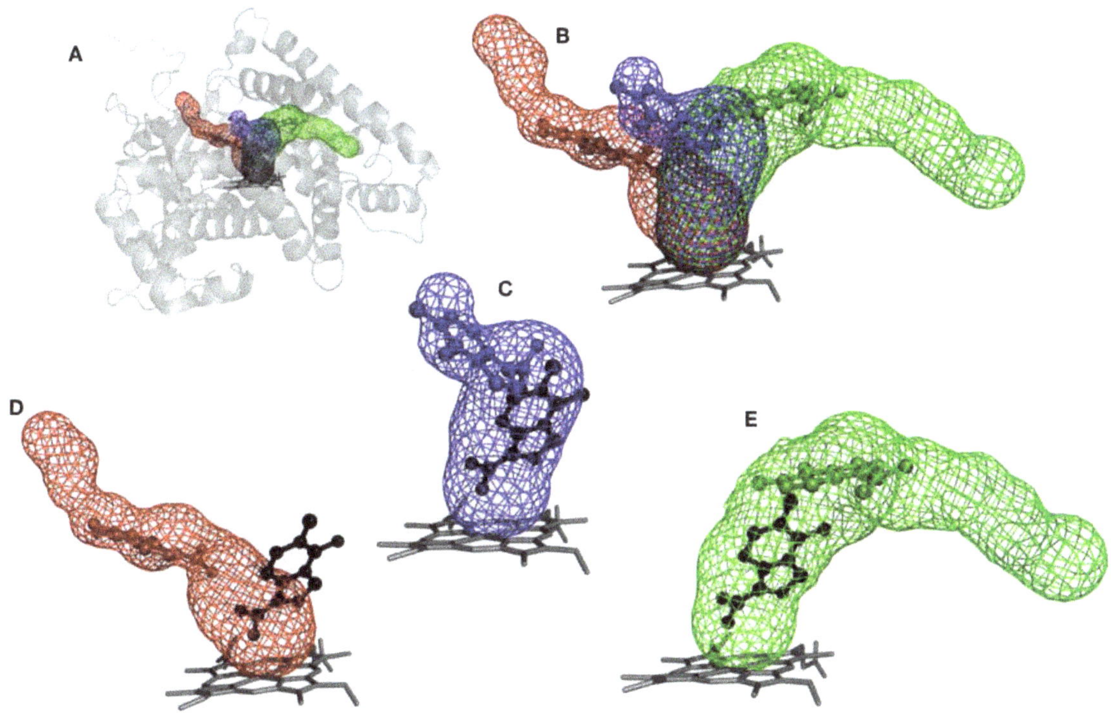

FIGURE 5 | Structure of cytochrome P450 17A1 with tunnels calculated using Caver and binding poses obtained by CaverDock. **(A)** Global view of tunnels—tunnel 1 (blue), tunnel 2A (red), tunnel 3 (green). **(B)** View of tunnels with no protein visualized. Each tunnel has the ligand bound in the minimum obtained from the CaverDock continuous trajectory calculation. **(C)** Tunnel 1 and minimum binding energy pose obtained from CaverDock (blue) and AutoDock Vina (black). **(D)** Tunnel 2A and minimum binding energy pose obtained by CaverDock (red) and AutoDock Vina (black). **(E)** Tunnel 3 and minimum binding energy pose obtained by CaverDock (green) and AutoDock Vina (black).

the previously published correlation 0.63 for the computed relative residence times from molecular dynamics simulations, t_{comp}, with the measured residence times t_{expt} ($t_{expt} = 1/k_{off}$), we confirmed that CaverDock is able to predict koff rates when HOLO structures are used with only a fraction of the computational effort.

We checked the previous findings from the HOLO dataset by simulating the complete set of inhibitors with the APO structure. We did not find any correlation in this case. This, together with no visible barriers in the CaverDock profiles and slow kinetic rates suggests conformational changes in the protein during the binding and unbinding of the inhibitor molecules. Essential conformational change is missing in the APO structure forcing the molecules to bind differently when simulated by CaverDock. Development of the new version of CaverDock that will be taking into account protein backbone dynamics is currently on-going in our laboratory.

Screening of Inhibitors

The purpose of this analysis was to test whether CaverDock (Filipovic et al., 2019; Vavra et al., 2019) could be used for virtual screening. After deciding on the targets and libraries of compounds to use, we analyzed the tunnels for both targets. First, we choose the tunnels according to their ranking given by Caver and information from the literature and then used CaverDock to move the ligands from the outside of the proteins to the active site. Next, we performed virtual screening with the same libraries and targets using AutoDock Vina. It is worth noting that there was a large difference in the exhaustiveness used between the two programs: an exhaustiveness of thirty was used with Autodock Vina, whereas an exhaustiveness of one was used with CaverDock to keep the run time as short as possible. We showed that CaverDock provided new insights into the receptor ligand affinity. We also showed that CaverDock was a computationally cheap method with low run times. We studied 5 tunnels in the two proteins: three tunnels in cytochrome P450 17A1 (**Figure 5**) and two tunnels in leukotriene A4 hydrolase/aminopeptidase (**Figure 6**). Tunnel 1 was much shorter than the other two tunnels studied in cytochrome P450 17A1 (**Table 2**). It also had a narrow mouth when compared to the rest of the tunnel, but it was still wider than tunnel 3. Tunnel 2A was the most sinuous tunnel of the three, with more twists than the other two tunnels. However, they were not as sharp as the turn in tunnel 3. Tunnel 3 had a sharp turn halfway through the tunnel. It was narrow at the entrance of the protein, but after the turn widened sufficiently to allow a bulky inhibitor like Abiraterone to bind to the heme-group, as in the crystal structure.

The tunnels are modeled with the drug Temozolomide in both the CaverDock (**Supplementary Video**) and AutoDock

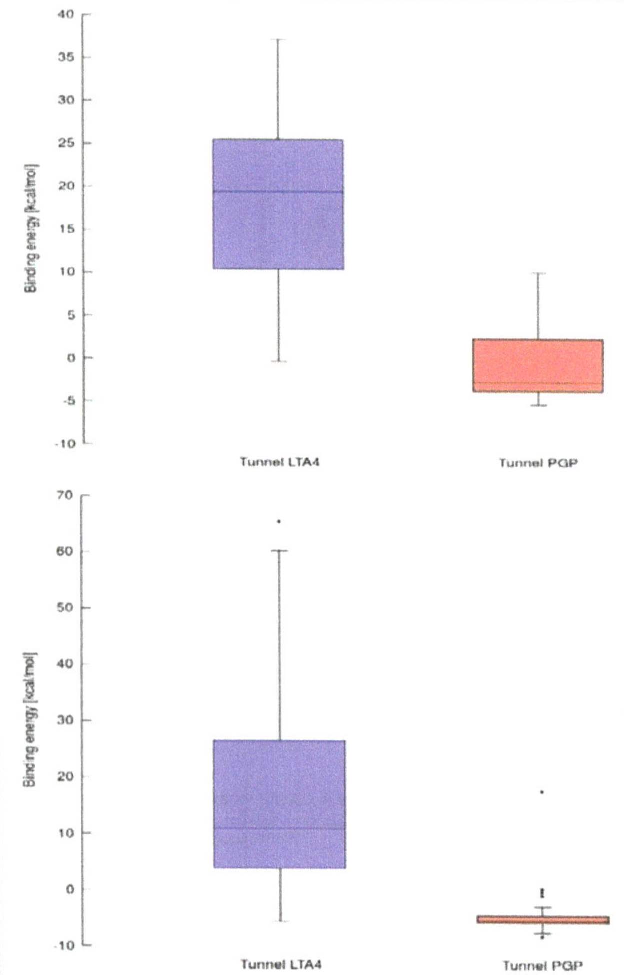

FIGURE 8 | Box and Whiskers plot representing the maxima (energy barriers) for continuous (up) and lower bound (down) trajectories obtained for leukotriene A4 hydrolase/aminopeptidase. Outlying values are indicated by circles.

case of the lower-bound calculation, once the drug encountered a bottleneck, it was allowed to flip in order to find a more suitable conformation on the other side of the bottleneck, while the point being dragged through the discs of the tunnel was kept constant (**Figure 8**). This trajectory always yielded a lower energy value for the barrier because, by definition, the bottleneck was easier to overcome. On the other hand, lower time demands and similar results make the lower bound calculation very powerful for virtual screening.

CONCLUSIONS

Our results demonstrate that CaverDock is applicable for screening of large libraries of potential inhibitors. It provides information on binding and unbinding processes. The tool estimates a profile of potential energies and calculates respective trajectories without the need for time-demanding molecular dynamics simulations. Setting up a calculation using CaverDock is simple and comprises five steps: (i) definition of a receptor, (ii) definition of the ligands, (iii) calculation of tunnels using Caver, (iv) screening of un/binding trajectories, and (v) data analysis. The tool is accompanied by a user manual that explains the setting up of calculations as well as troubleshooting. A standalone version of CaverDock with detailed documentation is available at https://loschmidt.chemi.muni.cz/caverdock/. The automated version of CaverDock is available via the web https://loschmidt.chemi.muni.cz/caverweb/.

The dynamics of side chains lining the protein tunnels and channels can be described to a certain level with the current implementation of CaverDock. Making residue side chains flexible increases calculation times but ultimately considers protein dynamics. We concluded that simulations employing a large number (>4) of flexible amino acid residues may cause undesirable steric clashes. Thus, we advise that results obtained with flexible residues should be interpreted carefully using biochemical intuition when analyzing calculated trajectories and energy profiles. Implementation of a more thorough protocol to address protein flexibility is on-going in our laboratory. CaverDock calculations can be extended to ensembles of protein structures. Particularly challenging is the trade-off between rigorous description of flexible systems and time demands connected with such calculations. Structural comparison of complexes obtained by CaverDock with those determined by crystallographic analysis revealed that we were able to predict the correct poses for a vast majority of inhibitors. The comparison of our profile of potential energies with the rates obtained by kinetic results yields a correlation of 0.53 whereas the more computational expensive molecular dynamics simulation had a correlation of 0.63. Prediction accuracy can be potentially improved by proper treatment of backbone flexibility.

Our study demonstrates that CaverDock is sufficiently fast to screen even large libraries of ligands. Calculation of rigid trajectories using 4 processors took on average 53 min per molecule with 90% successfully calculated cases. Bulky or very flexible ligands take more time, but some of these large ligands may not be able to access the active site via the studied access tunnels. Although it takes longer to perform a CaverDock calculation than a pure virtual screening of ligand binding to the active site with AutoDock Vina, CaverDock provides more data, which may be useful in rational drug design projects. Information on the bottlenecks and energy required for ligands to pass through these narrowed parts of the access tunnel could be useful for medicinal chemists. CaverDock was able to correctly identify tunnels in the proteins explored by the inhibitors included in our screening campaigns.

In summary, we have shown that CaverDock is a robust and ready-to-use software that can be employed in screening campaigns of important pharmacological targets. CaverDock analysis may be a useful complement to virtual screening campaigns carried out using traditional docking tools.

AUTHOR CONTRIBUTIONS

GP and OV carried out the computational work and wrote the manuscript. JF developed the software. DB and JD designed the study. All authors contributed to interpretation of the data, revision of the manuscript, and have given approval of its final version.

FUNDING

This work was supported by the Ministry of Education, Youth, and Sports of the Czech Republic (LQ1605, LM2015047, LM2015051, LM2015055, CZ.02.1.01/0.0/0.0/16_013/0001761) and the European Union (720776). Computational resources were provided by CESNET (LM2015042) and the CERIT Scientific Cloud (LM2015085).

REFERENCES

Bajorath, J. (2002). Integration of virtual and high-throughput screening. *Nat. Rev. Drug Discov.* 1:882. doi: 10.1038/nrd941

Berman, H. M., Westbrook, J., Feng, Z., Gilliland, G., Bhat, T. N., Weissig, H., et al. (2000). The protein data bank. *Nucleic Acids Res.* 28, 235–242. doi: 10.1093/nar/28.1.235

Bielska, E., Lucas, X., Czerwoniec, A., Kasprzak, J. M., Kaminska, K. H., and Bujnicki, J. M. (2014). Virtual screening strategies in drug design – methods and applications. *BioTechnologia* 92, 249–264. doi: 10.5114/bta.2011.46542

Bleicher, K. H., Böhm, H.-J., Müller, K., and Alanine, A. I. (2003). Hit and lead generation: beyond high-throughput screening. *Nat. Rev. Drug Discov.* 2, 369–378. doi: 10.1038/nrd1086

Bottegoni, G., Veronesi, M., Bisignano, P., Kacker, P., Favia, A. D., and Cavalli, A. (2016). Development and application of a virtual screening protocol for the identification of multitarget fragments. *ChemMedChem* 11, 1259–1263. doi: 10.1002/cmdc.201500521

Chang, D. T.-H., Oyang, Y.-J., and Lin, J.-H. (2005). MEDock: a web server for efficient prediction of ligand binding sites based on a novel optimization algorithm. *Nucleic Acids Res.* 33, W233–W238. doi: 10.1093/nar/gki586

Chaput, L., Martinez-Sanz, J., Saettel, N., and Mouawad, L. (2016). Benchmark of four popular virtual screening programs: construction of the active/decoy dataset remains a major determinant of measured performance. *J. Cheminform.* 8:56. doi: 10.1186/s13321-016-0167-x

Cheng, T., Li, Q., Zhou, Z., Wang, Y., and Bryant, S. H. (2012). Structure-based virtual screening for drug discovery: a problem-centric review. *AAPS J.* 14, 133–141. doi: 10.1208/s12248-012-9322-0

Chovancova, E., Pavelka, A., Benes, P., Strnad, O., Brezovsky, J., Kozlikova, B., et al. (2012). CAVER 3.0: a tool for the analysis of transport pathways in dynamic protein structures. *PLoS Comput. Biol.* 8:e1002708. doi: 10.1371/journal.pcbi.1002708

Clark, D. E. (2008). What has virtual screening ever done for drug discovery? *Expert Opin. Drug Discov.* 3, 841–851. doi: 10.1517/17460441.3.8.841

Clayton, G. M., Klein, D. J., Rickert, K. W., Patel, S. B., Kornienko, M., Zugay-Murphy, J., et al. (2013). Structure of the bacterial deacetylase LpxC bound to the nucleotide reaction product reveals mechanisms of oxyanion stabilization and proton transfer. *J. Biol. Chem.* 288, 34073–34080. doi: 10.1074/jbc.M113.513028

Čolović, M. B., Krstić, D. Z., Lazarević-Pašti, T. D., BondŽić, A. M., and Vasić, V. M. (2013). Acetylcholinesterase inhibitors: pharmacology and toxicology. *Curr. Neuropharmacol.* 11, 315–335. doi: 10.2174/1570159X11311030006

Cross, J. B., Thompson, D. C., Rai, B. K., Baber, J. C., Fan, K. Y., Hu, Y., et al. (2009). Comparison of several molecular docking programs: pose prediction and virtual screening accuracy. *J. Chem. Inf. Model.* 49, 1455–1474. doi: 10.1021/ci900056c

Cui, Y.-L., Xue, Q., Zheng, Q.-C., Zhang, J.-L., Kong, C.-P., Fan, J.-R., et al. (2015). Structural features and dynamic investigations of the membrane-bound cytochrome P450 17A1. *Biochim. Biophys. Acta* 1848, 2013–2021. doi: 10.1016/j.bbamem.2015.05.017

Cummings, M. D., DesJarlais, R. L., Gibbs, A. C., Mohan, V., and Jaeger, E. P. (2005). Comparison of automated docking programs as virtual screening tools. *J. Med. Chem.* 48, 962–976. doi: 10.1021/jm049798d

Devaurs, D., Bouard, L., Vaisset, M., Zanon, C., Al-Bluwi, I., Iehl, R., et al. (2013). MoMA-LigPath: a web server to simulate protein-ligand unbinding. *Nucleic Acids Res.* 41, W297–W302. doi: 10.1093/nar/gkt380

DeVore, N. M., and Scott, E. E. (2012). Structures of cytochrome P450 17A1 with prostate cancer drugs abiraterone and TOK-001. *Nature* 482, 116–119. doi: 10.1038/nature10743

Epps, D. E., and Vosters, A. F. (2002). The essential role of a free sulfhydryl group in blocking the cholesteryl site of cholesteryl ester transfer protein (CETP). *Chem. Phys. Lipids* 114, 113–122. doi: 10.1016/S0009-3084(01)00187-6

Espona-Fiedler, M., Soto-Cerrato, V., Hosseini, A., Lizcano, J. M., Guallar, V., Quesada, R., et al. (2012). Identification of dual mTORC1 and mTORC2 inhibitors in melanoma cells: prodigiosin vs. obatoclax. *Biochem. Pharmacol.* 83, 489–496. doi: 10.1016/j.bcp.2011.11.027

Fernández, A. (2014). Communication: chemical functionality of interfacial water enveloping nanoscale structural defects in proteins. *J. Chem. Phys.* 140:221102. doi: 10.1063/1.4882895

Filipovic, J., Vávra, O., Plhák, J., Bednar, D., Marques, S. M., Brezovsky, J., et al. (2019). CaverDock: a novel method for the fast analysis of ligand transport. *IEEE/ACM Trans. Comput. Biol. Bioinform.* doi: 10.1109/TCBB.2019.2907492. [Epub ahead of print].

Funk, C. D. (2001). Prostaglandins and leukotrienes: advances in eicosanoid biology. *Science* 294, 1871–1875. doi: 10.1126/science.294.5548.1871

Gattis, S. G., Hernick, M., and Fierke, C. A. (2010). Active site metal ion in UDP-3-O-((R)-3-hydroxymyristoyl)-N-acetylglucosamine deacetylase (LpxC) switches between Fe(II) and Zn(II) depending on cellular conditions. *J. Biol. Chem.* 285, 33788–33796. doi: 10.1074/jbc.M110.147173

Gerber, N. C., Rodriguez-Crespo, I., Nishida, C. R., and Ortiz de Montellano, P. R. (1997). Active site topologies and cofactor-mediated conformational changes of nitric-oxide synthases. *J. Biol. Chem.* 272, 6285–6290. doi: 10.1074/jbc.272.10.6285

Goldman, M., Wittelsberger, A., and De Magistris, M.-T. (2013). The innovative medicines initiative moves translational immunology forward. *Eur. J. Immunol.* 43, 298–302. doi: 10.1002/eji.201370024

Gomis-Rüth, F. X., Botelho, T. O., and Bode, W. (2012). A standard orientation for metallopeptidases. *Biochim. Biophys. Acta* 1824, 157–163. doi: 10.1016/j.bbapap.2011.04.014

Guallar, V., Lu, C., Borrelli, K., Egawa, T., and Yeh, S.-R. (2009). Ligand migration in the truncated hemoglobin-II from *Mycobacterium tuberculosis*: the role of G8 tryptophan. *J. Biol. Chem.* 284, 3106–3116. doi: 10.1074/jbc.M806183200

Haeggström, J. Z. (2004). Leukotriene A4 hydrolase/aminopeptidase, the gatekeeper of chemotactic leukotriene B4 biosynthesis. *J. Biol. Chem.* 279, 50639–50642. doi: 10.1074/jbc.R400027200

Haeggström, J. Z., Tholander, F., and Wetterholm, A. (2007). Structure and catalytic mechanisms of leukotriene A4 hydrolase. *Prostaglandins Other Lipid Mediat.* 83, 198–202. doi: 10.1016/j.prostaglandins.2007.01.006

Haeggström, J. Z., Wetterholm, A., Vallee, B. L., and Samuelsson, B. (1990). Leukotriene A4 hydrolase: an epoxide hydrolase with peptidase activity. *Biochem. Biophys. Res. Commun.* 173, 431–437. doi: 10.1016/S0006-291X(05)81076-9

Hanwell, M. D., Curtis, D. E., Lonie, D. C., Vandermeersch, T., Zurek, E., and Hutchison, G. R. (2012). Avogadro: an advanced semantic chemical editor, visualization, and analysis platform. *J. Cheminform.* 4:17. doi: 10.1186/1758-2946-4-17

Hernández-Ortega, A., Borrelli, K., Ferreira, P., Medina, M., Martínez, A. T., and Guallar, V. (2011). Substrate diffusion and oxidation in GMC oxidoreductases: an experimental and computational study on fungal aryl-alcohol oxidase. *Biochem. J.* 436, 341–350. doi: 10.1042/BJ20102090

Huang, Z., Wong, C. F., and Wheeler, R. A. (2008). Flexible protein-flexible ligand docking with disrupted velocity simulated annealing. *Proteins* 71, 440–454. doi: 10.1002/prot.21781

Jarzynski, 1997###Jarzynski, C. (1997). Nonequilibrium equality for free energy differences. *Phys. Rev. Lett.* 78, 2690–2693. doi: 10.1103/PhysRevLett.78.2690

Kabakov, A. E., Kudryavtsev, V. A., and Gabai, V. L. (2010). Hsp90 inhibitors as promising agents for radiotherapy. *J. Mol. Med.* 88, 241–247. doi: 10.1007/s00109-009-0562-0

Kaczor, A. A., Silva, A. G., Loza, M. I., Kolb, P., Castro, M., and Poso, A. (2016). Structure-based virtual screening for dopamine D2 receptor ligands as potential antipsychotics. *ChemMedChem* 11, 718–729. doi: 10.1002/cmdc.201500599

Kansy, M., Senner, F., and Gubernator, K. (1998). Physicochemical high throughput screening: parallel artificial membrane permeation assay in the description of passive absorption processes. *J. Med. Chem.* 41, 1007–1010. doi: 10.1021/jm970530e

Khatri, Y., Gregory, M. C., Grinkova, Y. V., Denisov, I. G., and Sligar, S. G. (2014). Active site proton delivery and the lyase activity of human CYP17A1. *Biochem. Biophys. Res. Commun.* 443, 179–184. doi: 10.1016/j.bbrc.2013.11.094

Kim, S., Thiessen, P. A., Bolton, E. E., Chen, J., Fu, G., Gindulyte, A., et al. (2016). PubChem substance and compound databases. *Nucleic Acids Res.* 44, D1202–D1213. doi: 10.1093/nar/gkv951

Kokh, D. B., Amaral, M., Bomke, J., Grädler, U., Musil, D., Buchstaller, H.-P., et al. (2018). Estimation of drug-target residence times by τ-random acceleration molecular dynamics simulations. *J. Chem. Theory Comput.* 14, 3859–3869. doi: 10.1021/acs.jctc.8b00230

Kollman, P. (1993). Free energy calculations: applications to chemical and biochemical phenomena. *Chem. Rev.* 93, 2395–2417. doi: 10.1021/cr00023a004

Kruse, A. C., Hu, J., Pan, A. C., Arlow, D. H., Rosenbaum, D. M., Rosemond, E., et al. (2012). Structure and dynamics of the M3 muscarinic acetylcholine receptor. *Nature* 482, 552–556. doi: 10.1038/nature10867

Kush, R., and Goldman, M. (2014). Fostering responsible data sharing through standards. *N. Engl. J. Med.* 370, 2163–2165. doi: 10.1056/NEJMp1401444

Lamb, M. L., and Jorgensen, W. L. (1997). Computational approaches to molecular recognition. *Curr. Opin. Chem. Biol.* 1, 449–457. doi: 10.1016/S1367-5931(97)80038-5

Lavecchia, A., and Di Giovanni, C. (2013). Virtual screening strategies in drug discovery: a critical review. *Curr. Med. Chem.* 20, 2839–2860. doi: 10.2174/09298673113209990001

Laverty, H., Gunn, M., and Goldman, M. (2012). Improving RandD productivity of pharmaceutical companies through public-private partnership: experiences from the Innovative Medicines Initiative. *Expert Rev. Pharmacoecon. Outcomes Res.* 12, 545–548. doi: 10.1586/erp.12.59

Law, V., Knox, C., Djoumbou, Y., Jewison, T., Guo, A. C., Liu, Y., et al. (2014). DrugBank 4.0: shedding new light on drug metabolism. *Nucleic Acids Res.* 42, D1091–D1097. doi: 10.1093/nar/gkt1068

Lee, P.-H., Kuo, K.-L., Chu, P.-Y., Liu, E. M., and Lin, J.-H. (2009). SLITHER: a web server for generating contiguous conformations of substrate molecules entering into deep active sites of proteins or migrating through channels in membrane transporters. *Nucleic Acids Res.* 37, W559–W564. doi: 10.1093/nar/gkp359

Li, J., Sun, L., Xu, C., Yu, F., Zhou, H., Zhao, Y., et al. (2012). Structure insights into mechanisms of ATP hydrolysis and the activation of human heat-shock protein 90. *Acta Biochim. Biophys. Sin.* 44, 300–306. doi: 10.1093/abbs/gms001

Lucas, M. F., and Guallar, V. (2012). An atomistic view on human hemoglobin carbon monoxide migration processes. *Biophys. J.* 102, 887–896. doi: 10.1016/j.bpj.2012.01.011

Madadkar-Sobhani, A., and Guallar, V. (2013). PELE web server: atomistic study of biomolecular systems at your fingertips. *Nucleic Acids Res.* 41, W322–W328. doi: 10.1093/nar/gkt454

Mangoni, M., Roccatano, D., and Di Nola, A. (1999). Docking of flexible ligands to flexible receptors in solution by molecular dynamics simulation. *Proteins* 35, 153–162.

Marques, S. M., Daniel, L., Buryska, T., Prokop, Z., Brezovsky, J., and Damborsky, J. (2017). Enzyme tunnels and gates as relevant targets in drug design. *Med. Res. Rev.* 37, 1095–1139. doi: 10.1002/med.21430

Morris, G. M., Huey, R., Lindstrom, W., Sanner, M. F., Belew, R. K., Goodsell, D. S., et al. (2009). AutoDock4 and AutoDockTools4: automated docking with selective receptor flexibility. *J. Comput. Chem.* 30, 2785–2791. doi: 10.1002/jcc.21256

Pagadala, N. S., Syed, K., and Tuszynski, J. (2017). Software for molecular docking: a review. *Biophys. Rev.* 9, 91–102. doi: 10.1007/s12551-016-0247-1

Ripphausen, P., Nisius, B., Peltason, L., and Bajorath, J. (2010). Quo vadis, virtual screening? A comprehensive survey of prospective applications. *J. Med. Chem.* 53, 8461–8467. doi: 10.1021/jm101020z

Rudberg, P. C., Tholander, F., Thunnissen, M. M. G. M., and Haeggström, J. Z. (2002). Leukotriene A4 hydrolase/aminopeptidase. Glutamate 271 is a catalytic residue with specific roles in two distinct enzyme mechanisms. *J. Biol. Chem.* 277, 1398–1404. doi: 10.1074/jbc.M106577200

Sanson, B., Colletier, J.-P., Xu, Y., Lang, P. T., Jiang, H., Silman, I., et al. (2011). Backdoor opening mechanism in acetylcholinesterase based on X-ray crystallography and molecular dynamics simulations. *Protein Sci.* 20, 1114–1118. doi: 10.1002/pro.661

Singh, S. P., and Konwar, B. K. (2012). Molecular docking studies of quercetin and its analogues against human inducible nitric oxide synthase. *Springerplus* 1:69. doi: 10.1186/2193-1801-1-69

Sousa, S. F., Cerqueira, N. M., Fernandes, P. A., and Ramos, M. J. (2010). Virtual screening in drug design and development. *Comb. Chem. High Throughput Screen.* 13, 442–453. doi: 10.2174/138620710791293001

Sterling, T., and Irwin, J. J. (2015). ZINC 15 – ligand discovery for everyone. *J. Chem. Inf. Model.* 55, 2324–2337. doi: 10.1021/acs.jcim.5b00559

Straatsma, T. P., and McCammon, J. A. (1992). Computational alchemy. *Annu. Rev. Phys. Chem.* 43, 407–435. doi: 10.1146/annurev.pc.43.100192.002203

Stsiapanava, A., Olsson, U., Wan, M., Kleinschmidt, T., Rutishauser, D., Zubarev, R. A., et al. (2014). Binding of Pro-Gly-Pro at the active site of leukotriene A4 hydrolase/aminopeptidase and development of an epoxide hydrolase selective inhibitor. *PNAS* 111, 4227–4232. doi: 10.1073/pnas.1402136111

Szul, T., Castaldi, P., Cho, M. H., Blalock, J. E., and Gaggar, A. (2016). Genetic regulation of expression of leukotriene A4 hydrolase. *ERJ Open Res.* 2:00058-2015. doi: 10.1183/23120541.00058-2015

Thunnissen, M. M., Nordlund, P., and Haeggström, J. Z. (2001). Crystal structure of human leukotriene A(4) hydrolase, a bifunctional enzyme in inflammation. *Nat. Struct. Biol.* 8, 131–135. doi: 10.1038/84117

Tomić, A., Berynskyy, M., Wade, R. C., and Tomić, S. (2015). Molecular simulations reveal that the long range fluctuations of human DPP III change upon ligand binding. *Mol. Biosyst.* 11, 3068–3080. doi: 10.1039/C5MB00465A

Totrov, M., and Abagyan, R. (2008). Flexible ligand docking to multiple receptor conformations: a practical alternative. *Curr. Opin. Struct. Biol.* 18, 178–184. doi: 10.1016/j.sbi.2008.01.004

Trott, O., and Olson, A. J. (2010). AutoDock Vina: improving the speed and accuracy of docking with a new scoring function, efficient optimization and multithreading. *J. Comput. Chem.* 31, 455–461. doi: 10.1002/jcc.21334

Vavra, O., Filipovic, J., Plhak, J., Bednar, D., Marques, S. M., Brezovsky, J., et al. (2019). CaverDock: a molecular docking-based tool to analyse ligand transport through protein tunnels and channels. *Bioinformatics* btz386. doi: 10.1093/bioinformatics/btz386. [Epub ahead of print].

Wang, S., Ma, J., Peng, J., and Xu, J. (2013). Protein structure alignment beyond spatial proximity. *Sci. Rep.* 3:1448. doi: 10.1038/srep01448

Yoshimoto, F. K., and Auchus, R. J. (2015). The diverse chemistry of cytochrome P450 17A1 (P450c17, CYP17A1). *J. Steroid Biochem. Mol. Biol.* 151, 52–65. doi: 10.1016/j.jsbmb.2014.11.026

Yu, X., Cojocaru, V., and Wade, R. C. (2013). Conformational diversity and ligand tunnels of mammalian cytochrome P450s. *Biotechnol. Appl. Biochem.* 60, 134–145. doi: 10.1002/bab.1074

Zhang, J. H., Chung, T. D., and Oldenburg, K. R. (1999). A simple statistical parameter for use in evaluation and validation of high throughput screening assays. *J. Biomol. Screen.* 4, 67–73. doi: 10.1177/108705719900400206

Zhang, T., Ozbil, M., Barman, A., Paul, T. J., Bora, R. P., and Prabhakar, R. (2015). Theoretical insights into the functioning of metallopeptidases and their synthetic analogues. *Acc. Chem. Res.* 48, 192–200. doi: 10.1021/ar500301y

7

Structure-Based and Molecular Modeling Studies for the Discovery of Cyclic Imides as Reversible Cruzain Inhibitors with Potent Anti-*Trypanosoma cruzi* Activity

Rafael A. A. Ferreira [1†], *Ivani Pauli* [2†], *Thiago S. Sampaio* [1], *Mariana L. de Souza* [2], *Leonardo L. G. Ferreira* [2], *Luma G. Magalhães* [2], *Celso de O. Rezende Jr.* [1], *Rafaela S. Ferreira* [3], *Renata Krogh* [2], *Luiz C. Dias* [1*] *and Adriano D. Andricopulo* [2*]

[1] *Instituto de Química, Universidade Estadual de Campinas, Campinas, Brazil,* [2] *Laboratório de Química Medicinal e Computacional, Centro de Pesquisa e Inovação em Biodiversidade e Fármacos, Instituto de Física de São Carlos, Universidade de São Paulo, São Carlos, Brazil,* [3] *Departamento de Bioquímica e Imunologia, Universidade Federal de Minas Gerais, Belo Horizonte, Brazil*

***Correspondence:**
Luiz C. Dias
ldias@unicamp.br
Adriano D. Andricopulo
aandrico@ifsc.usp.br

† *These authors have contributed equally to this work*

Chagas disease causes ~10,000 deaths each year, mainly in Latin America, where it is endemic. The currently available chemotherapeutic agents are ineffective in the chronic stage of the disease, and the lack of pharmaceutical innovation for Chagas disease highlights the urgent need for the development of new drugs. The enzyme cruzain, the main cysteine protease of *Trypanosoma cruzi*, has been explored as a validated molecular target for drug discovery. Herein, the design, molecular modeling studies, synthesis, and biological evaluation of cyclic imides as cruzain inhibitors are described. Starting with a micromolar-range cruzain inhibitor (**3a**, IC_{50} = 2.2 µM), this molecular optimization strategy resulted in the nanomolar-range inhibitor **10j** (IC_{50} = 0.6 µM), which is highly active against *T. cruzi* intracellular amastigotes (IC_{50} = 1.0 µM). Moreover, most compounds were selective toward *T. cruzi* over human fibroblasts, which were used as host cells, and are less toxic to hepatic cells than the marketed drug benznidazole. This study enabled the discovery of novel chemical diversity and established robust structure-activity relationships to guide the design of optimized cruzain inhibitors as new trypanocidal agents.

Keywords: Chagas disease, *Trypanosoma cruzi*, cruzain, SAR, medicinal chemistry, synthesis, inhibitors, molecular docking

INTRODUCTION

Caused by the protozoan *Trypanosoma cruzi* and endemic in 21 countries in Latin America, Chagas disease kills ~10,000 people each year[1]. This neglected tropical disease has reached non-endemic regions, affecting 8 million people worldwide and putting another 25 million at risk of infection[1]. The USA shows the greatest burden among non-endemic countries, with ~300,000 people estimated to be infected with *T. cruzi* (Pérez-Molina and Molina, 2018). In addition, Chagas disease is a major cause of infectious cardiomyopathy worldwide, contributing substantially to the global burden of cardiovascular disease (Bern, 2015; Cucunubá et al., 2016). Mortality and a

[1]https://www.who.int/chagas/en/

reduction in productivity of the affected populations significantly impact the economies of the endemic regions. These economic and social burdens can be translated in numbers that estimate losses of more than US $7.2 billion per year and ~243,600 disability-adjusted life years (DALYs) due to Chagas disease (GBD DALYs and HALE Collaborators, 2016; Arnal et al., 2019).

Even more than a century after the discovery of Chagas disease by Brazilian physician Carlos Chagas in 1909, current chemotherapy for this condition relies on two drugs only—benznidazole (**BZ**) and nifurtimox (Dias et al., 2014). These nitroheterocyclic compounds, which were identified between the mid-1960s and 1970s, are effective only when administered during the acute stage of the disease, a limitation that leaves millions of chronic chagasic patients without appropriate treatment (Molina et al., 2015). Moreover, benznidazole and nifurtimox cause severe adverse effects in up to 40% of patients, leading to poor adherence to treatment (Pérez-Molina and Molina, 2018). These drawbacks highlight the urgent need for the development of effective and safe drugs for the therapy of Chagas disease (Olivera et al., 2015; Ferreira and Andricopulo, 2019).

The enzyme cruzain (EC 3.4.22.51) is the main cysteine protease of *T. cruzi* and has been explored as a validated molecular target in Chagas disease drug discovery (McKerrow, 1999; Jose Cazzulo et al., 2001). It is expressed throughout the life cycle of *T. cruzi* and is involved in critical biological processes such as the interaction with host cells, parasite reproduction and evasion from the host immunologic system (Engel et al., 1998; Ferreira and Andricopulo, 2017). Cruzain has been validated as a molecular target for Chagas disease drug discovery based on genetic studies of *T. cruzi* and the ability of cruzain inhibitors to decrease parasite burden *in vivo* (Doyle et al., 2011; Ndao et al., 2014). These studies have recently supported the design and identification of several classes of cruzain inhibitors, including vinyl sulfones, triazoles, pyrimidines, thiosemicarbazones, chalcones, nitroalkenes, and benzimidazoles (Rogers et al., 2012; Ferreira et al., 2014; Avelar et al., 2015; Espíndola et al., 2015; Neitz et al., 2015; Latorre et al., 2016). The vinyl sulfone K777, which is a covalent cruzain inhibitor, showed promising results in preclinical efficacy tests; however, toxicity-related drawbacks prevented the compound from progressing into advanced clinical development (Ndao et al., 2014). The poor safety profile of K777 was associated with the irreversible mode of action of the compound. Following the failure of K777, the pursuit of novel cruzain inhibitors has recently focused on the design of reversible ligands. These investigations, along with the available structural data of cruzain bound with small molecule ligands, have been key to promoting the discovery of novel classes of inhibitors with improved safety profiles. Moreover, these data have enabled the integration of experimental and computational approaches into robust structure-based drug design (SBDD) campaigns that have been key to identifying novel chemical diversity to be explored in Chagas disease drug discovery.

MATERIALS AND METHODS

Molecular Docking

The three-dimensional structures of the designed cruzain inhibitors were constructed using the standard geometric parameters of SYBYL-X 2.1 (Certara, Princeton, NJ). Each compound was energetically minimized using the Tripos force field (Clark et al., 1989) and Powell conjugate gradient algorithm (Powell, 1977) with a convergence criterion of 0.05 kcal/mol.Å and Gasteiger-Hückel charges (Gasteiger and Marsili, 1980). The designed imide derivatives were docked into the cruzain catalytic site using GOLD 5.3 (Cambridge Crystallographic Data Centre, Cambridge, UK) (Jones et al., 1997). The X-ray structure of cruzain (PDB 3KKU, 1.28 Å) (Ferreira et al., 2010) was prepared by removing the water molecules and adding hydrogen atoms. The active site residues Cys25 and His162 were maintained as negatively charged and protonated, respectively. A sphere with a 10 Å radius centered on the sulfur atom of Cys25 was settled as the binding site. Compounds were docked by applying the GoldScore scoring function with a search efficiency of 200%. Visual analysis of the molecular docking-derived binding conformations was carried out with PyMOL 1.3 (Schrödinger, New York, NY) (Lill and Danielson, 2011).

Pro-Cruzain Expression, Activation, and Purification

Cruzain was expressed and purified using a modified version of a previously published protocol (Ferreira et al., 2014). *Escherichia coli* (M15) was preinoculated in Luria Bertani (LB) medium with ampicillin (100 µg/mL) and kanamycin (50 µg/mL) and kept overnight (37°C, 200 rpm). The preinoculum was diluted 10-fold in fresh LB medium (1 L) supplemented with 0.5 M NaCl, 0.2% glucose, 1 mM betaine, 0.5 M sorbitol, 100 µg/mL ampicillin and 50 µg/mL kanamycin, and incubated (37°C, 200 rpm). When the optical density (OD_{600}) reached 0.9, the culture was incubated at 47°C for 20 min to induce the expression of chaperones. Next, cruzain expression was induced by adding 0.2 mM isopropyl β-D-thiogalactopyranoside (IPTG), and the culture was kept overnight at 20°C. The cells were harvested by centrifugation (5,000 rpm, 30 min, 4°C) and suspended in 50 mL of lysis buffer (300 mM NaCl, 50 mM Tris-HCl, 1.6 mg/mL lysozyme, pH 8.0). The cells were then lysed by sonication (12 cycles of 30 s), and the suspension was centrifuged (9,000 rpm, 30 min, 4°C). The supernatant was collected, cruzain was precipitated by the addition of 35% ammonium sulfate (2 h), and this suspension was centrifuged (9,000 rpm, 30 min, 4°C). The precipitate was resuspended in lysis buffer and dialyzed to remove the ammonium sulfate. The soluble fraction of cruzain was purified by metal affinity chromatography using a Ni–NTA resin (Qiagen, Hilden, Germany). Contaminant proteins were removed using a washing buffer (300 mM NaCl, 50 mM Tris-HCl, 10 mM imidazole, pH 8.0). Next, cruzain was eluted with an increasing gradient of imidazole (25, 50, 75, 100, and 250 mM). The fractions containing cruzain were dialyzed in 0.1 M acetate buffer (1.5 L, pH 5.5) and concentrated to 0.5 mg/mL for subsequent activation.

Pro-cruzain was incubated in activation buffer (100 mM sodium acetate, 10 mM EDTA, 5 mM DTT, and 1 M NaCl, pH 5.5) at 37°C (Mott et al., 2010). The activation process was monitored at 30 min intervals by the cleavage of the substrate Z-Phe-Arg-AMC and confirmed by SDS-PAGE. Next, the mature enzyme was diluted 20-fold in binding buffer (20 mM sodium phosphate, 150 mM NaCl, pH 7.2) and incubated overnight with thiopropyl Sepharose 6B resin (GE Healthcare Life Sciences, Pittsburgh, PA) at 4°C. Cruzain was eluted using binding buffer supplemented with 20 mM DTT. Fractions containing the enzyme were stored at −80°C in 0.1 M sodium acetate (pH 5.5).

Cruzain Inhibition Assays

The catalytic activity of cruzain was monitored by cleavage of the fluorogenic substrate Z-Phe-Arg-aminomethyl coumarin (Z-Phe-Arg-AMC) as previously described (Ferreira et al., 2014). The enzyme kinetics assays were performed in 0.1 M sodium acetate buffer (pH 5.5) with 5 mM dithiothreitol (DTT) and 0.01% Triton X-100. The final concentrations of cruzain and substrate ($K_m = 1.6\,\mu M$) were 1.5 nM and 5.0 μM, respectively, except in the tests for the mechanism of inhibition, in which different substrate concentrations were used. The enzyme reaction was monitored for 5 min at 30°C in 96-well black flat bottom plates, and the activity was calculated based on the initial rates compared with a control (DMSO). Wavelengths of 355 nm for excitation and 460 nm for emission were used. IC_{50} values were independently determined by determining rate measurements for at least six inhibitor concentrations, each evaluated in triplicate. To determine the mechanism of inhibition, eight substrate concentrations and four inhibitor concentrations were used, each in triplicate. The mechanism of inhibition was determined by Lineweaver-Burk plots. SigmaPlot 10.0 (Systat Software Inc., Erkrath, Germany) was used to determine the IC_{50} values.

T. cruzi Intracellular Amastigote Assays

In vitro assays against *T. cruzi* were performed as described previously (Ferreira et al., 2014). The *T. cruzi* Tulahuen strain, which expresses the *E. coli* β-galactosidase gene *lacZ* (Buckner et al., 1996), was provided by Frederick S. Buckner (University of Washington, Seattle, WA). Stock solutions of the synthesized compounds were prepared in 100% DMSO. Epimastigotes were grown in liver infusion tryptone (LIT) supplemented with 10% fetal calf serum (FCS), penicillin and streptomycin (28°C). Metacyclogenesis from epimastigotes to trypomastigotes was induced by incubation of the epimastigotes in Grace's insect medium (Sigma-Aldrich, St. Louis, MO) supplemented with 10% FCS (28°C). HFF-1 human fibroblasts were seeded at 2×10^3/well (80 μL) in 96-well tissue culture plates in RPMI 1640 without phenol red supplemented with 10% FCS and incubated overnight (37°C, 5% CO_2). Next, trypomastigotes were added at 1.0×10^4/well (20 μL), and the plates were incubated (37°C, 5% CO_2). After 24 h, 3-fold serial dilutions (50 μL) of the synthesized compounds were added at concentrations ranging from 0.1 to 100 μM, and the plates were incubated (37°C, 5% CO_2). Each compound concentration was evaluated in triplicate. All plates included **BZ** (Sigma-Aldrich) as a positive control and untreated wells (100% growth) as a negative control. After 120 h, 50 μL of chlorophenol red β-D-galactopyranoside (CPRG, Sigma-Aldrich) and IGEPAL CA-630 (Sigma-Aldrich) (0.1%) was added to each well. The absorbance was measured at 570 nm in an automated microplate reader, and the data were transferred to SigmaPlot 10.0 (Systat Software Inc.) for IC_{50} value calculation.

Cytotoxicity in HFF-1 and HepG2 Cell Lines

The cytotoxicities of the compounds against HFF-1 fibroblasts and HepG2 hepatocytes were evaluated using the MTS tetrazolium assay (Promega, Madison, WI) (Barltrop et al., 1991). HFF-1 fibroblasts were seeded at 2×10^3/well in 96-well culture plates in RPMI 1640 without phenol red supplemented with 10% FCS and incubated overnight (37°C, 5% CO_2). HepG2 hepatocytes were seeded at 6×10^3/well in 96-well culture plates in DMEM (Cultilab, Campinas SP) supplemented with 10% FCS and incubated overnight (37°C, 5% CO_2). The compounds were added in 3-fold serial dilutions, and the plates were incubated at 37°C with 5% CO_2. Each compound concentration was evaluated in triplicate. All plates included doxorubicin (Sigma-Aldrich, St. Louis, MO) as a positive control and untreated wells (100% growth) as a negative control. After 72 h, 20 μL of MTS was added, and the plates were incubated for 4 h. The absorbance was measured at 490 nm in an automated microplate reader, and the data were transferred to SigmaPlot 10.0 (Systat Software Inc., Erkrath, Germany) for IC_{50} value calculation. The percent of nonviable cells was determined and compared to the negative control wells (100% growth).

Chemistry

All reactions were performed under an argon atmosphere with dry solvents and magnetic stirring unless stated otherwise. Dichloromethane (DCM) and triethylamine (Et_3N) were distilled from CaH_2. Tetrahydrofuran (THF) was distilled from sodium/benzophenone. Dimethyl formamide (DMF) was purchased from Sigma-Aldrich (anhydrous) and used without further purification. Yields refer to homogeneous materials obtained after purification of the reaction products by flash column chromatography using silica gel (200–400 mesh) or recrystallization. Analytical thin-layer chromatography was performed on silica-gel 60 and GF (5–40 μm thickness) plates, and visualization was accomplished using UV light, basic potassium permanganate staining or ninhydrin solution followed by heating. ^{1}H and proton-decoupled ^{13}C NMR spectra were acquired in $CDCl_3$, CD_3OD, or d_6-DMSO at 250 MHz (^{1}H) and 62.5 MHz (^{13}C) (Bruker DPX250), at 400 MHz (^{1}H) and 100 MHz (^{13}C) (Bruker Avance 400), at 500 MHz (^{1}H) and 125 MHz (^{13}C) (Varian Inova 500), or at 600 MHz (^{1}H) and 150 MHz (^{13}C) (Bruker Avance 600). Chemical shifts (δ) are reported in ppm using residual undeuterated solvent as an internal standard ($CDCl_3$ at 7.26 ppm, CD_3OD at 3.31 ppm, d_6-DMSO at 2.50 ppm, and TMS at 0.00 ppm for ^{1}H NMR spectra and $CDCl_3$ at 77.16 ppm, CD_3OD at 49.0 ppm, d_6-DMSO at 39.52 ppm for ^{13}C NMR spectra). Multiplicity data are reported as follows: s = singlet, d = doublet, t = triplet, q = quartet, br s = broad singlet, dd = doublet of doublets, dt = doublet of triplets, ddd = doublet of doublet of doublets and m = multiplet. The multiplicity is followed by the coupling constant(s) in Hz and integration. High-resolution mass spectrometry (HRMS) was measured using electrospray ionization (ESI) (Waters Xevo Q-TOF, Thermo LTQ-FT Ultra, or Thermo Q-Exactive) or electron ionization (EI) (GCT Premier, Waters).

General Procedures for the Preparation of Alcohols 2a-m

Method A: The aniline derivative containing the appropriate substituents was dissolved in dry dichloromethane (DCM) under an argon atmosphere with magnetic stirring. The solution was cooled to 0°C followed by the slow addition of acetoxyacetyl chloride (1.1 equivalents). The mixture was stirred for 5 min before the addition of zinc mesh 20 (0.1 equivalents) and removal of the ice bath, allowing the reaction to reach room temperature. The reaction mixture was monitored by thin layer chromatography (TLC), and after 30 min, total conversion was observed. Half of the initial volume of DCM was added to dilute the reaction mixture, and the zinc was removed by filtration. The supernatant was washed with an aqueous sodium bicarbonate solution. The organic phase was dried over magnesium sulfate ($MgSO_4$) and concentrated to dryness under vacuum. The product was purified by column chromatography on silica gel using a mixture of ethyl acetate/hexanes (50%) as the eluent. The obtained ester was dissolved in methanol at room temperature followed by the addition of solid potassium carbonate (K_2CO_3). The reaction mixture was stirred for 1 h and then quenched by the addition of ethyl acetate. The mixture was washed with aqueous saturated ammonium chloride (NH_4Cl) solution and brine. The resulting organic phase was dried over $MgSO_4$ and concentrated under reduced pressure. Purification was performed by column chromatography on silica gel using a mixture of ethyl acetate/hexanes (50%) as the eluent.

Method B: The aniline derivative containing the appropriate substituents was dissolved in dry DCM under an argon atmosphere with magnetic stirring. To the resulting solution, dry triethylamine (1.1 equivalents) and acetoxyacetyl chloride (1.1 equivalents) were added and stirring was maintained for 2 h to monitor the conversion by TLC. The mixture was then washed with saturated aqueous NH_4Cl solution and brine solution. The organic phase was dried over $MgSO_4$ and concentrated to dryness under vacuum. The obtained ester was dissolved in methanol at room temperature followed by the addition of solid potassium carbonate (K_2CO_3). The reaction mixture was stirred for 1 h and then quenched by the addition of ethyl acetate. The mixture was washed with aqueous saturated ammonium chloride (NH_4Cl) solution and brine. The resulting organic phase was dried over $MgSO_4$ and concentrated under reduced pressure. Purification was performed by column chromatography on silica gel using a mixture of ethyl acetate/hexanes (50%) as the eluent.

General Procedures for Production of Carboxylic Acids 1 and 9a-n

Method C: The appropriate cyclic anhydride and amino acid (1.1 equivalents) were dissolved in glacial acetic acid under an argon atmosphere. The mixture was magnetically stirred overnight followed by 4 h of reflux periodically monitored by TLC. After consumption of the cyclic anhydride, the reaction pot was cooled to room temperature. Acetic acid was removed in a rotary evaporator, and ice-cold water was added to the resulting slurry to generate a precipitate. Concentrated hydrochloric acid (HCl) was added, and the solid was collected by filtration, followed by high vacuum drying.

Method D: The appropriate cyclic anhydride and amino acid (1.1 equivalents) were added to a reaction flask containing toluene. To this suspension, TEA (0.1 equivalents) was added and a Dean-Stark apparatus was coupled to the system. The mixture refluxed for 4 h and cooled to room temperature. Toluene was removed in a rotary evaporator, and the residue was dissolved in ethyl acetate and washed twice with 1 M HCl. The organic phase was extracted with saturated aqueous sodium bicarbonate solution. The aqueous phase was acidified with HCl solution to pH 5.0 and extracted with ethyl acetate. The combined organic phases were dried over $MgSO_4$, concentrated under vacuum and used in the following step without further purification.

Method E: Leucine was dissolved in a 1:1 mixture of hydrobromic acid and water in an ice bath. Sodium nitrite (6.5 M aqueous solution) was added dropwise. The ice bath was removed, and the solution stirred at room temperature for 2.5 h. The acidic residues were removed under reduced pressure, and the remaining solution was extracted with diethyl ether 3 times. The combined organic phases were dried over $MgSO_4$ and concentrated under vacuum.

The residue was dissolved in DCM under an argon atmosphere. The solution was cooled in an ice bath and benzyl alcohol (1.1 equivalents), 1-ethyl-3-(3-dimethylaminopropyl) carbodiimide (EDC) (1.1 equivalents) and 4-dimethylaminopyridine (DMAP) (0.1 equivalents) were added. The ice bath was removed, and the mixture stirred for 5 h. Then, the reaction mixture was washed with saturated aqueous NH_4Cl solution and brine. The organic phase was dried over $MgSO_4$ and concentrated under vacuum. The product was purified by column chromatography on silica gel using a mixture of ethyl acetate/hexanes (50%) as the eluent.

A solution of the pure ester was prepared in acetonitrile under an argon atmosphere, and the appropriate cyclic amine was added (2.0 equivalents). To the resulting solution, cesium carbonate (1.1 equivalents) was added followed by stirring for 2 h. The solids were removed by filtration, and the solvent was removed under reduced pressure followed by redissolution in DCM and washing with water. The organic phase was dried over $MgSO_4$ and concentrated to dryness under vacuum. The product was purified by column chromatography on silica gel using a gradient from 0 to 4% methanol in DCM as the eluent.

The ester was dissolved in methanol, and 10% Pd/C was added (0.1 equivalents). The mixture stirred at room temperature under a hydrogen atmosphere (1 atm) for 30 min. The catalyst was removed by filtration over Celite®, and the solvent removed under reduced pressure to generate the pure carboxylic acid.

General Procedure for the Preparation of Compounds 3a-m and 10a-n

Method F: A solution of carboxylic acid in dry DCM was prepared, and the alcohol was added (1.1 equivalents). The solution was cooled in an ice bath followed by the addition of EDC (1.2 equivalents) and DMAP (0.1 equivalents). The solution was allowed to warm to room temperature and stirred for 4 h while monitoring periodically by TLC. The reaction mixture was washed with saturated aqueous NH_4Cl solution and brine. The organic phase was dried over $MgSO_4$ and concentrated under reduced pressure. The product was purified by column chromatography on silica gel using a mixture of ethyl acetate/hexanes (50%) as the eluent.

2-((3-chloro-4-methoxyphenyl)amino)-2-oxoethyl (2S)-2-(1,3-dioxo-1,3,3a,4,7,7a-hexahydro-2H-isoindol-2-yl)-4-methylpentanoate (3a)

Methods A and C followed by F

Very viscous liquid, 90% ^{1}H NMR (500 MHz, $CDCl_3$) δ 8.26 (sl, 1H); 7.83 (d, *J* = 2.5 Hz, 1H); 7.68 (dd, *J* = 9.0, 2.5 Hz, 1H); 6.90 (d, *J* = 9.0 Hz, 1H); 5.90 (m, 2H); 5.04 (d, *J* = 15.6 Hz, 1H); 4.88 (dd, *J* = 11.0, 4.4 Hz, 1H); 4.40 (d, *J* = 15.6 Hz, 1H); 3.89 (s, 3H); 3.23 (m, 2H); 2.65 (m, 2H); 2.27 (m, 2H); 2.08 (m, 1H); 1.94 (m, 1H); 1.41 (m, 1H); 0.93 (d, *J* = 6.6 Hz, 6H), ^{13}C NMR (125 MHz, $CDCl_3$) δ 180.4; 180.3; 168.1; 164.7; 151.9; 131.1; 127.8; 127.7; 122.3; 122.2; 119.4; 112.1; 63.4; 56.3; 51.0; 39.3; 39.2; 37.2; 24.7; 23.5; 23.4; 23.0; 20.9.

HRMS (ESI-Orbitrap): $[M+H]^+$ Calculated for $C_{23}H_{27}O_6N_2Cl$ 463.1617; found 463.1636.

2-((4-methoxyphenyl)amino)-2-oxoethyl (2S)-2-(1,3-dioxo-1,3,3a,4,7,7a-hexahydro-2H-isoindol-2-yl)-4-methylpentanoate (3b)

Methods B and C followed by F

Very viscous liquid, 88% ^{1}H NMR (250 MHz, DMSO) δ 9.78 (sl, 1H); 7.46 (d, *J* = 9.0 Hz, 1H); 6.89 (d, *J* = 9.0 Hz, 1H); 5.85 (m, 1H); 4.79 (dd, *J* = 11.1, 4.4 Hz, 1H); 4.63 (m, 2H); 3.72 (s, 3H); 3.24 (m, 2H); 2.39 (m, 2H); 2.20 (m, 2H); 1.99 (m, 1H); 1.77 (m, 1H); 1.34 (m, 1H); 0.84 (m, 6H), ^{13}C NMR (62.5 MHz, DMSO) δ 179.6; 179.5; 168.5; 164.3; 155.5; 131.3; 127.4; 120.4; 113.9; 63.4; 55.2; 50.2; 36.0; 24.1; 23.2; 23.0; 20.7.

HRMS (ESI-Orbitrap): $[M+H]^+$ Calculated for $C_{23}H_{28}O_6N_2$ 429.2026; found 429.2039.

2-((3-chlorophenyl)amino)-2-oxoethyl (2S)-2-(1,3-dioxo-1,3,3a,4,7,7a-hexahydro-2H-isoindol-2-yl)-4-methylpentanoate (3c)

Methods B and C followed by F

Very viscous liquid, 91% ^{1}H NMR (250 MHz, DMSO) δ 10.15 (m, 1H); 7.77 (m, 1H); 7.44 (m, 1H); 7.33 (m, 1H); 7.11 (m, 1H); 5.84 (m, 2H); 5.03 (m, 1H); 4.67 (m, 2H); 3,59 (m, 2H); 3.23 (m, 1H); 2.43 (m, 3H); 2.19 (m, 2H); 1.97 (m, 1H); 1.75 (m, 1H); 1.34 (m, 1H); 0.83 (m, 6H). ^{13}C NMR (62.5 MHz, DMSO) δ 179.6; 179.5; 179.4; 173.3; 173.2; 172.4; 169.2; 168.6; 165.7; 165.2; 139.8; 139.7; 133.2; 130.5; 127.5; 127.4; 125.0; 124.9; 123.4; 123.3; 118.8; 117.7; 63.4; 62.7; 52.3; 51.6; 51.5; 50.3; 50.2; 38.4; 36.1; 36.0; 25.3; 24.2; 24.1; 23.2; 23.1; 23.0; 20.7.

HRMS (ESI-Orbitrap): $[M+Na]^+$ Calculated for $C_{22}H_{25}O_5N_2ClNa$ 455.1350; found 455.1362.

2-oxo-2-(phenylamino)ethyl (2S)-2-(1,3-dioxo-1,3,3a,4,7,7a-hexahydro-2H-isoindol-2-yl)-4-methylpentanoate (3d)

Methods B and C followed by F

Very viscous liquid, 78% ^{1}H NMR (400 MHz, DMSO) δ 9.97 (s, 1H); 7.55 (m, 2H); 7.32 (m, 2H); 7.07 (m, 1H); 5.85 (m,2H); 4.79 (dd, *J* = 11.2, 4.4 Hz, 1H); 4.67 (m, 2H); 3.25 (m, 2H); 2.39 (m, 2H); 2.20 (dd, *J* = 14.9, 7.2 Hz, 2H); 2.03 (m, 1H); 1.77 (ddd, *J* = 14.2, 10.1, 4.5 Hz, 1H); 1.35 (m, 1H); 0.84 (dd, *J* = 7.6, 6.6 Hz, 6H). ^{13}C NMR (100 MHz, DMSO) δ 179.6; 168.5; 164.8; 138.2; 128.8; 127.4; 123.7; 119.3; 63.4; 50.2; 38.4; 36.0; 24.1; 23.2; 23.0; 20.7.

2-((4-fluorophenyl)amino)-2-oxoethyl (2S)-2-(1,3-dioxo-1,3,3a,4,7,7a-hexahydro-2H-isoindol-2-yl)-4-methylpentanoate (3e)

Methods B and C followed by F

Very viscous liquid, 82% ^{1}H NMR (250 MHz, DMSO) δ 10.02 (s, 1H); 7.56 (dd, *J* = 8.6, 5.0 Hz, 2H); 7.15 (t, *J* = 8.6 Hz, 2H); 5.84 (m, 2H); 4.79 (dd, *J* = 10.9, 4.3 Hz, 1H); 4.65 (m, 2H); 3.24 (m, 2H); 2.43 (m, 2H); 2.20 (m, 2H); 2.02 (m, 1H); 1.76 (m, 1H); 1.35 (m, 1H); 0.84 (m, 6H).

HRMS (ESI-Orbitrap): $[M+H]^+$ Calculated for $C_{22}H_{25}O_5N_2F$ 417.1826; found 417.1817.

2-((4-bromophenyl)amino)-2-oxoethyl (2S)-2-(1,3-dioxo-1,3,3a,4,7,7a-hexahydro-2H-isoindol-2-yl)-4-methylpentanoate (3f)

Methods B and C followed by F

Very viscous liquid, 84% ^{1}H NMR (250 MHz, DMSO) δ 10.13 (s, 1H); 7.53 (m, 4H); 5.84 (m, 2H); 4.78 (dd, *J* = 11.1, 4.5 Hz, 1H); 4.66 (m, 2H); 3.27 (m, 2H); 2.39 (m, 2H); 2.19 (m, 2H); 2.02 (m, 1H); 1.76 (m, 1H); 1.33 (m, 1H); 0.83 (m, 6H). ^{13}C NMR (62.5 MHz, DMSO) δ 179.7; 179.6; 168.6; 165.0; 137.7; 131.7; 127.6; 127.5; 121.3; 115.4; 63.4; 50.3; 36.0; 24.1; 23.2; 23.1; 20.8.

HRMS (ESI-Orbitrap): $[M+K]^+$ Calculated for $C_{22}H_{25}O_5N_2BrK$ 515.0577; found 515.0584.

2-((4-chlorophenyl)amino)-2-oxoethyl (2S)-2-(1,3-dioxo-1,3,3a,4,7,7a-hexahydro-2H-isoindol-2-yl)-4-methylpentanoate (3g)

Methods B and C followed by F

Very viscous liquid, 75% ^{1}H NMR (500 MHz, DMSO) δ 10.13 (s, 1H); 7.59 (m, 2H); 7.37 (m, 2H); 5.84 (m, 2H); 4.79 (dd, *J* = 11.2, 4.5 Hz, 1H); 4.67 (m, 2H); 3.24 (m, 2H); 2.39 (m, 2H); 2.20 (dd, *J* = 14.9, 7.4 Hz, 2H); 2.02 (m, 1H); 1.76 (ddd, *J* = 14.2, 10.1, 4.5 Hz, 1H); 1.35 (m, 1H); 0.84 (dd, *J* = 9.8, 6.7 Hz, 6H). ^{13}C NMR (125 MHz, DMSO) δ 179.6; 179.5; 168.5; 165.0; 137.2; 128.8; 127.5; 127.4; 127.3; 120.9; 63.4; 50.2; 38.5; 36.0; 24.1; 23.2; 23.0; 20.7.

HRMS (ESI-Orbitrap): $[M+H]^+$ Calculated for $C_{22}H_{26}O_5N_2Cl$ 433.1530; found 433.1507.

2-((4-hydroxyphenyl)amino)-2-oxoethyl (2S)-2-(1,3-dioxo-1,3,3a,4,7,7a-hexahydro-2H-isoindol-2-yl)-4-methylpentanoate (3h)

Methods B and C followed by F

Very viscous liquid, 84% ^{1}H NMR (250 MHz, DMSO) δ 10.05 (s, 1H); 7.57 (d, J = 8.8 Hz, 1H); 6.98 (d, J = 8.8 Hz, 1H); 5.80 (m, 2H); 4.88 (m, 1H); 4.66 (m, 1H); 3.24 (m, 1H); 2.40 (m, 2H); 2.19 (m, 2H); 1.98 (m, 1H); 1.77 (m, 1H); 1.35 (m, 1H); 0.85 (m, 6H).

2-(naphthalen-2-ylamino)-2-oxoethyl (2S)-2-(1,3-dioxo-1,3,3a,4,7,7a-hexahydro-2H-isoindol-2-yl)-4-methylpentanoate (3i)

Methods B and C followed by F

Very viscous liquid, 68% ^{1}H NMR (250 MHz, DMSO) δ 8.43 (s, 2H); 7.80 (m, 4H); 7.45 (m, 2H); 5.91 (m, 2H); 5.13 (d, J = 15.5 Hz, 1H); 4.92 (dd, J = 10.8, 4.5 Hz, 1H); 4.47 (d, J = 15.5 Hz, 1H); 3.23 (m, 2H); 2.68 (m, 2H); 2.22 (m, 3H); 1.97 (m, 1H); 0.95 (d, J = 6.5 Hz, 6H).

HRMS (ESI-Orbitrap): $[M+Na]^+$ Calculated for $C_{26}H_{28}O_5N_2Na$ 471.18959; found 471.18888.

2-((4-fluoro-3-nitrophenyl)amino)-2-oxoethyl (2S)-2-(1,3-dioxo-1,3,3a,4,7,7a-hexahydro-2H-isoindol-2-yl)-4-methylpentanoate (3j)

Methods A and C followed by F

Very viscous liquid, 84% ^{1}H NMR (400 MHz, $CDCl_3$) δ 8.72 (sl, 1H); 8.56 (dd, J = 6.6, 2.7 Hz, 1H); 8.20 (m, 1H); 7.27 (m, 1H); 5.92 (m, 2H); 5.07 (d, J = 15.8 Hz, 1H); 4.90 (dd, J = 10.7, 4.6 Hz, 1H); 4.46 (d, J = 15.7 Hz, 1H); 3.26 (m, 2H); 2.67 (m, 2H); 2.31 (m, 2H); 1.99 (m, 2H); 1.41 (m, 1H); 0.93 (d, J = 6.4 Hz, 6H), ^{13}C NMR (100 MHz, $CDCl_3$) δ 180.7; 180.5; 153.1; 150.5; 137.1; 137.0; 134.3; 134.2; 127.8; 127.6; 126.7; 126.6; 118.7; 118.5; 117.00; 116.97; 63.3; 51.1; 39.4; 39.3; 37.4; 29.6; 24.7; 23.6; 23.5; 23.0; 21.0.

HRMS (ESI-Orbitrap): $[M+Na]^+$ Calculated for $C_{22}H_{24}O_7N_3FNa$ 484.14095; found 484.14483.

2-((4-((tert-butoxycarbonyl)(methyl)amino)phenyl)amino)-2-oxoethyl (2S)-2-(1,3-dioxo-1,3,3a,4,7,7a-hexahydro-2H-isoindol-2-yl)-4-methylpentanoate (3k)

Methods A and C followed by F

Very viscous liquid, 90% ^{1}H NMR (500 MHz, $CDCl_3$) δ 7.74 (d, J = 8.5 Hz, 2H); 7.21 (d, J = 8.5 Hz); 5.90 (m, 2H); 5.05 (d, J = 15.9 Hz, 1H); 4.88 (dd, J = 11.0, 4.3 Hz, 1H); 4.41 (d, J = 15.3 Hz, 1H); 3.24 (s, 3H); 2.65 (m, 2H); 2.27 (m, 2H); 2.10 (m, 1H); 1.95 (m, 1H); 1.45 (s, 9H); 0.92 (d, J = 6.71 Hz, 6H), ^{13}C NMR (125 MHz, $CDCl_3$) δ 180.4; 180.3; 168.1; 164.8; 154.8; 140.2; 134.7; 127.72; 127.68; 125.9; 120.1; 80.2; 63.4; 51.0; 39.3; 39.2; 37.3; 37.2; 28.3; 24.7; 23.6; 23.5; 23.0; 20.9.

HRMS (ESI-Orbitrap): $[M+Na]^+$ Calculated for $C_{28}H_{37}O_7N_3Na$ 550.25237; found 550.25177.

2-((4-nitrophenyl)amino)-2-oxoethyl (2S)-2-(1,3-dioxo-1,3,3a,4,7,7a-hexahydro-2H-isoindol-2-yl)-4-methylpentanoate (3l)

Methods A and C followed by F

Very viscous liquid, 89% ^{1}H NMR (600 MHz, $CDCl_3$) δ 8.72 (sl, 1H); 8.24 (m, 2H); 8.03 (m, 2H); 5.91 (m, 2H); 5.10 (d, J = 15.8 Hz, 1H); 4.90 (dd, J = 11.0, 4.4Hz, 1H); 3.25 (m, 2H); 2.66 (m, 2H); 2.29 (m, 2H); 2.06 (m, 1H); 1.96 (m, 1H); 1.41 (m, 1H); 0.93 (d, J = 6.6 Hz, 6H), ^{13}C NMR (150 MHz, $CDCl_3$) δ 180.6; 180.5; 168.1; 165.7; 143.9; 143.4; 127.8; 127.7; 124.9; 119.6; 63.4; 51.1; 39.37; 39.35; 37.4; 24.7; 23.6; 23.5; 23.0; 21.0.

HRMS (ESI-Orbitrap): $[M+Na]^+$ Calculated for $C_{22}H_{25}O_7N_3Na$ 466.15902; found 466.15749.

2-((4-methoxy-2-nitrophenyl)amino)-2-oxoethyl (2S)-2-(1,3-dioxo-1,3,3a,4,7,7a-hexahydro-2H-isoindol-2-yl)-4-methylpentanoate (3m)

Methods A and C followed by F

Very viscous liquid, 98% ^{1}H NMR (500 MHz, $CDCl_3$) δ 10.51 (sl, 1H); 8.57 (d, J = 9.15 Hz, 1H); 7.66 (d, J = 2.9 Hz, 1H); 7.24 (dd, J = 9.3, 3.0 Hz, 1H); 5.92 (m, 2H); 4.95 (dd, J = 11.3, 4.4 Hz, 1H); 4.77 (m, 2H); 3.87 (s, 3H); 3.31 (m, 1H); 3.18 (m, 1H); 2.62 (m, 2H); 2.26 (m, 2H); 2.16 (m, 1H); 1.97 (m, 1H); 1.39 (m, 1H); 0.93 (dd, J = 6.6, 4.5 Hz, 6H), ^{13}C NMR (125 MHz, $CDCl_3$) δ 179.5; 179.43; 168.0; 165.0; 155.5; 137.7; 127.7; 127.6; 126.6; 124.0; 122.8; 108.8; 64.0; 55.8; 50.9; 39.2; 38.9; 36.7; 24.6; 23.6; 23.4; 23.0; 20.77.

HRMS (ESI-Orbitrap): $[M+Na]^+$ Calculated for $C_{23}H_{28}O_8N_3$ 474.19045; found 474.19131.

2-((3-chloro-4-methoxyphenyl)amino)-2-oxoethyl (S)-2-(1,3-dioxoisoindolin-2-yl)-4-methylpentanoate (10a)

Methods A and C followed by F

Very viscous liquid, 82% ^{1}H NMR (250 MHz, DMSO) δ 10.04 (sl, 1H); 7.92 (m, 4H); 7.69 (d, J = 2.4 Hz, 1H); 7.37 (dd, J = 8.9, 2.4 Hz, 1H); 7.10 (d, J = 9.0 Hz, 1H); 5.04 (dd, J = 11.2, 4.4 Hz, 1H); 4.72 (m, 2H); 3.81 (s, 3H); 2.24 (m, 1H); 1.93 (ddd, J = 14.0, 9.9, 4.5 Hz, 1H); 1.49 (m, 1H); 0.89 (m, 6H). ^{13}C NMR (62.5 MHz, DMSO) δ 169.1; 167.2; 164.6; 150.7; 135.0; 131.9; 131.0; 123.5; 121.0; 120.6; 119.2; 112.9; 63.4; 56.1; 49.9; 36.6; 24.5; 22.9; 20.8.

HRMS (ESI-Orbitrap): $[M+H]^+$ Calculated for $C_{23}H_{24}O_6N_2Cl$ 459.1323; found 459.1355.

2-((3-chloro-4-methoxyphenyl)amino)-2-oxoethyl (2S)-2-(1,3-dioxooctahydro-2H-isoindol-2-yl)-4-methylpentanoate (10b)

Methods A and C followed by F

Very viscous liquid, 91% ^{1}H NMR (500 MHz, $CDCl_3$) δ 8.32 (sl, 1H); 7.83 (d, J = 2.5 Hz, 1H); 7.68 (dd, J = 8.9, 2.6 Hz, 1H); 6.90 (d, J = 8.9 Hz, 1H); 5.08 (d, J = 15.6 Hz, 1H); 4.90 (dd, J = 10.9, 4.3 Hz, 1H); 4.45 (d, J = 15.6 Hz, 1H); 3.89 (s, 3H); 2.12 (ddd, J = 14.5, 10.7, 4.3 Hz, 1H); 1.98 (m, 2H); 1.85 (m, 2H); 1.77 (m, 1H); 1.47 (m, 4H); 1.36 (m, 1H); 0.96 (m, 6H). ^{13}C NMR (100 MHz, $CDCl_3$) δ 180.3; 179.4; 168.4; 164.7; 152.0; 131.1; 122.3; 119.5; 112.1; 63.5; 56.3; 50.5; 40.0; 39.8; 37.4; 25.0; 24.0; 23.3; 23.1; 21.6; 21.1.

HRMS (ESI-Orbitrap): $[M+Na]^+$ Calculated for $C_{23}H_{29}O_6N_2ClNa$ 487.19118; found 487.16025.

2-((3-chloro-4-methoxyphenyl)amino)-2-oxoethyl (S)-2-(2,5-dioxo-2,5-dihydro-1H-pyrrol-1-yl)-4-methylpentanoate (10c)

Methods A and D followed by F

Very viscous liquid, 46% ^{1}H NMR (400 MHz, $CDCl_3$) δ 8.12 (sl, 1H); 7.76 (d, J = 2.6 Hz, 1H); 7.62 (dd, J = 8.9, 2.6 Hz, 1H); 6.90 (d, J = 8.9 Hz, 1H); 6.84 (s, 2H); 5.04 (d, J = 15.5 Hz, 1H); 4.91 (dd, J = 11.4, 4.4 Hz, 1H); 4.47 (d, J = 15.5 Hz, 1H); 3.89 (s, 3H); 2.18 (ddd, J = 14.3, 11.2, 4.3 Hz, 1H); 1.98 (ddd, J = 14.3, 10.0, 4.3 Hz, 1H); 1.47 (m, 1H); 0.96 (dd, J = 6.6, 1.2 Hz, 6H). ^{13}C NMR (100 MHz, $CDCl_3$) δ 170.4; 168.4; 164.6; 152.1; 134.6; 130.9; 122.5; 122.4; 63.6; 56.3; 50.4; 38.0; 24.9; 23.0; 21.0.

2-((3-chloro-4-methoxyphenyl)amino)-2-oxoethyl (S)-2-(2,5-dioxopyrrolidin-1-yl)-4-methylpentanoate (10d)

Methods A and D followed by F

Very viscous liquid, 72% ^{1}H NMR (400 MHz, $CDCl_3$) δ 8.30 (sl, 1H); 7.79 (d, J = 2.6 Hz, 1H); 7.62 (dd, J = 8.9, 2.7 Hz, 1H); 6.89 (d, J = 8.9 Hz, 1H); 5.01 (d, J = 15.4 Hz, 1H); 4.94 (dd, J = 10.5, 4.8 Hz, 1H); 4.49 (d, J = 15.5 Hz, 1H); 3.88 (s, 3H); 2.86 (m, 4H); 2.05 (m, 2H); 1.45 (m, 1H); 0.96 (dd, J = 6.7, 4.6 Hz, 6H), ^{13}C NMR (100 MHz, $CDCl_3$) δ 177.2; 168.2; 164.7; 152.0; 131.0; 122.3; 119.6; 112.1; 63.4; 56.3; 50.9; 37.3; 28.2; 24.9; 22.9; 21.1.

HRMS (ESI-Orbitrap): $[M+Na]^+$ Calculated for $C_{19}H_{23}O_6N_2ClNa$ 433.11423; found 433.11424.

2-((3-chloro-4-methoxyphenyl)amino)-2-oxoethyl (S)-4-methyl-2-(3-methyl-2,5-dioxo-2,5-dihydro-1H-pyrrol-1-yl)pentanoate (10e)

Methods A and D followed by F

Very viscous liquid, 88% ^{1}H NMR (500 MHz, $CDCl_3$) δ 8.19 (sl, 1H); 7.78 (d, J = 2.5 Hz, 1H); 7.65 (dd, J = 8.9, 2.6 Hz, 1H); 6.90 (d, J = 9.0 Hz, 1H); 6.46 (d, J = 1.9 Hz, 1H); 5.04 (d, J = 15.6 Hz, 1H); 4.89 (dd, J = 11.4, 4.3 Hz, 1H); 4.45 (d, J = 15.6 Hz, 1H); 3.89 (s, 3H); 2.17 (m, 4H); 1.96 (m, 1H); 1.47 (m, 1H); 0.95 (dd, J = 6.7, 1.7 Hz, 6H), ^{13}C NMR (125 MHz, $CDCl_3$) δ 171.6; 170.5; 168.6; 164.6; 152.0; 146.3; 130.9; 127.8; 122.4; 122.3; 119.5; 112.1; 63.5; 56.3; 50.5; 38.1; 24.9; 23.0; 20.9; 11.2.

HRMS (ESI-Orbitrap): $[M+Na]^+$ Calculated for $C_{20}H_{23}O_6N_2ClNa$ 445.11369; found 445.11261.

2-((3-chloro-4-methoxyphenyl)amino)-2-oxoethyl (S)-2-(3,4-dichloro-2,5-dioxo-2,5-dihydro-1H-pyrrol-1-yl)-4-methylpentanoate (10f)

Methods A and D followed by F

Very viscous liquid, 27% ^{1}H NMR (500 MHz, $CDCl_3$) δ 7.85 (sl, 1H); 7.74 (d, J = 2.5 Hz, 1H); 7.59 (dd, J = 9.0, 2.5 Hz, 1H); 6.91 (d, J = 9.0 Hz, 1H); 5.02 (d, J = 15.4, 1H); 4.98 (dd, J = 11.4, 4.5 Hz, 1H); 4.52 (d, J = 15.4 Hz, 1H); 3.90 (s, 3H); 2.21 (m, 1H); 2.00 (m, 1H); 1.51 (m, 1H); 0.97 (dd, J = 6.5, 4.3 Hz, 6H), ^{13}C NMR (125 MHz, $CDCl_3$) δ 167.6; 164.1; 163.0; 152.3; 133.9; 130.6; 122.6; 122.4; 119.6; 112.2; 63.9; 56.4; 51.9; 37.9; 25.0; 23.0; 20.9.

HRMS (ESI-Orbitrap): $[M+Na]^+$ Calculated for $C_{19}H_{19}O_6N_2Cl_3Na$ 499.02009; found 499.02014.

2-((3-chloro-4-methoxyphenyl)amino)-2-oxoethyl 2-(1,3-dioxo-1,3,3a,4,7,7a-hexahydro-2H-isoindol-2-yl)acetate (10g)

Methods A and C followed by F

Very viscous liquid, 80% ^{1}H NMR (500 MHz, DMSO) δ 12.40 (sl, 1H); 9.89 (s, 1H); 7.75 (d, J = 2.6 Hz, 1H); 7.43 (dd, J = 8.9, 2.6 Hz, 1H); 7.11 (d, J = 9.0 Hz, 1H); 5.61 (m, 2H); 4.62 (m, 2H); 3.82 (s, 3H); 3.07 (m, 2H); 2.46 (m, 2H); 2.33 (m, 2H), ^{13}C NMR (125 MHz, DMSO) δ 174.6; 172.6; 165.3; 150.7; 132.0; 125.3; 124.9; 121.1; 120.6; 119.3; 112.9; 62.5; 56.2; 38.8; 38.6; 25.6; 25.2.

2-((3-chloro-4-methoxyphenyl)amino)-2-oxoethyl (2S)-2-(1,3-dioxo-1,3,3a,4,7,7a-hexahydro-2H-isoindol-2-yl)-3-phenylpropanoate (10h)

Methods A and D followed by F

Very viscous liquid, 87% ^{1}H NMR (250 MHz, $CDCl_3$) δ 8.26 (sl, 1H); 7.83 (d, J = 2.7 Hz, 1H); 7.71 (dd, J = 8.9, 2.6 Hz, 1H); 7.22 (m, 5H); 6.92 (d, J = 8.8 Hz, 1H); 5.70 (m, 2H); 5.12 (m, 2H); 4.42 (d, J = 15.5 Hz, 1H); 3.90 (s, 3H); 3.56 (m, 1H); 3.36 (dd, J = 14.3, 11.3 Hz, 1H); 2.99 (m, 2H); 2.48 (ddd, J = 15.8, 6.0, 2.9 Hz, 1H); 2.22 (m, 3H).

HRMS (ESI-Orbitrap): $[M+Na]^+$ Calculated for $C_{26}H_{25}O_6N_2ClNa$ 519.12988; found 519.12918.

$[\alpha]_D^{20}$ −24,0 (1, MeOH).

HPLC flow 3.5 mL/min, polarity hexane:ethyl acetate (60:40). Rt 16.76 min, area 97.10%; Rt 20.09 min, area 2.90%.

2-((3-chloro-4-methoxyphenyl)amino)-2-oxoethyl 2-(1,3-dioxo-1,3,3a,4,7,7a-hexahydro-2H-isoindol-2-yl)-3-phenylpropanoate ($10h_{rac}$)

Methods A and D followed by F

Very viscous liquid, 81% ^{1}H NMR (500 MHz, $CDCl_3$) δ 8.29 (sl, 1H); 7.84 (d, J = 2.2 Hz, 1H); 7.69 (dd, J = 8.8, 2.4 Hz, 1H); 7.24 (m, 3H); 7.13 (d, J = 7.1 Hz, 2H); 6.92 (d, J = 9.0 Hz, 1H); 5.70 (m, 2H); 5.12 (m, 2H); 4.43 (d, J = 15.6 Hz, 1H); 3.90 (s, 3H); 3.56 (dd, J = 14.3, 5.2 Hz, 1H); 3.35 (dd, J = 14.2, 11.5 Hz, 1H); 3.04 (m, 1H); 2.93 (m, 1H); 2.48 (ddd, J = 15.7, 6.05, 2.6 Hz, 1H); 2.29 (ddd, J = 15.8, 5.9, 3.0 Hz, 1H); 2.17 (m, 2H), ^{13}C NMR (125 MHz, $CDCl_3$) δ 180.2; 179.8; 167.3; 164.6; 152.0; 135.3; 131.0; 129.0; 128.6; 127.4; 127.21; 127.17; 122.33; 122.28; 119.5; 112.1; 63.4; 56.3; 53.2; 39.0; 38.9; 34.3; 23.11; 23.07.

HRMS (ESI-Orbitrap): $[M+Na]^+$ Calculated for $C_{26}H_{25}O_6N_2ClNa$ 519.12988; found 519.12965.

$[\alpha]_D^{20}$ 0 (1, MeOH).

HPLC flow 3.5 mL/min, polarity hexane:ethyl acetate (60:40). Rt 17.16 min, area 50.19%; Rt 20.49 min, area 49.81%.

2-((3-chloro-4-methoxyphenyl)amino)-2-oxoethyl (2R)-2-(1,3-dioxo-1,3,3a,4,7,7a-hexahydro-2H-isoindol-2-yl)-3-(naphthalen-2-yl)propanoate (10i)

Methods A and D followed by F

Very viscous liquid, 43% (for 2 steps) ^{1}H NMR (400 MHz, $CDCl_3$) δ 8.29 (sl, 1H); 7.85 (d, J = 2.7 Hz, 1H); 7.77 (m, 3H); 7.71 (dd, J = 8.9, 2.6 Hz, 1H); 7.54 (m, 1H); 7.46 (m, 2H); 7.29 (dd, J = 8.4, 1.8 Hz, 1H); 6.93 (d, J = 8.9 Hz, 1H); 5.48 (m, 2H); 5.26 (dd, J = 11.4, 5.4 Hz, 1H); 5.14 (d, J = 15.4 Hz, 1H); 4.44 (d, J = 15.4 Hz, 1H); 3.72 (dd, J = 14.3, 5.3 Hz, 1H); 3.54 (dd, J = 14.4, 11.4 Hz, 1H); 3.00 (ddd, J = 9.0, 7.6, 3.0 Hz, 1H); 2.87 (ddd, J = 9.0, 7.8; 2.7 Hz, 1H); 2.46 (ddd, J = 15.8, 6.4, 2.6 Hz, 1H); 2.22 (ddd, J = 15.8, 6.4, 3.0 Hz, 1H); 2.08 (m, 2H), ^{13}C NMR (100 MHz, $CDCl_3$) δ 180.2; 180.0; 167.4; 164.7; 152.1; 133.3;

132.8; 132.5; 131.1; 128.5; 128.1; 127.7; 127.4; 127.2; 127.0; 126.6; 126.3; 125.9; 122.5; 122.4; 119.6; 112.2; 63.5; 56.4; 53.2; 39.0; 38.9; 34.6; 23.1.

HRMS (ESI-Orbitrap): $[M+Na]^+$ Calculated for $C_{30}H_{27}O_6N_2ClNa$ 569.14553; found 569.14428.

2-((3-chloro-4-methoxyphenyl)amino)-2-oxoethyl (S)-2-(2,5-dioxo-2,5-dihydro-1H-pyrrol-1-yl)-3-phenylpropanoate (10j)

Methods A and D followed by F

Very viscous liquid, 23% ^{1}H NMR (500 MHz, $CDCl_3$) δ 8.17 (sl, 1H); 7.76 (d, $J = 2.6$ Hz, 1H); 7.66 (dd, $J = 8.9, 2.6$ Hz, 1H); 7.25 (m, 3H); 7.13 (m, 2H); 6.92 (d, $J = 8.9$ Hz, 1H); 6.69 (s, 2H); 5.10 (m, 2H); 4.50 (d, $J = 15.4$ Hz, 1H); 3.90 (s, 3H); 3.57 (dd, $J = 14.2, 5.2$ Hz, 1H); 3.38 (dd, $J = 14.2, 11.2$ Hz, 1H), ^{13}C NMR (125 MHz, $CDCl_3$) δ 170.1; 167.6; 164.5; 152.2; 135.5; 134.3; 130.9; 128.9; 128.8; 127.4; 122.5; 119.7; 112.2; 63.7; 56.4; 53.2; 35.4.

HRMS (ESI-Orbitrap): $[M+Na]^+$ Calculated for $C_{22}H_{19}O_6N_2ClNa$ 465.08239; found 465.08244.

2-((3-chloro-4-methoxyphenyl)amino)-2-oxoethyl (S)-4-methyl-2-(pyrrolidin-1-yl)pentanoate (10k)

Methods A and E followed by F

Very viscous liquid, 93% ^{1}H NMR (500 MHz, MeOD) δ 8.66 (sl, 1H); 7.57 (d, $J = 2.7$ Hz, 1H); 7.46 (dd, $J = 8.8, 2.5$ Hz, 1H); 6.88 (d, $J = 9.0$ Hz, 1H); 4.73 (m, 2H); 3.88 (s, 1H); 3.35 (dd, $J = 9.9, 4.6$ Hz, 1H); 2.73 (m, 2H); 2.63 (m, 2H); 1.80 (m, 5H); 1.58 (m, 2H); 0.96 (dd, $J = 8.5, 6.1$ Hz, 6H), ^{13}C NMR (125 MHz, MeOD) δ 171.3; 165.3; 152.2; 130.6; 122.7; 122.4; 120.0; 112.1; 65.1; 62.7; 56.3; 50.6; 39.0; 25.4; 23.4; 23.3; 21.9.

2-((3-chloro-4-methoxyphenyl)amino)-2-oxoethyl (S)-4-methyl-2-(piperidin-1-yl)pentanoate (10l)

Methods A and E followed by F

Very viscous liquid, 87% ^{1}H NMR (500 MHz, $CDCl_3$) δ 8.05 (sl, 1H); 7.56 (d, $J = 2.7$ Hz, 1H); 7.42 (dd, $J = 8.9, 2.6$ Hz, 1H); 6.90 (d, $J = 8.8$ Hz, 1H); 4.83 (d, $J = 15.6$ Hz, 1H); 4.63 (d, $J = 15.6$ Hz, 1H); 3.82 (s, 3H); 3.37 (dd, $J = 8.8, 5.7$ Hz, 1H); 2.59 (m, 4H); 1.60 (m, 7H); 1.44 (m, 2H); 0.94 (dd, $J = 9.1, 6.3$ Hz, 6H), ^{13}C NMR (125 MHz, $CDCl_3$) δ 170.8; 165.3; 152.4; 130.2; 123.0; 122.6; 120.1; 112.2; 66.5; 62.4; 56.4; 50.9; 36.6; 26.4; 25.3; 24.4; 22.8; 22.4.

HRMS (ESI-Orbitrap): $[M+Na]^+$ Calculated for $C_{20}H_{29}O_4N_2ClNa$ 419.17081; found 419.17050.

2-((3-chloro-4-methoxyphenyl)amino)-2-oxoethyl (S)-4-methyl-2-morpholinopentanoate (10m)

Methods A and E followed by F

Very viscous liquid, 75% ^{1}H NMR (500 MHz, $CDCl_3$) δ 7.96 (sl, 1H); 7.56 (d, $J = 2.6$ Hz, 1H); 7.38 (dd, $J = 8.8, 2.6$ Hz, 1H); 6.89 (d, $J = 8.9$ Hz, 1H); 4.76 (d, $J = 15.3$ Hz, 1H); 4.68 (d, $J = 15.3$ Hz, 1H); 3.88 (s, 3H); 3.68 (m, 4H); 3.40 (t, $J = 7.3$ Hz, 1H); 2.67 (m, 4H); 1.65 (m, 3H); 0.96 (dd, $J = 8.9, 6.1$ Hz, 6H), ^{13}C NMR (125 MHz, $CDCl_3$) δ 170.8; 165.0; 152.4; 130.1; 122.8; 122.6; 120.0; 112.2; 67.2; 65.8; 62.6; 56.3; 49.8; 36.8; 25.0; 22.6; 22.4.

HRMS (ESI-Orbitrap): $[M+Na]^+$ Calculated for $C_{19}H_{27}O_5N_2ClNa$ 421.15007; found 421.14966.

tert-butyl (S)-4-(1-(2-((3-chloro-4-methoxyphenyl)amino)-2-oxoethoxy)-4-methyl-1-oxopentan-2-yl)piperazine-1-carboxylate (10n)

Methods A and E followed by F

Very viscous liquid, 69% ^{1}H NMR (500 MHz, $CDCl_3$) δ 7.86 (sl, 1H); 7.56 (d, $J = 2.4$ Hz, 1H); 7.37 (dd, $J = 8.9, 2.4$ Hz, 1H); 6.89 (d, $J = 9.0$ Hz, 1H); 4.74 (d, $J = 15.3$ Hz, 1H); 4.67 (d, $J = 15.3$ Hz, 1H); 3.89 (s, 3H); 3.43 (m, 5H); 2.62 (m, 4H); 1.65 (m, 3H); 1.44 (s, 9H); 0.95 (dd, $J = 12.3, 5.9$ Hz, 6H), ^{13}C NMR (125 MHz, $CDCl_3$) δ 170.7; 164.9; 154.3; 152.4; 130.1; 122.8; 122.7; 120.0; 112.3; 79.8; 65.5; 62.6; 56.4; 49.3; 37.1; 28.4; 25.0; 22.5.

HRMS (ESI-Orbitrap): $[M+Na]^+$ Calculated for $C_{24}H_{36}O_6N_3ClNa$ 520.21848; found 520.21832.

General Procedure for the Preparation of Compounds 3k' and 10o

The esters, obtained through methods A and D or E followed by F, were dissolved in dry DCM, and a large excess of HCl (4 M solution in dioxane) was added. The resulting solution was stirred at room temperature for 4 h. The solvent mixture was removed under reduced pressure, and the residue was dissolved in DCM followed by crystallization from hexane.

2-((4-(methylamino)phenyl)amino)-2-oxoethyl 2-(1,3-dioxo-1,3,3a,4,7,7a-hexahydro-2H-isoindol-2-yl)-4-methylpentanoate (3k')

Very viscous liquid, 75% ^{1}H NMR (500 MHz, $CDCl_3$) δ 8.04 (sl, 1H); 7.53 (d, J =8.8 Hz, 2H); 6.60 (d, $J = 8.8$ Hz, 2H); 5.89 (m, 2H); 5.02 (d, $J = 15.3$ Hz, 1H); 4.87 (dd, $J = 11.1, 4.3$ Hz, 1H); 4.40 (d, $J = 15.4$ Hz, 1H); 3.72 (sl, 1H); 3.20 (m, 2H); 2.83 (s, 3H); 2.64 (m, 2H); 2.25 (m, 2H); 2.11 (m, 1H); 1.94 (m, 1H); 1.40 (m, 1H); 0.92 (d, $J = 6.6$ Hz, 6H), ^{13}C NMR (125 MHz, $CDCl_3$) δ 180.3; 180.1; 168.0; 164.3; 146.6; 127.7; 121.7; 112.5; 63.5; 51.1; 39.2; 37.1; 31.0; 24.8; 23.55; 23.48; 23.0; 20.9.

HRMS (ESI-Orbitrap): $[M+Na]^+$ Calculated for $C_{23}H_{29}O_5N_3FNa$ 450.19994; found 450.19913.

2-((3-chloro-4-methoxyphenyl)amino)-2-oxoethyl (S)-4-methyl-2-(piperazin-1-yl)pentanoate hydrochloride (10o)

Amorphous solid, 96% ^{1}H NMR (500 MHz, MeOD) δ 7.67 (m, 1H); 7.38 (m, 1H); 7.02 (m, 1H); 4.83 (m, 2H); 3.98 (m, 1H); 3.85 (s, 3H); 3.78 (m, 1H); 3.46 (m, 6H); 3.27 (m, 1H); 1.82 (m, 3H); 1.00 (dd, $J = 11.1, 6.2$ Hz, 6H), ^{13}C NMR (125 MHz, $CDCl_3$) δ 172.3; 170.5; 167.3; 167.2; 156.2; 153.9; 132.7; 123.9; 123.4; 121.4; 114.1; 74.4; 68.3; 66.9; 64.5; 64.4; 57.2; 47.8; 44.5; 44.0; 41.0; 38.2; 26.4; 26.1; 23.4; 23.1; 22.4; 22.2.

HRMS (ESI-Orbitrap): $[M+H]^+$ Calculated for $C_{19}H_{28}O_4N_3Cl$ 398.18466; found 398.18384.

General Procedure for the Preparation of Compounds 3l' and 3m'

The esters, obtained through methods A and D followed by F, were dissolved in methanol, followed by the addition of the catalyst Pd/C (10 wt%, 0.1 equivalents). The mixture stirred at room temperature under a hydrogen atmosphere (1 atm) for 4 h and then filtered through Celite®. The filtrate was concentrated in vacuum. The product was purified by column chromatography on silica gel using a mixture of ethyl acetate/hexanes (50%) as the eluent.

2-((4-aminophenyl)amino)-2-oxoethyl 2-(1,3-dioxo-1,3,3a,4,7,7a-hexahydro-2H-isoindol-2-yl)-4-methylpentanoate (3l')

Pale amorphous solid, 92% ^{1}H NMR (500 MHz, $CDCl_3$) δ 8.06 (sl, 1H); 7.51 (d, J = 8.7 Hz, 2H); 6.67 (d, J = 8.7 Hz, 2H); 5.89 (m, 2H); 5.03 (d, J = 15.4 Hz, 1H) 4.87 (dd, J = 11.0, 4.3 Hz, 1H); 4.40 (d, J = 15.4 Hz, 1H); 3.65 (sl, 2H); 3.20 (m, 2H); 2.64 (m, 2H); 2.26 (m, 2H); 2.10 (m, 1H); 1.94 (m, 1H); 1.40 (m, 1H); 0.92 (d, J = 6.6 Hz, 6H). ^{13}C NMR (125 MHz, $CDCl_3$) δ 180.4; 180.2; 168.1; 164.4; 143.4; 128.9; 127.7; 121.7; 115.3; 63.5; 51.1; 39.3; 37.1; 24.8; 23.58; 23.50; 23.1; 21.0.

HRMS (ESI-Orbitrap): $[M+Na]^+$ Calculated for $C_{22}H_{27}O_5N_3Na$ 436.18484; found 436.18421.

2-((2-amino-4-methoxyphenyl)amino)-2-oxoethyl 2-(1,3-dioxo-1,3,3a,4,7,7a-hexahydro-2H-isoindol-2-yl)-4-methylpentanoate (3m')

Light brown amorphous solid, 94% ^{1}H NMR (500 MHz, $CDCl_3$) δ 7.90 (sl, 1H); 7.08 (d, J = 8.5 Hz, 1H); 6.34 (m, 2H); 5.90 (m, 2H); 4.98 (d, J = 15.6 Hz, 1H); 4.87 (dd, J = 11.0, 4.3 Hz, 1H); 4.54 (d J = 15.4 Hz, 1H); 3.75 (s, 3H); 3.18 (m, 2H); 2.61 (m, 2H); 2.23 (m, 2H); 2.07 (m, 1H); 1.93 (m, 1H); 1.37 (m, 1H); 0.91 (dd, J = 6.6, 3.4 Hz, 6H). ^{13}C NMR (125 MHz, $CDCl_3$) δ 180.12; 180.09; 168.5; 165.6; 159.3; 142.8; 127.71; 127.71; 127.26; 115.5; 104.5; 102.6; 63.8; 55.3; 51.0; 39.21; 39.15; 37.1; 24.7; 23.50; 23.48; 23.0; 20.9.

HRMS (ESI-Orbitrap): $[M+Na]^+$ Calculated for $C_{23}H_{30}O_6N_3$ 444.21627; found 444.21738.

Procedure for the Preparation of N-(2-((3-chloro-4-methoxyphenyl)amino)-2-oxoethyl)-2-(1,3-dioxo-1,3,3a,4,7,7a-hexahydro-2H-isoindol-2-yl)-4-methylpentanamide (5)

2-(1,3-Dioxo-1,3,3a,4,7,7a-hexahydro-2*H*-isoindol-2-yl)-4-methylpentanoic acid **(1)** was dissolved in dichloromethane at room temperature. Oxalyl chloride (1.5 equivalents) and 0.1 mL of dimethyl formamide (DMF) were added to this solution as the catalyst. After 2 h, the solvent was removed under vacuum. The residue was dissolved in dichloromethane, and glycine (1.0 equivalents) was added, followed by the addition of triethylamine (2.2 equivalents).

The isolated product from the previous step was dissolved in dichloromethane at room temperature. Oxalyl chloride (1.5 equivalents) and 0.1 mL dimethyl formamide (DMF) were added to this solution as the catalyst. After 2 h, the solvent was removed under vacuum. The residue was dissolved in dichloromethane, and 3-chloro-4-methoxyaniline (1.0 equivalents) was added, followed by the addition of triethylamine (2.2 equivalents). The reaction stirred for an additional 2 h. The reaction mixture was washed with water and saturated aqueous NH_4Cl solution. The organic phase was dried over $MgSO_4$ and the solvent was removed under reduced pressure. The product was purified by column chromatography on silica gel using a mixture of ethyl acetate/hexanes (50%) as the eluent.

Amorphous solid, 78% ^{1}H NMR (250 MHz, DMSO) δ 9.68 (sl, 1H); 7.64 (d, J = 2.4 Hz, 1H); 7.39 (dd, J = 8.9, 2.4 Hz, 1H); 7.09 (d, J = 9.0 Hz, 1H); 5.86 (m, 2H) 4.65 (dd, J = 11.3, 4.3 Hz, 1H); 3.81 (sl, 3H); 3.18 (m, 2H); 2.39 (m, 2H); 2.11 (m, 3H); 1.79 (m, 1H); 1.29 (m, 1H); 0.83 (m, 6H). ^{13}C NMR (62.5 MHz, DMSO) δ 180.1; 179.8; 166.8; 150.8; 132.1; 127.7; 127.6; 122.0; 120.4; 120.2; 112.7; 56.2; 52.4; 36.2; 24.3; 23.4; 23.3; 23.1; 20.6.

Procedure for the Preparation of 2-((3-chloro-4-methoxyphenyl)amino)ethyl 2-(1,3-dioxo-1,3,3a,4,7,7a-hexahydro-2H-isoindol-2-yl)-4-methylpentanoate (7)

A solution of compound **1** in dry DCM was prepared, and alcohol **6** was added (1.1 equivalents). The solution was cooled in an ice bath followed by the addition of EDC (1.2 equivalents) and DMAP (0.1 equivalents). The solution was allowed to warm to room temperature and stirred for 4 h while monitoring periodically by TLC. The reaction mixture was washed with saturated aqueous NH_4Cl solution and brine. The organic phase was dried over $MgSO_4$ and concentrated under reduced pressure. The product was purified by column chromatography on silica gel using a mixture of ethyl acetate/hexanes (50%) as the eluent.

Pale oil, 62% ^{1}H NMR (500 MHz, $CDCl_3$) δ 6.82 (d, J = 8.7 Hz, 1H); 6.70 (d, J = 2.8 Hz, 1H); 6.51 (dd, J = 8.8, 2.8 Hz, 1H); 5.89 (m, 1H); 5.82 (m, 1H); 4.76 (dd, J = 11.3, 4.3 Hz, 1H); 4.43 (ddd, J = 11.1, 7.1, 3.9 Hz, 1H); 4.18 (m, 1H); 3.82 (m, 3H); 3.30 (m, 2H); 3.10 (m, 2H); 2.60 (m, 2H); 2.23 (m, 2H); 2.09 (m, 1H); 1.84 (m, 1H); 1.35 (m, 1H); 0.89 (dd, J = 8.8, 6.5 Hz, 6H). ^{13}C NMR (125 MHz, $CDCl_3$) δ 179.64; 179.61; 169.1; 147.6; 142.5; 127.7; 127.6; 123.4; 115.2; 114.2; 112.1; 64.0; 57.0; 51.2; 43.1; 39.0; 38.9; 36.7; 24.8; 23.43; 23.42; 23.1; 21.0. HRMS (ESI-Orbitrap) m/z [M + Na] calculated for $C_{23}H_{29}O_5N_2ClNa$ 471.16572; found 471.16522.

RESULTS AND DISCUSSION

In this work, we report the discovery of a series of reversible cruzain inhibitors showing promising trypanocidal activity and low toxicity. The imide derivative **3a** (**Figure 1A**), a reversible cruzain inhibitor that was previously identified from a virtual high-throughput screening (HTS) combined approach (Ferreira et al., 2010), was taken as the initial hit for molecular optimization. The SBDD strategy relied on the molecular docking-predicted binding mode of **3a** within the catalytic site of cruzain (**Figure 1B**). The enzyme-inhibitor interactions rely mainly on a hydrogen bonding network. The secondary amide oxygen fills the S3 subsite and interacts with the main chain nitrogen of Gly66. The secondary amide nitrogen in turn forms a hydrogen bond with the main chain carbonyl of Asp161, which lies at the interface between the S2 and S1' subsites. The ester carbonyl projects into the S1 subsite where it engages in a hydrogen bond with the side chain nitrogen of Gln19. One of the imide carbonyl oxygens forms

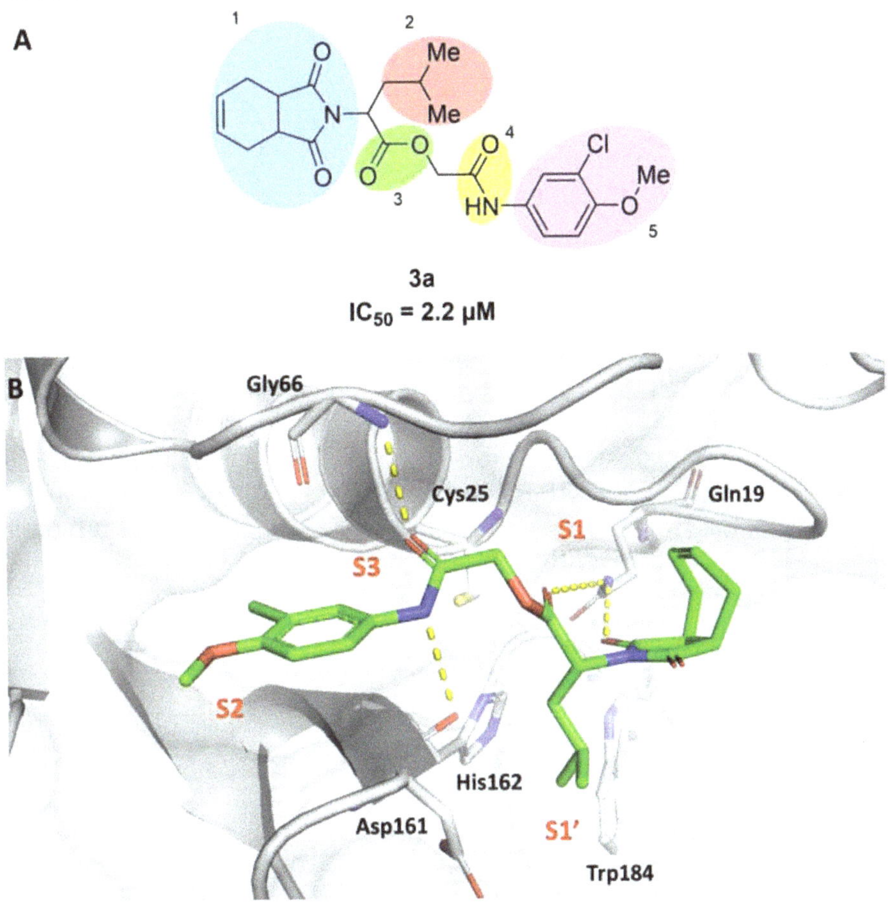

FIGURE 1 | (A) Compound **3a** was used as the initial hit for the design of imide derivatives as novel cruzain inhibitors with anti-T. cruzi activity. **(B)** Molecular docking-predicted binding conformation of compound **3a** within the active site of cruzain. Cruzain (PDB 3KKU, 1.28 Å) is depicted in cartoon and surface representations. Binding site residues (carbon in gray) and compound **3a** (carbon in green) are shown as sticks. Hydrogen bonds are shown as dashed lines. Cruzain subsites are labeled as S1, S1', S2, and S3.

a hydrogen bond with the side chain nitrogen of Gln19 at the S1 subsite. The 3-chloro-4-methoxyphenyl ring projects into the S2 subsite and the isobutyl fragment lies in S1'. Based on these findings, compound **3a** was divided into five fragments that underwent the molecular modifications that eventually led to the series of cruzain inhibitors described herein. The data gathered from the designed analogs were used to further improve the potency against both cruzain and *T. cruzi* and disclose the structure-activity relationships (SAR) enclosed in this dataset.

Synthesis of Imide Derivatives

The synthesis of the initial hit (**3a**) and analogs with modifications to the aromatic moiety is outlined in **Scheme 1**. The aromatic ring was manipulated by introducing electron withdrawing and donating groups and hydrogen bond donors and acceptors. Carboxylic acid **1** was coupled under Steglich-like conditions (Pande et al., 2014) with alcohols **2a-m** furnishing the intended esters **3a-m**. Ester **3k'** was obtained through deprotection of **3k** under acidic conditions, and compounds **3l'** and **3m'** were generated from the reduction of **3l** and **3m**, respectively.

Considering the low stability of the ester group in acidic and basic media, we synthesized a more stable analog with an amide group, as illustrated in **Scheme 2**. Initially, carboxylic acid intermediate **1** was transformed into an acyl chloride via reaction with oxalyl chloride. The acyl chloride was further used in a coupling reaction with glycine, producing intermediate **4**. Intermediate **4** was converted into an acyl chloride, using the same conditions previously mentioned, and coupled with 3-chloro-4-methoxyaniline to generate the target compound **5** (**Scheme 2A**). Compound **7** (**Scheme 2B**) was synthesized from 3-chloro-4-methoxyaniline with ethyl carbonate catalyzed by molecular sieves (Kinage et al., 2011) to produce **6**, followed by coupling with **1** using Steglich conditions.

Further analogs of compound **3a** were designed to explore modifications to the imide nucleus and the hydrophobic isobutyl region (R^1). The synthesis was performed according to **Scheme 3**

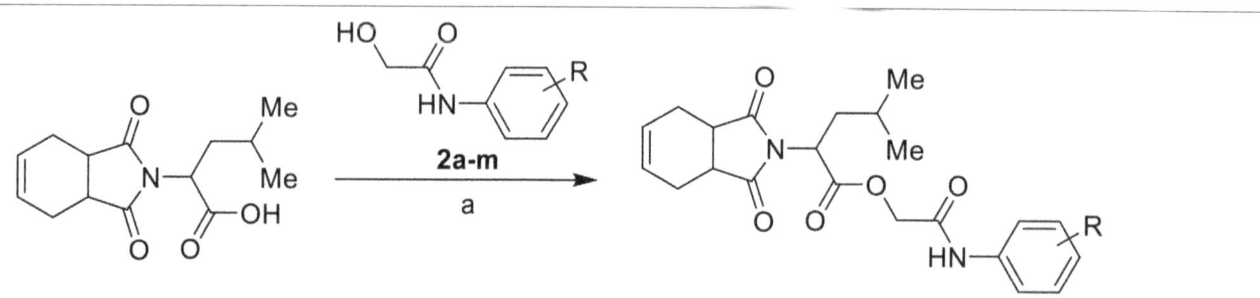

1

3a: R = *m*-chloro-*p*-methoxy
3b: R = *p*-methoxy
3c: R = *m*-chloro
3d: R = hydrogen
3e: R = *p*-fluoro
3f: R = *p*-bromo
3g: R = *p*-chloro
3h: R = *p*-hydroxy
3i: R = phenyl
3j: R = *p*-fluoro-*m*-nitro
3k: R = *p*-*N*-Boc-methylamino →(b) 3k':R = *p*-methylamino
3l: R = *p*-nitro →(c) 3l':R = *p*-amino
3m: R = *p*-methoxy-*o*-nitro →(c) 3m': R = *p*-methoxy-*o*-amino

SCHEME 1 | Synthesis of initial hit **3a** and analogs with modifications to the aromatic ring. Reagents and conditions: (a) CH_2Cl_2, **1**, EDC, DMAP (cat), rt, 4 h; (b) CH_2Cl_2, HCl (4 M in 1,4-dioxane), rt, 4 h; (c) MeOH, H_2 1 atm, 10% Pd/C, rt, 30 min.

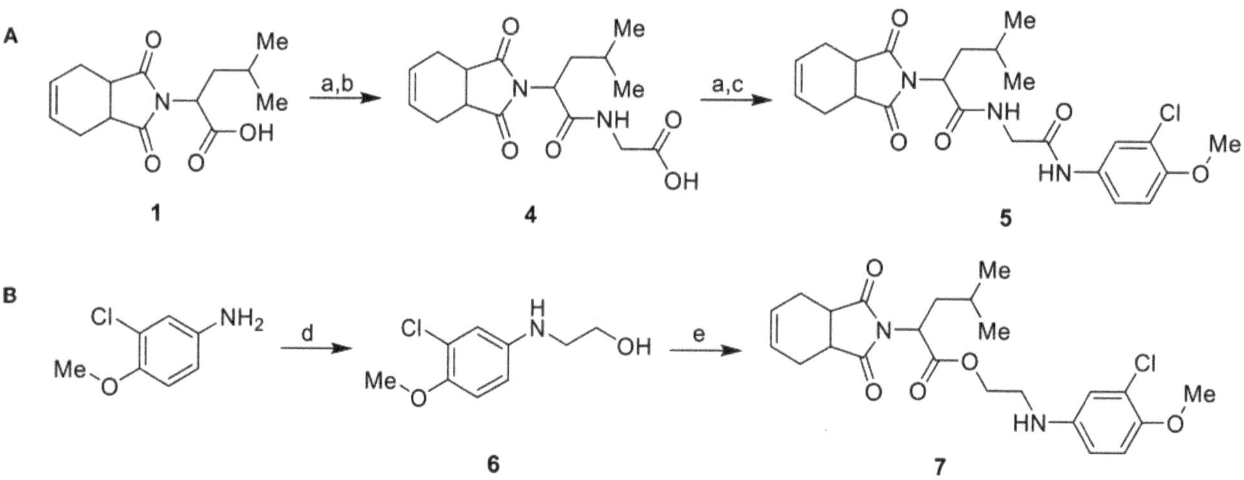

SCHEME 2 | Synthesis of analogs of the initial hit **3a** with modifications to the ester and amide functional groups. **(A)** Synthesis of compound **5** by coupling intermediate **4** with 3-chloro-4-methoxyaniline. **(B)** Synthesis of compound **7** by coupling compoud **6** with **1**. Reagents and conditions: (a) CH_2Cl_2, oxalyl chloride, DMF (cat), rt, 2 h; (b) CH_2Cl_2, glycine, Et_3N, rt, 2 h; (c) CH_2Cl_2, 3-chloro-4-methoxyaniline, Et_3N, rt, 2 h; (d) DMF, ethylene carbonate, molecular sieve 4 Å (cat), 150°C, 4 d; (e) CH_2Cl_2, **1**, EDC, DMAP (cat), rt, 4 h.

to evaluate the effects of changing the stereochemical and electronic features on the biological activity of the target compounds. Intermediates **9a-c** and **9g** were prepared according to a previously described procedure (Faghihi, 2008). A mixture of readily available *L*-amino acids and the corresponding cyclic anhydride in acetic acid stirred overnight, followed by 4 h of reflux to obtain carboxylic acids **9a-c** and **9g**. The synthesis of compounds **9d-f** and **9h-j** was carried out by refluxing in toluene with triethylamine as the catalyst. The stereocenter of the carboxylic acids was observed to have the absolute configuration of *R* (Pande et al., 2014). The amino acid side chains gave rise to hydrophobic fragments. Diazotization of *L*-leucine (Badiola et al., 2014) followed by bromoacid formation and subsequent nucleophilic substitution with the appropriate amines generated the amine nucleus in intermediates **9k-n**, presumably with an inverted configuration of the stereogenic center (*S*) due to inversion during the nucleophilic substitution reaction. Intermediates **9a-n** were coupled under Steglich conditions (Neises and Steglich, 1978) to produce the intended esters **10a-n**. Compound **10o** was produced by deprotection of the N-Boc analog (**10n**) under acidic conditions.

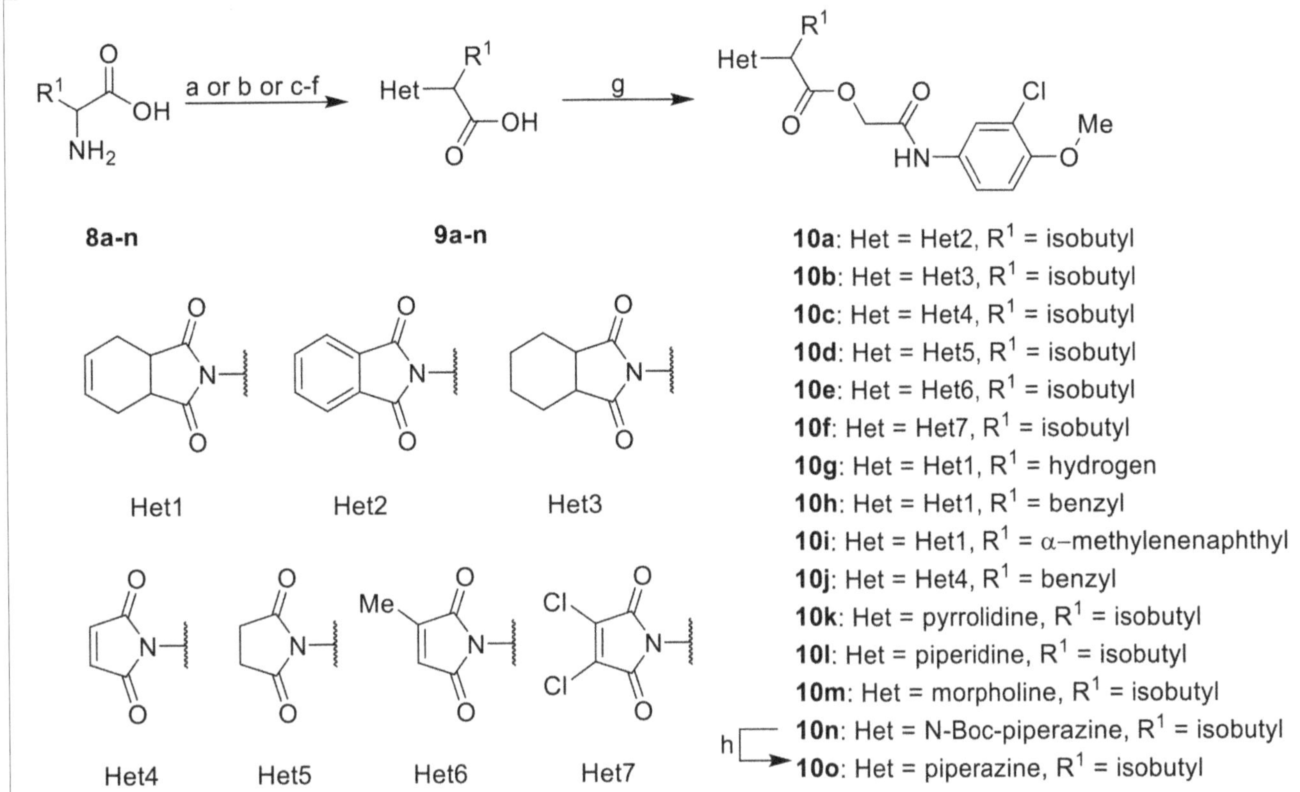

SCHEME 3 | Synthesis of analogs of compound **3a** with changes to the imide and isobutyl moieties. Reagents and conditions: (a) (for compounds **9a-c** and **9g**) AcOH, cyclic anhydride (correspondent to Het), rt, o.n., then reflux, 4 h; (b) (for compounds **9d-f**, **9h-j**) toluene, cyclic anhydride (corresponding to Het), Et_3N (cat), reflux, 3 h; (c) (for compounds **9k-n**) H_2O, HBr (48% v/v in H_2O), $NaNO_2$, 0°C to rt, 3 h; (d) CH_2Cl_2, BnOH, EDC, DMAP (cat), rt, 4 h; (e) MeCN, amine (corresponding to Het), Cs_2CO_3, rt – 60°C, 30 min – o.n.; (f) MeOH, H_2 1 atm, 10% Pd/C, rt, 30 min; (g) CH_2Cl_2, **2a**, EDC, DMAP (cat), rt, 4 h; (h) CH_2Cl_2, HCl (4 M in 1,4-dioxane), rt, 4 h.

Identification of Imide Derivatives as Cruzain Inhibitors

The activities of inhibitor **3a** (IC_{50} = 2.2 μM) and its analogs having modifications to the imide moiety against cruzain are shown in **Figure 2**. The incorporation of an aromatic ring into the imide ring to form an isoindoline-1,3-dione core in compound **10a** reduced the percent inhibition from 88 to 39% at an inhibitor concentration of 100 μM. In fact, compound **10a** assumes a completely different binding conformation, with the imide projecting into the S2 subsite. This causes the loss of key interactions with the enzyme as predicted by the molecular docking simulations (**Figure S1A**). The coupling of a saturated ring to the imide resulted in a 2-fold decrease in the potency of compound **10b** (IC_{50} = 4.2 μM) over **3a**. The addition of unsaturation to the unsubstituted imide yielded compound **10c** (IC_{50} = 2.3 μM), which was equipotent with respect to inhibitor **3a**. In fact, compound **10c** preserves the enzyme-inhibitor interactions observed for **3a**, however, the imide carbonyl oxygen is predicted to interact with the side chain nitrogen of Trp184 instead of Gln19. The predicted binding modes of analogs **10b** and **10c** are shown in **Figures S1B,C**, respectively). Withdrawing the unsaturation of the imide produced compound **10d** (IC_{50} = 12.0 μM), which was 6-fold less active than **3a**.

Following the positive result observed for compound **10c**, we designed compounds **10e** and **10f**, which have the imide nucleus incorporating an unsaturation but with two different substitution patterns. Compound **10e**, with a methyl substituent, was equipotent (IC_{50} = 2.5 μM) relative to **10c**, whereas compound **10f**, featuring two chlorine atoms as substituents, resulted in a 6-fold increase in potency (IC_{50} = 0.60 μM). Replacing the imide core with an amine (**10k**, **10l**, **10m**, **10n**, and **10o**) led to a significant drop in the activity of the compounds, highlighting the essentiality of the carbonyl groups. In fact, **Figure 1B** shows a hydrogen bond between one of the carbonyl groups and the side chain nitrogen of Gln19 at the S1 subsite. Replacing the imide group with other ring systems, such as pyrrolidine, piperidine, and morpholine, abrogated the biological activity of this series. The predicted binding conformations of **10k** and **10l** (pyrrolidine and piperidine derivatives, respectively) show that the lack of the imide carbonyl groups changes the binding pattern of these compounds compared to that observed for the active analogs. As shown in **Figure S2**, the isobutyl and cyclic amines do not interact with

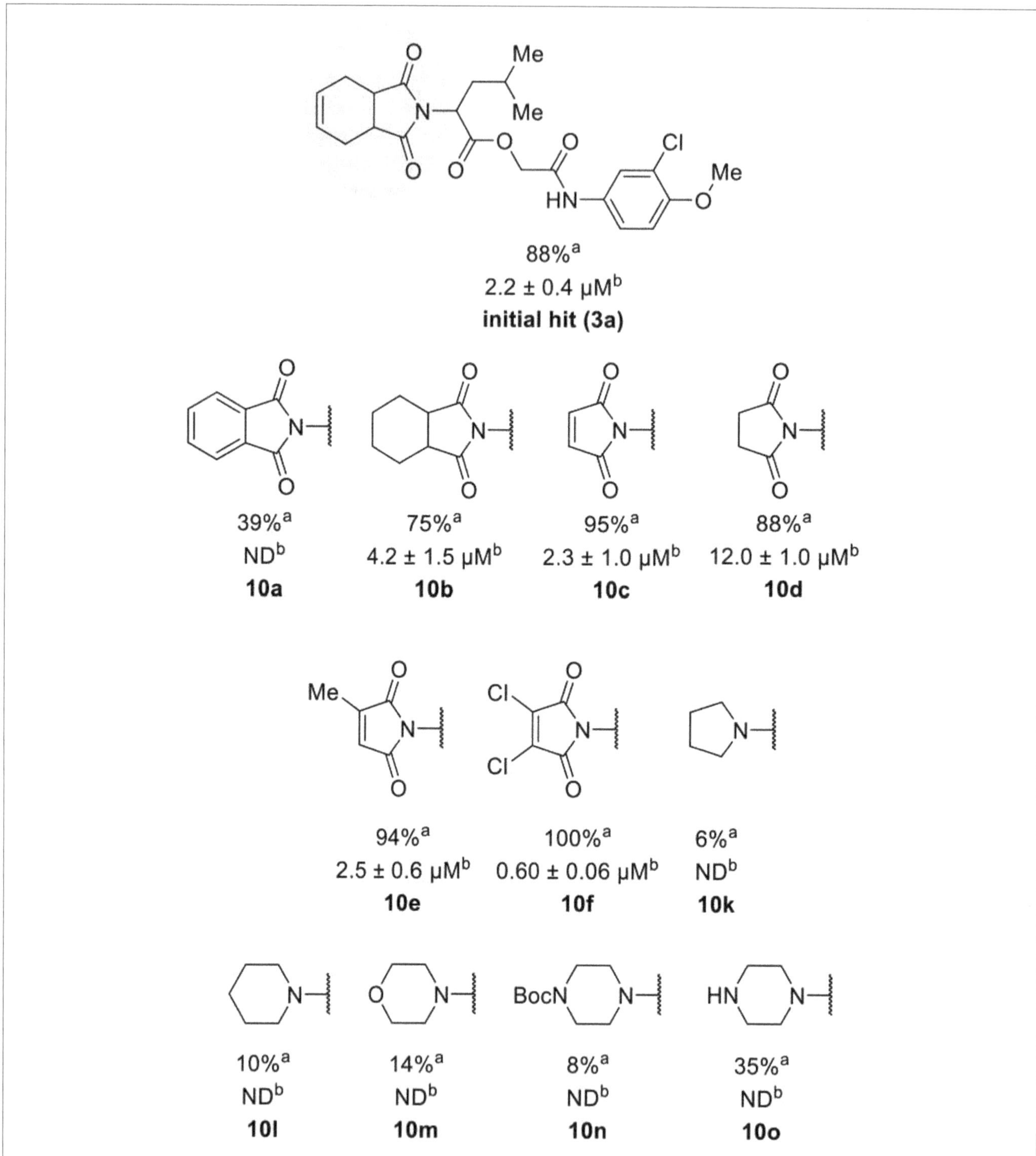

FIGURE 2 | Activity of the series of analogs featuring modifications in the imide nucleus against cruzain. [a]Percent inhibition against cruzain at 100 μM corresponding to the mean of three measurements. [b]IC_{50} values against cruzain, which were independently determined by obtaining rate measurements in triplicate for at least six inhibitor concentrations. The IC_{50} values represent the mean ± SD of three individual experiments. ND, IC_{50} not determined.

the S1' and S1 subsites as expected, and become exposed to the solvent.

The molecular optimization strategy also involved modifications to the hydrophobic (isobutyl) fragment of compound **3a** (**Figure 3A**). Removing the isobutyl group to obtain a methylene as the linker between the ester and the imide rendered the resulting compound inactive (**10g**). Bulky hydrophobic groups proved to be essential for interaction with

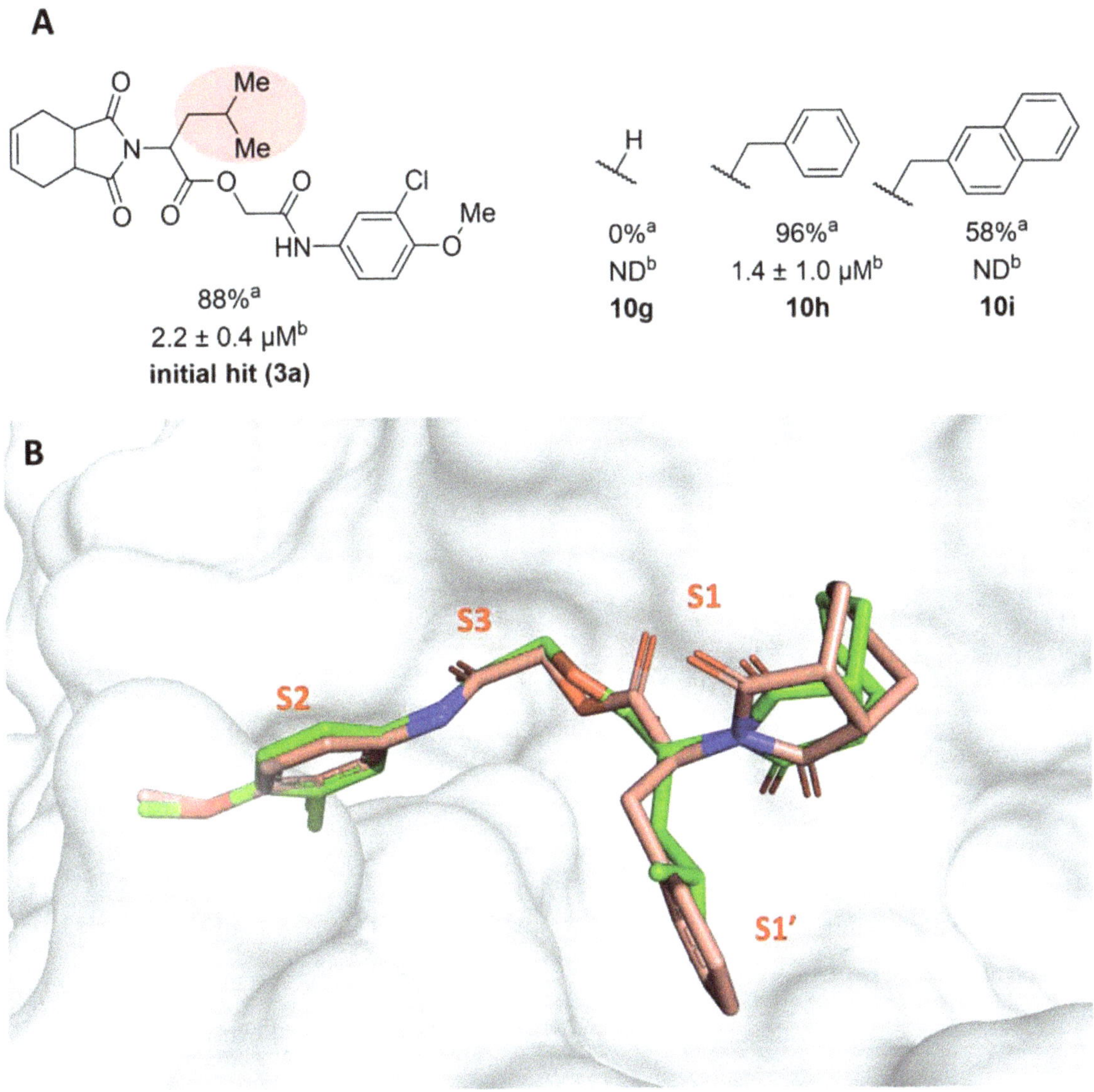

FIGURE 3 | (A) Results for modifications of the isobutyl fragment. [a]Percent inhibition against cruzain at 100 μM corresponding to the mean of three measurements. [b]IC_{50} values against cruzain, which were independently determined by obtaining rate measurements in triplicate for at least six inhibitor concentrations. The IC_{50} values correspond to the mean ± SD of three individual experiments. ND, IC_{50} not determined. **(B)** Superposition of the molecular docking-predicted binding conformation of compounds **3a** (carbon in green) and compound **10 h** (carbon in salmon). Cruzain (PDB 3KKU, 1.28 Å) is depicted in surface representation. Inhibitors **3a** and **10 h** are shown as sticks. Cruzain subsites are labeled as S1, S1', S2, and S3.

the S1' subsite. Replacing the isobutyl with a methylene led to a completely different binding pattern from that observed for the active compounds. The docking algorithm was unable to place the imide into S1 and the aromatic ring into S2, which rendered compound **10g** inactive (**Figure S3A**). Replacement of the isobutyl by the bulkier and planar benzyl group increased the potency by 2-fold (**10h**, $IC_{50} = 1.4\,\mu M$) compared to compound **3a**. This activity improvement can be reasoned to be a result of the better complementarity of the benzyl group with the S1' subsite of the enzyme (**Figure 3B**). Replacing the benzyl with the bulkier methylene naphthyl moiety led to compound **10i**, which was significantly less active, suggesting the ideal volume of a benzyl ring to occupy the S1' subsite. In fact, the naphthyl group of analog **10i** projects into the S2 subsite, which can be the driving force for the percent inhibition value (58%) determined for this compound since S2 usually accommodates bulky hydrophobic groups (**Figure S3B**). However, this modification caused the imide to lose its interaction with S1, which is a key driving force for the activity of this series.

To probe the relevance of the ester and amide groups for the activity of cruzain inhibitors, compounds **5** and **7** were prepared (**Figure 4A**). Replacing the ester with an amide, resulting in compound **5**, caused a reduction in the percent inhibition from 88 to 38%. Converting the amide carbonyl

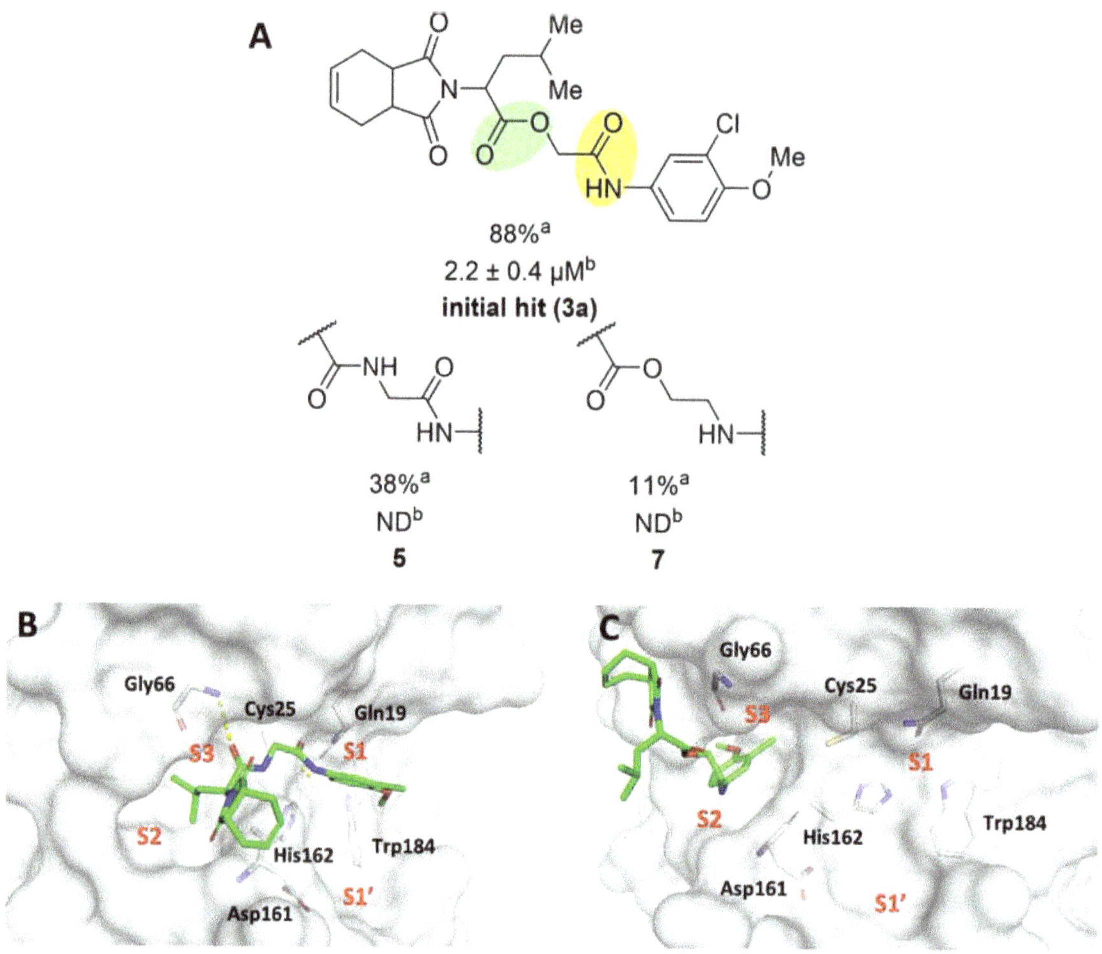

FIGURE 4 | (A) Results for the modifications to the ester and secondary amide functions. [a]Percent inhibition against cruzain at 100 μM corresponding to the mean of three measurements. [b]IC_{50} values against cruzain, which were independently determined by obtaining rate measurements in triplicate for at least six inhibitor concentrations. The IC_{50} values correspond to the mean ± SD of three individual experiments. ND: IC_{50} not determined. **(B)** Molecular docking predicted binding mode of compound **5**. **(C)** Predicted binding mode of compound **7**. Cruzain (PDB 3KKU, 1.28 Å) is depicted in surface representation. Binding site residues (carbon in gray) and inhibitors (carbon in green) are shown as sticks. Hydrogen bonds are shown as dashed lines. Cruzain subsites are labeled as S1, S1', S2, and S3.

into a methylene decreased the biological activity even further, as observed for compound **7** (11% inhibition). As illustrated in **Figure 1B**, the amide oxygen of compound **3a** is predicted to form a hydrogen bond with the main chain nitrogen of Gly66 and the ester carbonyl interacts with Gln19. The loss of these interactions may be one of the reasons for the significant activity drop observed for compound **7**. In fact, modifying the ester and amide groups significantly changed the binding mode of both compounds **5** and **7** (**Figures 4B,C**, respectively) compared to that of the active analogs. Compound **5**, which had the two carbonyl groups preserved, forms a hydrogen bond with Gly66 at S3, which can be reasoned as the cause of its higher percent inhibition value (38%) compared to that of analog **7** (11%). Notwithstanding, the imide of both compounds is exposed to the solvent and no interaction with S1' is observed, which are critical detrimental features of analogs **5** and **7**.

The leverage of the 3-chloro-4-methoxyphenyl moiety on cruzain activity was assessed by modifying the substitution pattern of the aromatic ring (**Figure 5**). Removing either chlorine or methoxyphenyl led to the less active compounds **3b** (IC_{50} = 13.9 μM) and **3c** (IC_{50} = 40.1 μM), respectively. Compound **3b** retains the key polar interactions with the enzyme, however, the lack of the chlorine prevents an optimal interaction with the S2 pocket, which is known to be essential for potent cruzain inhibition as reported previously (Ferreira et al., 2014) (**Figure S4A**). The effect of removing the methoxy group from the S2-interacting aromatic ring proved to be more detrimental to activity than the removal of the chlorine. In fact, compound **3c** was predicted to lose most of the key polar interactions with the enzyme (**Figure S4B**), which resulted in a poorly active compound (IC_{50} = 40.1 μM). The unsubstituted phenyl derivative (**3d**) was 8-fold less active (IC_{50} = 16.7 μM) than the parent 3-chloro-4-methoxyphenyl compound (**3a**). Additional

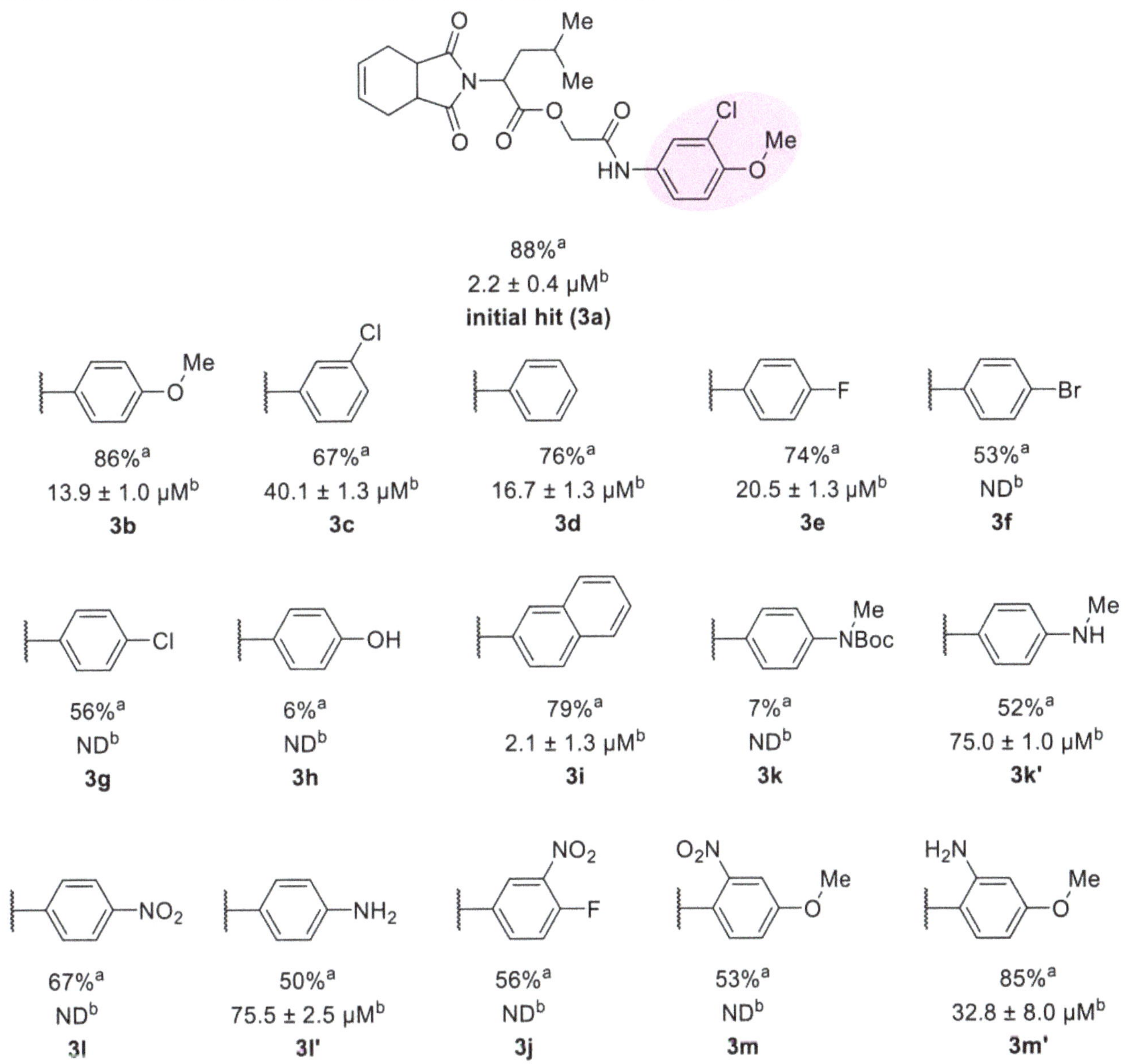

FIGURE 5 | Results for the modifications to the aromatic ring. [a]Percent inhibition against cruzain at 100 μM corresponding to the mean of three measurements. [b]IC_{50} values against cruzain, which were independently determined by obtaining rate measurements in triplicate for at least six inhibitor concentrations. The IC_{50} values correspond to the mean ± SD of three individual experiments. ND, IC_{50} not determined.

manipulations, such as introducing hydrogen bond donors and acceptors and replacing the chlorine or changing its position, led to poorly active or inactive compounds (**3e-h**, **3k**, **3k'**, **3l**, **3l'**, **3j**, **3m**, and **3m'**). **Figures S4** and **S5** show that a suboptimal interaction between the aromatic ring and the S2 subsite lead to the loss of most, if not all, polar contacts that proved to be important for activity. The exception was compound **3i**, with naphthyl replacing the phenyl as the S2-interacting aromatic system (**Figure S5D**). This is consistent with the binding mode of these compounds, which shows that the aromatic moiety interacts with the S2 subsite (**Figure 1B**). The S2 subsite, which is mostly composed of hydrophobic amino acids, can accommodate bulky groups, as shown in our previous work on benzimidazole derivatives (Ferreira et al., 2014). Such groups can therefore promote an optimum interaction with the S2 subsite, leading to more potent cruzain inhibitors.

Since all compounds described so far were obtained from enantiopure amino acids, we next evaluated how the absolute configuration influences the activity against cruzain. To this end, the racemic form of compound **10h** was prepared ($\mathbf{10h}_{rac}$). The synthesis of $\mathbf{10h}_{rac}$ was achieved by the same procedure presented in **Scheme 3**, using *DL*-phenylalanine instead of *L*-phenylalanine. Chiral column HPLC and optical rotation analyses confirmed that all reactions did not lead to racemization when *L*-phenylalanine was used as the starting material. These analyses also confirmed that the racemic compound was obtained when *DL*-phenylalanine was used as the starting material. The racemate (**10h**$_{rac}$) exhibited an IC_{50} value of 1.16 μM against cruzain, while compound **10h** had an IC_{50} of 1.4 μM. The very close IC_{50} values obtained for both the racemate and the enantiopure compound demonstrated that the absolute configuration of the stereocenter is not relevant to the activity of this series of compounds.

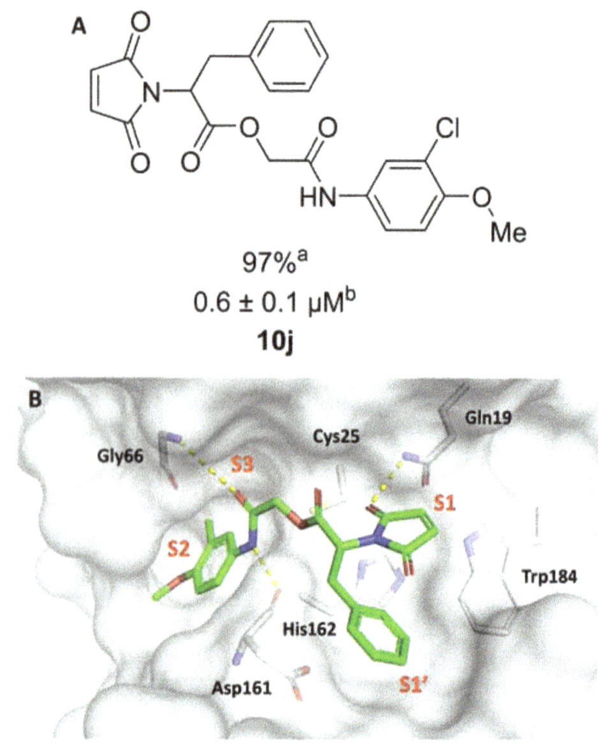

FIGURE 6 | (A) Modifications to the imide nucleus and hydrophobic fragment. [a]Percent inhibition against cruzain at 100 μM corresponding to the mean of three measurements. [b]IC_{50} values against cruzain, which were independently determined by obtaining rate measurements in triplicate for at least six inhibitor concentrations. The IC_{50} values correspond to the mean ± SD of three individual experiments. ND, IC_{50} not determined. **(B)** Molecular docking predicted binding mode of compound **10j**. Cruzain (PDB 3KKU, 1.28 Å) is depicted in surface representation. Binding site residues (carbon in gray) and inhibitors (carbon in green) are shown as sticks. Hydrogen bonds are shown as dashed lines. Cruzain subsites are labeled as S1, S1', S2, and S3.

In the next molecular optimization step, we combined the best fragments from all five regions of initial hit **3a**. This strategy produced the most active compound (**10j**, IC_{50} = 0.6 μM) among the synthesized analogs, which was 4-fold more active than compound **3a** (**Figure 6A**). Compound **10j** conserves the same binding mode of the other active compounds in this series, forming the key intermolecular interactions with the S1, S1', S2, and S3 subsites. The S1' and S2 subsites are optimally filled with the benzyl and 3-chloro-4-methoxyphenyl rings, respectively. A hydrogen bond is formed between the amide oxygen and Gly66, and the imide carbonyl interacts with Gln19 (**Figure 6B**).

The aim of this study was to identify new imide derivatives as competitive cruzain inhibitors. Considering the competitive nature of hit compound **3a**, the synthesized analogs were expected to follow the same behavior. Hence, we conducted further studies to establish the mechanism of inhibition of compounds **10h** and **3i**. The competitive mechanism of these compounds was corroborated by the Lineweaver–Burk plots shown in **Figure 7**. As expected for competitive inhibitors, the maximum velocity ($1/V_{max}$, intersections with the *y*-axis) remained unchanged with increasing inhibitor concentrations [I], while the apparent Michaelis–Menten constant ($K_M^{app} = -1/K_M$, intersections with the *x*-axis) increased with escalating [I].

Discovery of Novel Trypanocidal Agents

The biological activity of 22 compounds was evaluated against *T. cruzi* intracellular amastigotes along with **BZ** (**Tables 1–3**). Several compounds showed trypanocidal activity similar to or superior to that of **BZ** (IC_{50} = 3.0 μM). The data in **Table 1** show that the hit compound **3a**, despite being a potent cruzain

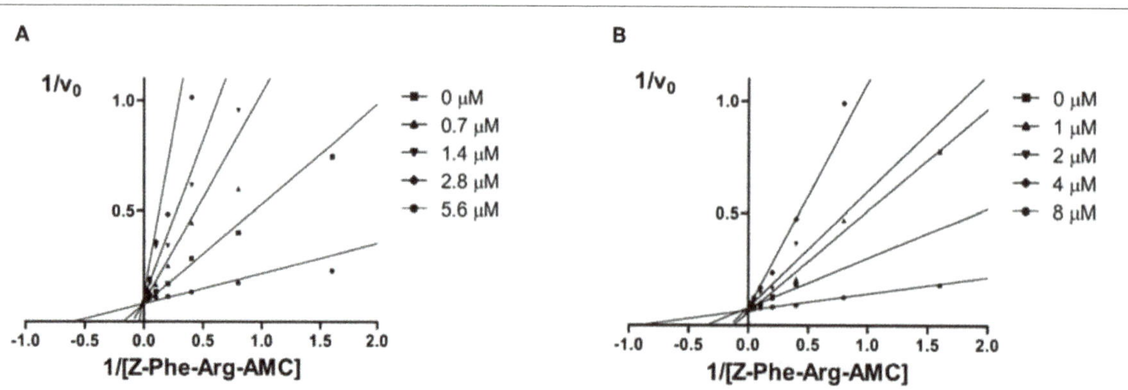

FIGURE 7 | Double reciprocal *Lineweaver-Burk* plots for compounds **10 h (A)** and **3i (B)**. Each curve denotes to a different inhibitor concentration.

TABLE 1 | Cruzain inhibition and trypanocidal activity of compounds with modifications to the imide nucleus.

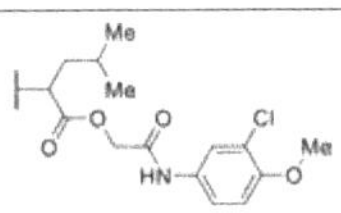

Compound	Structure	IC_{50} cruzain (μM)[a]	IC_{50} *T. cruzi* (μM)[b]
Initial hit (3a)	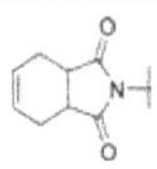	2.2 ± 0.4	>100
10b	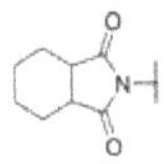	4.2 ± 1.5	>100
10c	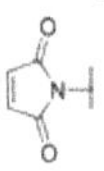	2.3 ± 1.0	0.9 ± 0.3
10d	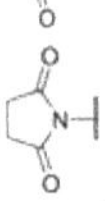	12.0 ± 1.0	18.5 ± 3.1
10e	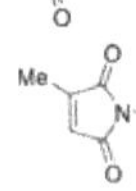	2.5 ± 0.6	1.2 ± 0.3
10f	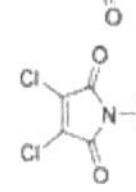	0.6 ± 0.1	2.0 ± 0.7
10k	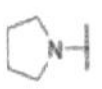	ND	>100
10l	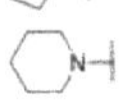	ND	11.6 ± 2.4
10m	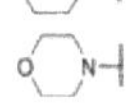	ND	1.8 ± 0.4
10n	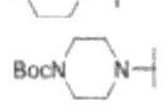	ND	1.6 ± 0.5
10o	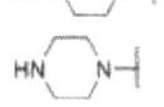	ND	1.7 ± 0.5
BZ	-	ND	3.0 ± 0.6

[a]IC_{50} values against cruzain were independently determined by obtaining rate measurements in triplicate for at least six inhibitor concentrations. The values represent the mean ± SD of three individual experiments. [b]IC_{50} values against T. cruzi represent the mean ± SD of two individual experiments. ND, not determined.

TABLE 2 | Cruzain inhibition and trypanocidal activity of compounds with modifications to the hydrophobic fragment and the amide function.

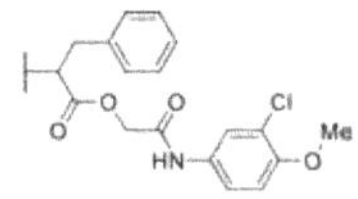

Compound	Structure	IC_{50} cruzain (μM)[a]	IC_{50} *T. cruzi* (μM)[b]
10h	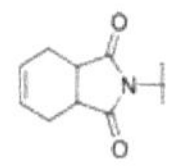	1.4 ± 0.8	>100
10j	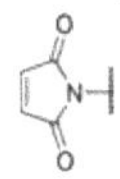	0.6 ± 0.1	1.0 ± 0.3
7	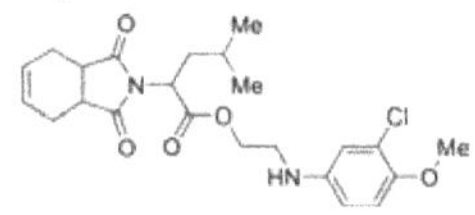	ND	1.5 ± 0.4

[a]IC_{50} values against cruzain were independently determined by obtaining rate measurements in triplicate for at least six inhibitor concentrations. The values represent the mean ± SD of three individual experiments. [b]IC_{50} values against T. cruzi represent the mean ± SD of two individual experiments. ND, not determined.

TABLE 3 | Cruzain inhibition and trypanocidal activity of compounds with modifications to the aromatic ring.

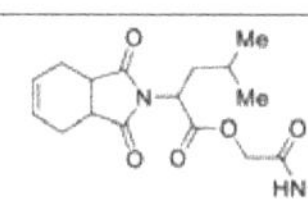

Compound	Structure	IC_{50} cruzain (μM)[a]	IC_{50} *T. cruzi* (μM)[b]
3k	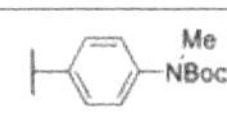	ND	3.9 ± 0.9
3k'	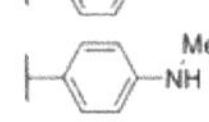	75.0 ± 1.0	>100
3l	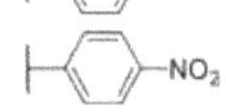	ND	>100
3l'	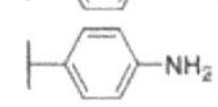	75.5 ± 2.5	>100
3m'	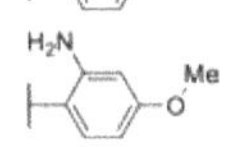	32.0 ± 8.0	>100
3d	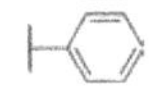	16.7 ± 1.3	>100
3e	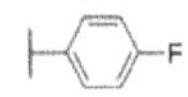	20.5 ± 1.3	>100
3i	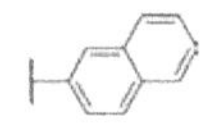	2.1 ± 1.3	32.8 ± 4.9

[a]IC_{50} values against cruzain were independently determined by obtaining rate measurements in triplicate for at least six inhibitor concentrations. The values represent the mean ± SD of three individual experiments. [b]IC_{50} values against T. cruzi represent the mean ± SD of two individual experiments. ND, not determined.

inhibitor, was not active against the parasite. The same behavior was observed for compound **10b**, which differs from **3a** only by the absence of a double bond in the ring coupled to the imide. Compounds having the imide with unsaturation and without the coupled six-membered ring showed promising trypanocidal activity (**10c**, **10e,** and **10f**, IC_{50} values of 0.9, 1.2 and 2 μM, respectively).

Compounds lacking the imide carbonyl groups (**10l-10o**), although inactive against cruzain, were active against *T. cruzi.* Compound **10k**, in which the imide was replaced with a pyrrolidine, was inactive against both cruzain and *T. cruzi.* Replacing pyrrolidine with piperidine, a larger heterocycle, resulted in compound **10l**, which was moderately active against the parasite (IC_{50} = 11.6 μM). Introducing an additional heteroatom in the 6-membered cycle, whether nitrogen or oxygen, generated remarkably active compounds (**10m**, **10n,** and **10o**, IC_{50} values of 1.8, 1.6, and 1.7, respectively). These results indicate that these cyclic amines exert their trypanocidal activity by modulating a molecular target other than cruzain.

Table 2 shows the data for compounds modified on the hydrophobic fragment and the amide group. Replacing the isobutyl with a benzyl group resulted in compound **10h**, which, although active against cruzain, was inactive against the parasite. Notwithstanding, the benzyl group in compound **10j** combined with the maleimide fragment generated the most active compound against both *T. cruzi* (IC_{50} = 1.0 μM) and cruzain (IC_{50} = 0.6 μM). Compound **7**, in which the amide carbonyl was removed, displayed the opposite behavior to that of compound **10h**, i.e., **7** was active against *T. cruzi* but inactive on cruzain.

As shown in **Table 3**, except for compounds **3k** and **3i**, modifications to the aromatic ring were unfavorable for activity against both *T. cruzi* and cruzain.

Figure 8 illustrates an SAR scheme for the synthesized imide derivatives. Following our initial approach, compound **3a** was divided into five fragments, and the most relevant SARs were identified. In short, the imide function, although required for cruzain inhibition, is not essential for activity against *T. cruzi*. Benzyl is the ideal hydrophobic fragment for activity against cruzain and is tolerable regarding the activity against *T. cruzi*. Replacement of the 3-chloro-4-methoxyphenyl fragment is, in general, unfavorable for activity against *T. cruzi* and cruzain. Removal of the ester group is unfavorable for activity against cruzain, while the replacement of the secondary amide proved to be tolerable regarding the trypanocidal activity. The gathered data showed a lack of a direct correlation between the phenotypic and target-based results for some compounds; this was expected to some degree given the complexity of the intracellular environment and issues related to transport across membranes. For other compounds, however, the target-based and phenotypic data are clearly correlated. Compounds **10c**, **10e**, **10f**, and **10g**, for instance, besides being active against the enzyme, proved to be potent trypanocidal agents.

In vitro Toxicity and Selectivity

The cytotoxicity of the synthesized analogs was assessed using HFF-1 human fibroblasts and HepG2 human hepatocytes (**Table 4**). The selectivity index (SI) was calculated as the ratio between the CC_{50} values for the human cells and the IC_{50} values for *T. cruzi*. In general, the designed compounds demonstrated no significant toxicity against HFF-1 and HepG2 cells. Three compounds showed SI values for HFF-1 fibroblasts comparable or superior to that of **BZ** (SI >33): **10m** (SI >55), **7** (SI >66) and **3k** (SI >25). It is worth noting that these compounds were active against *T. cruzi*. Another aspect worth mentioning is that the most cytotoxic compounds (**10c**, **10e**, and **10j**) are Michael acceptors, which is a possible reason for their cytotoxicity. With respect to cytotoxicity to HepG2 cells, most compounds produced higher SI values than that of **BZ**, particularly those that are highly active against *T. cruzi*: **10c** (SI = 36.6), **10f** (SI >32), **10m** (SI >35), **10o** (SI = 30.6), **10j** (SI = 67), and **7** (SI = 42).

CONCLUSION

The SBDD strategy applied herein, comprising synthetic organic chemistry, molecular docking, enzyme kinetics and phenotypic assays, resulted in the discovery of potent, reversible and non-peptidic cruzain inhibitors with remarkable trypanocidal activity. The success of this experimental-computational molecular optimization approach can be illustrated by compound **10j**, the most potent cruzain inhibitor (IC_{50} = 0.6 μM), which is significantly more active than initial hit **3a** (IC_{50} = 2.2 μM). One of the most potent cruzain inhibitors reported to date, compound **10j** represents a new chemical class among the known inhibitors of this enzyme. Furthermore, compound **10j** shows trypanocidal activity (IC_{50} = 1.0 μM) that is 3-fold higher than that of the clinically used drug **BZ** (IC_{50} = 3.0 μM). Other promising compounds are **10c**, **10f**, **10m**, **10n**, **10o**, **10j**, **7** and **3k**, which showed trypanocidal activity comparable to that of **BZ** and SI values (HFF-1/*T. cruzi*) >10.

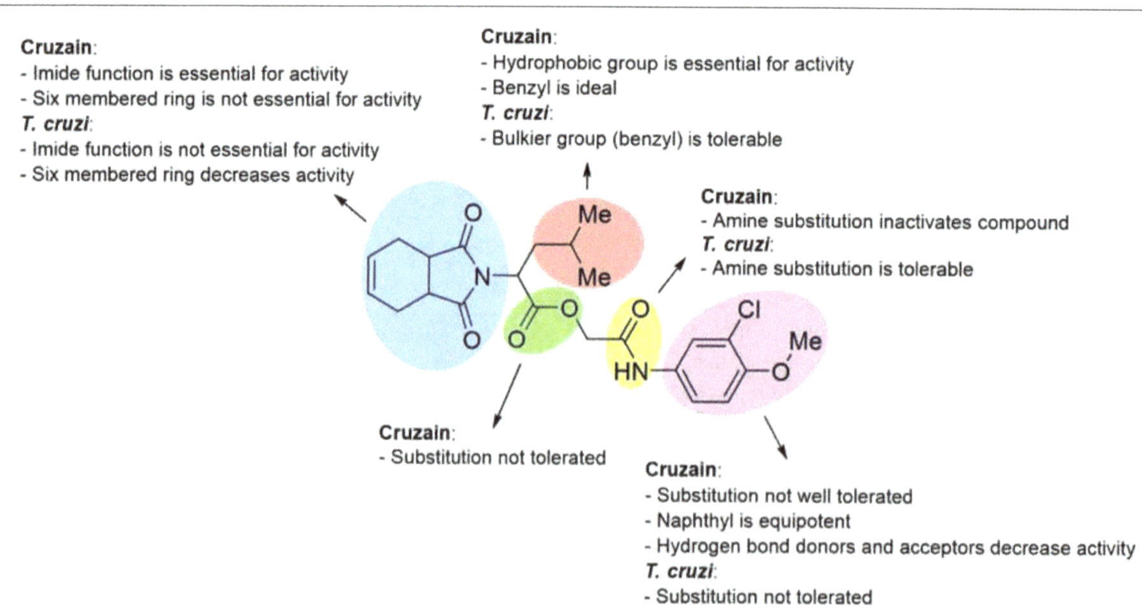

FIGURE 8 | SAR scheme for both cruzain and *T. cruzi*. Compound **3a** was used as the reference structure.

TABLE 4 | Comparison of the trypanocidal activity with cytotoxicity data obtained for HFF-1 and HepG2 cells.

Compound	IC_{50} *T. cruzi* (μM)[a]	CC_{50} HFF-1 (μM)[b]	SI HFF-1/*T. cruzi*[c]	CC_{50} HepG2 (μM)[b]	SI HepG2/*T. cruzi*[c]
BZ	3.0 ± 0.6	>100	>33	>64	>21
10c	0.9 ± 0.3	12 ± 1	13.3	33 ± 5	36.6
10d	18.5 ± 3.1	>100	>5	>64	>3
10e	1.2 ± 0.3	4.8 ± 0.5	4	5 ± 1	4.2
10f	2.0 ± 0.7	33 ± 9	16.5	>64	>32
10l	11.6 ± 2.4	>100	>8	>64	>5
10m	1.8 ± 0.4	> 100	>55	>64	>35
10n	1.6 ± 0.5	32 ± 5	20	27 ± 2	16.9
10o	1.7 ± 0.5	32 ± 3	18.8	52 ± 7	30.6
10j	1.0 ± 0.3	15.7 ± 0.8	15.7	67 ± 8	67
7	1.5 ± 0.4	>100	>66	63 ± 8	42
3k	3.9 ± 0.9	>100	>25	>64	>16
3i	32.8 ± 4.9	>100	>3	45 ± 8	1.4
Doxorubicin	–	0.21 ± 0.09	–	0.4 ± 0.1	–

[a]*T. cruzi intracellular amastigote assay. Data represent the mean ± SD of two independent assays.* [b]*Cytotoxicity assay. Data represent the mean ± SD of two independent assays.* [c]*Selectivity index (SI), CC_{50}/IC_{50}.*

The target-based results enabled the identification of relevant SARs, which allowed the uncovering of pivotal structural aspects that drive the enzyme-inhibitor molecular recognition and the activity of the investigated compounds. Moreover, these findings provide substantial insights into the design of reversible cruzain inhibitors, which can be useful to surmount the drawbacks associated with irreversible ligands. An important aspect to remark is the *in vitro* toxicity profile of some compounds, which indicates that they may be safer than the drugs currently available for the treatment of Chagas disease. In a context characterized by a lack of therapeutic innovation and serious safety and efficacy issues, the cruzain inhibitors described herein can be explored as novel chemical matter in forthcoming Chagas disease drug discovery campaigns.

AUTHOR CONTRIBUTIONS

RAF: conceptualization, writing, molecular design, and organic synthesis. IP: conceptualization, writing, molecular design, and enzyme kinetics. TS: organic synthesis. CR: organic synthesis. MS: molecular design and enzyme kinetics. RSF: conceptualization, molecular design, and enzyme kinetics. LM and RK: *in vitro* experiments. LF: writing, molecular design, and *in vitro* experiments. LD: conceptualization, supervision, organic synthesis, and writing. AA: conceptualization, supervision, molecular design, and writing.

FUNDING

The National Council for Scientific and Technological Development (CNPq), Brazil, the Coordination for the Improvement of Higher Education Personnel (CAPES), Brazil, and the São Paulo Research Foundation (FAPESP), Brazil, grants 2013/07600-3 and 2011/13789-6, for financial support and postdoctoral fellowship (grant 158926/2014-5).

REFERENCES

Arnal, A., Waleckx, E., Rico-Chávez, O., Herrera, C., Dumonteil, E. (2019). Estimating the current burden of Chagas disease in Mexico: A systematic review and meta-analysis of epidemiological surveys from 2006 to 2017. *PLoS Negl. Trop. Dis.* 13:e0006859. doi: 10.1371/journal.pntd.0006859

Avelar, L. A., Camilo, C. D., de Albuquerque, S., Fernandes, W. B., Gonçalez, C., Kenny, P. W., et al. (2015). Molecular design, synthesis and trypanocidal activity of dipeptidyl nitriles as cruzain inhibitors. *PLoS Negl. Trop. Dis.* 7:e0003916. doi: 10.1371/journal.pntd.0003916

Badiola, E., Fiser, B., Gómez-Bengoa, E., Mielgo, A., Olaizola, I., Urruzuno, I., et al. (2014). Enantioselective construction of tetrasubstituted stereogenic carbons through Brønsted base catalyzed michael reactions: α'-hydroxy enones as key enoate equivalent. *J. Am. Chem. Soc.* 136, 17869–17881. doi: 10.1021/ja 510603w

Barltrop, J. A., Owen, T. C., Cory, A. H., and Cory, J. G. (1991). 5-(3-carboxymethoxyphenyl)-2-(4,5-dimethylthiazolyl)-3-(4-sulfophenyl)tetrazolium, inner salt (MTS) and related analogs of 3-(4,5-dimethylthiazolyl)-2,5-diphenyltetrazolium bromide (MTT) reducing to purple water-soluble formazans as cell-viability indicators. *Bioorg. Med. Chem. Lett.* 1, 611–614. doi: 10.1016/S0960-894X(01)81162-8

Bern, C. (2015). Chagas' disease. *N. Engl. J. Med.* 373, 456–466. doi: 10.1056/NEJMra1410150

Buckner, F. S., Verlinde, C. L., La Flamme, A. C., and Van Voorhis, W. C. (1996). Efficient technique for screening drugs for activity against *Trypanosoma cruzi* using parasites expressing beta-galactosidase. *Antimicrob. Agents Chemother.* 40, 2592–2597. doi: 10.1128/AAC.40.11.2592

Clark, M., Cramer III, R. D., and Van Opdenbosch, N. (1989). Validation of the general purpose tripos 5.2 force field. *J. Comput. Chem.* 10, 982–1012. doi: 10.1002/jcc.540100804

Cucunubá, Z. M., Okuwoga, O., Basáñez, M. G., and Nouvellet, P. (2016). Increased mortality attributed to Chagas disease: a systematic review and meta-analysis. *Parasit. Vectors* 9:42. doi: 10.1186/s13071-016-1315-x

Dias, J. C., Coura, J. R., and Yasuda, M. A. (2014). The present situation, challenges, and perspectives regarding the production and utilization of effective drugs against human Chagas disease. *Rev. Soc. Bras. Med. Trop.* 47, 123–125. doi: 10.1590/0037-8682-0248-2013

Doyle, P. S., Zhou, Y. M., Hsieh, I., Greenbaum, D. C., McKerrow, J. H., and Engel, J. C. (2011). The *Trypanosoma cruzi* protease cruzain mediates immune evasion. *PLoS Pathog.* 7:e1002139. doi: 10.1371/journal.ppat.10 02139

Engel, J. C., Doyle, P. S., Palmer, J., Hsieh, I., Bainton, D. F., and McKerrow, J. H. (1998). Cysteine protease inhibitors alter Golgi complex ultrastructure and function in *Trypanosoma cruzi*. *J. Cell Sci.* 111, 597–606.

Espíndola, J. W., Cardoso, M. V., Filho, G. B., Oliveira, E., Silva, D. A., Moreira, D. R., et al. (2015). Synthesis and structure-activity relationship study of a new series of antiparasitic aryloxyl thiosemicarbazones inhibiting *Trypanosoma cruzi* cruzain. *Eur. J. Med. Chem.* 101, 818–835. doi: 10.1016/j.ejmech.2015.06.048

Faghihi, K. (2008). New optically active poly(amide-imide)s based on N,N′-(pyromellitoyl)-bis-L-amino acid and 1,3-bis(4-aminophenoxy) propane: synthesis and characterization. *J. Appl. Polym. Sci.* 109, 74–81. doi: 10.1002/app.27675

Ferreira, L. G., and Andricopulo, A. D. (2017). Targeting cysteine proteases in trypanosomatid disease drug discovery. *Pharmacol. Ther.* 180, 49–46. doi: 10.1016/j.pharmthera.2017.06.004

Ferreira, L. L. G., and Andricopulo, A. D. (2019). Drugs and vaccines in the 21st century for neglected diseases. *Lancet Infect. Dis.* 19, 125–127. doi: 10.1016/S1473-3099(19)30005-2

Ferreira, R. S., Dessoy, M. A., Pauli, I., Souza, M. L., Krogh, R., Sales, A. I., et al. (2014). Synthesis, biological evaluation, and structure-activity relationships of potent noncovalent and nonpeptidic cruzain inhibitors as anti-*Trypanosoma cruzi* agents. *J. Med. Chem.* 6, 2380–2392. doi: 10.1021/jm 401709b

Ferreira, R. S., Simeonov, A., Jadhav, A., Eidam, O., Mott, B. T., Keiser, M. J., et al. (2010). Complementarity between a docking and a high-throughput screen in discovering new cruzain inhibitors. *J. Med. Chem.* 53, 4891–4905. doi: 10.1021/jm100488w

Gasteiger, J., and Marsili, M. I. (1980). Iterative partial equalization of orbital electronegativity - a rapid access to atomic charges. *Tetrahedron* 36, 3219–3228. doi: 10.1016/0040-4020(80)80168-2

GBD DALYs and HALE Collaborators. (2016). Global, regional, and national disability-adjusted life-years (DALYs) for 315 diseases and injuries and healthy life expectancy (HALE), 1990-2015: a systematic analysis for the Global Burden of Disease Study. *Lancet* 388, 1603–1658. doi: 10.1016/S0140-6736(16) 31460-X

Jones, G., Willett, P., Glen, R. C., Leach, A. R., and Taylor, R. (1997). Development and validation of a genetic algorithm for flexible docking. *J. Mol. Biol.* 267, 727–748. doi: 10.1006/jmbi.1996.0897

Jose Cazzulo, J., Stoka, V., and Turk, V. (2001). The major cysteine proteinase of *Trypanosoma cruzi*: a valid target for chemotherapy of Chagas disease. *Curr Pharm Des.* 7, 1143–1156. doi: 10.2174/1381612013397528

Kinage, A. K., Upare, P. P., Shivarkar, A. B., and Gupte, S. P. (2011). Highly regio-selective synthesis of β-amino alcohol by reaction with aniline and propylene carbonate in self solvent system over large pore zeolite catalyst. *GSC* 1, 76–84. doi: 10.4236/gsc.2011.13013

Latorre, A., Schirmeister, T., Kesselring, J., Jung, S., Joh,é, P., Hellmich, U. A., et al. (2016). Dipeptidyl nitroalkenes as potent reversible inhibitors of cysteine proteases rhodesain and cruzain. *ACS Med. Chem. Lett.* 7, 1073–1076. doi: 10.1021/acsmedchemlett. 6b00276

Lill, M. A., and Danielson, M. L. (2011). Computer-aided drug design platform using PyMOL. *J. Comput. Aided Mol. Des.* 1, 13–19. doi: 10.1007/s10822-010-9395-8

McKerrow, J. H. (1999). Development of cysteine protease inhibitors as chemotherapy for parasitic diseases: insights on safety, target validation, and mechanism of action. *Int. J. Parasitol.* 29, 833–837. doi: 10.1016/S0020-7519(99)00044-2

Molina, I., Salvador, F., Sánchez-Montalv,á, A., Treviño, B., Serre, N., Sao Avilés, A., et al. (2015). Toxic profile of benznidazole in patients with chronic chagas disease: risk factors and comparison of the product from two different manufacturers. *Antimicrob. Agents Chemother.* 59, 6125–6123. doi: 10.1128/AAC.04660-14

Mott, B. T., Ferreira, R. S., Simeonov, A., Jadhav, A., Ang, K. K., Leister, W., et al. (2010). Identification and optimization of inhibitors of Trypanosomal cysteine proteases: cruzain, rhodesain, and TbCatB. *J. Med. Chem.* 53, 52–60. doi: 10.1021/jm901069a

Ndao, M., Beaulieu, C., Black, W. C., Isabel, E., Vasquez-Camargo, F., Nath-Chowdhury, M., et al. (2014). Reversible cysteine protease inhibitors show promise for a Chagas disease cure. *Antimicrob. Agents Chemother.* 2, 1167–1178. doi: 10.1128/AAC.01855-13

Neises, B., and Steglich, W. (1978). Simple method for the esterification of carboxylic acids. *Angew.Chem.* 17, 522–524. doi: 10.1002/anie.197 805221

Neitz, R. J., Bryant, C., Chen, S., Gut, J., Caselli, E. H., Ponce, S., et al. (2015). Tetrafluorophenoxymethyl ketone cruzain inhibitors with improved pharmacokinetic properties as therapeutic leads for Chagas' disease. *Bioorg. Med. Chem. Lett.* 21, 4834–4837. doi: 10.1016/j.bmcl.2015.06.066

Olivera, M. J., Cucunubá, Z. M., Álvarez, C. A., and Nicholls, R. S. (2015). Safety profile of nifurtimox and treatment interruption for chronic chagas disease in colombian adults. *Am. J. Trop. Med. Hyg.* 93, 1224–1230. doi: 10.4269/ajtmh.15-0256

Pande, S. V., Utale, P. S., Gholse, S. B., Tekade, P. V., and Patil, S. G. (2014). Synthesis and antibacterial evaluation of carboxamide derivatives of amino acids. *Pharm. Chem. J.* 48, 29–33. doi: 10.1007/s11094-014-1040-8

Pérez-Molina, J. A., and Molina, I. (2018). Chagas disease. *Lancet* 391, 82–94. doi: 10.1016/S0140-6736(17)31612-4

Powell, M. J. D. (1977). Restart procedures for conjugate gradient method. *Math. Program.* 12, 241–254. doi: 10.1007/BF01593790

Rogers, K. E., Keränen, H., Durrant, J. D., Ratnam, J., Doak, A., Arkin, M. R., et al. (2012). Novel cruzain inhibitors for the treatment of Chagas' disease. *Chem. Biol. Drug Des.* 3, 398–405. doi: 10.1111/j.1747-0285.2012. 01416.x

8

Vienna LiverTox Workspace—A Set of Machine Learning Models for Prediction of Interactions Profiles of Small Molecules with Transporters Relevant for Regulatory Agencies

Floriane Montanari†, Bernhard Knasmüller, Stefan Kohlbacher, Christoph Hillisch, Christine Baierová, Melanie Grandits and Gerhard F. Ecker*

Pharmacoinformatics Research Group, Department of Pharmaceutical Chemistry, University of Vienna, Vienna, Austria

***Correspondence:**
Melanie Grandits
melanie.grandits@univie.ac.at

†Present address:
Floriane Montanari,
Department of Digital Technologies,
Bayer AG, Berlin, Germany

Transporters expressed in the liver play a major role in drug pharmacokinetics and are a key component of the physiological bile flow. Inhibition of these transporters may lead to drug-drug interactions or even drug-induced liver injury. Therefore, predicting the interaction profile of small molecules with transporters expressed in the liver may help medicinal chemists and toxicologists to prioritize compounds in an early phase of the drug development process. Based on a comprehensive analysis of the data available in the public domain, we developed a set of classification models which allow to predict—for a small molecule—the inhibition of and transport by a set of liver transporters considered to be relevant by FDA, EMA, and the Japanese regulatory agency. The models were validated by cross-validation and external test sets and comprise cross validated balanced accuracies in the range of 0.64–0.88. Finally, models were implemented as an easy to use web-service which is freely available at https://livertox.univie.ac.at.

Keywords: Vienna LiverTox Workspace, web service, machine learning, ABC-transporter, OATP-transporter, toxicity, classification models

INTRODUCTION

Membrane transporters expressed in the liver play different, but interconnected roles: on the one hand, basolateral transporters pick up xenobiotics, and endogenous molecules from the portal vein to the liver, or excrete their substrates into the blood. Apical transporters, on the other hand, take care of the flux toward the bile duct network (**Figure 1**). Three main types of substrates are of interest with respect to liver toxicity: drugs, which enter the hepatocytes at the first hepatic pass or at the elimination stage; bilirubin, a product of the degradation of the heme; and bile salts, which circulate between the gastro-intestinal tract, and the liver.

Additionally, to the enzyme family of cytochromes, also the transporters expressed in the liver are crucial for a fully functional organ. Some of them are e.g., involved in the bilirubin cycle: OATP1B1 and OATP1B3 uptake bilirubin into the hepatocytes (Briz et al., 2003), where glucuronidation takes place. MRP2 then excretes the bilirubin conjugate to the bile (Kamisako et al., 1999). At the basolateral membrane, MRP3 might also excrete it back to the sinusoidal blood (Keppler, 2014). As a result, inhibition of the uptake OATP transporters or of MRP2 may

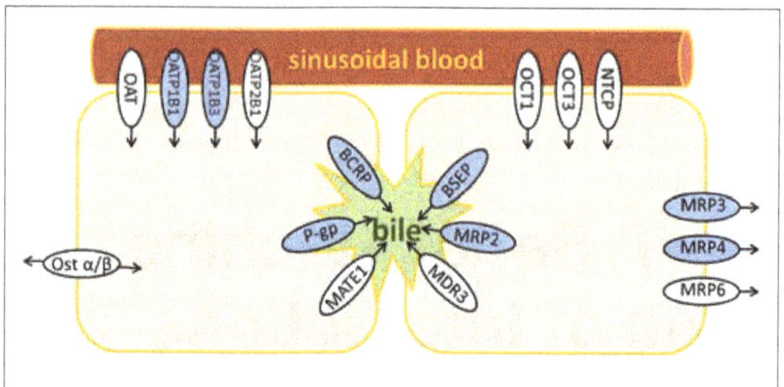

FIGURE 1 | Main hepatic transporters. In blue, transporters for which predictive models (inhibition and/or transport) are available in the Vienna LiverTox Workspace.

lead to the accumulation of bilirubin (conjugated or not) in the blood, which is referred to as hyperbilirubinemia. Conjugated hyperbilirubinemia is a marker of hepatobiliary injury (Dufour et al., 2000; Ozer et al., 2008; Padda et al., 2011), and predicting it may allow to flag compounds that could cause liver injury.

Bile acids are synthesized in the liver by catabolism of cholesterol and then excreted to the bile by the active bile salt export pump (BSEP) and by the multidrug resistance-associated protein 2 (MRP2) (Meier and Stieger, 2002). Bile salts have a pronounced detergent effect, which explains their toxicity when they accumulate in the liver (Attili et al., 1986). For their transport in the bile duct, bile salts form mixed micelles with phospholipids of the outer leaflet of the membrane. The multidrug resistance protein 3 (MDR3) allows lipid flopping at the apical membrane of the hepatocyte, and its function is necessary to avoid bile duct toxicity (Nicolaou et al., 2012). After reaching the intestine via the bile flow, bile acids are reabsorbed into the portal vein, and taken up again into the hepatocytes by the sodium taurocholate co-transporting polypeptide (NTCP) (Stieger, 2011). Impairment of bile flow leading to a toxic accumulation of bile salts in the hepatocytes might lead to drug-induced cholestasis, which is one of the main causes of drug-induced liver injury (DILI) (Padda et al., 2011).

Apart from playing a role in proper bile flow and bilirubin elimination, liver transporters also transport drugs that will then be metabolized and excreted. At this stage, drugs can inhibit different transporters and cause drug-drug interactions (König et al., 2013) (in case of co-administered inhibitor and substrate) or liver injury (by disrupting the bile flow for example). This is why predicting the inhibition and the substrate profile for liver transporters might be useful in identifying potentially problematic compounds. In addition, the Food and Drugs administration recommends experimental testing of the interactions between drugs and transporters (especially P-gp, BCRP, OATP1B1, and OATP1B3) to identify potential drug-drug interactions (U.S. Department of Health Human Services Food Drug Administration Center for Drug Evaluation Research, 2012). Thus, it definitely would be of value to have a suite of computational models available which allow the fast and easy assessment of compounds for their interaction profile with transporters expressed in the liver.

Here, we present the Vienna LiverTox Workspace, a web server for the prediction of interactions with liver transporters as well as selected liver toxicity endpoints. To the best of our knowledge, it is the first time that such an ensemble of predictive models for hepatotoxicity and liver transport is made available to the public. The predictions are made by individual machine learning models built on publicly available data for each target of interest.

Abbreviations: ADME-Tox, absorption distribution metabolism excretion toxicity; BCRP, breast cancer resistance protein; BSEP, bile salt export pump; DILI, drug-induced liver injury; ECFP, extended connectivity fingerprint, MDR1, multidrug resistance protein 1; MDR3, multidrug resistance protein 3; MRP2, multidrug resistance-associated protein 2; MRP3, multidrug resistance-associated protein 3; MRP4, multidrug resistance-associated protein 4; NTCP, sodium taurocholate co-transporting polypeptide; OATP1B1, organic anion transporting polypeptide 1B1; OATP1B3, organic anion transporting polypeptide 1B3; P-gp, P-glycoprotein; SMILES, simplified molecular input line entry system.

METHODS

Data Curation

The datasets for the training and testing of the models were collected from different sources (online tools as well as publications). The data were cleaned by using an in-house system combining the molecular operating environment (MOE 2014.09) (Molecular Operating Environment, 2014) wash option and the Atkinson Standardiser (https://github.com/flatkinson/standardiser). This approach was used for some of the datasets and for others the cleaning procedure of already published papers were used (Pinto et al., 2012; Kotsampasakou et al., 2015). In general, duplicates were removed from the dataset, including pairs of stereoisomers. Further, if these compounds share the same class label, one of the compounds was kept. A detailed list of references as well as the number of compounds revealed after the preprocessing of the data is given in **Table S1**. In the sections Transporter Models and Hepatotoxicity Models, the data curation as well as the model generation for the specific endpoints is given. The datasets are available in the Supplementary Material (**Data Sheet 2**).

Transporter Models

The web service allows for the prediction of interactions between a small molecule and eight different liver transporters (**Figure 1**, transporters marked in blue). The lack of publicly available data for the other transporters explains the absence of respective models in the Vienna LiverTox Workspace.

All the models predicting whether a compound will be a substrate of a transporter (BCRP, P-gp, BSEP, MRP2, and MRP3) were built upon a dataset correlating expression levels of 47 ABC-transporters with drug toxicity, which can then be used to infer transported vs. non-transported compounds (Szakács et al., 2004). For the transport inhibition models (BCRP, P-gp, BSEP, MRP3, MRP4, OATP1B1, and OATP1B3) the datasets were collected from literature and, if necessary, manually aggregated. In both cases, the models predict a binary outcome: the query compound is a substrate or not, or an inhibitor or not.

For chemistry encoding of the compounds, we used circular fingerprints or 2D molecular descriptors as implemented in

TABLE 1 | Overview of the parameters used for the models.

	Descriptors	Trainings set	Algorithm
INHIBITION			
P-gp (MDR1)	ECFP8-like fingerprints	Broccatelli et al., 2011	SVM
BSEP	Molecular descriptors	Warner et al., 2012 Dawson et al., 2012 Morgan et al., 2010	Naïve bayes
BCRP	ECFP8-like fingerprints	Montanari and Ecker, 2014	Logistic regression
MRP3	Molecular descriptors	Köck et al., 2014	BayesNet
MRP4	Molecular descriptors	Köck et al., 2014	AdaBoost (MetaCost)
OATP1B1	Molecular descriptors	De Bruyn et al., 2013	BayesNet
OATP1B3	Molecular descriptors	De Bruyn et al., 2013	BayesNet
TRANSPORT			
P-gp (MDR1)	Molecular descriptors	Szakács et al., 2004	Rotation Forest (MetaCost)
BSEP			SVM (MetaCost)
BCRP			k-nearest neighbors (MetaCost)
MRP2			
MRP3			
TOXICITY			
Hyperbilirubinemia	ECFP8-like fingerprints	Liu et al., 2011	SVM (MetaCost)
Cholestasis	Molecular descriptors	SIDER v2 database (Kuhn et al., 2010, 2016)	Tree model (MetaCost)
Drug-induced liver injury (DILI)	Molecular descriptors	Various sources*	Random Forest

*see https://livertox.univie.ac.at/ for a detailed list.

RDKit version 2015.03.1 (https://www.rdkit.org/). Different machine learning algorithms were applied and the one giving the best cross-validation results was kept as final model. Especially for the transport prediction, a heavy class imbalancy (most of the drugs in the training set were non-substrates) was noted, which was handled by MetaCost (Domingos, 1999). The exact methodology and cross-validation performance for each individual transporter model is described in the documentation available at https://livertox.univie.ac.at, and an overview is given in **Table 1**. In some cases, external test sets were collected from Metrabase (Mak et al., 2015) or from recent publications (time-split evaluation).

Hepatotoxicity Models

Three models in the web service can be used to assess human liver damage potentially caused by a test compound: hyperbilirubinemia, cholestasis, and drug-induced liver injury (DILI).

For hyperbilirubinemia, 835 compounds were taken from Kotsampasakou et al. (2017a) and the modeling methodology was kept as in Kotsampasakou et al. (2017b): ECFP-like fingerprints were computed with RDKit (https://www.rdkit.org/), then a combination of feature selection, MetaCost, and support vector machines with RBF kernel was used for learning. The cholestasis model uses data from Kotsampasakou and Ecker (2017) and a combination of MetaCost and a tree algorithm to predict whether a compound is likely to cause cholestasis or not. Finally, the DILI model is based on a 966-compound dataset carefully compiled from literature (Kotsampasakou et al., 2017c). RDKit molecular descriptors and a random forest of 500 trees are used for modeling.

Web Service Implementation

The Vienna LiverTox Workspace has been implemented as Python/php based web service. It consists of two parts, namely the backend and the frontend. The backend consists of a docker image which runs the machine learning models on an input SD-File. It consists of a Python Flask server (https://palletsprojects.com/p/flask/) which processes the requests from the frontend. Each request consists of one or more input molecules and a list of models to run the predictions on. The frontend, also a docker image, is based on the CakePHP framework (https://cakephp.org/) and is responsible for the user interface (UI), which sends the request to the backend and displays the results. The web service provides, after a login, the possibility to upload a SD File of 10 compounds. The service can also be used without logging in but then it is only possible to draw and predict a single molecule. JSME (Bienfait and Ertl, 2013) is used as drawing tool. The web service runs on an Ubuntu Linux based server with two twelve-core Intel Xeon 64bit processors and 128 GB RAM, and is hosted at the University of Vienna by the Pharmacoinformatics Research Group.

The models use the RDKit library (https://www.rdkit.org/) (version 2015.03.1) for computing the descriptors and handling the chemistry aspects, while the Weka (Hall et al., 2009) (version 3.7.11) and scikit-learn (Pedregosa et al., 2011) (version 0.14.1) libraries are used to train and run the predictive models. The models also include a compound cleaning step, implemented with the Atkinson Standardiser (https://github.com/flatkinson/standardiser) (**Figure 2**).

The steps performed during model building and a test compound prediction are shown in **Figure 2**. In both cases, the compound is standardized and the molecular descriptors are calculated. In the case of the model generation, this allows the training of the model and its development (left workflow). For the prediction of a test compound, the descriptors are passed to the available model to predict its class affiliation (right workflow).

In general, the output of the model gives, in addition to the class prediction, the actual score. This score is a numerical value between 0 and 1, and roughly corresponds to a probability of being active (inhibitor, substrate, or toxic compound). Therefore, a value close to 1 indicates substrate/inhibitor/toxic properties, a value close to 0 annotates for non-substrates/non-inhibitors/non-toxic.

Applicability Domain

The Applicability Domain (AD) is used to validate the reliability of a given prediction model. It defines whether a dataset of interest is in or out of domain, meaning if it falls within the chemical space of the model or not. If it is out of Domain, the prediction cannot be regarded as reliable.

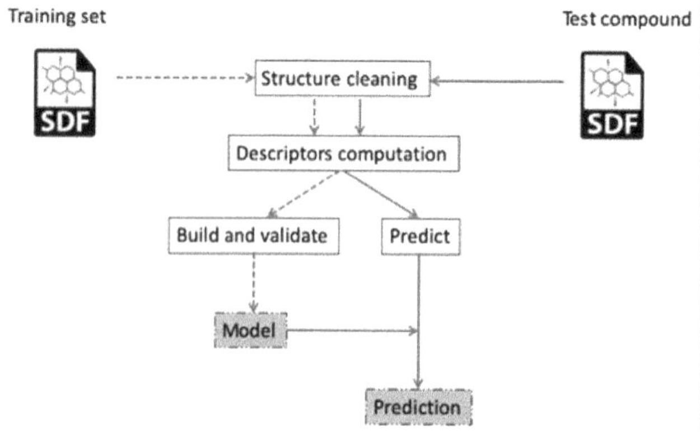

FIGURE 2 | General steps to build a model (left workflow, dotted line) or predict a property for a test compound (right workflow, solid line). Figure adapted from Carrió et al. (2015) published in Journal of Cheminformatics is licensed under CC BY 4.0 (https://creativecommons.org/licenses/by/4.0/).

In our study, an Applicability Domain model, using the approach of Sahigara et al. (2013), was created for each transporter with the respective training set. RDKit descriptors were used as molecule representation. This approach combines the classical, widely used k-Nearest Neighbor (k-NN) method with a probability density function estimation. It uses three stages to determine the reliable space of a prediction model. First, a set of thresholds is defined depending on the diverse densities of the training set by considering the 15 k-nearest neighbors using Euclidean distances. This allows the AD to consider a dense and sparse training region (The threshold defines if a test sample can be reliable predicted). In a next step a decision rule is derived to filter out outlier molecules. Finally, the reliability of the AD is tested by looking at the model statistics and prediction errors. This feature is not yet implemented in the Web service, but will be available soon.

RESULTS

Model Results

The performance of the models was estimated by calculating statistical performance metrics using a 10-fold cross-validation. The results are provided in **Table 2**. The overall accuracy, corresponding to the rate of correct predictions, ranges from 0.59 to 0.87. Also, the sensitivity of the models was calculated (0.57–0.85). This parameter gives the number of actual positives that are correctly identified and is expressed by the number of true positives divided by the number of positive predictions. Further, the number of actual negatives was determined by the

TABLE 2 | Performance metrics of the transporter models.

	Accuracy	Sensitivity	Specificity	Balanced accuracy	MCC	ROC AUC
INHIBITION						
P-gp (MDR1)	0.87	0.85	0.90	0.88	0.76	0.94
BSEP	0.85	0.77	0.87	0.82	0.60	0.91
BCRP	0.83	0.77	0.87	0.82	0.64	0.90
MRP3	0.82	0.75	0.87	0.81	0.62	0.86
MRP4	0.73	0.86	0.65	0.76	0.49	0.74
OATP1B1	0.77	0.71	0.78	0.75	0.34	0.80
OATP1B3	0.81	0.78	0.81	0.80	0.35	0.81
TRANSPORT						
P-gp (MDR1)	0.81	0.81	0.81	0.81	0.44	0.85
BSEP	0.71	0.65	0.72	0.69	0.28	0.69
BCRP	0.73	0.57	0.75	0.66	0.20	0.71
MRP2	0.70	0.60	0.72	0.66	0.27	0.73
MRP3	0.72	0.60	0.74	0.67	0.28	0.72
TOXICITY						
Hyperbilirubinemia	0.67	0.64	0.67	0.66	0.20	0.69
Cholestasis	0.59	0.72	0.56	0.64	0.22	0.64
Drug-induced liver injury (DILI)	0.65	0.72	0.58	0.65	0.30	0.70

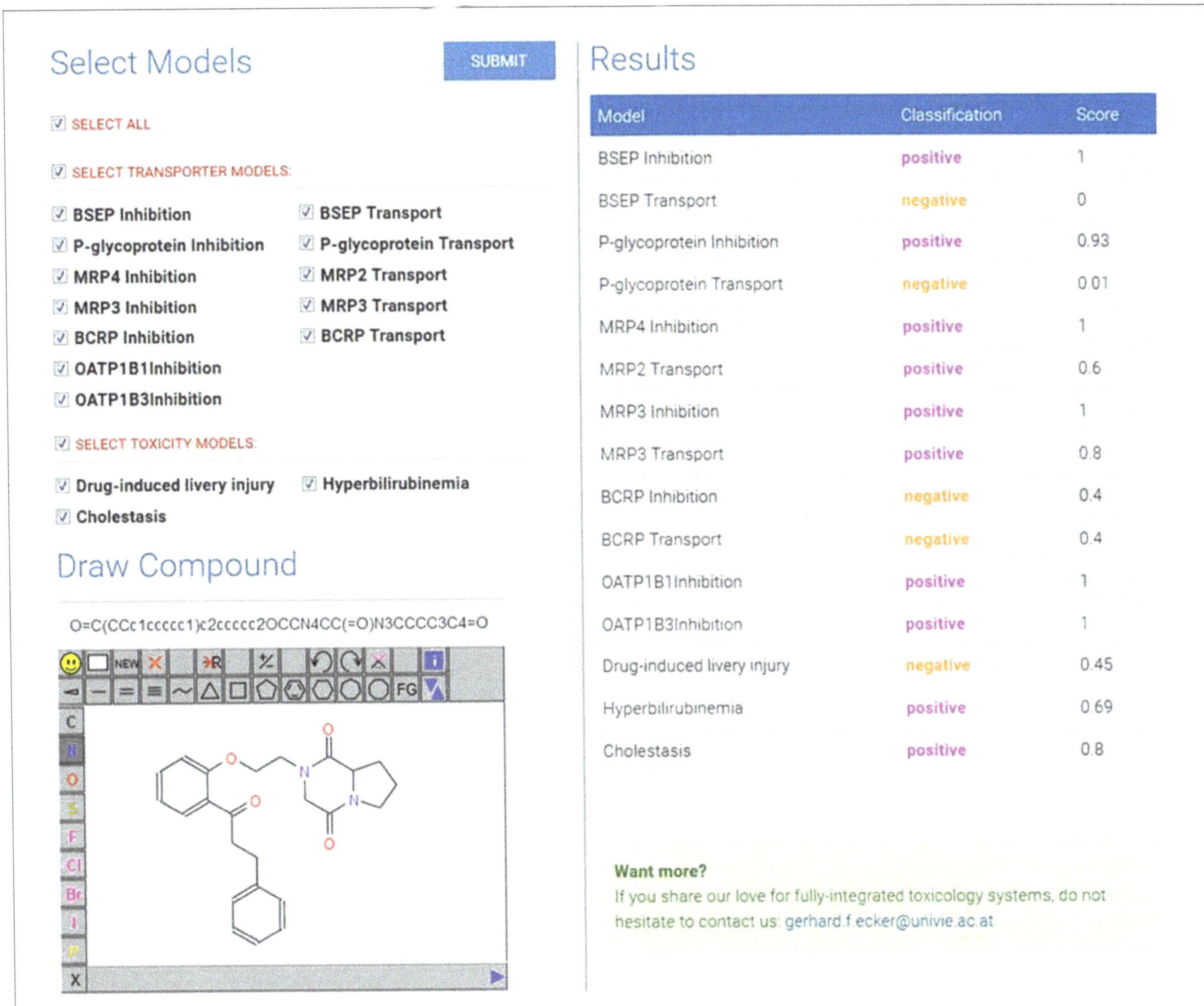

FIGURE 3 | Overview of the web service interface. On the left side, test compound is drawn and desired models are selected. On the right side, results table with the predictions and model scores.

number of true negatives divided by the number of negative predictions. The so-called specificity ranges from 0.56 to 0.90. To estimate a metric for the quality of the models, the Matthews correlation coefficient (MCC) and the Area under the Receiver Operating Characteristics curve (ROC AUC) were determined. The MCC is a number between −1 and 1 where 0 indicates a prediction equal to a random prediction and 1 indicates a perfect prediction, whereas −1 is a complete miss. The scores for our models are in the range of 0.20–0.76. The ROC AUC measures the ability of the model to distinguish between negatives and positives, while a higher value indicates a better performance. In the models provided on the Vienna LiverTox Workspace the ROC AUC ranges from 0.64 to 0.94. Furthermore, if data was available, the models were also validated with one or more external test sets. For more details see the documentation on the website.

Use Case: Prediction of Liver Interaction for a Propafenone Analog

In this section, we briefly detail how predictions can be generated for a given compound using the LiverTox web service. In first instance, the compound is drawn or its SMILES string is pasted in the Molecule Editor (Bienfait and Ertl, 2013). Then the models can be selected on the left panel, either one by one or all at the same time (**Figure 3**, left side).

By clicking on the SUBMIT button, the data is sent to the backend server where the predictions are running. Upon completion of the calculations, a table listing the different models and corresponding outputs will appear (**Figure 3**, right side). The second column in the results table corresponds to the binary classification, while the third column "Score" gives the actual output of the model, which corresponds to a probability of being active. For example, for BCRP inhibition and transport

TABLE 3 | Comparison of existing free online tools to predict ADME-Tox properties of compounds.

Web service	Transporters predictions	CYP450 predictions	Hepatotox. predictions	Batch prediction	Run time for 1 compound
ProTox-II (Drwal et al., 2014)	No	No	No	Yes (max. 100)	<5 s
BioZyne (Levatić et al., 2013)	P-gp	No	No	Not for free	~5 s
QSAR DB (http://qsar.food.dtu.dk/)	No	Yes	No	Yes	N.A.
pkCSM (Pires et al., 2015)	P-gp	Yes	Yes	Yes (max. 100)	<5 s for 30 models
Lazar (Maunz et al., 2013)	No	No	No	No	~10 s for 6 models
Vienna LiverTox Workspace	P-gp, BSEP, BCRP, MRP2, MRP3, MRP4, OATP1B1, OATP1B3	No	Yes	Not for free	~30 s for 15 models

and for DILI, the output score is close to 0.5 (which is the threshold used to separate predicted actives from predicted inactives), which indicates an uncertainty of these three models for the particular query compound. Propafenone derivatives are frequently reported as inhibitors of P-gp, and indeed the P-gp inhibition model predicts this particular one to be an inhibitor with a high score (0.93).

The Transporters selected for this web service were chosen based on their importance for regulatory agencies such as FDA, EMA and the Japanese regulatory agency. They recommend or in some cases request these proteins to be routinely tested in inhibition—and substrate studies of new drugs.

DISCUSSION

Many systems already exist to predict *in silico* activities or properties of small molecules. **Table 3** compares freely available ones with our own web service in terms of model offer, submission and run time. For example, ProTox-II predicts oral drug toxicity in rodents (lethal dose LD_{50} and a category of toxicity between 1 and 6) using similarity to compounds with known LD_{50} and recognition of toxic fragments (Drwal et al., 2014). BioZyne proposes exclusively one model for P-gp transport prediction based on the same dataset as ours (Szakács et al., 2004; Levatić et al., 2013). It uses a Support Vector Machine classifier for the prediction of P-gp substrates. The Danish (Q)SAR Database contains pre-calculated properties combined from more than 200 models from both commercial and free tools (http://qsar.food.dtu.dk/). Predictions for environmental toxicity, blood-brain barrier permeation, cytochrome interactions, or human genotoxicity are available. Unfortunately, new predictions for compounds that are not part of the database cannot be made. PkCSM is another web service for predicting pharmacokinetics properties of compounds (Pires et al., 2015). Models such as P-gp inhibition and transport, blood-brain barrier permeation, interaction with cytochromes, renal clearance, or even liver toxicity are available.

In general, our models for the inhibitors show a better performance especially when looking at the correct prediction of the positives. The prediction of true negatives is for the inhibitor and transporter models quite similar which can be explained by the availability of more negatives if the training set is unbalanced. This is especially the case for the substrate models. The quality of the prediction (MCC) is higher for the inhibition models of P-gp, BSEP, BCRP, and MRP3 since the available dataset is more balanced. In comparison, the three toxicity models show a poorer performance due to the complexity of these endpoints and especially for hyperbilirubinemia and cholestasis which shows also a lack of positives.

CONCLUSION

We have presented the Vienna LiverTox Workspace, a web service dedicated to the prediction of liver toxicity and interactions between small molecules and liver transporters. It is easy to use, fast, web browser agnostic, and well-documented. Thanks to its modular system, it will be easy to integrate new models in the future, as well as re-implement existing models in case new training data becomes available. We hope that our models will help researchers to flag potentially dangerous compounds and shed light on the relationships between liver transporters and toxicity.

AUTHOR CONTRIBUTIONS

FM, SK, CH, and MG developed the models. BK, CB, and MG implemented the web service. MG and GE supervised the study. FM and MG wrote the majority of the manuscript. All authors contributed to refining the manuscript.

FUNDING

We gratefully acknowledge financial support provided by the Austrian Science Fund, grant #F03502 (SFB35), and by the Innovative Medicines Initiative Joint Undertaking under grant agreement n°115002 (eTOX).

REFERENCES

Attili, A. F., Angelico, M., Cantafora, A., Alvaro, D., and Capocaccia, L. (1986). Bile acid-induced liver toxicity: relation to the hydrophobic-hydrophilic balance of bile acids. *Med. Hypotheses* 19, 57–69. doi: 10.1016/0306-9877(86)90137-4

Bienfait, B., and Ertl, P. (2013). JSME: a free molecule editor in JavaScript. *J. Cheminform.* 5:24. doi: 10.1186/1758-2946-5-24

Briz, O., Serrano, M. A., MacIas, R. I. R., Gonzalez-Gallego, J., and Marin, J. J. G. (2003). Role of organic anion-transporting polypeptides, OATP-A, OATP-C and OATP-8, in the human placenta-maternal liver tandem excretory pathway for foetal bilirubin. *Biochem. J.* 371, 897–905. doi: 10.1042/bj20030034

Broccatelli, F., Carosati, E., Neri, A., Frosini, M., Goracci, L., Oprea, T. I., et al. (2011). A novel approach for predicting P-glycoprotein (ABCB1) inhibition using molecular interaction fields. *J. Med. Chem.* 54, 1740–1751. doi: 10.1021/jm101421d

Carrió, P., López, O., Sanz, F., and Pastor, M. (2015). eTOXlab, an open source modeling framework for implementing predictive models in production environments. *J. Cheminform.* 7:8. doi: 10.1186/s13321-015-0058-6

Dawson, S., Stahl, S., Paul, N., Barber, J., and Kenna, J. G. (2012). *In vitro* inhibition of the bile salt export pump correlates with risk of cholestatic drug-induced liver injury in humans. *Drug Metab. Dispos.* 40, 130–8. doi: 10.1124/dmd.111.040758

De Bruyn, T., van Westen, G. J. P., IJzerman, A. P., Stieger, B., de Witte, P., Augustijns, P. F., et al. (2013). Structure-based identification of OATP1B1/3 inhibitors. *Mol. Pharmacol.* 83, 1257–1267. doi: 10.1124/mol.112.084152

Domingos, P. (1999). "MetaCost: a general method for making classifiers cost-sensitive," in *Proceedings of the Fifth ACM SIGKDD International Conference on Knowledge Discovery and Data Mining* (New York), 155–164. doi: 10.1145/312129.312220

Drwal, M. N., Banerjee, P., Dunkel, M., Wettig, M. R., and Preissner, R. (2014). ProTox: a web server for the *in silico* prediction of rodent oral toxicity. *Nucleic Acids Res.* 42, W53–W58. doi: 10.1093/nar/gku401

Dufour, D. R., Lott, J. A., Nolte, F. S., Gretch, D. R., Koff, R. S., and Seeff, L. B. (2000). Diagnosis and monitoring of hepatic injury. II. Recommendations for use of laboratory tests in screening, diagnosis, and monitoring. *Clin. Chem.* 46, 2050–68.

Hall, M., Frank, E., Holmes, G., Pfahringer, B., Reutemann, P., and Witten, I. H. (2009). The WEKA data mining software: an update. *SIGKDD Explor. Newsl.* 11, 10–18. doi: 10.1145/1656274.1656278

Kamisako, T., Leier, I., Cui, Y., König, J., Buchholz, U., Hummel-Eisenbeiss, J., et al. (1999). Transport of monoglucuronosyl and bisglucuronosyl bilirubin by recombinant human and rat multidrug resistance protein 2. *Hepatology* 30, 485–490. doi: 10.1002/hep.510300220

Keppler, D. (2014). The roles of MRP2, MRP3, OATP1B1, and OATP1B3 in conjugated hyperbilirubinemia. *Drug Metab. Dispos.* 42, 561–565. doi: 10.1124/dmd.113.055772

Köck, K., Ferslew, B. C., Netterberg, I., Yang, K., Urban, T. J., Swaan, P. W., et al. (2014). Risk factors for development of cholestatic drug-induced liver injury: inhibition of hepatic basolateral bile acid transporters multidrug resistance-associated proteins 3 and 4. *Drug Metab. Dispos.* 42, 665–74. doi: 10.1124/dmd.113.054304

König, J., Müller, F., and Fromm, M. F. (2013). Transporters and drug-drug interactions: important determinants of drug disposition and effects. *Pharmacol. Rev.* 65, 944–966. doi: 10.1124/pr.113.007518

Kotsampasakou, E., Brenner, S., Jäger, W., and Ecker, G. F. (2015). Identification of novel inhibitors of organic anion transporting polypeptides 1B1 and 1B3 (OATP1B1 and OATP1B3) using a consensus vote of six classification models. *Mol. Pharm.* 12, 4395–4404. doi: 10.1021/acs.molpharmaceut.5b00583

Kotsampasakou, E., and Ecker, G. F. (2017). Predicting drug-induced cholestasis with the help of hepatic transporters—an *in silico* modeling approach. *J. Chem. Inf. Model.* 57, 608–615. doi: 10.1021/acs.jcim.6b00518

Kotsampasakou, E., Escher, S. E., and Ecker, G. F. (2017a). Curated human hyperbilirubinemia data and the respective OATP1B1 and 1B3 inhibition predictions. *Data Br.* 11, 204–207. doi: 10.1016/j.dib.2017.02.009

Kotsampasakou, E., Escher, S. E., and Ecker, G. F. (2017b). Linking organic anion transporting polypeptide 1B1 and 1B3 (OATP1B1 and OATP1B3) interaction profiles to hepatotoxicity—The hyperbilirubinemia use case. *Eur. J. Pharm. Sci.* 100, 9–16. doi: 10.1016/j.ejps.2017.01.002

Kotsampasakou, E., Montanari, F., and Ecker, G. F. (2017c). Predicting drug-induced liver injury: the importance of data curation. *Toxicology* 389, 139–145. doi: 10.1016/j.tox.2017.06.003

Kuhn, M., Campillos, M., Letunic, I., Jensen, L. J., and Bork, P. (2010). A side effect resource to capture phenotypic effects of drugs. *Mol. Syst. Biol.* 6:343. doi: 10.1038/msb.2009.98

Kuhn, M., Letunic, I., Jensen, L. J., and Bork, P. (2016). The SIDER database of drugs and side effects. *Nucleic Acids Res.* 44, D1075–D1079. doi: 10.1093/nar/gkv1075

Levatić, J., Curak, J., Kralj, M., Šmuc, T., Osmak, M., and Supek, F. (2013). Accurate models for P-gp drug recognition induced from a cancer cell line cytotoxicity screen. *J. Med. Chem.* 56, 5691–5708. doi: 10.1021/jm400328s

Liu, Z., Shi, Q., Ding, D., Kelly, R., Fang, H., and Tong, W. (2011). Translating clinical findings into knowledge in drug safety evaluation - drug induced liver injury prediction system (DILIps). *PLoS Comput. Biol.* 7:e1002310. doi: 10.1371/journal.pcbi.1002310

Mak, L., Marcus, D., Howlett, A., Yarova, G., Duchateau, G., Klaffke, W., et al. (2015). Metrabase: a cheminformatics and bioinformatics database for small molecule transporter data analysis and (Q)SAR modeling. *J. Cheminform.* 7:31. doi: 10.1186/s13321-015-0083-5

Maunz, A., Gütlein, M., Rautenberg, M., Vorgrimmler, D., Gebele, D., and Helma, C. (2013). Lazar: a modular predictive toxicology framework. *Front. Pharmacol.* 4:38. doi: 10.3389/fphar.2013.00038

Meier, P. J., and Stieger, B. (2002). Bile salt transporters. *Annu. Rev. Physiol.* 64, 635–661. doi: 10.1146/annurev.physiol.64.082201.100300

Molecular Operating Environment (2014). *Molecular Operating Environment.* Available at: https://www.chemcomp.com/

Montanari, F., and Ecker, G. F. (2014). BCRP inhibition: from data collection to ligand-based modeling. *Mol. Inform.* 33, 322–331. doi: 10.1002/minf.201400012

Morgan, R. E., Trauner, M., van Staden, C. J., Lee, P. H., Ramachandran, B., Eschenberg, M., et al. (2010). Interference with bile salt export pump function is a susceptibility factor for human liver injury in drug development. *Toxicol. Sci.* 118, 485–500. doi: 10.1093/toxsci/kfq269

Nicolaou, M., Andress, E. J., Zolnerciks, J. K., Dixon, P. H., Williamson, C., and Linton, K. J. (2012). Canalicular ABC transporters and liver disease. *J. Pathol.* 226, 300–315. doi: 10.1002/path.3019

Ozer, J., Ratner, M., Shaw, M., Bailey, W., and Schomaker, S. (2008). The current state of serum biomarkers of hepatotoxicity. *Toxicology* 245, 194–205. doi: 10.1016/j.tox.2007.11.021

Padda, M. S., Sanchez, M., Akhtar, A. J., and Boyer, J. L. (2011). Drug-induced cholestasis. *Hepatology* 53, 1377–1387. doi: 10.1002/hep.24229

Pedregosa, F., Varoquaux, G., Gramfort, A., Michel, V., Thirion, B., Grisel, O., et al. (2011). Scikit-learn: machine learning in python. *J. Mach. Learn. Res.* 12, 2825–2830.

Pinto, M., Trauner, M., and Ecker, G. F. (2012). An *in silico* classification model for putative ABCC2 substrates. *Mol. Inform.* 31, 547–553. doi: 10.1002/minf.201200049

Pires, D. E. V., Blundell, T. L., and Ascher, D. B. (2015). pkCSM: predicting small-molecule Pharmacokinetic And Toxicity Properties Using Graph-Based Signatures. *J. Med. Chem.* 58, 4066–4072. doi: 10.1021/acs.jmedchem.5b00104

Sahigara, F., Ballabio, D., Todeschini, R., and Consonni, V. (2013). Defining a novel k-nearest neighbours approach to assess the applicability domain of a QSAR model for reliable predictions. *J. Cheminform.* 5:27. doi: 10.1186/1758-2946-5-27

Stieger, B. (2011). "The role of the sodium-taurocholate cotransporting polypeptide (NTCP) and of the bile salt export pump (BSEP) in physiology and pathophysiology of bile formation," in *Handbook of Experimental Pharmacology* (Berlin; Heidelberg: Springer), 205–259. doi: 10.1007/978-3-642-14541-4_5

Szakács, G., Annereau, J.-P., Lababidi, S., Shankavaram, U., Arciello, A., Bussey, K. J., et al. (2004). Predicting drug sensitivity and resistance:

profiling ABC transporter genes in cancer cells. *Cancer Cell* 6, 129–37. doi: 10.1016/j.ccr.2004.06.026

U.S. Department of Health and Human Services Food and Drug Administration Center for Drug Evaluation and Research (2012). *Guidance for Industry. Drug Interaction Studies Study Design, Data Analysis, Implications for Dosing, and Labeling Recommendations.* Rockville, MD.

Warner, D. J., Chen, H., Cantin, L.-D., Kenna, J. G., Stahl, S., Walker, C. L., et al. (2012). Mitigating the inhibition of human bile salt export pump by drugs: opportunities provided by physicochemical property modulation, *in silico* modeling, and structural modification. *Drug Metab. Dispos.* 40, 2332–41. doi: 10.1124/dmd.112.047068

9

A Pilot Study of All-Computational Drug Design Protocol: From Structure Prediction to Interaction Analysis

*Yifei Wu, Lei Lou and Zhong-Ru Xie**

Computational Drug Discovery Laboratory, School of Electrical and Computer Engineering, College of Engineering, University of Georgia, Athens, GA, United States

Correspondence:
Zhong-Ru Xie
paulxie@uga.edu

Speeding up the drug discovery process is of great significance. To achieve that, high-efficiency methods should be exploited. The conventional wet-bench methods hardly meet the high-speed demand due to time-consuming experiments. Conversely, *in silico* approaches are much more efficient for drug discovery and design. However, *in silico* approaches usually serve as a supportive role in research processes. To fully exert the strength of computational methods, we propose a protocol which integrates various *in silico* approaches, from *de novo* protein structure prediction to ligand-protein interaction simulation. As a proof of concept, human SK2/calmodulin complex was used as a target for validation. First, we obtained a predicted structure of SK2/calmodulin and predicted binding sites which were consistent with the literature data. Then we investigated the ligand-protein interaction via virtual mutagenesis, flexible docking, and binding affinity calculation. As a result, the binding energies of mutants have similar trends compared with the EC_{50} values ($R = 0.6$ for NS309 in V481 mutants). The results indicate that our protocol can be applied to the drug design of structure unknown proteins. Our study also demonstrates that the integration of *in silico* approaches is feasible and it facilitates the acceleration of new drug discovery.

Keywords: ligand-protein docking, molecular dynamics simulation, computational drug discovery, SK2, structural prediction, binding site prediction, virtual mutation, pharmaceutical industry

1. INTRODUCTION

To discover a new drug is an urgent but time-consuming process (Zhou et al., 2016; Gómez-Bombarelli et al., 2018). In the process of new drug development, *in silico* approaches have been successfully exploited to perform multiple simulations, such as selecting drug candidates from a database via high throughput virtual screening (Aparna et al., 2014; de Ruyck et al., 2016; Vilar et al., 2016; Imam and Gilani, 2017). The application of *in silico* approaches not only speeds up new drug discovery, but also collects related information, reveals the mechanisms and proposes new hypotheses. Compared to bench research, computational experiments perform high-efficiency simulations which considerably reduce the research time and the cost of experiments (Abel et al., 2017). However, in most cases, *in silico* approaches played an assisting role in the process. In this study, we propose an all-computational protocol integrating multiple *in silico* approaches to simulate the entire drug discovery process from *de novo* protein structure prediction to drug-protein interaction disclosure.

Up to now, reliable *in silico* approaches, such as molecular dynamics simulation (MD simulation) and machine learning (Durrant and McCammon, 2011; Lavecchia, 2015; Mortier et al., 2015), have been increasingly developed and applied in finding new drugs and optimizing them for treatment of diseases. However, most research projects only use one single *in silico* approach. For instance, the homology models of CIB2, a calcium- and integrin- binding protein, were constructed based on CIB1 structures using SWISS-MODEL server (Waterhouse et al., 2018). Based on the models, the way how the point mutations affect the affinities of calcium- and integrin-binding were predicted and then validated by *in vitro* experiments (Riazuddin et al., 2012). Besides, the results of ligand-protein docking were used to test the substrate specificity of OCT-1 and OCT-2 (organic cation transporter) to guide the following *in vivo* experimental validation (Papaluca and Ramotar, 2016). These works simply employed the *in silico* approaches as supportive methods, which did not sufficiently leverage the high-speed advantages of computational methods. Integrating the established *in silico* researches into an all-computation pipeline and producing validated good results is a milestone in the "omics" era.

Human small conductance calcium-activated (SK2) ion channels, consisted of SK2 subunits and calmodulin molecule, have been proved to be therapeutic targets for treatment of neuronal diseases, such as Parkinson's and amyotrophic lateral sclerosis (ALS) (Bond et al., 2005; Lu et al., 2009). The crystalized structures of human SK2 bound with Riluzole, an approved drug for ALS (Romano et al., 2015), and an analog [pdb (Berman et al., 2003) ligand ID: 658] of the SK2 activator CyPPA, an anti-ataxic agent (Herrik et al., 2012), have been released recently. It was also reported that ligands of two different chemical classes, Riluzole and its analog NS309, and CyPPA and its analogs, all bind to the same binding site where the interface of SK2 and calmodulin is. In addition, two key residues in the binding site were mutated to investigate how different mutations affect the potency of two ligands (Cho et al., 2018). As a proof of concept, we chose SK2 as the target to examine the protocol we proposed. Hence, in this study, we basically repeated the entire procedure of the previous study of Cho et al. (2018) with consecutive *in silico* approaches and compared our results with those of the bench experiments. We first constructed the human SK2/calmodulin model (PSK2) using SWISS-MODEL server and docked the ligands Riluzole and CyPPA analog 1 (PDB ligand ID: 658, see section 2.1), onto the predicted binding site. The predicted site is consistent with the reported results (Cho et al., 2018). Then the residues V481 and A477 in the binding pocket were virtually mutated and the mutation effects were assessed via binding energies (MM-GBSA ΔG_{Bind}) calculation. The results show that the binding energies of mutants have similar trends compared with the EC_{50} (the concentration of a drug that gives half-maximal response) values ($R = 0.6$ for NS309 in V481 mutants). Overall, our results suggest that this protocol of *in silico* approach can provide a systematic prediction on the unknown structures of proteins and potential drugs, and they also demonstrate the ability of *in silico* approaches to speed up the new drug design process.

2. MATERIALS AND METHODS

2.1. Protein Structure Preparation

Having a determined or predicted structure of the drug target protein is the first prerequisite of structure-based drug design. To prove the all-computational protocol is valid, we started our process from structure prediction. To predict the structure of SK2 and calmodulin from *Homo sapiens*, its amino acid sequence was obtained from the UniProt website (uniprot ID: Q9H2S1). Then we uploaded the sequence onto the SWISS-MODEL server, the most widely-used and reliable structure prediction server, to build a structure model (Bienert et al., 2016; Waterhouse et al., 2018) and selected the 3-D complex structure of *Rattus norvegicus* SK2 ion channels with NS309 (PDB ID: 4J9Z) (Zhang et al., 2013) as the template of structure prediction. 4J9Z was downloaded from RCSB's Protein Data Bank (Berman et al., 2003), and the predicted structure of SK2 and calmodulin were combined in Maestro (11.5 version, Schrodinger). To test the accuracy of modeling, we uploaded the predicted protein structure and the crystalized complex structure of human SK2 and calmodulin with Riluzole (PDB ID: 5V02) onto Zhang's web server (Zhang and Skolnick, 2005) to calculate the TM-align score. 5V02 was downloaded from RCSB's Protein Data Bank. In addition, site-directed mutants were constructed using the Mutate Residue function of Maestro.

A PDB structure of the target protein cannot be directly used in molecular docking without preprocessing. In most of the cases, a PDB file does not include the information of hydrogens, the (potential) charges of atoms, or the bond orders between any two atoms. In addition, the protein structures may be determined with a missing fragment(s), a low resolution or alternate positions, or under an unnatural condition, for example, low or high pH values. To make sure molecular docking can simulate the binding between ligands and the target protein correctly and precisely, the protein and ligand preparation is necessary. The wild-type and mutant (predicted) protein structures to be used for docking were processed by protein preparation wizard in Maestro (Sastry et al., 2013). The workflow of protein preparation contains three steps as follows: (1) Preprocess: assigning bond orders, adding hydrogens, creating zero-order bonds to metals, creating disulfide, filling in missing side chains using Prime, deleting waters beyond 5.00 Å from het groups (to keep the water molecules which may form hydrogen-bond bridges between the protein and the ligand and remove those cannot form hydrogen-bond bridges) and generating het states using Epik ($pH = 7.0 \pm 2.0$) (Shelley et al., 2007); (2) Optimization: setting $pH = 7.0$ and performing optimization; (3) Minimization: this step was performed using the OPLS3 force field (Harder et al., 2015). The converge heavy atoms to root-mean-square deviation (RMSD) is 0.30 Å.

2.2. Ligand Preparation

The 3-D molecular structures of Riluzole and NS309 were obtained from the PubChem database (Kim et al., 2018). The 3-D molecular structures of CyPPA analog 1 ((4-chloro-phenyl)-[2-(3,5-dimethyl-pyrazol-1-yl)-pyrimidin-4-yl]-amine) and analog 2 (4-chloro-phenyl)-[2-(3,5-dimethyl-pyrazol-1-yl)-6-methyl-pyrimidin-4-yl]-amine) were built in Maestro (11.5 version, Schrodinger) based on a previous study (Cho et al., 2018). All the compounds were prepared using OPLS3 force field in Ligprep panel in Maestro (Sastry et al., 2013; Harder et al., 2015). The preparation process included converting 2D structures to 3D ones, adding hydrogens, computing correct partial charges, and optimizing the structures.

2.3. Binding Site Prediction

Knowing the potential ligand binding site(s) is also an important prerequisite prior to molecular docking. There are many well-developed binding site prediction methods and servers (Xie and Hwang, 2015); however, the predictions produced by different methods may disagree with each other. Therefore, researchers usually compare the prediction results produced by different methods to find the consensus among all predictions. In our study, binding site prediction process was completed using the LISE web server (http://lise.ibms.sinica.edu.tw/applet/) (Xie and Hwang, 2012), which is reported to have the highest accuracy (80–90% for a soluble protein), and the binding site prediction tool, Sitemap, in Maestro, which we used in the docking procedure after this step. The SK2 predicted structure was uploaded onto the LISE web server for binding site prediction. The top three predictions from LISE were then downloaded and imported into Maestro. Meanwhile, in Maestro, SiteMap (Halgren, 2007, 2009) predicted five ligand binding sites. After comparing the results obtained using two prediction methods, we used the consensus region to define the docking grid box.

2.4. Ligand-Protein Docking

In order to predict the details of the interaction between ligands and the target protein and to estimate their binding affinities (see section 2.5), ligand docking was conducted the extra-precision (XP) mode in Maestro. Maestro has three precision options for docking including high throughput virtual screening (HTVS), standard precision (SP), and extra precision (XP). Users can choose an option based on their need or the computational load. After the ligands and the target proteins were processed using Ligprep and protein preparation, respectively, a receptor grid box was generated according to the results of binding site prediction. The size of the receptor grid box was set as default. To investigate the interaction of the protein and ligands, Induced Fit Docking (IFD) (Farid et al., 2006; Sherman et al., 2006a,b; Clark et al., 2016) was performed in Maestro. Using the IFD, the Ligprep outputs were imported and docked to the target protein. The standard protocol was applied to generate up to 20 poses. The force field was OPLS3. Under the prime refinement tab, the conformations of binding site residues within 5 Å (default value) of the ligand were refined. In the Glide redocking process, the energy of each protein/ligand complex structure and the number of top structures were set as the default settings. The XP mode was used for all IFD process.

2.5. MM-GBSA Calculation

The binding energy (ΔG_{Bind}) between a protein and a ligand reflects how stable they bind to each other and how a point mutation affects the ligand binding. Therefore, we examined if our model can correctly predict the trend of binding affinity changes of the mutations on the target protein. In this study, ΔG_{Bind} were estimated using the Prime MM-GBSA module in Maestro (Greenidge et al., 2012). In MM-GBSA panel, the pose viewer files of docked complex were uploaded. The solvation model was VSGB and the force field was OPLS3 (Li et al., 2011). Prime MM-GBSA ΔG_{Bind} was calculated using this equation:

$$\Delta G_{Bind} = E_{complex}(\text{minimized}) - [E_{ligand}(\text{minimized}) + E_{receptor}(\text{minimized})] \quad (1)$$

Where ΔG_{Bind} is binding free energy and $E_{complex}$(minimized), E_{ligand}(minimized), and $E_{receptor}$(minimized) are minimized energies of receptor-ligand complex, ligand and receptor, respectively.

2.6. Virtual Mutation

Based on the literature, valine 481 (V481) of SK2 is a crucial residue which forms the hydrophobic core between SK2 and calmodulin (Cho et al., 2018). To investigate the impacts of V481 mutations in the binding pocket using *in silico* approaches, we first implemented the site-directed mutagenesis in Maestro. The V481 was virtually mutated to alanine, serine, threonine, aspartate, or phenylalanine. Then NS309 and CyPPA analog 2 were docked onto the mutated binding site of PSK2 using IFD and the binding free energies were calculated using MM-GBSA to reveal the effects of mutated residues.

Alanine 477 (A477) is another vital residue in the binding pocket (Cho et al., 2018). We exploited the same method mentioned above to virtually mutate A477 to isoleucine, leucine, valine, serine, threonine, arginine, and aspartate, docked NS309 and CyPPA analog 2 onto the mutated binding site of PSK2 and calculated the binding free energies using MM-GBSA.

2.7. Molecular Dynamics Simulation

The molecular dynamics (MD) simulations were performed using GROMACS version 2018.1 and CHARMM36 all-atom force field (March 2019) (Vanommeslaeghe et al., 2010, 2012; Vanommeslaeghe and MacKerell, 2012; Yu et al., 2012; Gutiérrez et al., 2016). The starting coordinates of each protein-ligand complex were obtained from docking experiments. Then we defined a dodecahedral unit cell and filled it with water molecules. After adding ions, the complex was minimized for 50,000 steps of steepest descent minimization. Next, the complex was equilibrated using an NVT ensemble (constant Number of particles, Volume, and Temperature) and NPT ensemble (the Number of particles, Pressure, and Temperature). The target temperature for equilibration was 300 K. At last, the simulations were performed for 30 ns. After the MD simulations, we calculated the RMSD of the residues which were mentioned in the previous research in four trajectories (Cho et al., 2018). Then, we selected four time points of two residues: I100 on protein-NS309 complex (15,000, 18,000, 24,000, and 30,000 ps) and D64 on protein-CyPPA analog 1 (2,610, 6,000, 15,000, and 21,000 ps). Finally, four conformations of both residues were converted into PDB files and were superposed using PyMol.

3. RESULTS

3.1. Structure Prediction of Human SK2/Calmodulin Complex

The structure of human SK2/calmodulin was generated using template-based modeling on the SWISS-MODEL server (**Figure 1A**). Based on the structure of SK2/calmodulin from *Rattus norvegicus* (PDB ID: 4J9Z), the structure models were predicted using the amino acid sequences of human SK2 and calmodulin. Additionally, the loop (residue A403 to residue D413, the "intrinsically disordered fragment"—IDF), which had not been determined in structure of human SK2/calmodulin complex (PDB: 5V02), was obtained in the predicted model (**Figure 1A**). It suggests that the predicted structure can be used to supplement the crystallized structure.

To test the accuracy of the predicted model, we used TM-align server to calculate the TM-align score (Zhang and Skolnick, 2005). The predicted models were aligned with 5V02, and the TM-align scores of SK2 and calmodulin are 0.99124 and 0.89215. These TM-align scores show that the structure of human SK2/calmodulin complex has been accurately predicted.

3.2. Binding Site Prediction

To determine the binding pocket in SK2/calmodulin complex, the Sitemap and LISE were exploited to predict binding sites (Halgren, 2007, 2009; Xie and Hwang, 2012). The top three predicted results from LISE were overlapped with the results of Sitemap. After the comparison, we found that there was only one consensus. Then we selected this binding site to generate receptor grid for docking. To verify the accuracy of binding site prediction, we also overlapped the predicted binding site with that of 5V02 (**Figure 1B**). Notably, the predicted binding site is the same binding site of Riluzole in 5V02, which suggests that this binding site is the potential binding site for the ligands. Hence, the *in silico* approaches successfully predict the accurate binding site.

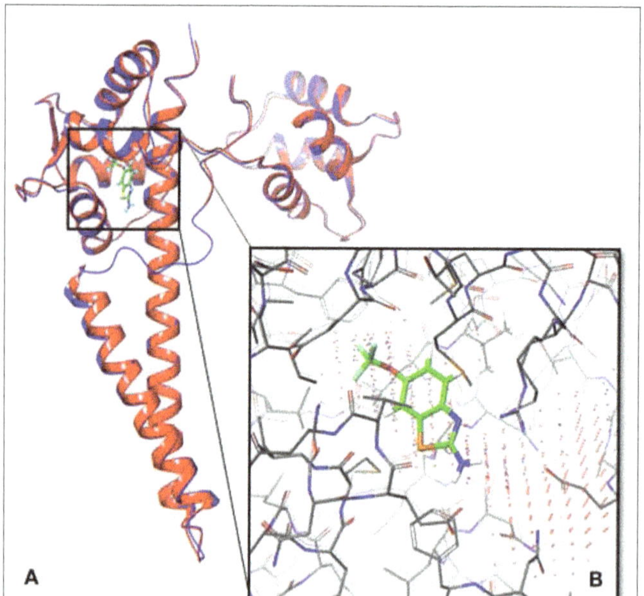

FIGURE 1 | Overlapped structures of the predicted model of human SK2 ion channels and 5V02. **(A)** The predicted structure of human SK2 ion channels (PSK2) in blue overlapped with its crystallized structure (5V02) in red. The structure of a missing loop (IDF) near the ligand binding pocket in 5V02/5V03 has also been predicted. The green compound was Riluzole, which was the ligand in 5V02. **(B)** The predicted binding sites (Blue dots represent the results from Sitemap; red dots represent the results from LISE) overlapped with the Riluzole binding site in 5V02.

3.3. Molecular Docking

Based on the previous study (Cho et al., 2018), the interface of SK2 and calmodulin can be bound by Riluzole, NS309, CyPPA analog 1, and analog 2. To investigate whether we can obtain the same results using *in silico* approaches, we first docked Riluzole and CyPPA analog 1 onto the predicted model (PSK2) via IFD (Induced Fit Docking) in Maestro, and redocked these ligands onto the determined structures (5V02 and 5V03) and calculated the binding energies as the control. Then we calculated the binding energies using MM-GBSA to estimate the binding affinities (Greenidge et al., 2012). As a result, the MM-GBSA ΔG_{Bind} of PSK2 with Riluzole and CyPPA analog 1 are −40.19 and −56.11 kcal/mol, respectively. As indicated in **Table 1**, those results of PSK2 are compatible to the results of 5V02 and 5V03, which demonstrate that accurate results can be obtained using *in silico* approaches. Additionally, the docking pose of PSK2 with Riluzole is almost identical with that in 5V02 (**Figure 2A**, the RMSD between the ligand of crystal structure and docking poses on 5V02 or PSK2 is 0.43 or 0.72 Å), which indicates that the simulated result from IFD can obtain accurate data in comparison with the results of crystallization. In **Figure 2B**, the coordinates of docked and native ligands are almost the same even though the poses of two ligands are not completely overlapped (the RMSD between the ligand of crystal structure and docking poses on 5V03 or PSK2 is 1.59 or 0.87 Å). Analyzing the docking results, Riluzole and CyPPA analog 1 interact with residues in both SK2 and calmodulin (**Figure 3**). The interacting residues in the binding site are mostly hydrophobic residues. As CyPPA analogs are larger molecules, they interact with more residues. Compared the list of interacting residues (**Table S1**), our results are almost identical to those of the previous study (Cho et al., 2018). The discrepancy may be because Maestro analyzes the interactions between ligands and the protein based on the interaction energy and the previous

TABLE 1 | MM-GBSA ΔG_{Bind} of ligands bound to crystallized structures and predicted structures.

Protein	Ligand	MM-GBSA ΔG_{Bind} (kcal/mol)
5V02	Riluzole	−40.83
5V03	CyPPA analog 1	−62.72
PSK2	Riluzole	−40.19
PSK2	NS309	−49.97
PSK2	CyPPA analog 1	−56.11
PSK2	CyPPA analog 2	−64.84

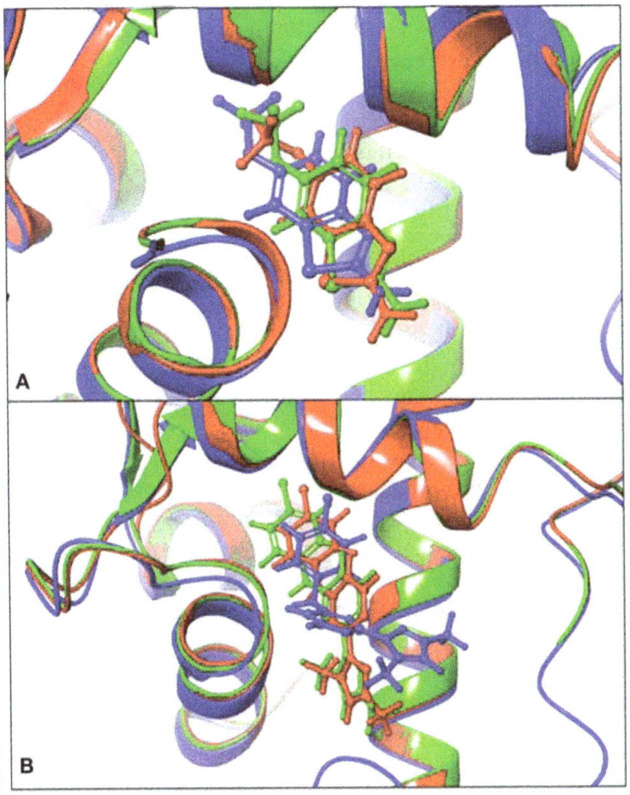

FIGURE 2 | Comparison of the docked poses and the native structures. **(A)** Comparison of the docking results on the PSK2 in blue color, the docking results on 5V02 in green color, and determined structures 5V02 in red color; The blue-colored Riluzole is the docked pose on the PSK2, the green-colored Riluzole is the docked pose on 5V02, and the red-colored Riluzole is the determined structure in 5V02; **(B)** Comparison of the docking results on the PSK2 in blue color, the docking results on 5V03 in green color, and determined structure 5V03 in red color; The blue-colored CyPPA analog 1 is the docked pose on the PSK2, the green-colored CyPPA analog 1 is the docked pose on 5V03 and the red-colored CyPPA analog 1 is the determined structure in 5v03.

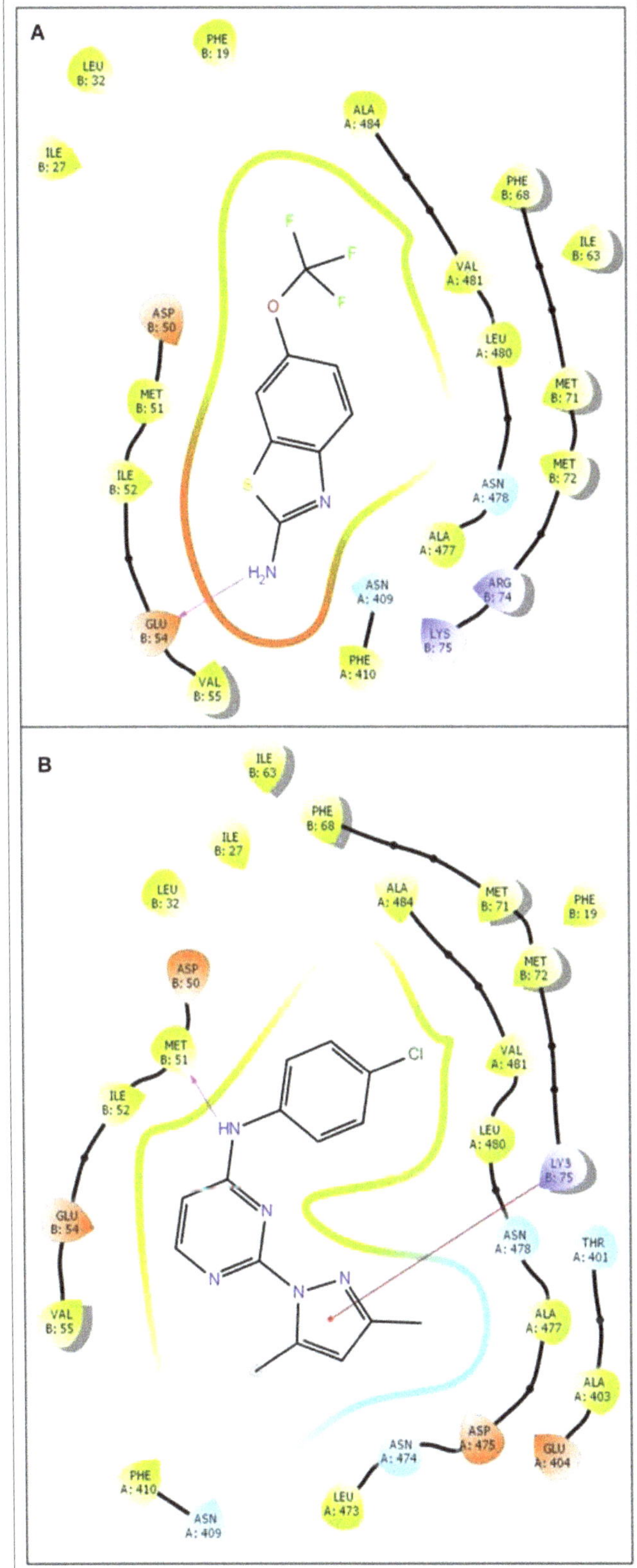

FIGURE 3 | 2D ligand-protein interaction of Riluzole **(A)** and CyPPA analog 1 **(B)** at PSK2 binding site. The pink arrow is referred to hydrogen bond. The red line is referred to Pi-cation interaction.

study (Cho et al., 2018) simply lists the residues within 5 Å of either ligand. According to the docking results of PSK2 with Riluzole and CyPPA analog 1, we docked NS309 and CyPPA analog 2 on the same binding site using the same methods mentioned above (**Figure 4** and **Figure S1**). The binding affinities MM-GBSA ΔG_{Bind} are showed in **Table 1**. The MM-GBSA ΔG_{Bind} values of CyPPA analog 1 and CyPPA analog 2 on the PSK2 are more negative than those of the other ligands, which suggests that CyPPA analog 1 and CyPPA analog 2 are promising drug candidates.

To verify the ligand-induced perturbations, NMR spectrum was used to identify residues with significant chemical shifts in previous experiments (Cho et al., 2018). With computational approaches, we ran MD simulations for each protein-ligand complex to simulate the conformational changes after the binding of ligands. A previous research reports that the residues on EF hands of calmodulin had conformational changes due to the ligand binding (Cho et al., 2018). Therefore, we calculated

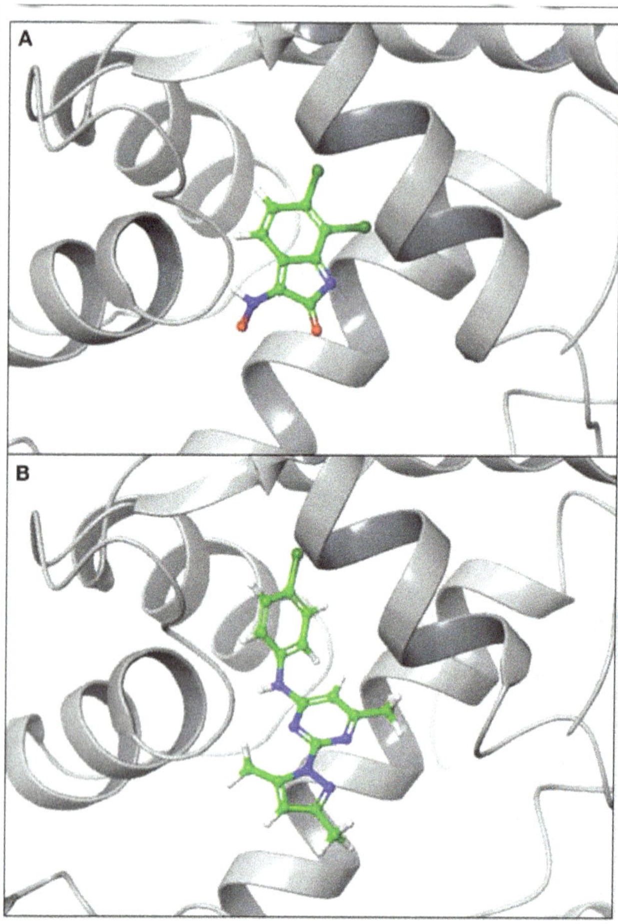

FIGURE 4 | Docking poses of SK2 predicted structure with NS309 **(A)** and CyPPA analog 2 **(B)**.

RMSD for those residues. According to the results of RMSD, we compared four trajectories of each residue and superposed their different poses at different time points. As a result, we found I100, on the complex of NS309, had obvious perturbations on four time points (**Figure 5** and **Figure S2**). In addition, D64 which was a critical residue for calcium sensing, also showed dramatically conformational changing on the complex structure of PSK2 and CyPPA analog 1 (**Figure 6** and **Figure S3**). Hence, the different poses of those residues demonstrated that the ligand could induce the perturbations of the calmodulin, which was consistent with the conclusion in the previous research (Cho et al., 2018).

3.4. Virtual Mutations at V481 and A477 in the Binding Pocket

The results of a previous study (Cho et al., 2018) show that the site-directed mutations on the key residues V481 and A477 in the binding site result in changes in the binding affinities. To validate that the *in silico* approach can simulate and predict the impacts of these mutations, we performed the virtual mutation experiments, docked the ligands on all mutants, and calculated the corresponding binding energies of each mutant. The MM-GBSA ΔG_{Bind} of V481 mutants are shown in **Table 2**. To verify the accuracy of *in silico* approaches, the Pearson's correlation coefficients between MM-GBSA ΔG_{Bind} and EC_{50} were calculated ($R = 0.6$ for NS309 in V481 mutants). **Table 2** indicates that substitutions with small side chains (V481S) or a charged amino acid (V481D) significantly decrease the binding affinities of NS309. Conversely, the binding affinity of NS309 in PSK2 V481F is close to that in wild-type. The results above are consistent with the conclusion in literature, that is, this position requires a non-charged residue with a bigger side chain (Cho et al., 2018).

Similarly, we find that CyPPA analog 2 in PSK2 V481F mutant with large aromatic side chains also shows a close binding affinity compared to that in PSK2 WT (**Table 2**), which demonstrates a good correlation between calculated binding affinities and EC_{50}. The mutants with small side chains (V481A and V481S) or a charged amino acid (V481D) also shows the relatively lower binding affinities of CyPPA analog 2. Those results demonstrate that the simulation results are compatible with the data from biological experiments. The consistent conclusion has successfully proved that the all-computational protocol can be widely applied in future biomedical research.

In **Table 3**, all PSK2 A477 mutants have slightly lower NS309 potency than that of PSK2 WT and the predicted binding affinities MM-GBSA ΔG_{Bind} have similar results. According to the results in literature (Cho et al., 2018), CyPPA analog 2 should exhibit shifted potencies at PSK2 A477L, PSK2 A477V, PSK2 A477S, PSK2 A477T, PSK2 A477R, and PSK2 A477D, but not at PSK2 A477I. However, in **Table 3**, the MM-GBSA ΔG_{Bind} of PSK2 A477I is not different from those of other mutants. As an isoleucine has a long side chain, different rotamers may largely change the estimated binding affinities. Performing an MD simulation may be a good solution to optimize the structures of mutants and improve the docked poses and estimated binding energies.

4. DISCUSSION

In the field of new drug discovery, research efficiency is particularly essential. On one hand, the speed of new drug development is of great importance to patients, especially the ones with fatal diseases such as cancers or acute infectious diseases (Shi et al., 2015). Statistics show that there will be around 1.7 million new cancer cases and 600 thousands cancer deaths in the United States in 2019 (Siegel et al., 2019). This race against time has always been a huge challenge for the researchers in this field. On the other hand, to bring a new drug to the market from compound identification to final FDA approval usually costs up to billions of dollars (Cleary et al., 2018). Therefore, the time and cost-efficient virtual process of drug development will benefit many pharmaceutical companies and our society. *In silico* approaches which can save considerable amount of research time and cost should be applied to drug design. With the rapid development of computer science and engineering, the availability and accuracy of *in silico* approaches have been constantly improving. Although many progresses have been made in utilizing *in silico* approaches to simulate certain biological experiments, the whole experimental processes completed in the virtual way from protein structure simulation

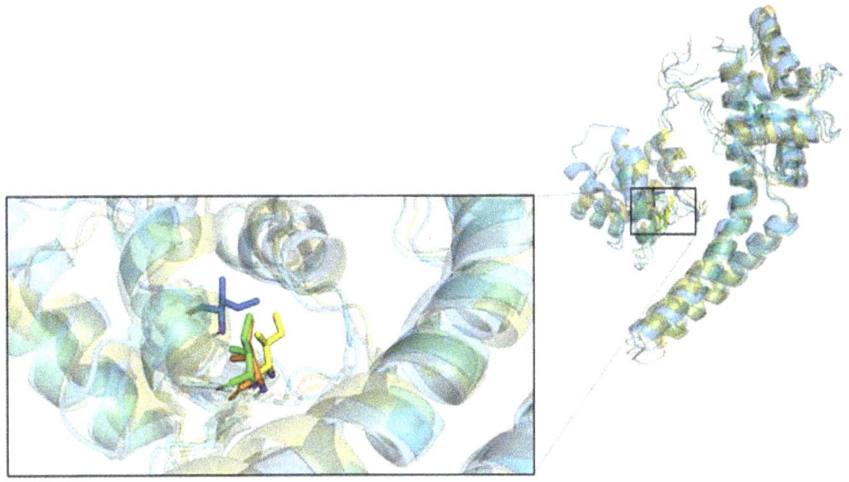

FIGURE 5 | Superposition of four conformations of I100 at four time points on the simulation trajectory of the complex of PSK2 and NS309.

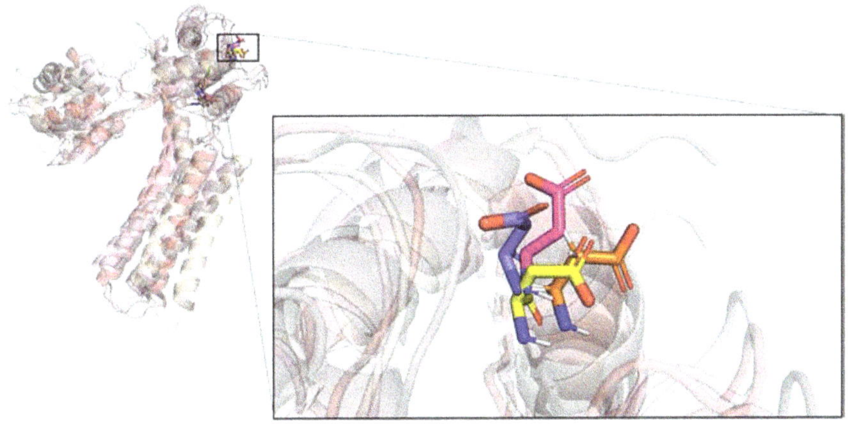

FIGURE 6 | Superposition of four conformations of D64 at four time points on the simulation trajectory of the complex of PSK2 and CyPPA analog 1.

TABLE 2 | EC_{50} and MM-GBSA ΔG_{Bind} of NS309 and CyPPA analog 2 bound to the V481 mutants.

Protein	NS309		CyPPA analog 2	
	EC_{50} (μM)	MM-GBSA ΔG_{Bind} (kcal/mol)	EC_{50} (μM)	MM-GBSA ΔG_{Bind} (kcal/mol)
WT	1.1	−49.97	2.5	−64.84
V481A	4.3	−54.28	>250	−29.05
V481S	5.1	−32.65	>250	−49.94
V481T	1.2	−32.77	46.6	−49.97
V481D	7.4	−25.97	>250	−46.75
V481F	0.8	−57.77	3.3	−64.09

TABLE 3 | EC_{50} and MM-GBSA ΔG_{Bind} of NS309 and CyPPA analog 2 bound to the A477 mutants.

Protein	NS309		CyPPA analog 2	
	EC_{50} (μM)	MM-GBSA ΔG_{Bind} (kcal/mol)	EC_{50} (μM)	MM-GBSA ΔG_{Bind} (kcal/mol)
WT	1.1	−49.97	2.5	−67.14
A477I	2.0	−37.26	2.0	−47.89
A477L	1.7	−24.71	99.0	−37.60
A477V	2.0	−39.67	>250	−45.63
A477S	3.0	−36.65	>250	−46.05
A477T	2.0	−23.36	>250	−51.04
A477R	2.1	−31.24	>250	−51.50
A477D	3.9	−30.94	>250	−49.71

to protein-drug interaction characterization has never been achieved before.

In this study, we proposed a protocol of integration of *in silico* approaches to simulate the process from protein structure determination to key residues mutagenesis and characterization. To validate this strategy, we selected the human SK2 ion channels as our target protein. With successful prediction, we obtained accurate protein structures (TM-align score >0.5) and the same binding site as the crystallized structure. Furthermore, the docking poses of Riluzole and CyPPA analog 1 are consistent with the ligand bound conformations in the crystallized structures. We also successfully reproduced similar effects of site-directed mutagenesis on the ligand binding, which demonstrated great potential of the integration of *in silico* approaches. However, the purpose of integrating *in silico* approaches is not to completely replace biological experiments but to speed up the drug discovery process with the continuous and automatic computational process.

A possible reason why an all-computation protocol of drug design has not been proposed and implemented is the inaccuracy or uncertainty of prediction results might accumulate in the sequential computational pipeline. However, the state-of-the-art bioinformatics algorithms, software or servers have been highly accurate in many cases so that it is time to integrate them into a fully computational process or even a fully automatic process. This is the first study to demonstrate the feasibility of an all-computational protocol in drug design. To achieve the ultimate goal of "automatic" drug discovery, more online servers or computational algorithms like PROCHECK (Laskowski et al., 1993), which can be used to assess or estimate the reliability of prediction results generated by each *in silico* approach, need to be developed. Despite its innovative approach, there are a few limitations of this study. First, the accuracy of protein structure prediction relies on the methods and/or templates. In our research, we selected the SK2/calmodulin from *Rattus norvegicus* (PDB ID: 4J9Z) as the template to build protein structure on SWISS MODEL, whose results are more accurate than the results from other webservers (data not shown). Hence, a reliable tool or method is critical to the accuracy of the final simulated results. Second, the binding affinity changes are hard to be precisely reproduced, especially those of the mutants, because considering possible conformational changes on target proteins is still the biggest challenge of docking. This suggests that MD simulation which can simulate the conformational changes should be used to further improve the precision of the predictions.

In conclusion, this work established and demonstrated an integrated protocol of *in silico* approaches for the first time. Its applicability can be potentially extended beyond the characterizing of SK2 ion channels to investigating other proteins with unknown structures, such as the Alzheimer's disease related proteins (Fitzpatrick et al., 2017; Hatami et al., 2017), which are also treatment targets of neural degenerative diseases. Although there are challenges to the *in silico* approaches, our work still paves a new way toward an automatic procedure of drug design.

AUTHOR CONTRIBUTIONS

YW carried out the research, analyzed the data, and drafted the manuscript. LL analyzed the data. Z-RX conceived the project, guided the research, and revised the manuscript. All authors read and approved the final manuscript.

FUNDING

This work has been supported by a start-up grant from the College of Engineering, University of Georgia.

ACKNOWLEDGMENTS

The authors would like to acknowledge Dr. Gareth Young and Dr. Shenping Liu for kindly providing their experimental data (EC_{50}), and Dr. Wen-Ching Chan, Xingzi Yuan, Hsin-Tzu Wang, Jane Hua, and Crystal Zhu for the useful suggestions on editing this manuscript.

REFERENCES

Abel, R., Mondal, S., Masse, C., Greenwood, J., Harriman, G., Ashwell, M. A., et al. (2017). Accelerating drug discovery through tight integration of expert molecular design and predictive scoring. *Curr. Opin. Struct. Biol.* 43, 38–44. doi: 10.1016/j.sbi.2016.10.007

Aparna, V., Dineshkumar, K., Mohanalakshmi, N., Velmurugan, D., and Hopper, W. (2014). Identification of natural compound inhibitors for multidrug efflux pumps of *Escherichia coli* and pseudomonas aeruginosa using *in silico* high-throughput virtual screening and *in vitro* validation. *PLoS ONE* 9:e101840. doi: 10.1371/journal.pone.0101840

Berman, H. M., Bourne, P. E., Westbrook, J., and Zardecki, C. (2003). "The protein data bank," in *Protein Structure*, ed D. Chasman (Boca Raton, FL: CRC Press), 394–410. doi: 10.1201/9780203911327.ch14

Bienert, S., Waterhouse, A., de Beer, T. A., Tauriello, G., Studer, G., Bordoli, L., et al. (2016). The swiss-model repository—new features and functionality. *Nucleic Acids Res.* 45, D313–D319. doi: 10.1093/nar/gkw1132

Bond, C. T., Maylie, J., and Adelman, J. P. (2005). Sk channels in excitability, pacemaking and synaptic integration. *Curr. Opin. Neurol.* 15, 305–311. doi: 10.1016/j.conb.2005.05.001

Cho, L. T.-Y., Alexandrou, A. J., Torella, R., Knafels, J., Hobbs, J., Taylor, T., et al. (2018). An intracellular allosteric modulator binding pocket in SK2 ion channels is shared by multiple chemotypes. *Structure* 26, 533–544. doi: 10.1016/j.str.2018.02.017

Clark, A. J., Tiwary, P., Borrelli, K., Feng, S., Miller, E. B., Abel, R., et al. (2016). Prediction of protein–ligand binding poses via a combination of induced fit docking and metadynamics simulations. *J. Chem. Theory Comput.* 12, 2990–2998. doi: 10.1021/acs.jctc.6b00201

Cleary, E. G., Beierlein, J. M., Khanuja, N. S., McNamee, L. M., and Ledley, F. D. (2018). Contribution of NIH funding to new drug approvals 2010–2016. *Proc. Natl. Acad. Sci. U.S.A.* 115, 2329–2334. doi: 10.1073/pnas.1715368115

de Ruyck, J., Brysbaert, G., Blossey, R., and Lensink, M. F. (2016). Molecular docking as a popular tool in drug design, an *in silico* travel. *Adv. Appl. Bioinform. Chem.* 9:1. doi: 10.2147/AABC.S105289

Durrant, J. D., and McCammon, J. A. (2011). Molecular dynamics simulations and drug discovery. *BMC Biol.* 9:71. doi: 10.1186/1741-7007-9-71

Farid, R., Day, T., Friesner, R. A., and Pearlstein, R. A. (2006). New insights about herg blockade obtained from protein modeling, potential energy mapping, and docking studies. *Bioorg. Med. Chem.* 14, 3160–3173. doi: 10.1016/j.bmc.2005.12.032

Fitzpatrick, A. W., Falcon, B., He, S., Murzin, A. G., Murshudov, G., Garringer, H. J., Crowther, R. A., et al. (2017). Cryo-em structures of tau filaments from Alzheimer's disease. *Nature* 547:185. doi: 10.1038/nature23002

Gómez-Bombarelli, R., Wei, J. N., Duvenaud, D., Hernández-Lobato, J. M., Sánchez-Lengeling, B., Sheberla, D., et al. (2018). Automatic chemical design using a data-driven continuous representation of molecules. *ACS Cent. Sci.* 4, 268–276. doi: 10.1021/acscentsci.7b00572

Greenidge, P. A., Kramer, C., Mozziconacci, J.-C., and Wolf, R. M. (2012). MM/GBSA binding energy prediction on the PDBbind data set: successes, failures, and directions for further improvement. *J. Chem. Inf. Model.* 53, 201–209. doi: 10.1021/ci300425v

Gutiérrez, I. S., Lin, F.-Y., Vanommeslaeghe, K., Lemkul, J. A., Armacost, K. A., Brooks, C. L. III., et al. (2016). Parametrization of halogen bonds in the charmm general force field: improved treatment of ligand–protein interactions. *Bioorg. Med. Chem.* 24, 4812–4825. doi: 10.1016/j.bmc.2016.06.034

Halgren, T. (2007). New method for fast and accurate binding-site identification and analysis. *Chem. Biol. Drug Des.* 69, 146–148. doi: 10.1111/j.1747-0285.2007.00483.x

Halgren, T. A. (2009). Identifying and characterizing binding sites and assessing druggability. *J. Chem. Inf. Model.* 49, 377–389. doi: 10.1021/ci800324m

Harder, E., Damm, W., Maple, J., Wu, C., Reboul, M., Xiang, J. Y., et al. (2015). OPLS3: a force field providing broad coverage of drug-like small molecules and proteins. *J. Chem. Theory Comput.* 12, 281–296. doi: 10.1021/acs.jctc.5b00864

Hatami, A., Monjazeb, S., Milton, S., and Glabe, C. G. (2017). Familial Alzheimer's disease mutations within the amyloid precursor protein alter the aggregation and conformation of the amyloid-β peptide. *J. Biol. Chem.* 292, 3172–3185. doi: 10.1074/jbc.M116.755264

Herrik, K. F., Redrobe, J. P., Holst, D., Hougaard, C., Nielsen, K. S., Nielsen, A. N., et al. (2012). CyPPA, a positive SK3/SK2 modulator, reduces activity of dopaminergic neurons, inhibits dopamine release, and counteracts hyperdopaminergic behaviors induced by methylphenidate1. *Front Pharmacol.* 3:11. doi: 10.3389/fphar.2012.00011

Imam, S. S., and Gilani, S. J. (2017). Computer aided drug design: a novel loom to drug discovery. *Org. Med. Chem.* 1, 1–6. doi: 10.19080/OMCIJ.2017.01.555567

Kim, S., Chen, J., Cheng, T., Gindulyte, A., He, J., He, S., et al. (2018). Pubchem 2019 update: improved access to chemical data. *Nucleic Acids Res.* 47, D1102–D1109. doi: 10.1093/nar/gky1033

Laskowski, R. A., MacArthur, M. W., Moss, D. S., and Thornton, J. M. (1993). Procheck: a program to check the stereochemical quality of protein structures. *J. Appl. Crystallogr.* 26, 283–291. doi: 10.1107/S0021889892009944

Lavecchia, A. (2015). Machine-learning approaches in drug discovery: methods and applications. *Drug Discov. Today* 20, 318–331. doi: 10.1016/j.drudis.2014.10.012

Li, J., Abel, R., Zhu, K., Cao, Y., Zhao, S., and Friesner, R. A. (2011). The VSGB 2.0 model: a next generation energy model for high resolution protein structure modeling. *Proteins* 79, 2794–2812. doi: 10.1002/prot.23106

Lu, L., Timofeyev, V., Li, N., Rafizadeh, S., Singapuri, A., Harris, T. R., et al. (2009). α-actinin2 cytoskeletal protein is required for the functional membrane localization of a Ca2+-activated K+ channel (SK2 channel). *Proc. Natl. Acad. Sci. U.S.A.* 106, 18402–18407. doi: 10.1073/pnas.0908207106

Mortier, J., Rakers, C., Bermudez, M., Murgueitio, M. S., Riniker, S., and Wolber, G. (2015). The impact of molecular dynamics on drug design: applications for the characterization of ligand–macromolecule complexes. *Drug Discov. Today* 20, 686–702. doi: 10.1016/j.drudis.2015.01.003

Papaluca, A., and Ramotar, D. (2016). A novel approach using *C. elegans* DNA damage-induced apoptosis to characterize the dynamics of uptake transporters for therapeutic drug discoveries. *Sci. Rep.* 6:36026. doi: 10.1038/srep36026

Riazuddin, S., Belyantseva, I. A., Giese, A. P., Lee, K., Indzhykulian, A. A., Nandamuri, S. P., et al. (2012). Alterations of the CIB2 calcium-and integrin-binding protein cause usher syndrome type 1J and nonsyndromic deafness DFNB48. *Nat. Genet.* 44, 1265–1271. doi: 10.1038/ng.2426

Romano, S., Coarelli, G., Marcotulli, C., Leonardi, L., Piccolo, F., Spadaro, M., et al. (2015). Riluzole in patients with hereditary cerebellar ataxia: a randomised, double-blind, placebo-controlled trial. *Lancet Neurol.* 14, 985–991. doi: 10.1016/S1474-4422(15)00201-X

Sastry, G. M., Adzhigirey, M., Day, T., Annabhimoju, R., and Sherman, W. (2013). Protein and ligand preparation: parameters, protocols, and influence on virtual screening enrichments. *J. Comput. Aided Mol. Des.* 27, 221–234. doi: 10.1007/s10822-013-9644-8

Shelley, J. C., Cholleti, A., Frye, L. L., Greenwood, J. R., Timlin, M. R., and Uchimaya, M. (2007). Epik: a software program for pK a prediction and protonation state generation for drug-like molecules. *J. Comput. Aided Mol. Des.* 21, 681–691. doi: 10.1007/s10822-007-9133-z

Sherman, W., Beard, H. S., and Farid, R. (2006a). Use of an induced fit receptor structure in virtual screening. *Chem. Biol. Drug Des.* 67, 83–84. doi: 10.1111/j.1747-0285.2005.00327.x

Sherman, W., Day, T., Jacobson, M. P., Friesner, R. A., and Farid, R. (2006b). Novel procedure for modeling ligand/receptor induced fit effects. *J. Med. Chem.* 49, 534–553. doi: 10.1021/jm050540c

Shi, J., Wang, E., Milazzo, J. P., Wang, Z., Kinney, J. B., and Vakoc, C. R. (2015). Discovery of cancer drug targets by CRISPR-Cas9 screening of protein domains. *Nat. Biotechnol.* 33, 661–667. doi: 10.1038/nbt.3235

Siegel, R. L., Miller, K. D., and Jemal, A. (2019). Cancer statistics, 2019. *CA Cancer J. Clin.* 69, 7–34. doi: 10.3322/caac.21551

Vanommeslaeghe, K., Hatcher, E., Acharya, C., Kundu, S., Zhong, S., Shim, J., et al. (2010). Charmm general force field: a force field for drug-like molecules compatible with the charmm all-atom additive biological force fields. *J. Comput. Chem.* 31, 671–690. doi: 10.1002/jcc.21367

Vanommeslaeghe, K., and MacKerell, A. D. Jr. (2012). Automation of the CHARMM general force field (CGenFF) I: bond perception and atom typing. *J. Chem. Inf. Model.* 52, 3144–3154. doi: 10.1021/ci300363c

Vanommeslaeghe, K., Raman, E. P., and MacKerell, A. D. Jr. (2012). Automation of the charmm general force field (CGenFF) II: assignment of bonded parameters and partial atomic charges. *J. Chem. Inf. Model.* 52, 3155–3168. doi: 10.1021/ci3003649

Vilar, S., Quezada, E., Uriarte, E., Costanzi, S., Borges, F., Viña, D., et al. (2016). Computational drug target screening through protein interaction profiles. *Sci. Rep.* 6:36969. doi: 10.1038/srep36969

Waterhouse, A., Bertoni, M., Bienert, S., Studer, G., Tauriello, G., Gumienny, R., et al. (2018). Swiss-model: homology modelling of protein structures and complexes. *Nucleic Acids Res.* 46, W296–W303. doi: 10.1093/nar/gky427

Xie, Z.-R., and Hwang, M.-J. (2012). Ligand-binding site prediction using ligand-interacting and binding site-enriched protein triangles. *Bioinformatics* 28, 1579–1585. doi: 10.1093/bioinformatics/bts182

Xie, Z.-R., and Hwang, M.-J. (2015). "Methods for predicting protein–ligand binding sites," in *Methods Mol. Biol.*, ed A. Kukol (New York, NY: Springer), 383–398.

Yu, W., He, X., Vanommeslaeghe, K., and MacKerell, A. D. Jr. (2012). Extension of the charmm general force field to sulfonyl-containing compounds and its utility in biomolecular simulations. *J. Comput. Chem.* 33, 2451–2468. doi: 10.1002/jcc.23067

Zhang, M., Pascal, J. M., and Zhang, J.-F. (2013). Unstructured to structured transition of an intrinsically disordered protein peptide in coupling Ca2+-sensing and SK channel activation. *Proc. Natl. Acad. Sci. U.S.A.* 110, 4828–4833. doi: 10.1073/pnas.1220253110

Zhang, Y., and Skolnick, J. (2005). TM-align: a protein structure alignment algorithm based on the TM-score. *Nucleic Acids Res.* 33, 2302–2309. doi: 10.1093/nar/gki524

Zhou, W., Wang, Y., Lu, A., and Zhang, G. (2016). Systems pharmacology in small molecular drug discovery. *Int. J. Mol. Sci.* 17:246. doi: 10.3390/ijms17020246

10

In silico Design of Novel HIV-1 NNRTIs Based on Combined Modeling Studies of Dihydrofuro[3,4-d]pyrimidines

Yanming Chen [1], Yafeng Tian [1], Ya Gao [1], Fengshou Wu [1], Xiaogang Luo [1,2], Xiulian Ju [1] and Genyan Liu [1]*

[1] Key Laboratory for Green Chemical Process of Ministry of Education, Hubei Key Laboratory of Novel Reactor and Green Chemical Technology, School of Chemical Engineering and Pharmacy, Wuhan Institute of Technology, Wuhan, China,
[2] School of Materials Science and Engineering, Zhengzhou University, Zhengzhou, China

***Correspondence:**
Genyan Liu
liugenyan@yahoo.com;
liugenyan@wit.edu.cn

A novel series of dihydrofuro[3,4-d]pyrimidine (DHPY) analogs have recently been recognized as promising HIV-1 non-nucleoside reverse transcriptase (RT) inhibitors (NNRTIs) with potent antiviral activity. To better understand the pharmacological essentiality of these DHPYs and design novel NNRTI leads, in this work, a systematic *in silico* study was performed on 52 DHPYs using three-dimensional quantitative structure–activity relationship (3D-QSAR), molecular docking, virtual screening, absorption-distribution-metabolism-excretion (ADME) prediction, and molecular dynamics (MD) methods. The generated 3D-QSAR models exhibited satisfactory parameters of internal validation and well-externally predictive capacity, for instance, the q^2, R^2, and r_{pred}^2 of the optimal comparative molecular similarity indices analysis model were 0.647, 0.970, and 0.751, respectively. The docking results indicated that residues Lys101, Tyr181, Tyr188, Trp229, and Phe227 played important roles for the DHPY binding. Nine lead compounds were obtained by the virtual screening based on the docking and pharmacophore model, and three new compounds with higher docking scores and better ADME properties were subsequently designed based on the screening and 3D-QSAR results. The MD simulation studies further demonstrated that the newly designed compounds could stably bind with the HIV-1 RT. These hit compounds were supposed to be novel potential anti-HIV-1 inhibitors, and these findings could provide significant information for designing and developing novel HIV-1 NNRTIs.

Keywords: HIV-1 non-nucleoside reverse transcriptase inhibitors (NNRTIs), dihydrofuro[3,4-d]pyrimidines, virtual screening, molecular docking, rational drug design

INTRODUCTION

Acquired immune deficiency syndrome (AIDS) caused by human immunodeficiency virus (HIV) is one of the most widely spread infectious diseases worldwide. There is no effective drug or vaccine that could cure AIDS absolutely at present. According to the report from the Joint United Nations Program on HIV/AIDS, there were approximately 36.9 million people living with HIV worldwide in 2018, and neighboring 1.8 million new cases and 0.94 million AIDS-related deaths

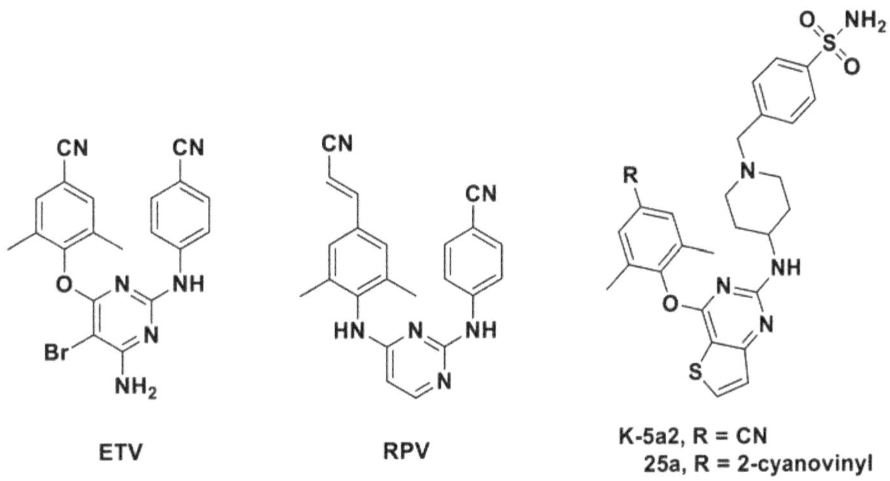

FIGURE 1 | Chemical structures of diarylpyrimidines (DAPYs).

in 2017[1]. Two main types of HIV (HIV-1 and HIV-2) have been identified currently. HIV-1 is widely spread throughout the world, whereas HIV-2 has correspondingly poor transmission (Vasavi et al., 2019; Wang et al., 2019). In the fight against HIV-1, highly active antiretroviral therapy (HAART) has been considered to be a relatively successful and effective therapy in controlling HIV-1 epidemics (Chen et al., 2011; Wang et al., 2018).

HIV-1 reverse transcriptase (RT), as one of the most important enzymes that convert the single-stranded RNAs into double-stranded DNAs, is vital to restrain HIV-1 replication and a prime target for antiviral research (Esposito et al., 2012). Inhibitors of the HIV-1 RT are divided into nucleoside RT inhibitors (NRTIs) and non-nucleoside RT inhibitors (NNRTIs), and the latter binds to an allosteric site that is located about 10 Å distance from the polymerizing processing site (Zhan et al., 2009). NNRTIs have become an indispensable portion of HAART regimen due to its potent antiviral activity, high specificity, and low cytotoxicity. However, single mutations such as K103N, Y181C, V106A, and L100I in the binding site of the HIV-1 RT might result in decreased inhibitory potencies of NNRTIs, and a double mutation (K103N+Y181C) was more frequently discovered in the process of treating with NNRTIs (Das et al., 2008).

Six HIV-1 NNRTIs including nevirapine, delavirdine, efavirenz, etravirine (ETV), rilpivirine (RPV), and doravirine have been approved by US Food and Drug Administration for clinical use to date (Namasivayam et al., 2019). ETV and RPV (**Figure 1**), which belong to diarylpyrimidine (DAPY) derivatives that were recognized as one of the most effective families of NNRTIs, have attracted considerable attention due to their excellent potency against HIV-1 wild-type and mutant strains. However, the low solubility and unsatisfactory oral bioavailability of these analogs restrict their clinical usage in some respects (Gu et al., 2019). Thus, novel NNRTIs with improved pharmacokinetic profiles have been urged to design and discover.

Recently, Kang et al. (2016, 2017) have designed and synthesized a series of thiophene[3,2-d]pyrimidine derivatives, among which compounds **K-5a2** and **25a** (**Figure 1**) were two representative HIV-1 NNRTIs, exhibiting more drug-like pharmacokinetic properties and greater inhibitory activities compared to nevirapine and efavirenz. Compound **25a** also exhibited better inhibition against HIV-1 mutant strains than ETV and RPV. However, compound **K-5a2** did not display excellent activity against K103N+Y181C mutant HIV-1 strains (Kang et al., 2017; Yang et al., 2018). Further structural modification on **K-5a2** and **25a** using six alicyclic-fused pyrimidine rings led to a series of dihydrofuro[3,4-d]pyrimidine (DHPY) derivatives with potent anti-HIV activity (**Table 1**) (Kang et al., 2019).

To date, there are many computer-aided drug design methods applied in designing and developing novel HIV-1 inhibitors (Almerico et al., 2007). For example, the three-dimensional quantitative structure–activity relationship (3D-QSAR) and pharmacophore models were utilized to learn about structural characteristics of HIV-1 NNRTIs in our previous studies (Liu et al., 2018; Wan et al., 2018). The multivariate statistical procedures, containing principal component and discriminant analysis, could be as credible methods to predict the activities of HIV-1 inhibitors by taking advantage of the vast anti-HIV data (Almerico et al., 2003, 2006). The molecular docking and molecular dynamics (MD) simulation were often used to understand the binding conformations of ligands in the active sites of HIV-1-related proteins. Furthermore, a comparative analysis with the combination of docking and multivariate methods was used to study the drug resistance of HIV-1 inhibitors and to further design new compounds with appropriate structural features (Almerico et al., 2008).

[1]UNAIDS. *UNAIDS Data 2018*, Available online at: http://www.unaids.org/en/resources/documents/2018/unaids-data-2018

TABLE 1 | Chemical structures of DHPYs and their actual and predicted activities as HIV-1 NNRTIs.

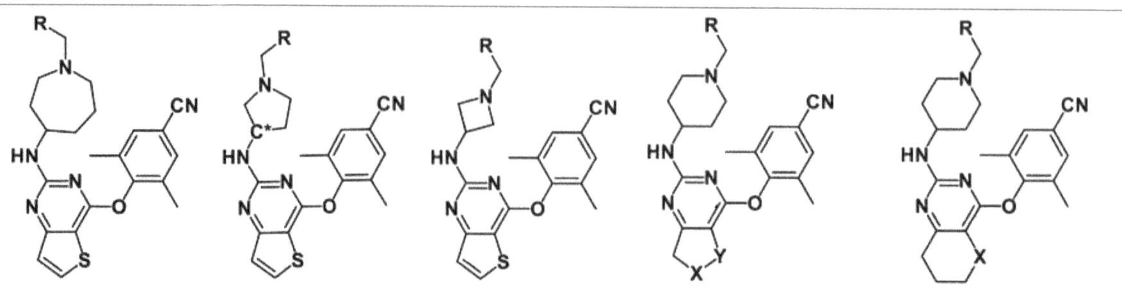

compounds 01-04; compounds 05-09: *C= (R), compounds 10-13: *C= (S); compounds 14-18; compounds 19-24: X=C Y=S, compounds 25-29: X=S Y=C, compounds 30-35: X=O Y=C, compounds 36-41: X=C Y=C; compounds 42-47: X=C, compounds 48-52: X=S

No.	*R*	EC$_{50}$ (nM)	Actual pEC$_{50}$	CoMFA Predicted pEC$_{50}$	CoMFA Residual	CoMSIA Predicted pEC$_{50}$	CoMSIA Residual
01[b]	4-SO$_2$NH$_2$-Ph	2.20	8.658	8.728	0.070	8.672	0.014
02	3-CONH$_2$-Ph	10.3	7.987	8.043	0.056	8.014	0.027
03	4-SO$_2$CH$_3$-Ph	9.98	8.001	7.919	−0.082	7.992	−0.009
04[a]	4-pyridinyl	31.7	7.499	7.528	0.029	7.392	−0.107
05[b]	4-SO$_2$NH$_2$-Ph	8.69	8.061	8.046	−0.015	8.076	0.015
06	4-CONH$_2$-Ph	10.4	7.983	8.042	0.059	8.025	0.042
07	3-CONH$_2$-Ph	41.3	7.384	7.360	−0.024	7.365	−0.019
08	4-SO$_2$CH$_3$-Ph	13.9	7.857	7.923	0.066	7.860	0.003
09[a]	4-pyridinyl	16.0	7.796	7.500	−0.296	7.830	0.034
10	4-SO$_2$NH$_2$-Ph	104	6.983	7.083	0.100	7.004	0.021
11	4-CONH$_2$-Ph	55.7	7.254	7.164	−0.090	7.242	−0.012
12	4-SO$_2$CH$_3$-Ph	50.7	7.295	7.214	−0.081	7.275	−0.020
13[b]	4-pyridinyl	16.7	7.777	7.843	0.066	7.781	0.004
14	4-SO$_2$NH$_2$-Ph	4.53	8.344	8.251	−0.093	8.335	−0.009
15	4-CONH$_2$-Ph	4.76	8.322	8.317	−0.005	8.304	−0.018
16	3-CONH$_2$-Ph	8.95	8.048	7.954	−0.094	8.053	0.005
17[a]	4-SO$_2$CH$_3$-Ph	207	6.684	6.860	0.176	7.329	0.645
18[b]	4-pyridinyl-Ph	2.21	8.656	8.690	0.034	8.680	0.024
19	4-SO$_2$NH$_2$-Ph	4.3	8.367	8.468	0.101	8.467	0.100
20[a]	4-CONH$_2$-Ph	4.8	8.319	8.490	0.171	8.328	0.009
21	4-SO$_2$CH$_3$-Ph	5.9	8.229	8.197	−0.032	8.238	0.009
22[b]	4-pyridinyl	2.6	8.585	8.613	0.028	8.637	0.052
23[a]	4-NO$_2$-Ph	8.0	8.097	8.103	0.006	8.226	0.129
24	3-CONH$_2$-Ph	27.7	7.558	7.500	−0.058	7.547	−0.011
25[a]	4-SO$_2$NH$_2$-Ph	37.2	7.429	7.494	0.065	7.263	−0.166
26[a,b]	4-SO$_2$Me-Ph	3.8	8.420	8.406	−0.014	7.714	−0.706
27	4-NO$_2$-Ph	11.5	7.939	7.902	−0.037	7.898	−0.041
28	4-NH$_2$-Ph	8.4	8.076	7.889	−0.187	8.067	−0.009
29	4-NHSO$_2$Me-Ph	11.2	7.951	8.043	0.092	7.987	0.036
30	4-SO$_2$NH$_2$-Ph	2.8	8.553	8.562	0.009	8.543	−0.010
31[b]	4-CONH$_2$-Ph	1.6	8.796	8.768	−0.028	8.812	0.016
32	4-SO$_2$CH$_3$-Ph	1.9	8.721	8.677	−0.044	8.629	−0.092
33	4-pyridinyl	2.3	8.638	8.701	0.063	8.736	0.098
34	4-NO$_2$-Ph	7.4	8.131	8.075	−0.056	8.178	0.047
35[a]	3-CONH$_2$-Ph	7.8	8.108	7.971	−0.137	8.238	0.130
36[b]	4-SO$_2$NH$_2$-Ph	1.1	8.959	8.867	−0.092	8.941	−0.018
37	4-CONH$_2$-Ph	6.1	8.215	8.387	0.172	8.270	0.055

(Continued)

TABLE 1 | Continued

				CoMFA		CoMSIA	
No.	***R***	**EC_{50} (nM)**	**Actual pEC_{50}**	**Predicted pEC_{50}**	**Residual**	**Predicted pEC_{50}**	**Residual**
38[a]	4-SO_2CH_3-Ph	4.9	8.310	8.603	0.293	8.479	0.169
39	4-pyridinyl	1.8	8.745	8.642	−0.103	8.452	−0.293
40	4-NO_2-Ph	14.5	7.839	7.953	0.114	7.858	0.019
41[a]	3-$CONH_2$-Ph	2.0	8.699	8.060	−0.639	8.437	−0.262
42	4-SO_2NH_2-Ph	6.0	8.222	8.145	−0.077	8.169	−0.053
43[b]	4-$CONH_2$-Ph	6.0	8.222	8.182	−0.040	8.218	−0.004
44[a]	4-SO_2CH_3-Ph	8.0	8.097	8.278	0.181	8.308	0.211
45	4-pyridinyl	8.6	8.066	8.033	−0.033	8.188	0.122
46	4-NO_2-Ph	77.4	7.111	7.330	0.219	7.106	−0.005
47[a]	3-$CONH_2$-Ph	6.5	8.187	7.792	−0.395	8.369	0.182
48[b]	4-SO_2NH_2-Ph	2.7	8.569	8.588	0.019	8.540	−0.029
49	4-$CONH_2$-Ph	3.0	8.523	8.523	0.000	8.434	−0.089
50	4-SO_2CH_3-Ph	3.9	8.409	8.453	0.044	8.451	0.042
51	4-NO_2-Ph	8.6	8.066	8.024	−0.042	8.056	−0.010
52[a]	3-$CONH_2$-Ph	5.1	8.292	8.087	−0.205	8.429	0.137

[a] *Test set compounds used for 3D-QSAR models.*
[b] *The compounds used for pharmacophore models.*
CoMFA, comparative molecular field analysis; CoMSIA, comparative molecular similarity indices analysis; DHPY, dihydrofuro[3,4-d]pyrimidine; NNRTIs, non-nucleoside reverse transcriptase inhibitors.

To further explore the essential structural and pharmacological features of the novel DHPYs as HIV-1 NNRTIs in this study, the combination of 3D-QSAR models, molecular docking, and MD simulation was applied to analyze the 3D-QSARs of these DHPYs and their binding modes in the HIV-1 RT. We also utilized the pharmacophore- and docking-based virtual screening to obtain some hit compounds from ZINC database and subsequently designed new potential NNRTIs according to the screening and 3D-QSAR results. Molecular docking and MD simulations were utilized to identify the binding of these new NNRTIs and the stabilization of the protein–ligand complexes.

MATERIALS AND METHODS

Preparation of Small Molecules

A total of 52 DHPY derivatives were collected from the published literature (Kang et al., 2019) for performing the molecular modeling study. Their structures, EC_{50}, and corresponding pEC_{50} ($-\log EC_{50}$) values were listed in **Table 1**. All compounds were stretched by SYBYL-X 2.1 (Tripos Inc., St. Louis, USA) running on Windows 7 workstation and minimized with Gasteiger–Hückel charges, the termination of 0.005 kcal/(mol·Å) and max iterations of 1,000 by Powell method. Other parameters were set to default values.

Three-Dimensional Quantitative Structure–Activity Relationship Model

The 3D-QSAR model could help to find a significant correlation between the biological activities of drug molecules and their structures (Borisa and Bhatt, 2015). In this study, comparative molecular field analysis (CoMFA) and comparative molecular similarity indices analysis (CoMSIA) methods were used to construct 3D-QSAR models. All compounds were randomly divided into a training set (39 compounds) to generate CoMFA and CoMSIA models and a test set (13 compounds) to confirm the reliability of the generated models (**Table 1**). The number of test set compounds should be kept in the range from 1/4 to 1/3 of the total compounds. Compound **36** with the highest activity was used as a template, and all training set compounds were superimposed on it by the common skeleton alignment (**Figure 2A**).

For generating a reasonable model, the internal predictive ability was evaluated by partial least squares (PLS) regression method using the SAMPLS. The leave-one-out (LOO) cross-validation procedure was applied to determine the optimum number of components (ONC) and the highest cross-validation correlation coefficient (Q^2) (Bush and Nachbar, 1993), and non-cross-validated analysis was applied to compute the non-cross-validated correlation coefficient (R^2), standard error of estimate (SEE), and the Fisher test values (F) (Li et al., 2014). External validation parameters were also essential for further assessing the predictive capability of 3D-QSAR models, such as r_0^2, k, $r_0^{'2}$, and $k^{'}$. r_0^2, and k were the corresponding correlation coefficient and the slope value of linear regression equation, respectively, for predicted vs. actual activities when the intercept was set to zero, and $r_0^{'2}$ and $k^{'}$ were for actual vs. predicted activities, respectively. In addition, r_m^2, $r_m^{'2}$, Δr_m^2, $\overline{r_m^2}$, and the root mean square error (RMSE) as traditional data were also calculated to appraise the predictive ability. A model, which met the requirements of $[(r^2 - r_0^2)/r^2]$ or $[(r^2 - r_0^{'2})/r^2] < 0.1, 0.85 \leq k \leq 1.15$ or $0.85 \leq k^{'} \leq 1.15$, $\Delta r_m^2 < 0.2$ and $\overline{r_m^2} > 0.5$, especially

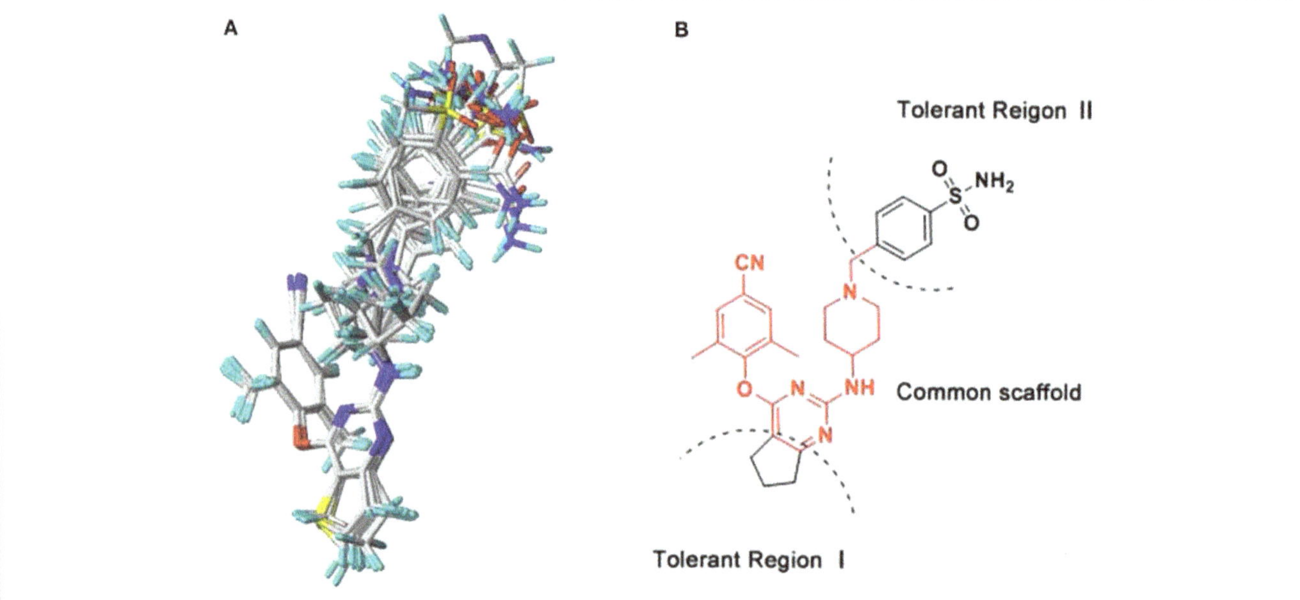

FIGURE 2 | The molecular alignment using compound **36** as a template. **(A)** The alignment results of the training set compounds used for the three-dimensional quantitative structure–activity relationship (3D-QSAR) models. **(B)** The chemical structure of compound **36**, and the red region represents the common scaffold.

the predictive correlation ${r_{pred}}^2 > 0.6$, would be deemed to possess well-predictive capability and reliability (Caballero, 2010; Ojha et al., 2011; Roy et al., 2016). The parameters were calculated according to our previous studies (Wang et al., 2018; Gao et al., 2019; Liu et al., 2019).

Pharmacophore Model

Ten compounds (**Table 1**) with high activities and diverse structures were selected to generate pharmacophore model using Genetic Algorithm with Linear Assignment of Hypermolecular Alignment of Database (GALAHAD) module in SYBYL-X 2.1. GALAHAD method mainly contained two steps. The ligands are neatly aligned to each other in internal coordinate space, and then the produced conformations as rigid bodies are aligned in Cartesian space. In the process of running GALAHAD, the parameters of population size, max generation, and molecules required to hit were automatically set according to the experiment activity data. Finally, 20 models with diverse parameters including SPECIFICITY, N_HITS, STERICS, HBOND, and Mol_Qry were generated.

In order to further validate the ability of the pharmacophore model, a decoy set method was used for evaluating the generated model. The decoy set database was comprised of 6,234 inactive compounds downloaded from the DUD-E database (http://dud.docking.org/) (Mysinger et al., 2012) and 42 active compounds from **Table 1** except the compounds used for constructing the pharmacophore model. The enrichment factor (EF) and Güner–Henry (GH) scores were considered as metrics to assess the reliability of the pharmacophore models. The GH score took the percent yield of actives in a hit list (%Y, recall) and the percent ratio of actives in a database (%A, precision) into account. While the GH score is ranging 0.6–1, the pharmacophore model would be regarded as a rational model (Kalva et al., 2014).

$$\%Y = H_a/H_t \times 100\% \quad (1)$$

$$\%A = H_a/A \times 100\% \quad (2)$$

$$EF = (H_a/H_t)/(A/D) \quad (3)$$

$$GH = (H_a\,(3A + H_t))/(4AH_t) \times (1 - (H_t - H_a)/(D - A)) \quad (4)$$

where H_a is the number of active molecules in the hit list, H_t is the hit compounds from the decoy set database, A is the total number of active compounds in the database, and D is the sum of the database.

Molecular Docking

The crystal structures of wild-type HIV-1 RT (PDB ID: 6C0J) and K103N/Y181C mutant RT (PDB ID: 6C0R) were downloaded from the Protein Data Bank and were used for the docking study. While preparing the two proteins, hydrogen atoms were added after the crystallographic ligands were extracted and all water molecules except for W936 were removed. In order to verify the rationality and reliability of the docking method, the extracted ligands (**K-5a2** and **25a**) were first redocked into the corresponding active site using the Surflex-Dock Geom module of SYBYL-X 2.1 with default parameters. All compounds were then docked into the binding pocket as the same pattern. Twenty conformations with different scores were produced for each docked compound, and the highest-score conformation of each compound was chosen for further study.

Virtual Screening

The selected GALAHAD model was converted into a UNITY query for virtual screening from ZINC database, and the "Flex search" was employed to serve as query type. Lipinski's rule of five as the primary filter was utilized to further decrease screened compounds. The QFIT score, whose value was between 0 and 100, reflected how closely the hit compounds matched with query. In consideration of the time and accuracy of screening, two ways of molecular docking including Surflex-Dock and Surflex-Dock Geom were implemented to verify the potential hit compounds obtained from the pharmacophore-based screening.

ADME Analysis

ADME properties are essential for selecting and evaluating lead candidates. The online tool Swiss ADME (http://www.swissadme.ch/index.php) was applied to calculate the pharmacokinetic properties of new NNRTI candidates, such as lipophilicity, water solubility, and blood–brain barrier (BBB) permeability (Daina et al., 2017). The synthetic accessibility was also predicted by the score from 1 to 10, in which a score of 1 suggested the synthetic route was relatively easy and a score closer to 10 indicated the compound had complex structure and was tough to be synthesized.

Molecular Dynamics Simulation

To further explore the dynamics protein–ligand interactions, 10 ns MD simulations were performed on compound **36** and newly designed inhibitors using GROMACS2016.5 software with AMBER 99SB force field. Before starting MD simulation, several important procedures should be performed to generate a steady environment. First, it was very momentous to generate the topology file of ligand by a acpype tool, which was on the basis of Python. Second, a 12 Å × 12 Å × 12 Å cubic box full of water models (transferable intermolecular potential with 3 points) was set to create the aqueous environment for the whole system. Nine chloride ions were added into the box for the sake of keeping the state of charge neutrality. In order to satisfy a tolerance of 10 kJ/mol, the steepest descent method for 50,000 steps was carried out for minimization without constraint to avoid possible collision between atoms. NVT at 300 K using V-rescale for 100 ps and NPT at 1 atm pressure using Parrine–Rahman for 100 ps were successively equilibrated to maintain proper temperature and pressure for the system. At last, the 10 ns MD simulation was run and the simulation step length was defined as 2 fs.

RESULTS AND DISCUSSION

Statistical Analysis of the Comparative Molecular Field Analysis and Comparative Molecular Similarity Indices Analysis Models

The classical parameters of the CoMFA and CoMSIA models were summarized in **Table S1**. In general, the q^2 and R^2 should be more than 0.5 and 0.9, respectively, and the *SEE* and *F*-value should be rational. As for the CoMSIA models, there were different combinations of five fields as shown in **Table S1**. The model generated by the combination of the steric (S), electrostatic (E), hydrogen-bond acceptor (A), hydrogen-bond donor (D), and hydrophobic (H) fields was the optimal CoMSIA model because of its satisfactory q^2, R^2, *SEE*, F, and r_{pred}^2 values. The

TABLE 2 | External validation results of the CoMFA and CoMSIA models.

Validation parameters	RMSE	MAE	r^2	r_0^2	$r_0'^2$	$\frac{r^2-r_0^2}{r^2}$	k	k′	r_m^2	$r_m'^2$	Δr_m^2	$\overline{r_m^2}$
CoMFA	0.263	1.608	0.750	0.746	0.709	0.006	1.007	0.992	0.700	0.597	0.103	0.648
CoMSIA	0.302	0.549	0.655	0.653	0.533	0.004	0.996	1.003	0.622	0.426	0.196	0.524

CoMFA, comparative molecular field analysis; CoMSIA, comparative molecular similarity indices analysis; RMSE, root mean square error; MAE, mean absolute error.

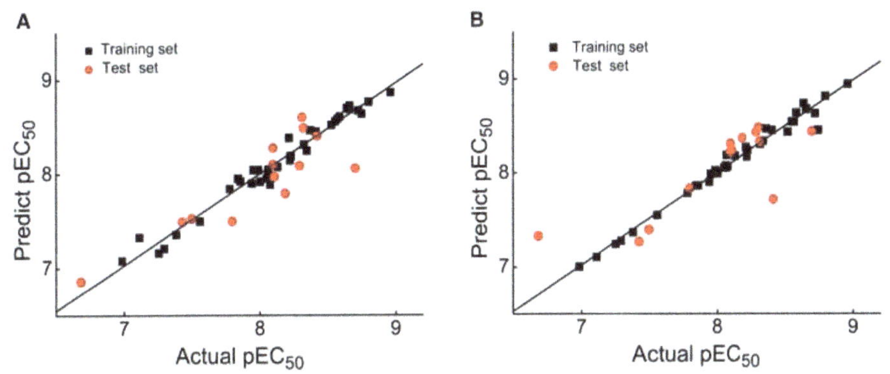

FIGURE 3 | Plots of actual vs. predicted pEC_{50} values of all dihydrofuro[3,4-d]pyrimidines (DHPYs) based on the comparative molecular field analysis (CoMFA) **(A)** and comparative molecular similarity indices analysis (CoMSIA) **(B)** models.

contributions of S, E, A, D, and H fields were 4.1, 19.7, 29, 33.4, and 13.8%, respectively, indicating that A and D fields played more important roles. The q^2 of the CoMFA and CoMSIA models were 0.647 and 0.735, respectively, which indicated that both models were rational. The R^2 values of the CoMFA and CoMSIA models were 0.970 and 0.982, respectively, and the r_{pred}^2 values were 0.751 and 0.672, respectively, suggesting that both models had excellent predictive abilities. In addition, it was common for the CoMFA and CoMSIA models that the E field contribution was more than the S field contribution, which illustrated that the E field could be more significant than the S field in the effect on compound activity.

External validation parameters could further confirm the reasonability of the constructed CoMFA and CoMSIA models. As shown in **Table 2**, all external validation results of the CoMFA and CoMSIA models were in the rational range, for example, the $\overline{r_m^2}$ values of the CoMFA and CoMSIA model were 0.648 and 0.524, respectively. The statistical results of **Table S1** and **Table 2** proved that the generated 3D-QSAR models were reliable and possessed excellent predictive capacity. **Figure 3** showed the plots of actual vs. predicted pEC_{50} values for all compounds based on the CoMFA and CoMSIA models. All compounds were evenly distributed in the two sides of the trend lines, which indicated that the 3D-QSAR models had excellent abilities to predict the activities of DHPYs. The predictive capacity of the CoMFA model seems to be better than that of the CoMSIA model.

Contour Maps of the Comparative Molecular Field Analysis and Comparative Molecular Similarity Indices Analysis Models

The contour maps of the CoMFA and CoMSIA models could visually provide significant information for the QSARs of

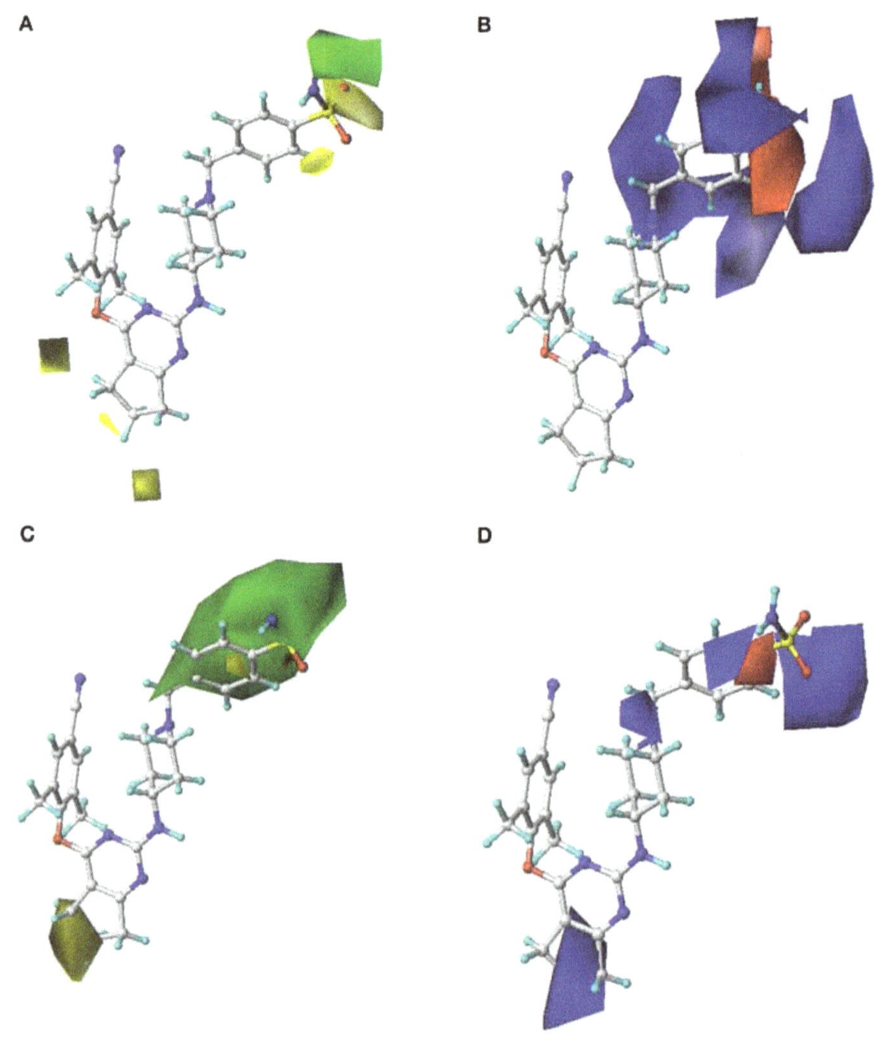

FIGURE 4 | Contour maps of steric and electrostatic fields with compound **36** as a reference in the comparative molecular field analysis (CoMFA) **(A,B)** and comparative molecular similarity indices analysis (CoMSIA) **(C,D)** models.

DHPYs. Compound **36** with the highest activity was utilized as a reference molecule to analyze the contour maps of both models. As shown in **Figure 2B**, the structure of compound **36** consisted of the common scaffold, Tolerant Regions I and II.

Figure 4 showed the S and E field contour maps of the CoMFA and CoMSIA models. In the S field, the green contour indicates that a bulky substituent at this position is beneficial for the activity, whereas a yellow block corresponds to a region where a small group is favorable for the activity. For the E field, a blue contour means that introduction of electropositive groups in this region may improve the biological activity, whereas the red contour indicates that electronegative groups may be beneficial for the activity. As can be seen from **Figures 4A,C**, the S field contours of the CoMFA model were consistent with those of the CoMSIA model. The yellow contour in the Tolerant Region I indicated that a relatively small group at this region would be beneficial for enhancing the activity, which might explain why the actual activities of compounds **30–41** were greater than those of compounds **25–29**. On the other hand, in the Tolerant Region II, there was a green contour at the terminal, suggesting that introduction of a bulky group was more favorable, which was in agreement with the activity orders: **18** (pyridine-4-yl-Ph) > **14** (4-SO_2NH_2-Ph) > **17** (4-SO_2CH_3-Ph), **19** (4-SO_2NH_2-Ph) > **21** (4-SO_2CH_3-Ph) > **23** (4-NO_2-Ph), and **42** (4-SO_2NH_2-Ph) > **44** (4-SO_2CH_3-Ph) > **46** (4-NO_2-Ph). At the *para-position* of the benzene ring of Tolerant Region II, two yellow contours indicated that small substituents here might be favorable for the activity, for instance, **3** (4-SO_2CH_3-Ph) > **2** (3-$CONH_2$-Ph) > **4** (pyridine-4-yl), **8** (4-SO_2CH_3-Ph) > **9** (pyridine-4-yl), **31** (4-$CONH_2$-Ph) > **33** (pyridine-4-yl). In **Figures 4B,D**, it can be clearly observed that a big blue contour was located at the terminal of Tolerant Region II, indicating that the positively charged group might be beneficial for the activity, such as **1** (4-SO_2NH_2-Ph) > **3** (4-SO_2CH_3-Ph), **15** (4-$CONH_2$-Ph) > **17** (4-SO_2CH_3-Ph), and **19** (4-SO_2NH_2-Ph) > **21** (4-SO_2CH_3-Ph). In addition, a red contour was located at the *para-position* of the benzene ring of Tolerant Region II, indicating that electronegative groups were beneficial for the antiviral activity at this position.

The H, D, and A field contour maps of the CoMSIA models were shown in **Figure 5**. In the H field, yellow contours represent the favorable zone of hydrophobic groups, whereas white contours show the unfavorable zone of hydrophobic groups. As shown in **Figure 5A**, a huge white near Tolerant Region I indicated that this place was appropriate to introduce hydrophobic groups. In addition, there was a white contour at the benzene ring of Tolerant Region II, which illustrated that hydrophobic substituents here were beneficial. The H field results were in good consistency with those of the previous study (Kang et al., 2019) that DHPYs with hydrophobic groups at corresponding positions exhibited promising activities. As for the D field, cyan suggests hydrogen-bond donor groups are useful for enhancing the activity, whereas purple is opposite. In **Figure 5B**, a cyan contour close to the linker atom of the pyrimidine ring and the right wing showed that the hydrogen-bond donor might be helpful for the activity at this position. There was also a cyan contour at the terminal of Tolerant Region II, indicating that hydrogen-bond donor groups were beneficial here, for example, **28** (4-NH_2-Ph) > **27** (4-NO_2-Ph). A purple contour near the para-position of the benzene ring of Tolerant Region II manifested that the place might not be suitable for hydrogen-bond donor groups, such as **1** (4-SO_2NH_2-Ph) > **2** (3-$CONH_2$-Ph). In the A field, beneficial and unbeneficial contour of hydrogen-bond acceptors are colored in magenta and red, respectively. In **Figure 5C**, a red contour at the terminal of Tolerant Region II signified that the hydrogen-bond acceptors at this position were disadvantageous for the activity, and two magenta contours at the para-position of the benzene ring of Tolerant Region II illustrated that the hydrogen-bond acceptor was advantageous. In short, introduction of hydrogen-bond acceptors at the para-position of the benzene ring of Tolerant Region II and hydrogen-bond donors at the terminal of Tolerant Region II might be advantageous for the inhibitory activity.

In a word, the contour maps of 3D-QSAR models presented that a small and/or hydrophobic group in Tolerant Region I;

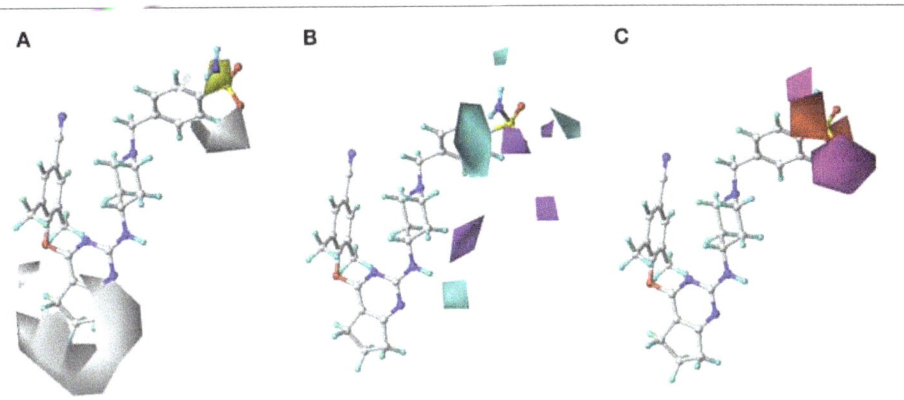

FIGURE 5 | Contour maps of hydrophobic **(A)**, hydrogen-bond donor **(B)**, and hydrogen-bond acceptor **(C)** fields in the optimal comparative molecular similarity indices analysis (CoMSIA) model.

a small, electronegative and/or hydrogen-bond accepter group at the *para-position* of the benzene ring of Tolerant Region II; and/or a bulky, electropositive and/or hydrogen-bond donor group at the terminal of Tolerant Region II would be favorable for increasing the activity, respectively.

Pharmacophore Model

The statistical parameters of 20 pharmacophore models generated by GALAHAD were listed in **Table S2**. As for pharmacophore models, it could be served as the query for a UNITY flex search only if the SPECIFITY value was more than 5. The identical value of the PARETO column indicated that all models were statistically equivalent. In general, a good pharmacophore model should have small ENERGY and high SPECIFITY, N_HITS, STERICS, and MOL_QRY (Caballero, 2010). Among 20 models, model_20 was regarded as the optimal model by the comprehensive consideration of the abovementioned parameters.

The pharmacophore features of the best GALAHAD Model_20 were displayed in **Figure 6**, including three hydrophobic centers (HYs, cyan), four hydrogen-bond acceptor atoms (AAs, green), and one hydrogen-bond donor atom (DAs, magenta). All features were located in the left and middle structures of DHPYs. One of the hydrogen-bond acceptor atom at the connecting atom of the left ring indicated that hydrogen-bond acceptor groups might increase the inhibitory activities at this position, which was consistent with our previous study (Wan et al., 2018). The other hydrogen-bond acceptor atoms were located at the nitrogen atoms of the pyrimidine ring and the cyano group of the left benzene ring. Moreover, the hydrophobic center of the left phenyl ring was located at the hydrophobic pocket of the HIV-1 RT, which was also in good consistency with our previous studies (Wan et al., 2018). The right linker atom was the hydrogen-bond donor atom, which suggested that the hydrogen-bond donor atom at this position was likely to improve the anti-HIV-1 activities, which was in good agreement with the 3D-QSAR results.

For the optimal pharmacophore, there were 70 compounds screened from the decoy database, and 42 of them were active molecules. In addition, the calculated values of %Y, %A, EF, and GH were 60%, 100%, 89.66, and 0.70, respectively, which met the requirements that the EF value should be more than 1 and the GH value should be in the range from 0.6 and 1. These statistical results indicated that model_20 had excellent abilities of recognizing the false positives and distinguishing the

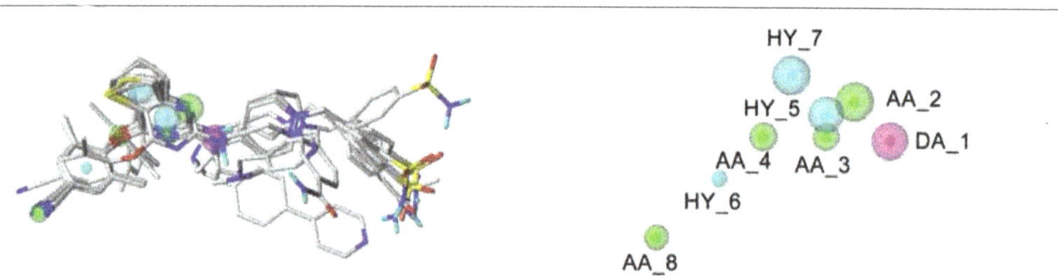

FIGURE 6 | The best pharmacophore model with the alignment of 10 training set compounds. The model includes four hydrogen-bond acceptor atoms (green), three hydrophobic centers (cyan), and one hydrogen-bond donor atom (magenta).

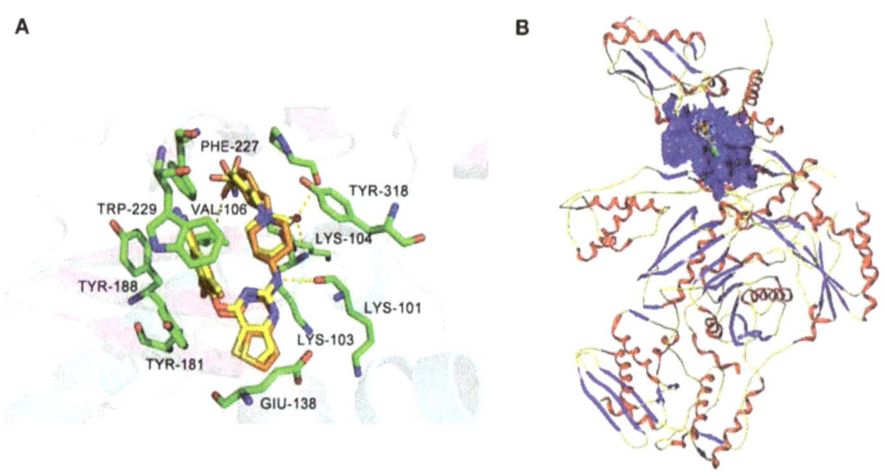

FIGURE 7 | The redocked results of **K-5a2** in the binding pocket of the HIV-1 reverse transcriptase (RT) (PDB: 6C0J). **(A)** The superimposition of the cognate **K-5a2** (yellow) and the redocked **K-5a2** (orange). **(B)** The blue region represents the surface of the binding pocket.

similar structures of active and inactive compounds from the database. Thus, model_20 could be used for the next virtual screening studies.

Molecular Docking

Molecular docking was performed to investigate the binding modes of DHPYs at the active site of the HIV-1 RT. To validate the reliability of the molecular docking method, the cognate ligand (**K-5a2**) was redocked into the binding pocket of the HIV-1 RT (PDB: 6C0J), and the result was shown in **Figure 7A**. The original crystallographic and redocked conformations were almost superposition, and the root mean square deviation (RMSD) value between them for all atoms was 0.38 Å, which suggested that the docking method and used parameters were reasonable (Khan et al., 2010). As seen from **Figure 7A**, the two ligands adopted a similar binding pattern, in which the left benzene ring was located at the hydrophobic region consisting of residues Tyr181, Tyr188, Trp229, Phe227, and Val106 and could form π-π stacking interactions with the aromatic residues of them. In addition, it was noteworthy that the two ligands not only formed hydrogen-bond interactions with residues Lys101, Lys104, and Val106, respectively, but also interacted with residues Lys103 and Pro236 *via* a network of hydrogen bonds by a water molecule (W936). Those results were in good consistency with previous reports (Yang et al., 2018; Kang et al., 2019). At the same time, the hydrogen bond formed between the C = O of Lys101 and the NH of the right linker atom indicated that hydrogen-bond donor atoms were beneficial in the place, which was a good agreement with the results of pharmacophore and 3D-QSAR models. As shown in **Figure 7B**, 52 DHPYs embedded in the binging pocket by the similar *U*-shaped conformations, suggesting the accuracy of the docking method.

Virtual Screening

To discover and design novel HIV-1 NNRTI leads, a multistage-filtered virtual screening was performed based on the constructed pharmacophore model and the established molecular docking method (**Figure 8**). First, a total of 19,740 compounds were obtained from ZINC database by the pharmacophore-based virtual screening and the restriction with Lipinski's rule of five. Then, 3,451 compounds were selected on the basis of the QFIT score of more than 50. In order to enhance the efficiency and accuracy of docking screening, the preliminary docking by Surflex-Dock and the second round docking by Surflex-Dock Geom were performed. The results indicated that only 20 compounds met the requirements simultaneously. In view of the predicted ADME properties of the screened 20 compounds, nine compounds were selected to regard as NNRTI hits, whose structures and docking scores were shown in **Table 3**. Furthermore, the interactions between the screened compounds and the HIV-1 RT were shown in **Table S3**. Nine screened compounds formed hydrophobic interactions with residues Tyr181, Tyr188, Phe227, Trp229, and Val106 and π-π stacking interactions with the aromatic residues of them. Except for ZINC_91409938, which formed a hydrogen-bond network with the residues Pro236 and Lys103 by a water molecule (W936), the screened compounds also formed

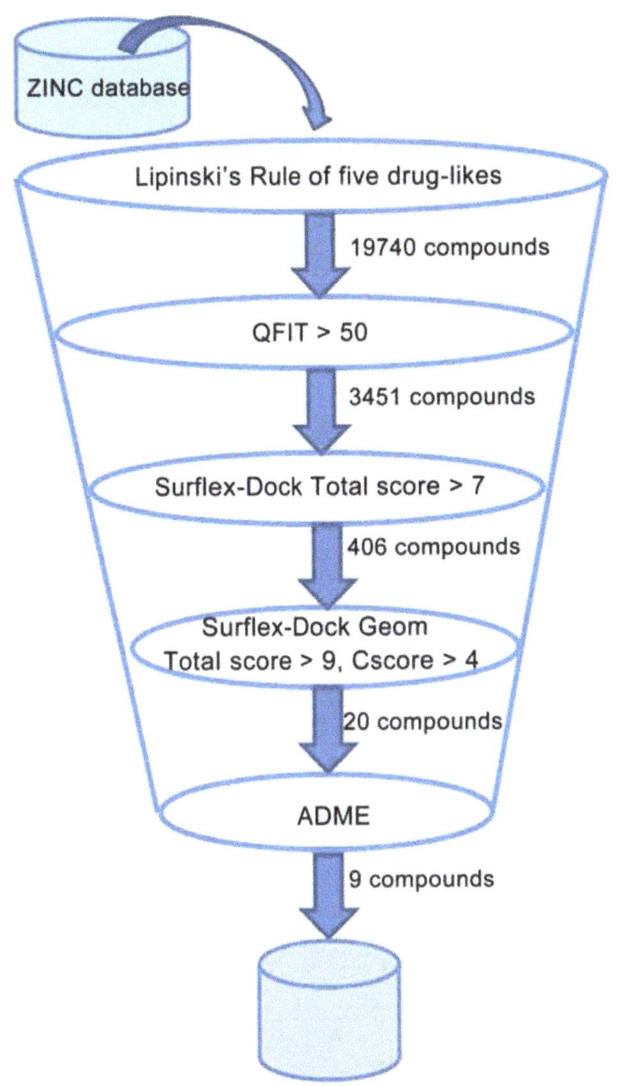

FIGURE 8 | Representation of the overall virtual screening process.

hydrogen bonds with the key residues Lys101 and Glu138. The docking results indicated that nine screened compounds might be potential NNRTIs.

Newly Designed Non-nucleoside Reverse Transcriptase Inhibitors

According to the structural characteristics of DHPYs and the results of the 3D-QSAR models and molecular docking, we further designed three new compounds (**N1**, **N2,** and **N3**; **Table 4**) using ZINC_73709240 as a lead compound. The 3D-QSAR contour maps indicated that the hydrogen-bond acceptor at the *para-position* of the benzene ring of Tolerant Region II and the hydrogen-bond donor at the terminal of Tolerant Region II were favorable to the inhibitory activity. Therefore, we designed compounds **N1**, **N2,** and **N3** by adding amide or

TABLE 3 | Chemical structures and docking scores of the screened hit compounds as novel HIV-1 NNRTIs from ZINC database.

Compound No.	Structure	Docking score
ZINC_57841658	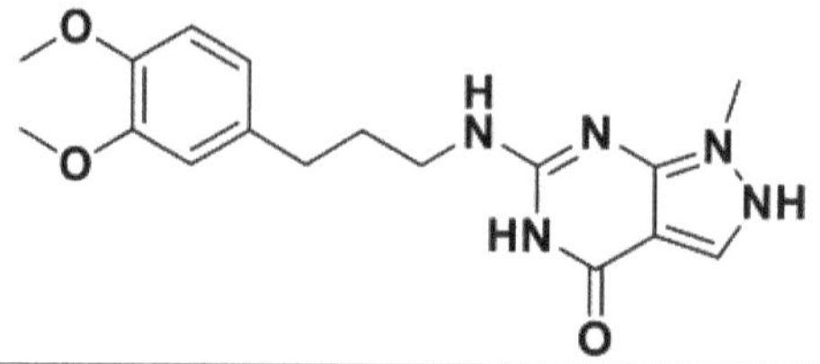	9.43
ZINC_60381334	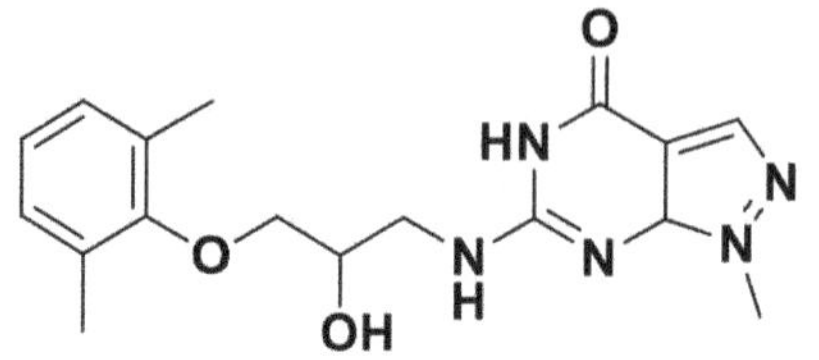	9.02
ZINC_63070905	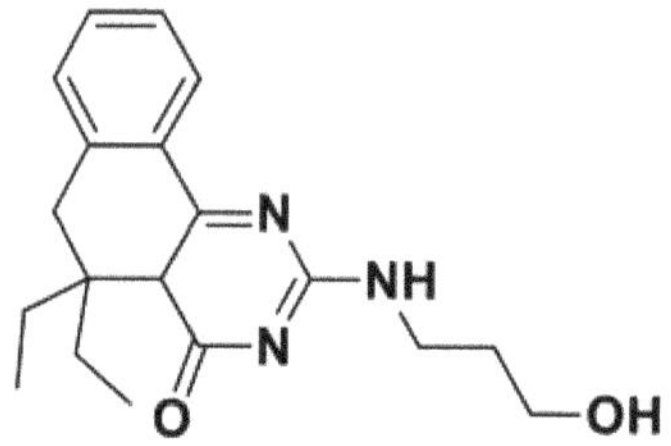	9.56
ZINC_69532225	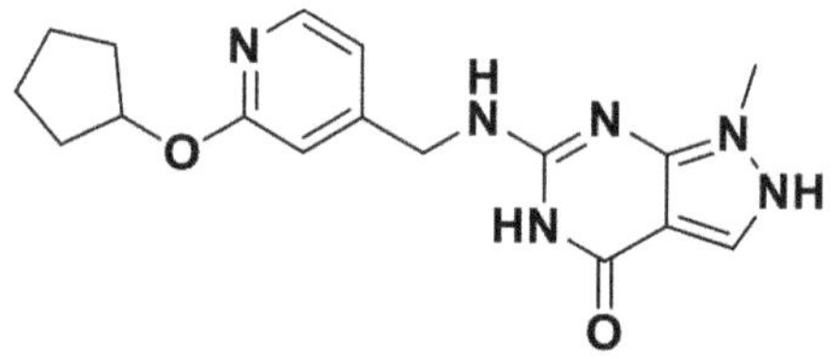	9.12
ZINC_71894576	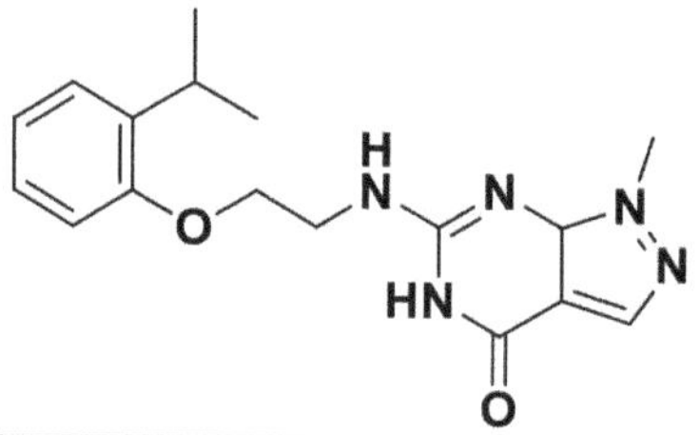	9.00
ZINC_73709240	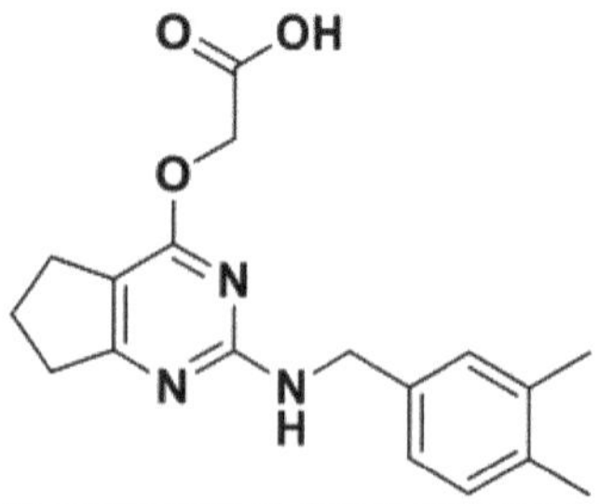	9.64
ZINC_89506228	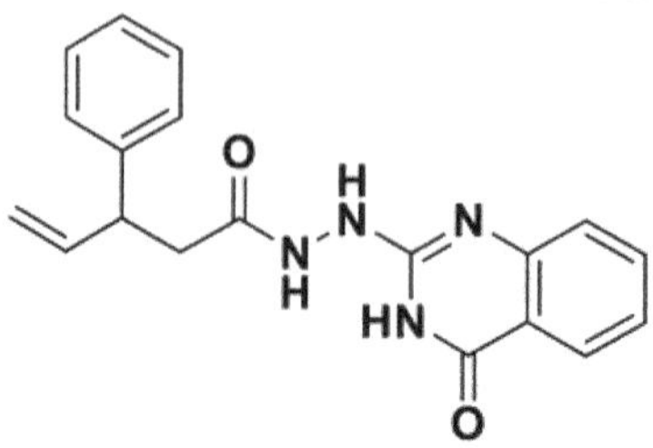	9.29

(Continued)

TABLE 3 | Continued

Compound No.	Structure	Docking score
ZINC_91409938	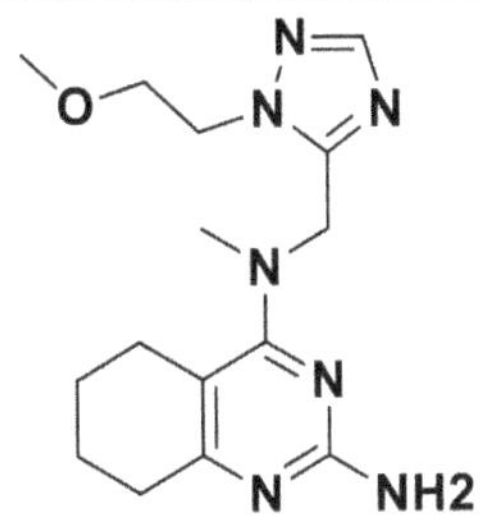	9.30
ZINC_97995063	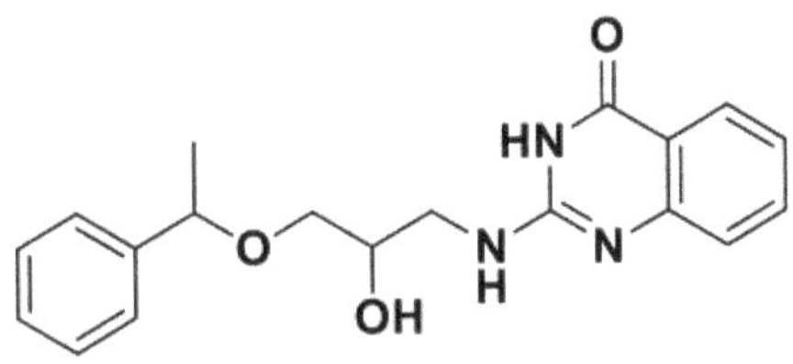	9.22

NNRTIs, non-nucleoside reverse transcriptase inhibitors.

TABLE 4 | Chemical structures and docking scores of the newly designed HIV-1 NNRTIs.

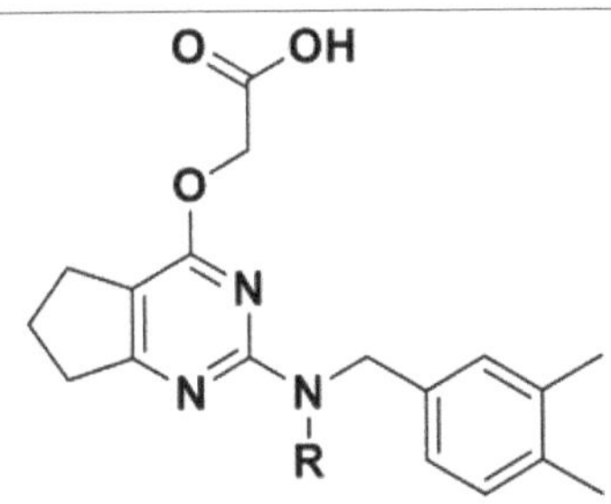

Compound No.	R	Docking score	
		Wild-type HIV-1 RT	Mutant HIV-1 RT (K103N+Y181C)
N1	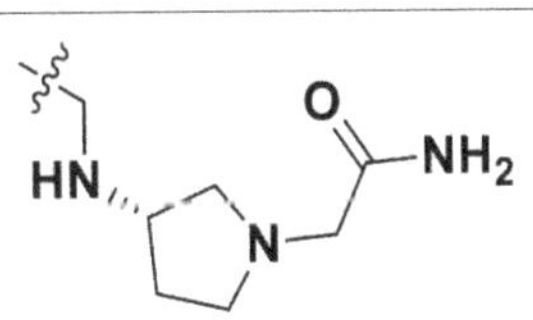	13.83	10.60
N2	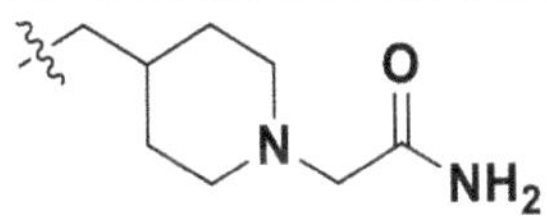	12.59	12.03
N3	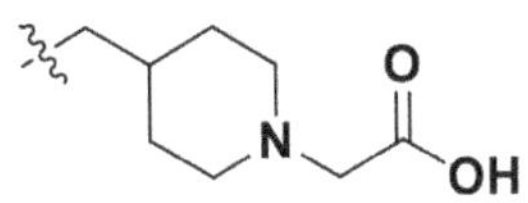	12.93	12.88

NNRTIs, non-nucleoside reverse transcriptase inhibitors; RT, reverse transcriptase.

carboxyl groups as hydrogen-bond donors or acceptors at these positions (**Table 4**).

All designed compounds were then docked into the binding site of HIV-1 RT by Surflex-Dock Geom method. The docking scores of compounds **N1**, **N2,** and **N3** were 13.83, 12.59, and 12.93, respectively, and higher than that of compound **36** (11.86), suggesting that the interactions between the newly designed compounds and the protein might be more stable. As shown

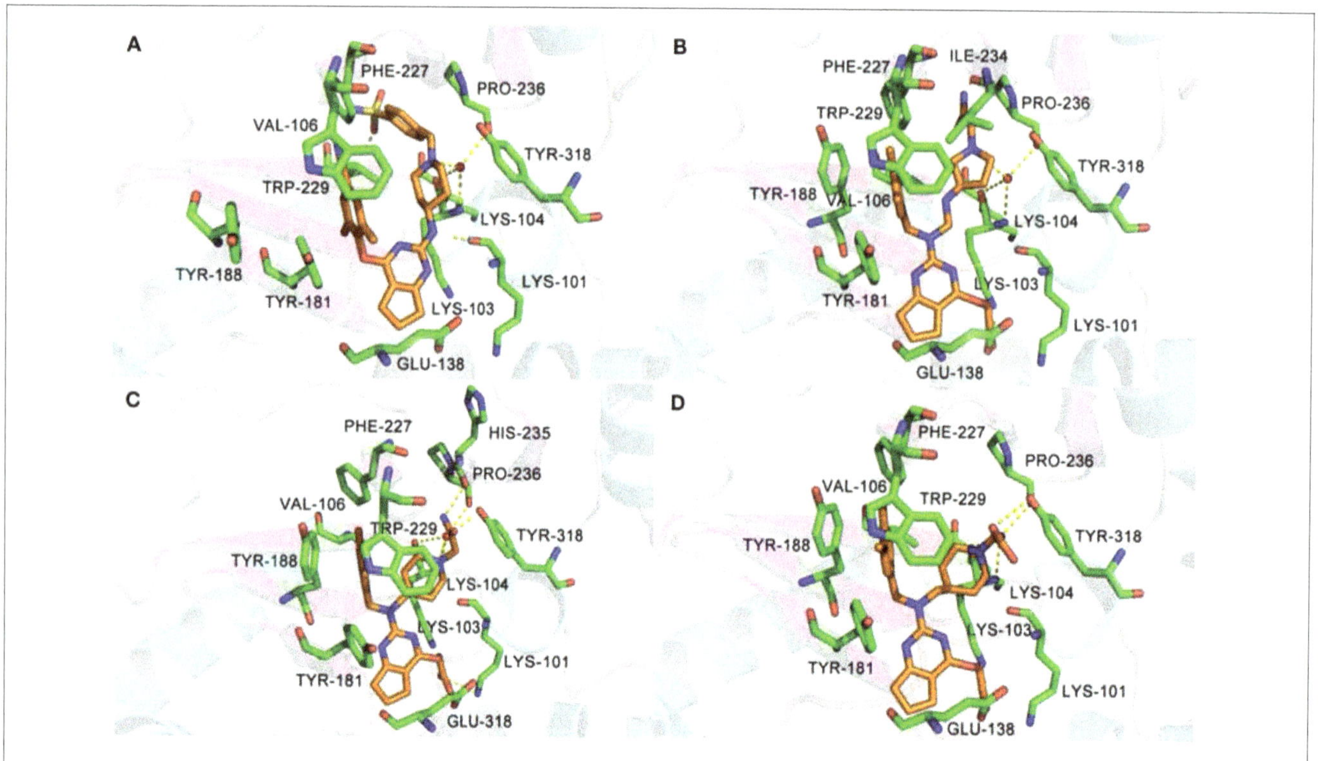

FIGURE 9 | The docked results of compounds **36 (A)**, **N1 (B)**, **N2 (C)**, and **N3 (D)** in the binding pocket of wild-type HIV-1 reverse transcriptase (RT) (PDB: 6C0J).

in **Figure 9**, the binding modes of compounds **N1**, **N2,** and **N3** with the protein were basically similar to that of compound **36**. The left wings of four ligands were all located in the hydrophobic region and formed π-π stacking interactions with residues Tyr181, Tyr188, Trp229, and Phe227, and the positive nitrogen of their right wing formed hydrogen-bond networks with Lys103 and Pro236 through a water molecule (W936), which was in good agreement with the docking results. However, there were some differences for four compounds in terms of protein–ligand interactions. As for compound **36**, it formed three hydrogen bonds with Lys101 (Lys101-O…H-N-, 2.8 Å) and Val106 (Val106-NH…O=C, 3.0 Å; -O…H-N-, 2.7 Å), which was consistent with the redocked results of **K-5a2**. As can be seen from **Figures 9A,B**, compounds **N1** and **N3** not only formed hydrogen bonds with Glu138 and Lys103 but also had hydrogen bonds with Ile234 and/or Tyr318. Another finding was that five hydrogen bonds were formed between residues Glu138, Lys103, Lys101, Tyr318, and His235 with compound **N2**. The docking results revealed that the four compounds interacted with key amino acid residues (Lys101 and Glu138), and several new hydrogen bonds between three newly designed compounds and residues Lys103, Ile234, Tyr318, and His235 were found. These results suggested that compounds **N1**, **N2,** and **N3** might be the potential inhibitors with improving anti-HIV-1 activities.

To further explore whether the newly designed compounds could inhibit mutant HIV-1 RT, they were also docked into the mutant (K103N+Y181C) RT (PDB ID: 6C0R) (**Figure S1**; **Table 4**). The co-crystallizing ligand (**25a**) of 6C0R as a reference compound was also redocked into the binding site as displayed in **Figure S1A**. Kang et al. (2017) reported that the inhibitory activity of compound **25a** (EC_{50} = 5.5 ± 0.81 nM) against the K103N+Y181C mutant RT was better than that of RPV (EC_{50} = 11 ± 1.9 nM). Our docking results indicated that compound **25a** formed four hydrogen bonds with residues Lys101, Val106, Lys104, and Tyr188, respectively, and the π-π stacking and/or hydrophobic interactions were also found with residues Trp229, Phe227, and Tyr188. In addition, the residue Tyr183 played an important role in the binding site of the mutant RT and could offset the loss of π-stacking and hydrophobic interactions between inhibitors and residue Tyr181 as it was mutated to Cys181 (Das et al., 2008).

The docking scores of three hit compounds were relatively high (**Table 4**), especially compounds **N2** and **N3**, whose docking scores were higher than **25a** (12.02), indicating that the newly designed molecules might have better inhibitory activity against the mutant RT. It was observed that the hydrogen bond with residue Lys101, π-π stacking, and hydrophobic interactions still existed for three complexes (**Figure S1**). However, the difference was that compounds **N1**, **N2**, and **N3** could form a direct hydrogen bond with the mutated residue Asn103, which indicated that these designed molecules could bind well in the binding pocket with mutations. These docking results demonstrated that the three hit compounds might have the ability to inhibit the HIV-1 RT mutant. However, the actual anti-HIV activities of the three hits are necessary to be identified in future studies.

TABLE 5 | Predicted absorption-distribution-metabolism- excretion (ADME) parameters and drug-like properties of compound **36** and the newly designed inhibitors (**N1–3**).

Properties	Parameters	Compounds			
		36	**N1**	**N2**	**N3**
Physicochemical Properties	MW[a] (g/mol)	532.66	482.58	481.59	482.57
	Rotatable bonds	7	11	10	10
	HBA	8	8	7	8
	HBD	2	3	2	2
	TPSA[b]	142.61	133.91	121.88	116.09
Lipophilicity	iLOGP	3.82	3.29	3.38	3.60
	XLOGP3	4.17	0.04	0.92	1.57
	WLOGP	4.33	0.63	1.72	2.32
	MLOGP	2.06	0.44	1.42	1.82
	Silicos IT logP	3.51	2.08	3.09	3.33
	Consensus logP	3.58	1.30	2.11	2.53
Water Solubility	ESOL Class	MS[c]	S[d]	S	S
	Ali Class	PS[e]	S	S	S
	Silicos IT Class	PS	MS	MS	MS
Pharmacokinetics	GI[f] absorption	low	high	high	high
	BBB[g] permeat	No	No	No	No
	CYP1A2 inhibitor	No	No	No	No
	CYP2C19 inhibitor	Yes	No	No	No
	CYP2C9 inhibitor	Yes	No	No	No
	CYP2D6 inhibitor	Yes	No	Yes	Yes
	CYP3A4 inhibitor	Yes	No	Yes	Yes
Druglikeness	Lipinski violations	1	0	0	0
	Ghose violations	2	2	2	2
	Egan violations	1	1	0	0
	Muegge violations	1	1	0	0
	Bioavailability Score	0.55	0.55	0.55	0.56
Medicinal Chemistry	PAINS[h] alerts	0	0	0	0
	Brenk alerts	0	1	0	0
	Leadlikeness violations	2	2	1	2
	Synthetic accessibility	4.68	4.68	4.12	4.10

[a] *Molecular weight.*
[b] *Total polar surface area.*
[c] *Moderately soluble.*
[d] *Soluble.*
[e] *Poorly soluble.*
[f] *Gastrointestinal.*
[g] *Blood–brain barrier.*
[h] *Pan assay interference compounds.*

ADME Analysis

ADME prediction studies were carried out for compound **36** and three newly designed NNRTIs (**N1**, **N2,** and **N3**). The results were depicted in **Table 5**. In this program, five inhibitors of cytochrome P450 (CYP) enzymes were predicted. CYPs, which primarily mediated oxidation of various compounds and participated in physiological and pathophysiological processes, were the major phase I drug-metabolizing enzymes and responsible for metabolism of about 75% of all marketed drugs (Moroy et al., 2012). In the family of CYP enzymes, the CYP3A4 was the most important enzyme on account of metabolizing ~50% of all drugs by itself, and the CYP2C9 enzyme mainly metabolizes several clinically used drugs such as celecoxib and diclofenac (Daly et al., 2017). As shown in **Table 5**, compounds **N1**, **N2,** and **N3** could be easier to be metabolized compared with compound **36.** In addition, three newly designed compounds showed high human gastrointestinal absorption (HIA), indicating that they might have a high chance of brain penetration (Li et al., 2019). The topological polar surface area (TPSA) values of compound **N1** and **N3** were in the range from 20 to 130 Å^2, which suggested that they possessed good transport properties *in vivo*. Notably, the synthetic accessibilities of designed compounds were lower than 5, suggesting that they were relatively easy to be synthesized. On the whole, the

ADME properties of the three newly designed compounds were superior to that of compound **36**, especially in pharmacokinetics, druglikeness, and medicinal chemistry properties. Thus, the three newly designed compounds might be supposed to have good pharmacokinetics properties.

Molecular Dynamics Simulation

As for newly designed molecules, their stability of protein–ligand interactions should be taken into account. Thus, 10 ns MD simulations were performed for four complex systems, 6C0J-36, 6C0J-N1, 6C0J-N2, and 6C0J-N3, respectively. The RMSD values of backbone atoms for the four complexes were displayed in **Figure 10A**. During the 10 ns MD simulations, the RMSD values of the four systems were relatively stable and were lower than 0.3 nm. **Figure 10B** showed the RMSD values of the four ligands during 10 ns MD simulations. The four ligands had similar fluctuations and reached equilibrium at approximately 0.5 ns. The root mean square fluctuation (RMSF) profiles of the four complexes (**Figures 10C,D**) also exhibited similar trends during the MD simulations. It should be pointed out that the key residues, Lys101 of chain A and Glu138 of chain B, had relatively lower RMSF values. As shown in **Figure 10E**, the radius of gyration (Rg) values, which could explain the compactness of the protein throughout simulation, basically maintained at about 3.5 nm, indicated that greater changes of the conformations of protein did not take place. In addition,

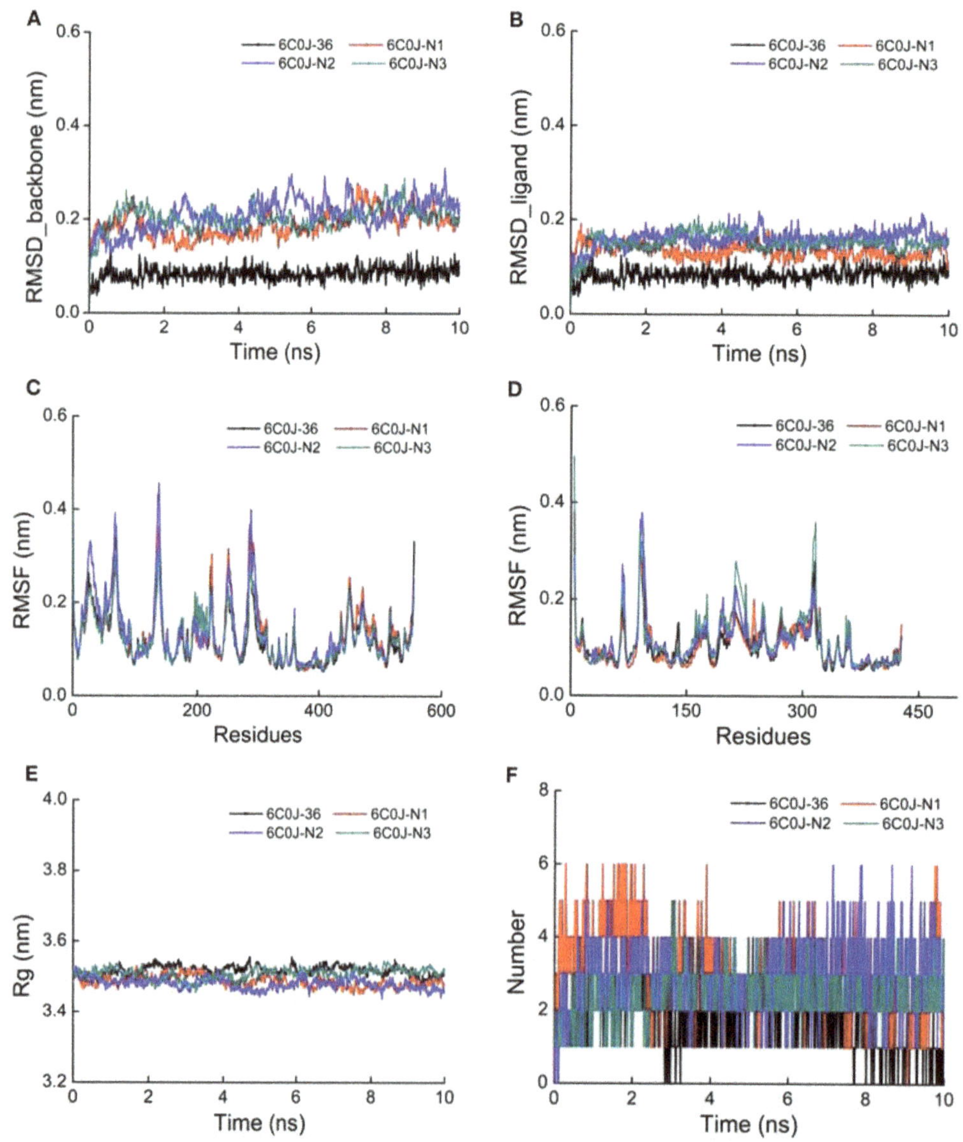

FIGURE 10 | The 10 ns molecular dynamics (MD) results of compounds **36**, **N1**, **N2**, and **N3** in wild-type HIV-1 reverse transcriptase (RT). **(A)** Root mean square deviation (RMSD) values of backbone atoms of the protein. **(B)** RMSD values of the ligands. **(C)** Root mean square fluctuation (RMSF) values of the chain A. **(D)** RMSF values of the chain B. **(E)** Radius of gyration (Rg) values of backbone atoms. **(F)** The total number of hydrogen bonds between the ligands and the protein.

the intermolecular hydrogen bonds could be used to analyze the protein–ligand interaction. As shown in **Figure 10F**, the hydrogen-bond numbers of 6C0J-36, 6C0J-N1, 6C0J-N2, and 6C0J-N3 complexes were 1-2, 1-6, 1-6, and 2-5 over the 10 ns simulations, respectively, which suggested that all newly designed compounds might be more stable than compound **36**. The MD simulation results revealed that four protein–ligand complexes could maintain a relative stability in the dynamic simulation and three newly designed compounds might have more interactions with the HIV-1 RT than compound **36**. These were in good consistency with the docking results.

In the same pattern, 10 ns MD simulations were also carried out for three protein–ligand complexes (6C0R-N1, 6C0R-N2, and 6C0R-N3) to further study whether they still could remain stable in the dynamic environment. The results were shown in **Figure S2**. The RMSD values of protein backbones of the three complexes were displayed in **Figure S2A**, and it can be clearly seen that they basically reached stability after 5 ns and were below 0.4 nm. The RMSD values of the three ligands were also stable (**Figure S2B**). **Figures S2C,D** were the RMSF plots of chains A and B, respectively, which showed that the residues of the three complexes fluctuated in the same trend, indicating that they had great stability. In addition, the Rg values just slightly floated within 3.5 nm from **Figure S2E**, indicating that the proteins had good compactness. The number of hydrogen bonds was also essential to verify the stability. As shown in **Figure S2F**, the hydrogen-bond numbers of compounds **N1**, **N2**, and **N3** were 2-4, 1-5, and 2-5 over the 10 ns MD, respectively, suggesting that the three compounds could tightly bind to the mutant RT. The abovementioned results revealed that the three complexes could keep stable during MD simulations and the three designed compounds could interact well with the mutant HIV-1 RT. However, the experimental activities of the three new hits against wild-type and mutant HIV-1 strains remain to be studied.

CONCLUSION

In conclusion, 52 DHPYs were collected to construct the CoMFA and CoMSIA models, which exhibited rationally statistical parameters and good predictive ability. These models well-explained the 3D-QSARs of these DHPY and provided useful information for designing new HIV-1 NNRTIs. The optimal pharmacophore model containing eight features was in agreement with the 3D-QSAR results. The docking results revealed that Lys101 was the key amino acid residue, and the hydrophobic and π-π stacking interactions with Tyr181, Tyr188, Trp229, and Phe227 also played key roles for the anti-HIV activity of DHPYs. Nine lead compounds were obtained by the pharmacophore-based and docking-based virtual screening as well as ADME prediction. Three novel inhibitors were designed by modifying the structure of the screened compound ZINC_73709240 according to the 3D-QSAR and docking results. Three newly designed inhibitors showed good stability and strong interactions not only in the wild-type RT but also in the K103N/Y181C RT mutant based on the docking and MD simulation results. The ADME prediction indicated that compounds **N1**, **N2,** and **N3** might possess desirable drug-like properties. However, further study on synthesis and anti-HIV activities of the three newly designed hits is necessary. We expect that the screened and designed compounds could be served as lead candidates of novel HIV-1 NNRTIs.

AUTHOR CONTRIBUTIONS

GL and YC proposed the research idea and designed the experiment. YC performed the experiment. YC, FW, YT, and YG analyzed the data. YC, XL, XJ, and GL wrote the manuscript. All authors revised and approved the manuscript.

FUNDING

This work was supported by the National Natural Science Foundation of China (No. 21807082), the Hubei Provincial Natural Science Foundation of China (No. 2017CFB121), and the Hubei Provincial Department of Education of China (No. Q20171503).

REFERENCES

Almerico, A. M., Lauria, A., Tutone, M., Diana, P., Barraja, P., Montalbano, A., et al. (2003). A multivariate analysis on non-nucleoside HIV-1 reverse transcriptase inhibitors and resistance induced by mutation. *QSAR Comb. Sci.* 22, 984–996. doi: 10.1002/qsar.200330834

Almerico, A. M., Tutone, M., Ippolito, M., and Lauria, A. (2007). Molecular modelling and QSAR in the discovery of HIV-1 integrase inhibitors. *Curr. Comput. Aid. Drug Des.* 3, 214–233. doi: 10.2174/157340907781695468

Almerico, A. M., Tutone, M., and Lauria, A. (2008). Docking and multivariate methods to explore HIV-1 drug-resistance: a comparative analysis. *J. Comput. Aid. Mol. Des.* 22, 287–297. doi: 10.1007/s10822-008-9186-7

Almerico, A. M., Tutone, M., Lauria, A., Diana, P., Barraja, P., Montalbano, A., et al. (2006). A multivariate analysis of HIV-1 protease inhibitors and resistance induced by mutation. *J. Chem. Inf. Model.* 46, 168–179. doi: 10.1021/ci050139z

Borisa, A., and Bhatt, H. (2015). 3D-QSAR (CoMFA, CoMFA-RG, CoMSIA) and molecular docking study of thienopyrimidine and thienopyridine derivatives to explore structural requirements for aurora-B kinase inhibition. *Eur. J. Pharm. Sci.* 79, 1–12. doi: 10.1016/j.ejps.2015.08.017

Bush, B. L., and Nachbar, R. B. (1993). Sample-distance partial least squares: PLS optimized for many variables, with application to CoMFA. *J Comput. Aid. Mol. Des.* 7, 587–619. doi: 10.1007/BF00124364

Caballero, J. (2010). 3D-QSAR (CoMFA and CoMSIA) and pharmacophore (GALAHAD) studies on the differential inhibition of aldose reductase by flavonoid compounds. *J. Mol. Graph. Model.* 29, 363–371. doi: 10.1016/j.jmgm.2010.08.005

Chen, X. W., Zhan, P., Li, D. Y., Clercq, E. D., and Liu, X. Y. (2011). Recent advances in DAPYs and related analogues as HIV-1 NNRTIs. *Curr. Med. Chem.* 18, 329–376. doi: 10.2174/092986711794839142

Daina, A., Michielin, O., and Zoete, V. (2017). SwissADME: a free web tool to evaluate pharmacokinetics, drug-likeness and medicinal chemistry friendliness of small molecules. *Sci. Rep.* 7:42717. doi: 10.1038/srep42717

Daly, A. K., Rettie, A. E., Fowler, D. M., and Miners, J. O. (2017). Pharmacogenomics of CYP2C9: functional and clinical considerations. *J. Pers. Med.* 8:1. doi: 10.3390/jpm8010001

Das, K., Bauman, J. D., Clark, A. D., Frenkel, Y. V., Lewi, P. J., Shatkin, A. J., et al. (2008). High-resolution structures of HIV-1 reverse transcriptase/TMC278 complexes: strategic flexibility explains potency against resistance mutations. *PNAS.* 105, 1466–1471. doi: 10.1073/pnas.0711209105

Esposito, F., Corona, A., and Tramontano, E. (2012). HIV-1 reverse transcriptase still remains a new drug target: structure, function, classical inhibitors, and new inhibitors with innovative mechanisms of actions. *Mol. Biol. Int.* 2012:586401. doi: 10.1155/2012/586401

Gao, Y., Chen, Y. M., Tian, Y. F., Zhao, Y. L., Wu, F. S., Luo, X. G., et al. (2019). *In silico* study of 3-hydroxypyrimidine-2,4-diones as inhibitors of HIV RT-associated RNase H using molecular docking, molecular dynamics, 3D-QSAR, and pharmacophore models. *New J. Chem.* 43, 17004–170017. doi: 10.1039/C9NJ03353J

Gu, S. X., Xiao, T., Zhu, Y. Y., Liu, G. Y., and Chen, F. E. (2019). Recent progress in HIV-1 inhibitors targeting the entrance channel of HIV-1 non-nucleoside reverse transcriptase inhibitor binding pocket. *Eur. J. Med. Chem.* 174, 277–291. doi: 10.1016/j.ejmech.2019.04.054

Kalva, S., Azhagiya Singam, E. R., Rajapandian, V., Saleena, L. M., and Subramanian, V. (2014). Discovery of potent inhibitor for matrix metalloproteinase-9 by pharmacophore based modeling and dynamics simulation studies. *J. Mol. Graph. Model.* 49, 25–37. doi: 10.1016/j.jmgm.2013.12.008

Kang, D. W., Fang, Z. J., Huang, B. S., Lu, X. Y., Zhang, H., Xu, H., et al. (2017). Structure-based optimization of thiophene[3,2-d]pyrimidine derivatives as potent HIV-1 non-nucleoside reverse transcriptase inhibitors with improved potency against resistance-associated variants. *J. Med. Chem.* 60, 4424–4443. doi: 10.1021/acs.jmedchem.7b00332

Kang, D. W., Fang, Z. J., Li, Z. Y., Huang, B. S., Zhang, H., Lu, X. Y., et al. (2016). Design, synthesis, and evaluation of thiophene[3,2-d]pyrimidine derivatives as HIV-1 non-nucleoside reverse transcriptase inhibitors with significantly improved drug resistance profiles. *J. Med. Chem.* 59, 7991–8007. doi: 10.1021/acs.jmedchem.6b00738

Kang, D. W., Zhang, H., Wang, Z., Zhao, T., Ginex, T., Luque, F. J., et al. (2019). Identification of dihydrofuro[3,4-d]pyrimidine derivatives as Novel HIV-1 non-nucleoside reverse transcriptase inhibitors with promising antiviral activities and desirable physicochemical properties. *J. Med. Chem.* 62, 1484–1501. doi: 10.1021/acs.jmedchem.8b01656

Khan, K. M., Wadood, A., Ali, M., Zia, U., Ul-Haq, Z., Lodhi, M. A., et al. (2010). Identification of potent urease inhibitors via ligand- and structure-based virtual screening and *in vitro* assays. *J. Mol. Graph. Model.* 28, 792–798. doi: 10.1016/j.jmgm.2010.02.004

Li, M., Wei, D., Zhao, H., and Du, Y. (2014). Genotoxicity of quinolones: substituents contribution and transformation products QSAR evaluation using 2D and 3D models. *Chemosphere* 95, 220–226. doi: 10.1016/j.chemosphere.2013.09.002

Li, Q., Zhang, C., and Ren, Y. (2019). Molecular modeling technology studies of novel pyrazoylethylbenzamide derivatives as selective orexin receptor 1 antagonists. *J. Taiwan Inst. Chem. Eng.* 100, 1–17. doi: 10.1016/j.jtice.2019.03.018

Liu, G. Y., Wan, Y. L., Wang, W. J., Fang, S., Gu, S. X., and Ju, X. L. (2019). Docking-based 3D-QSAR and pharmacophore studies on diarylpyrimidines as non-nucleoside inhibitors of HIV-1 reverse transcriptase. *Mol. Divers.* 23, 107–121. doi: 10.1007/s11030-018-9860-1

Liu, G. Y., Wang, W. J., Wan, Y. L., Ju, X. L., and Gu, S. X. (2018). Application of 3D-QSAR, pharmacophore, and molecular docking in the molecular design of diarylpyrimidine derivatives as HIV-1 nonnucleoside reverse transcriptase inhibitors. *Int. J. Mol. Sci.* 19:1436. doi: 10.3390/ijms19051436

Moroy, G., Martiny, V. Y., Vayer, P., Villoutreix, B. O., and Miteva, M. A. (2012). Toward *in silico* structure-based ADMET prediction in drug discovery. *Drug Discov. Today.* 17, 44–55. doi: 10.1016/j.drudis.2011.10.023

Mysinger, M. M., Carchia, M., Irwin, J. J., and Shoichet, B. K. (2012). Directory of useful decoys, enhanced (DUD-E): better ligands and decoys for better benchmarking. *J. Med. Chem.* 55, 6582–6594. doi: 10.1021/jm300687e

Namasivayam, V., Vanangamudi, M., Kramer, V. G., Kurup, S., Zhan, P., Liu, X., et al. (2019). The journey of HIV-1 non-nucleoside reverse transcriptase inhibitors (NNRTIs) from lab to clinic. *J. Med. Chem.* 62, 4851–4883. doi: 10.1021/acs.jmedchem.8b00843

Ojha, P. K., Mitra, I., Das, R. N., and Roy, K. (2011). Further exploring r_m^2 metrics for validation of QSPR models. *Chemom. Intell. Lab. Syst.* 107, 194–205. doi: 10.1016/j.chemolab.2011.03.011

Roy, K., Das, R. N., Ambure, P., and Aher, R. B. (2016). Be aware of error measures. Further studies on validation of predictive QSAR models. *Chemom. Intell. Lab. Syst.* 152, 18–33. doi: 10.1016/j.chemolab.2016.01.008

Vasavi, C. S., Tamizhselvi, R., and Munusami, P. (2019). Exploring the drug resistance mechanism of active site, non-active site mutations and their cooperative effects in CRF01_AE HIV-1 protease: molecular dynamics simulations and free energy calculations. *J. Biomol. Struct. Dyn.* 37, 2608–2626. doi: 10.1080/07391102.2018.1492459

Wan, Y. L., Tian, Y. F., Wang, W. J., Gu, S. X., Ju, X. L., and Liu, G. Y. (2018). *In silico* studies of diarylpyridine derivatives as novel HIV-1 NNRTIs using docking-based 3D-QSAR, molecular dynamics, and pharmacophore modeling approaches. *RSC Adv.* 8, 40529–40543. doi: 10.1039/C8RA06475J

Wang, R., Xu, K., and Shi, W. (2019). Quinolone derivatives: potential anti-HIV agent-development and application. *Arch. Pharm.* 352:e1900045. doi: 10.1002/ardp.201900045

Wang, W. J., Tian, Y. F., Wan, Y. L., Gu, S. X., Ju, X. L., Luo, X. G., et al. (2018). Insights into the key structural features of N1-ary-benzimidazols as HIV-1 NNRTIs using molecular docking, molecular dynamics, 3D-QSAR, and pharmacophore modeling. *Struct. Chem.* 30, 385–397. doi: 10.1007/s11224-018-1204-3

Yang, Y., Kang, D. W., Nguyen, L. A., Smithline, Z. B., Pannecouque, C., Zhan, P., et al. (2018). Structural basis for potent and broad inhibition of HIV-1 RT by thiophene[3,2-d]pyrimidine non-nucleoside inhibitors. *Elife* 7:e36340. doi: 10.7554/eLife.36340

Zhan, P., Liu, X. Y., and Li, Z. Y. (2009). Recent advances in the discovery and development of novel HIV-1 NNRTI platforms: 2006-2008 update. *Curr. Med. Chem.* 16, 2876–2889. doi: 10.2174/092986709788803231

11

Identification of Novel 3-Hydroxy-pyran-4-One Derivatives as Potent HIV-1 Integrase Inhibitors Using *in silico* Structure-Based Combinatorial Library Design Approach

Hajar Sirous [1†], *Giulia Chemi* [2†], *Sandra Gemma* [2], *Stefania Butini* [2], *Zeger Debyser* [3], *Frauke Christ* [3], *Lotfollah Saghaie* [4], *Simone Brogi* [5*], *Afshin Fassihi* [4*], *Giuseppe Campiani* [2*] and *Margherita Brindisi* [6]

[1] Bioinformatics Research Center, School of Pharmacy and Pharmaceutical Sciences, Isfahan University of Medical Sciences, Isfahan, Iran, [2] Department of Biotechnology, Chemistry and Pharmacy, Department of Excellence 2018-2022, University of Siena, Siena, Italy, [3] Molecular Medicine, K.U. Leuven and IRC KULAK, Leuven, Belgium, [4] Department of Medicinal Chemistry, Faculty of Pharmacy, Isfahan University of Medical Sciences, Isfahan, Iran, [5] Department of Pharmacy, University of Pisa, Pisa, Italy, [6] Department of Pharmacy, Department of Excellence 2018-2022, University of Naples Federico II, Naples, Italy

***Correspondence:**
Simone Brogi
simone.brogi@unipi.it
Afshin Fassihi
fassihi@pharm.mui.ac.ir
Giuseppe Campiani
campiani@unisi.it

† These authors have contributed equally to this work

We describe herein the development and experimental validation of a computational protocol for optimizing a series of 3-hydroxy-pyran-4-one derivatives as HIV integrase inhibitors (HIV INIs). Starting from a previously developed micromolar inhibitors of HIV integrase (HIV IN), we performed an in-depth investigation based on an *in silico* structure-based combinatorial library designing approach. This method allowed us to combine a combinatorial library design and side chain hopping with Quantum Polarized Ligand Docking (QPLD) studies and Molecular Dynamics (MD) simulation. The combinatorial library design allowed the identification of the best decorations for our promising scaffold. The resulting compounds were assessed by the mentioned QPLD methodology using a homology model of full-length binary HIV IN/DNA for retrieving the best performing compounds acting as HIV INIs. Along with the prediction of physico-chemical properties, we were able to select a limited number of drug-like compounds potentially displaying potent HIV IN inhibition. From this final set, based on the synthetic accessibility, we further shortlisted three representative compounds for the synthesis. The compounds were experimentally assessed *in vitro* for evaluating overall HIV-1 IN inhibition, HIV-1 IN strand transfer activity inhibition, HIV-1 activity inhibition and cellular toxicity. Gratifyingly, all of them showed relevant inhibitory activity in the *in vitro* tests along with no toxicity. Among them **HPCAR-28** represents the most promising compound as potential anti-HIV agent, showing inhibitory activity against HIV IN in the low nanomolar range, comparable to that found for Raltegravir, and relevant potency in inhibiting HIV-1 replication and HIV-1 IN strand transfer activity. In summary, our results outline **HPCAR-28** as a useful optimized hit for the potential treatment of HIV-1 infection by targeting HIV IN.

Keywords: 3-hydroxy-pyran-4-one, HIV-1 integrase inhibitors (HIV-1 INIs), *in silico* combinatorial library design, side chain hopping, hit compounds optimization

INTRODUCTION

HIV-1 integrase (IN) represents an attractive target in anti-HIV drug design mainly due to its specificity. Accordingly, HIV-1 IN does not have a functional equivalent in humans and plays a unique role in establishing irreversible and productive viral infections (Debyser et al., 2002; Delelis et al., 2008). This viral key enzyme catalyzes the insertion of proviral DNA, derived from reverse transcription of HIV-1 RNA, into the genome of the host-infected cells. The insertion is achieved through a two-step enzymatic process which starts with endonucleolytic cleavage of a terminal dinucleotide (GT) from each 3′-end of the proviral DNA (termed "3′-processing"), followed by a second reaction, known as "strand transfer" (ST), involving a concerted nucleophilic attack, by the reactive 3′-OH ends of the viral processed DNA to the host chromosomal DNA. As a result, a the covalent joining of the two DNA strands is observed (Chiu and Davies, 2004; Pommier et al., 2005). Both reactions are accomplished by the catalytic core domain of HIV-1 IN which contains two divalent metal ion cofactors (Mg^{2+}). These metal ions are coordinated by three catalytic carboxylate residues: Asp_{64}, Asp_{116}, and Glu_{152} (DDE triad) within the enzyme active site (Dyda et al., 1994; Neamati et al., 2002).

Targeting the metal cofactors within the active site of a viral metal-activated enzyme like HIV-1 IN has emerged as an attractive and validated strategy for the development of novel anti-HIV agents (Rogolino et al., 2012). With this aim, a metal binding pharmacophore model has been exploited for the design of diverse HIV-1 integrase inhibitors (HIV-1 INIs) as depicted in **Figure 1A**. This model is represented by two distinctive structural features: (1) a planar metal binding group (MBG), able to interact with the metal centers within the IN active site, and (2) a pendent aromatic or hetero-aromatic hydrophobic moiety located in close proximity of the MBG (Kawasuji et al., 2006a,b; Johns and Svolto, 2008). Continuous efforts in exploiting this pharmacophore model have culminated in the design and subsequent FDA approval of three INIs for clinical use as effective anti-HIV drugs: Raltegravir (**RLT**), Elvitegravir (**EVG**), and Dolutegravir (**DTG**) in 2007, 2012, and 2013, respectively (**Figure 1B**; Rowley, 2008; Sato et al., 2009; Katlama and Murphy, 2012).

A variety of MBGs have been extensively studied to design innovative and effective INIs (Liao et al., 2010; Di Santo, 2014). Recently, we were particularly interested in taking advantage of the 3-hydroxy-4-pyranone (HP) scaffold for the development of novel HIV-1 INIs due to its application as MBG in the design of several inhibitors of numerous Zn^{2+}, Mg^{2+}, Mn^{2+}, and Cu^{2+} dependent proteins. Accordingly, HP derivatives represent an impressive class of heterocyclic ligands with strong bidentate chelating capacity toward metal ions (Santos et al., 2012; Rostami et al., 2015; Sirous et al., 2015). As a first example of the potential of this structural template in HIV-IN inhibition, a series of HP compounds featuring a unique C-2 carboxamide moiety, namely 3-hydroxyl-pyran-4-one-2-carboxamide derivatives (HPCARs), were rationally designed and recently reported by us (**Figure 2**; Sirous et al., 2019). The proposed chemotypes were characterized by a chelating triad motif effectively coordinating the two metals according to the pharmacophore shared by INIs. Moreover, an aromatic backbone attached to the amide portion through a linker (substituted benzyl and phenylethyl moieties) was considered for providing the essential interactions with the hydrophobic pocket of the enzyme. Most of these HPCAR analogs offered favorable inhibitory potencies in both enzymatic and cell-based antiviral assays with low micromolar IC_{50} values. In particular, the substitution at the *para* position of the aromatic phenyl ring led to the identification of two halo-benzyl derivatives **HPb** and **HPd** (**Figure 2**) as promising lead HIV-1 IN inhibitors with IC_{50} values of 0.37 and 0.7 μM, respectively (Sirous et al., 2019).

In our quest for the search of innovative and effective INIs and considering the above-mentioned findings, we decided to design novel optimized derivatives exploiting the HPCAR chemotype. In this study, we performed the replacement of the pendant aromatic portion with other heterocyclic moieties in order to maintain the strong hydrophobic interactions within the HIV-1 IN binding site, with the possibility to explore additional functional groups for maximizing the contacts that could further stabilize the binding mode of the novel derivatives, leading to compounds with improved activity against HIV-1 IN. Accordingly, in the present study, an *in silico* protocol combining a combinatorial library design procedure coupled to extensive molecular docking studies and physico-chemical properties prediction was developed in a step-filtering approach to identify novel INIs with improved potency with respect to the HPCAR derivatives. The employed screening workflow for designing new HIV-1 INIs with suitable potency and satisfactory physico-chemical properties is illustrated in **Figure 3**. Considering the importance of the aromatic portion of INIs for their binding to both the viral DNA bases, and the hydrophobic pocket within the catalytic core of IN enzyme (Kawasuji et al., 2006b), many efforts were made for replacing the hydrophobic aromatic side chains (substituted benzyl and phenylethyl moieties) to generate a virtual combinatorial library of HP-based core derivatives. Accordingly, using side chain

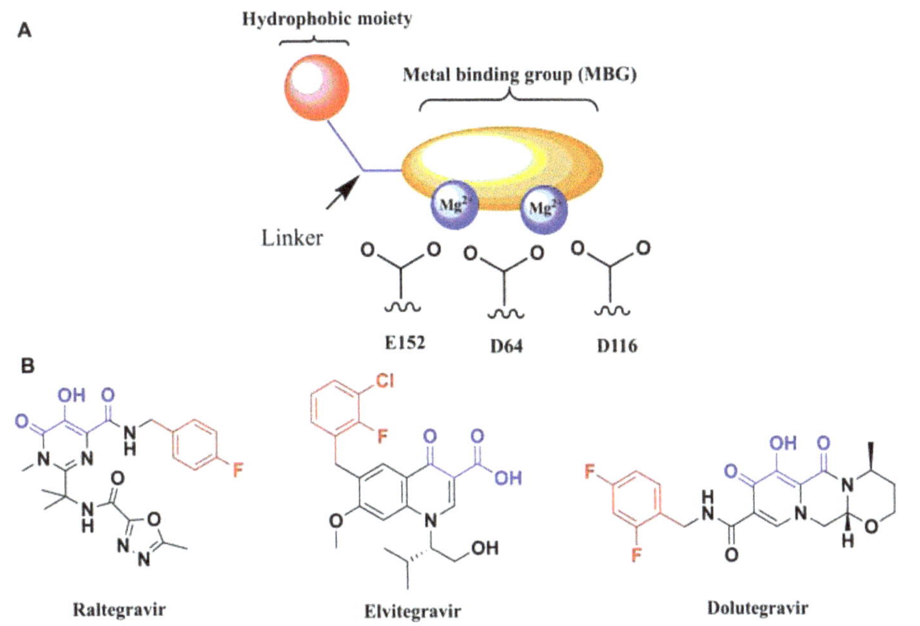

FIGURE 1 | (A) Graphical depiction of the pharmacophore model for HIV-1 INIs. **(B)** Chemical structure of the FDA approved HIV-1 INIs. Atoms in blue are part of MBG of the molecules able to chelate the two metal ions. The hydrophobic aromatic moiety of each compound is highlighted in red.

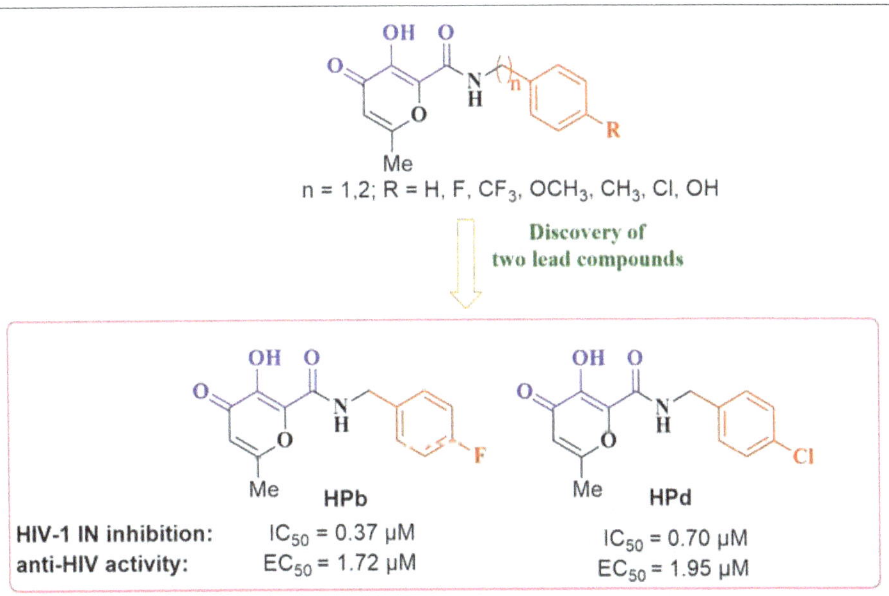

FIGURE 2 | General structure of 3-hydroxy-4-pyranone (HP) based inhibitors previously designed in our laboratory and two halogenated derivatives identified as lead compounds. The proposed chemotype satisfies minimal pharmacophore features for HIV-1 IN inhibition: the metal chelating triad (blue) and terminal hydrophobic benzyl group (red). The most promising HP compounds are shown with the IC_{50} and EC_{50} values for IN inhibitory and anti-HIV activities.

hopping strategy, various cyclic and heterocyclic fragments were attached to the defined position of the HP core in order to find the ideal sidechains with the highest predicted binding affinity for the IN active site. Finally, for validating the computational approach three representative hit candidates identified from this screening workflow were selected, further studied by molecular dynamics (MD) simulations in order to gain additional information about their mechanism of action as INIs, synthesized and submitted to biological evaluation for their HIV-1 IN inhibitory and anti-HIV-1 activities.

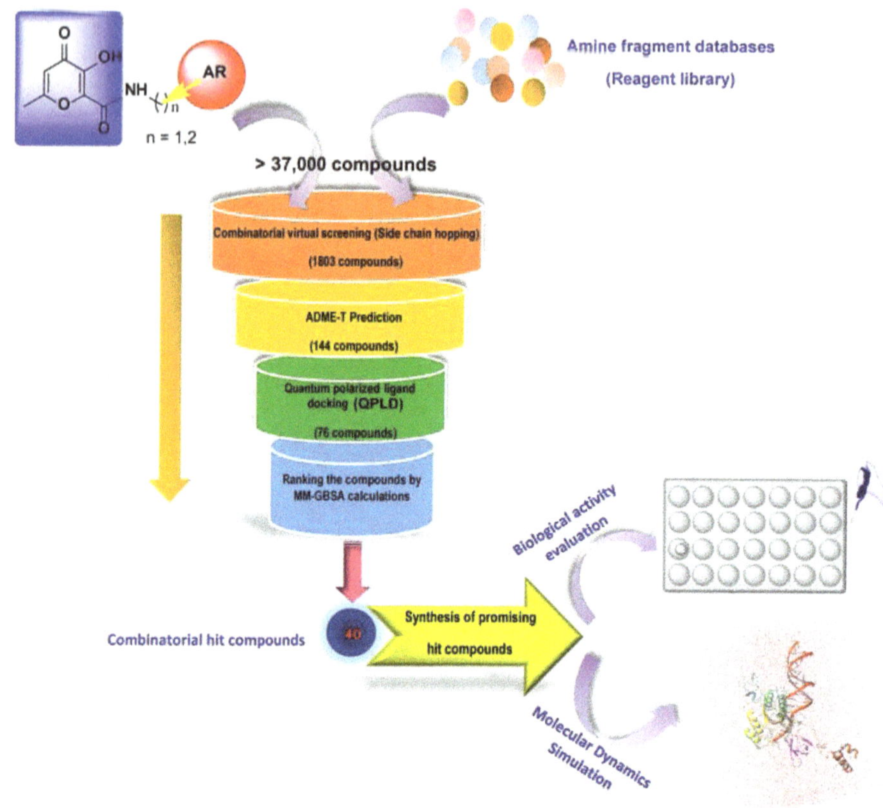

FIGURE 3 | Screening workflow employed in the present study for the *in silico* rational design of new HPCAR derivatives. The core of HPCAR was marked in a blue box. The hydrophobic fragment, AR group, is depicted as a red circle. During combinatorial library screening, diverse sets of fragments were provided from reagent file libraries and attached to the main core at the defined attach positions. The attach position in the scaffold structure is indicated as a yellow vector.

MATERIALS AND METHODS

Computational Details

Ligand Preparation

The 3D structure of the two investigated HPCAR derivatives (substituted with benzyl and phenylethyl moieties) were built by the 3D-sketcher module in Maestro suite (Maestro, version 9.2; Schrödinger, LLC, New York, NY, 2011). Molecular energy minimization of the structures was performed in MacroModel environment using the OPLS-AA 2005 as force field (Jorgensen et al., 1996; Kaminski et al., 2001). GB/SA model was utilized in order to simulate the solvent effects applying "no cut-off" for non-bonded interactions (Still et al., 1990). PRCG method with 1,000 maximum iterations and 0.001 gradient convergence threshold was employed. The same protocol was applied to the novel designed compounds obtained by the combinatorial screening (144 molecules) before submitting them to QPLD procedure. Furthermore, all the compounds were accurately prepared with LigPrep application implemented in Maestro suite (Gasser et al., 2015). Finally the most probable ionization state of the compounds was retrieved by Chemicalize (https://chemicalize.com/) as already reported by us (Brogi et al., 2018).

Protein Preparation

Computational studies were conducted using our recently described theoretical model of full-length HIV-1 IN in complex with viral DNA and Mg^{2+} cofactors (Sirous et al., 2019). The model was subjected to Protein Preparation Wizard protocol implemented in Maestro. This protocol allowed us to obtain a reasonable starting structure of the protein for molecular modeling calculations by a series of computational steps as described (Cappelli et al., 2013; Brogi et al., 2017a,b). Finally, the refined HIV-1 IN model was used for further computational studies.

Generation of Combinatorial Hits

"Combinatorial library enumeration" option available in CombiGlide (CombiGlide, version 2.7; Schrödinger, LLC: New York, 2011), a combinatorial screening software distributed by Schrödinger, was used to carry out structure-based combinatorial library design studies. This software provides the tools for accelerating the lead optimization process, helping in the generation of libraries of optimized derivatives to be selected for the further synthesis. In this direction, two HPCAR derivatives containing methylene and ethylene linkers between the chelating region and the aromatic moiety, identified from our previous studies (Sirous et al., 2019), were selected as main cores. For each investigated compound, a side chain hopping strategy was successfully applied for replacing the hydrophobic side chain, of the selected main cores, with different aromatic or heteroaromatic fragments as shown in **Figure 3**. This method employs the reagent files, chosen by the operator, as a source of fragments with various structures. The following steps are used to generate a new combinatorial library of ligands.

Reagents Preparation

In this step of CombiGlide workflow, a library of reagents containing diverse sets of fragments was built. The elements of this library can be selected from the available databases or generated by the operator. In fact, in the presented work, in addition to the reagent libraries provided by Maestro software, other reagent libraries with different aromatic groups were downloaded from Zinc fragment database (Irwin and Shoichet, 2005; Irwin et al., 2012) as SDF file format and submitted to the reagent preparation facility in the CombiGlide environment. Then the tasks in the reagent preparation process are: (i) the selection of the source of reagent structures; (ii) the selection of a reagent type (a functional group), and finally (iii) the structural conversion from the 2D structure to the 3D one. The selection of a reagent type was done considering the bond that will be replaced in accordance to the functional group formed when the reagent is added to the core. In this context, primary amine set was selected as reagent type. The detailed description of this reagent type is provided in **Table 1**. Concerning this reagent type, R represents the part of reagent that was kept in the process of combinatorial library generation. The bond that was broken to attach the reagent to the core was marked with a line crossing the bond. After running reagent preparation job, the output structure file in .bld format, containing properly prepared reagents, was used in the combinatorial screening process by CombiGlide.

Defining the Core and Attachments

The core is the structural element that is maintained throughout the combinatorial experiment. The attachment positions for each core were defined and the previously prepared reagents file was associated with each attachment point. The attachment point comprises bonds from the core structure that will be replaced in the build process. Considered the role of the hydrophobic side chain of the investigated HPCAR derivatives in binding both the viral DNA and the hydrophobic pocket within IN active site (Sirous et al., 2019), the replacement of benzyl and phenethyl amine moieties with different amine fragments from the reagents file, with other hydrophobic moieties, was performed.

TABLE 1 | Detailed description of predefined functional group type selected in the reagents preparation step of combinatorial library design.

Structure of reagent type	Name of reagent type	Definition of R
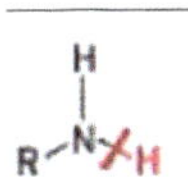	Amine_Primary_General_N_H	R can be alkyl, aryl. R cannot have a carbonyl carbon attached to the nitrogen of the amine.

Setting Up CombiGlide Docking Calculations

The docking step represents the main step of the combinatorial screening process in which a series of docking calculations are performed to screen out molecules that do not have satisfactory docking scores. In fact, on a core with a constant structure, CombiGlide attaches sidechains at defined positions of the core, and performs a docking calculation of the resulting compounds into the active site of HIV-1 IN, to assess the potential affinity of the new compounds. The grid box for the docking calculation was centered on the centroid between the two Mg^{2+} ions which roughly represents the center of the active site. The cubic grid box was adjusted based on a size capable of accommodating ligands with a length 15 Å. As part of grid generation procedure, metal constraints for the receptor grids were also applied. The other options and parameters in this step were set as default and then docking of the library members into the homology modeled HIV-1 IN active site was performed using the extra precision method (XP) in CombiGlide docking. At the end of the process a focused combinatorial library of more than 37,000 compounds was obtained for each studied core-containing molecule. The total structures obtained from combinatorial screening were sorted on the basis of their GlideScore (Glide, Version 5.7, Schrödinger, LLC, New York, NY, 2011; Friesner et al., 2004). The compounds with the better XP Glide scores compared with the corresponding core-containing molecules were selected for further studies. The interactions of these compounds, into HIV-1 IN active site, were assessed by using ligand-interaction diagram implemented in Maestro suite and visualized by PyMOL (PyMOL Molecular Graphics System, Version 1.6-alpha, Schrödinger, LLC, New York, NY, 2013).

Molecular Properties Prediction

The molecules selected from *in silico* combinatorial screening were evaluated using a series of filtering criteria for drug-like properties. In this regard, QikProp application (QikProp, version 3.4, Schrödinger, LLC, New York, NY, 2011) implemented in the Maestro suite was used for ADME-T properties predictions (Rostami et al., 2015; Zaccagnini et al., 2017). This step was performed to select compounds from each library with appropriate physico-chemical properties using the range values recommended by QikProp. Especially, Lipinski's rules of five, membrane permeability, lipophilicity, cardiotoxicity, or potential interaction with *h*ERG K^+ channel were considered as important criteria and investigated for filtering (Lipinski et al., 2001). Default settings were employed for these calculations. The compounds derived from the above-mentioned calculation were evaluated for their potential capability to behave as "Pan Assay Interference Compounds" (PAINS). This calculation was performed by means of FAFDrugs4.0 (http://fafdrugs4.mti.univ-paris-diderot.fr/) (Lagorce et al., 2008, 2011; Vallone et al., 2018; Brindisi et al., 2019). PAINS compounds are chemical compounds that tend to display activity against a wide range of targets by nonspecific interactions or by altering the results of the biological tests. The compounds containing this kind of moieties, that are often present in PAINS compounds, could be false positive hits and in general should be removed from the designed series (Baell and Holloway, 2010).

Quantum Polarized Ligand Docking (QPLD)

In order to narrow down the number of the potential INIs and for improving the reliability of the protocol, the quantum polarized ligand docking (QPLD) calculations were performed for the resulting compounds with satisfactory physico-chemical properties. These compounds were docked into the modeled HIV-1 IN using QPLD protocol implemented in Schrödinger 2011 (Schrödinger Suite 2011: QM-Polarized Ligand Docking protocol; Glide, Version 5.7, Schrödinger, LLC, New York, NY, 2011; Jaguar, version 7.8, Schrödinger LLC, New York, NY, 2011; QSite version 5.7, Schrödinger LLC, New York, NY, 2011) (Irwin et al., 2012). This step was added to improve the accuracy of classical docking calculation. In fact, this procedure aims to improve the partial charges on ligand atoms by replacing them with charges derived from quantum mechanical calculations on the ligand in the field of the receptor (Paolino et al., 2018). Within the QPLD framework, the ligand atoms are treated at the Quantum Mechanical (QM) level, whereas the IN enzyme including the Mg^{2+} ions as Molecular Mechanical (MM) region are described using the OPLS force field parameters. In this way, the same grid file previously employed in the CombiGlide step was used. The best docked compounds obtained from the previous CombiGlide docking calculations followed by the evaluation of the physico-chemical properties, were selected in the ligand option. In the first step of the QPLD calculation, compounds were initially docked into the active site of IN enzyme. The initial docking calculations were carried out using Glide standard precision (SP) docking protocol, generating 5 poses per docked molecule. In the second step, the polarizable ligand charges induced by the protein field were calculated with QSite software which is coupled with Jaguar quantum mechanics engine (Jaguar, version 7.8, Schrödinger LLC, New York, NY, 2011). In this regard, the QM charge calculations of the best scoring poses for each ligand were carried out using density functional theory (DFT) method with the B3LYP/6-31G*/LACVP* basis set within the protein environment defined by the OPLS-2005 force field. Finally, the ligands with modified partial charges were redocked into the IN active site using Glide XP mode of docking considering 10 poses for each ligand. The potential inhibitors were selected based on the lower values of XP GlideScore and the key interactions between the ligand and HIV-1 IN active site.

Ligand Binding Energy Calculations

The best docked pose of ligands selected from previous QPLD calculations were subjected to a subsequent analysis with MM-GBSA process implemented in Prime software (Prime, version 3.0, Schrödinger LLC, New York, NY, 2011) (Brindisi et al., 2015). This method was employed to predict binding affinity and relative free-binding energy (ΔG_{bind}) between ligands and HIV-1 IN with further accuracy. The MM-GBSA approach combines MM energies with a continuum solvent generalized Born (GB) model for polar solvation and with a solvent-accessible surface area (SASA) for non-polar solvation term. In this way, the best ligand poses were subjected to energy minimization by local optimization feature in the Prime. During this process, the ligand strain energy was also considered. Ligand binding energies were calculated using the OPLS-2005 force field and generalized-Born/surface area continuum solvent model as previously reported by us (Brindisi et al., 2015, 2016; Maquiaveli et al., 2016; Brogi et al., 2017a; Vallone et al., 2018).

Molecular Dynamics Simulation

MD simulations studies were performed by means of Desmond 4.8 academic version, provided by D. E. Shaw Research ("DESRES"), using Maestro as graphical interface (Desmond Molecular Dynamics System, version 4.8, D. E. Shaw Research, New York, NY, 2016. Maestro-Desmond Interoperability Tools, version 4.8, Schrödinger, New York, NY, 2016). The calculation was performed using the Compute Unified Device Architecture (CUDA) API (Nickolls et al., 2008) employing two NVIDIA GPU (Brindisi et al., 2019). The calculation was performed on a system comprising 72 Intel Xeon E5-2695 v4@2.10 GHz processors and two NVIDIA GeForce 1070 GTX GPU. The complexes **HPCAR-28**/IN, **HPCAR-89**/IN, and **HPCAR-142**/IN were prepared by Protein Preparation Wizard protocol. The complexes were positioned into an orthorhombic box filled with water (TIP3P model). OPLS_2005 force field was used in MD calculation. The physiological concentration of monovalent ions (0.15 M) was simulated by adding Na^+ and Cl^- ions. Constant temperature (300 K) and pressure (1.01325 bar) were employed with NPT (constant number of particles, pressure, and temperature) as ensemble class. RESPA integrator (Humphreys et al., 1994) was used in order to integrate the equations of motion, with an inner time step of 2.0 fs for bonded interactions and nonbonded interactions within the short-range cut-off. Nose-Hoover thermostats (Hoover, 1985) were used to maintain the constant simulation temperature, and the Martyna-Tobias-Klein method (Martyna et al., 1994) was used to control the pressure. Long-range electrostatic interactions were evaluated adopting particle-mesh Ewald method (PME). The cut-off for van der Waals and short-range electrostatic interactions was set at 9.0 Å. The equilibration of the systems was performed with the default protocol provided in Desmond, which consists of a series of restrained minimizations and MD simulations used to slowly relax the system. By following this protocol, a single trajectory of 100 ns was obtained. We performed five independent MD runs for each mentioned complex with an aggregate simulation time of 0.5 μs to provide more reliable results. The trajectory files were investigated by simulation interaction diagram tools, simulation quality analysis and simulation event. The described applications were used to generate all plots regarding MD simulations analysis included in the manuscript as reported in the Results and Discussion section.

Chemistry

All reactants and reagents were purchased from Alfa Aesar and Sigma–Aldrich as "synthesis grade." Chemical reactions were monitored by analytical thin-layer chromatography (TLC) using several solvent systems with different polarity on Merck Silica Gel 60 F_{254} (0.040–0.063 mm) with detection by UV. Merck Silica Gel 60 (0.040–0.063 mm) was used for column chromatography. ^{1}H NMR and ^{13}C NMR spectra were recorded on a Varian 300 MHz (USA) spectrometer using the residual signal of the deuterated solvent as internal standard. Splitting patterns of signals are indicated as singlet (s), doublet (d), triplet (t), multiplet (m), broad (br), and doublet of doublet (dd). The values of chemical shifts (δ) are reported in ppm and coupling constants (*J*) in hertz (Hz). Electrospray ionization-mass spectrometric (ESI-MS) were acquired with an Agilent 1100 series LC/MSD spectrometer equipped with a multimode ion source and by using methanol as solvent.

3-(Benzyloxy)-6-Methyl-4-oxo-4H-Pyran-2-Carboxylic Acid, BPCA

This key carboxylic acid intermediate was prepared according to a previously reported procedure (Sirous et al., 2019).

Procedures for the Synthesis of Amine Fragments AM (1–3)

With the aim of synthesizing the representative hit candidates, three kinds of different amine fragments were applied for amide coupling with the carboxylic acid functional group of intermediate **BPCA**. The required amine compounds were synthesized using the following methods.

Procedure for the Preparation of (3-Fluoro-5-(pyridin-2-yl)phenyl)methanamine (AM-1)

3-Fluoro-5-(pyridin-2-yl)benzonitrile (3)

Starting from 2-bromopyridine **1**, a Suzuki coupling with (3-cyano-5-fluorophenyl)boronic acid **2** catalyzed by tetrakis (triphenylphosphine) palladium (0) provided the phenyl-pyridine derivative **3**. In this reaction tetrakis was generated *in situ* from palladium (II) acetate and triphenylphosphine (Tan et al., 2014). To a vigorously stirred yellowish solution of palladium (II) acetate (0.28 g, 1.26 mmol, 0.2 eq) and triphenylphosphine (1.66 g, 6.33 mmol, 1 eq) in 4 mL dioxane/water (3:1), a premixed solution of 2-bromopyridine **1** (1.00 g, 6.33 mmol, 1 eq) in dioxane (50 mL), and a solution of potassium carbonate (2.62 g, 19 mmol, 3 eq) in water (28 mL) was added. The reaction mixture was allowed to stir for 15 min under N_2. This step was followed by the drop-wise addition of a solution of (3-cyano-5-fluorophenyl)boronic acid **2** (1.15 g, 6.96 mmol, 1.1 eq) in 8 mL dioxane/water (4:1) via a syringe. After the final addition, the reaction mixture was refluxed at 100°C in an oil bath under N_2. The progression of the reaction was monitored by TLC. The reaction was completed after 24 h. After that, the reaction mixture was cooled down to the room temperature and subsequently filtered through a short Celite pad. The filter cake was washed with dichloromethane (25 mL). The filtrate solution was diluted with water and extracted with dichloromethane (3 × 100 mL). The organic layers were combined, dried over sodium sulfate, filtered and then evaporated *in vacuo* to yield a crude product. The crude product was purified by flash chromatography on silica gel, eluting with 9:1 petroleum ether: ethyl acetate, to give **3** as a white solid (Tan et al., 2014). Yield: 64%, ^{1}H NMR (300 MHz, $CDCl_3$) δ (ppm): 8.75 (1H, d, *J* = 6.25 Hz, C6′-H), 8.42 (1H, d, *J* = 6.00 Hz, C4-H), 7.80 (2H, s, C6-H, and C2-H), 7.62–7.72 (1H, m, C4′-H), 7.22–7.40 (2H, m, C3′-H and C5′-H).

(3-Fluoro-5-(pyridin-2-yl)phenyl)methanamine (AM-1)

Dry $NiCl_2$ was prepared from hydrated $NiCl_2$. In this way, $NiCl_2 \bullet 6H_2O$ was used after drying in an oven at 250°C until its color turned from green to golden yellow. Then, it was powdered and stored in a vacuum desiccator for reaction. In a typical procedure (Caddick et al., 2003), nitrile compound **3** (0.2 g, 1.00 mmol, 1 eq) and anhydrous nickel (II) chloride (0.13 g, 1 mmol, 1 eq) were dissolved in dry ethanol (8 mL). Then, sodium borohydride (0.11 g, 3 mmol, 3 eq) was cautiously added in three portions to the vigorously stirred reaction mixture at room temperature. A black precipitate appeared during the addition of $NaBH_4$. When the addition of $NaBH_4$ was completed, stirring was continued and the progress of the reaction was monitored by TLC. After the complete disappearance of the nitrile compound in almost 15 min, the reaction mixture was filtered through a Celite pad. The filtered nickel boride precipitate was washed with ethanol (10 mL). The filtrate was collected, diluted with water (30 mL), and extracted with ethyl acetate (3 × 30 mL). The organic phase was combined, dried over sodium sulfate, filtered and concentrated on a rotary vacuum evaporator to afford a crude product. The crude product was purified by flash chromatography on silica gel, eluting with 4:1 chloroform:methanol to give the corresponding amine compound **AM-1** as a white solid (Caddick et al., 2003). Yield: 65%, ^{1}H NMR (300 MHz, DMSO-d_6) δ (ppm): 8.66 (2H, s, NH_2), 8.12 (1H, d, *J* = 6Hz, C6′-H), 7.69–7.98 (3H, m, Ar), 7.59–7.70 (1H, br, C4′-H), 7.20–7.40 (2H, m, C3′-H and C5′-H), 4.76 (2H, s, CH_2NH_2).

Procedure for the Preparation of (3-(2-methyl-1H-imidazol-4-yl)phenyl)methanamine (AM-2)

4,5-Dibromo-2-methyl-1H-imidazole (5)

2-Methyl-1*H*-imidazole **4** (10 g, 0.122 mol) was dissolved in 300 mL chloroform and cooled to the temperature between 0 and −5°C using salty ice bath. 48.66 g (15.60 mL, 0.305 mol) bromine was added to the reaction mixture drop-wise via a dropping funnel over 20 min. The reaction mixture was allowed to stir at room temperature. The progression of the reaction was monitored by TLC. The reaction was completed after 20 h. During this time, the reaction product precipitated as an orange solid. In the next step, the reaction mixture was cooled to 0°C in a salty ice bath and 250 mL of NaOH (2 N) was added drop-wise to the reaction mixture in order to quench unreacted bromine. The orange precipitate was filtered off and washed with water, dried *in vacuo* at 40°C for 12 h to give the yellow solid of **5** (Alonso-Alija et al., 2003). Yield: 43%, ^{1}H NMR (300 MHz, DMSO-d_6) δ (ppm): 8.68 (1H, brs, NH), 2.39 (3H, s, CH_3).

4-Bromo-2-methyl-1H-imidazole (6)

4,5-Dibromo-2-methyl-1*H*-imidazole **5** (5.0 g, 20.84 mmol) was suspended with sodium sulfite (80 g, 635 mmol) in 200 mL water and 100 mL ethanol. The suspension was refluxed at 100°C in an oil bath. The progression of the reaction was monitored by TLC. The reaction was completed after 48 h and the reaction mixture was extracted with ethyl acetate (3 × 100 mL). The organic phases were collected, dried over sodium sulfate, filtered and then evaporated *in vacuo* to yield a white solid as pure product **6** (Alonso-Alija et al., 2003). Yield: 75%, ^{1}H NMR (300 MHz, DMSO-d_6) δ (ppm): 12.00 (1H, brs, NH), 7.05 (1H, d, J = 1.80 Hz, C5-H), 2.21 (3H, s, CH_3).

3-(2-Methyl-1H-imidazol-4-yl)benzonitrile (8)

Nitrile compound **8** was synthesized according to same Suzuki procedure described for the preparation of compound **3** (Tan et al., 2014). Briefly, starting from a solution of palladium (II) acetate (0.42 g, 1.86 mmol, 0.2 eq) and triphenylphosphine (2.44 g, 9.32 mmol, 1 eq) in 6 mL dioxane/water (5:1), a solution of bromo-imidazole derivative **6** (1.5 g, 9.32 mmol, 1 eq) in dioxane (70 mL), a solution of potassium carbonate (3.87 g, 28 mmol, 3 eq) in water (40 mL) and a solution of (3-cyanophenyl) boronic acid **7** (1.51 g, 10.252 mmol, 1.1 eq) in 10 mL dioxane/water (5:1) were used in Sequence. Crude product was purified by flash chromatography on silica gel using 3:1 petroleum ether: ethyl acetate as the eluent to yield **8** as a white solid (Tan et al., 2014). Yield: 70%, ^{1}H NMR (300 MHz, DMSO-d_6) δ (ppm): 11.95 (1H, brs, NH), 8.10 (1H, s, C2′-H), 8.00 (1H, d, J = 9.40 Hz, C6′-H), 7.45–7.68 (3H, m, C5-H, C4′-H, C5′-H), 2.20 (3H, s, CH_3). ESI-MS (+) m/z (%): 183.9 $[M+H]^+$ (100).

(3-(2-Methyl-1H-imidazol-4-yl)phenyl)methanamine (AM-2)

Amine compound **AM-2** was synthesized according to the same procedure described for reduction of nitrile **3** to the corresponding primary amine **AM-1** (Caddick et al., 2003). In this way, starting from nitrile compound **8** (0.5 g, 2.73 mmol, 1 eq), 0.353 gr (2.73 mmol, 1 eq) of anhydrous nickel (II) chloride, and 0.31 g (8.19 mmol, 3 eq) sodium borohydride were used. The purification was performed via silica flash column chromatography using 4:1 chloroform: methanol as the eluent to yield the corresponding amine product **AM-2** as a white solid (Caddick et al., 2003). Yield: 61%, ^{1}H NMR (300 MHz, DMSO-d_6) δ (ppm): 11.72 (1H, brs, NH), 7.70–8.50 (5H, m, C5-H, C2′-H, C4′-H, C5′-H and C6′-H), 3.70 (2H, s, CH_2NH_2), 2.25 (3H, s, CH_3).

Procedure for the Preparation of (3-(1H-pyrrol-1-yl)phenyl)methanamine (AM-3)

3-(1H-Pyrrol-1-yl)benzonitrile (11)

Phenylpyrrole **11** was synthesized through a Clauson–Kaas reaction with 3-aminobenzonitrile **9** (Chatzopoulou et al., 2013). To a solution of 3-aminobenzonitrile **9** (1.00 g, 8.46 mmol, 1 eq) in 15.0 mL of 1,4-dioxane, 2,5-dimethoxytetrahydrofuran **10** (1.23 g, 9.306 mmol, 1.1 eq) dissolved in 7.0 mL of 1,4-dioxane were added. The reaction mixture was refluxed for 5 min, and then 3 mL of hydrochloric acid 5 N was added drop-wise. The reaction mixture was refluxed for 25 min until the reaction was completed. After cooling to room temperature, water was added to the reaction mixture. The reaction mixture was extracted with dichloromethane (3 × 50 mL). The organic layer was dried over anhydrous sodium sulfate, filtered, and concentrated *in vacuo*. Flash chromatography on silica gel, eluting with 4:1 petroleum ether: ethyl acetate, afforded compound **11** as an amorphous white solid (Chatzopoulou et al., 2013). Yield: 82%, ^{1}H NMR (300 MHz, $CDCl_3$) δ (ppm): 7.48–7.52 (4H, m, Ar), 7.08 (2H, t, J = 3.00 Hz, C2′-H, C5′-H), 6.79 (2H, t, J = 3.00 Hz, C3′-H, C4′-H).

(3-(1H-Pyrrol-1-yl)phenyl)methanamine (AM-3)

Amine compound **AM-3** was synthesized according to the same procedure described for the reduction of nitrile **3** to the corresponding primary amine **AM-1** (Caddick et al., 2003). In this way, starting from nitrile **11** (0.5 g, 2.97 mmol, 1 eq), 0.385 g (2.97 mmol, 1 eq) of anhydrous nickel (II) chloride, and 0.337 g (8.91 mmol, 3 eq) sodium borohydride were used. The purification was performed via silica column chromatography using 4:1 chloroform: methanol as the eluent to yield the corresponding amine **AM-3** as a white solid (Caddick et al., 2003). Yield: 75%, ^{1}H NMR (300 MHz, DMSO-d_6) δ (ppm): 7.52 (1H, s, C_2-H), 7.27–7.42 (4H, m, 3H: C3-H, C4-H and C5-H; 1H: C2′-H), 7.18 (1H, d, J = 4.40 Hz, C5′-H), 6.24 (2H, s, C3′-H, C4′-H), 3.77 (2H, s, CH_2NH_2).

General Procedure for the Synthesis of 3-(benzyloxy)-6-methyl-N-(Substituted benzyl)-4-oxo-4H-pyran-2-carboxamide Derivatives, BPCAR

To a vigorously stirred suspension of intermediate **BPCA** (100 mg, 0.38 mmol, 1 eq) in dry dichloromethane (8 mL), 1-ethyl-3-(3-dimethylaminopropyl) carbodiimide hydrochloride (EDCI) (72.5 mg, 0.38 mmol, 1 eq) was added and the mixture was stirred for 30 min under N_2 to provide a clear yellow solution. Then, *N*-hydroxysuccinimide (NHS) (43.7 mg, 0.38 mmol, 1 eq) was added to the stirring solution and the mixture was allowed to stir for 3 h under N_2 to produce the activated ester **12** as reported in the Chemistry details in the Result and Discussion section. After this step and complete consumption of the starting material **BPCA**, desired prepared amine fragment (1.5 eq) was added to the reaction mixture. The reaction was stirred at room temperature for 3 days under N_2. During this time, the progression of the reaction was monitored by TLC. Then, the reaction mixture was poured into a separatory funnel and the dichloromethane layer was washed with water (2 × 20 mL). The organic phase was collected, dried over anhydrous sodium sulfate, filtered, and concentrated *in vacuo* to yield a crude solid. The obtained solid was purified via silica flash column chromatography to give the desired carboxamide product as a pure substance (Sheehan et al., 1965; Sirous et al., 2019).

3-(Benzyloxy)-N-(3-fluoro-5-(pyridin-2-yl)benzyl)-6-methyl-4-oxo-4H-pyran-2-carboxamide (BPCAR-28)

Carboxamide derivative **BPCAR-28** was prepared according to the general procedure, using amine compound **AM-1** (115 mg, 0.57 mmol, 1.5 eq). The purification of the crude product using silica flash column chromatography, eluting with 1:1 petroleum ether: ethyl acetate solution, afforded the carboxamide product

BPCAR-28 as a white solid. Yield: 44%, ^{1}H NMR (300 MHz, $CDCl_3$) δ (ppm): 8.74 (1H, d, J = 5.5 Hz, C6′-H), 8.18(1H, brs, $NHCH_2$), 7.88 (1H, d, J = 5.5 Hz, Ar: C4-H), 7.76 (2H, s, Ar: C2-H and C6-H), 7.18–7.40 (6H, m, 5H: $OCH_2C_6H_5$; 1H: C4′-H), 7.02–7.16 (2H, m, C3′-H and C5′-H), 6.24 (1H, s, C5-H), 5.36 (2H, s, OCH_2-C_6H_5), 4.44 (2H, d, J = 8.00 Hz, $NHCH_2$-C_6H_4), 2.38 (3H, s, 6-CH_3).

3-(Benzyloxy)-6-methyl-N-(3-(2-methyl-1H-imidazol-4-yl)benzyl)-4-oxo-4H-pyran-2-carboxamide (BPCAR-89)

Carboxamide derivative **BPCAR-89** was prepared according to the general procedure, using amine compound **AM-2** (0.107 g, 0.57 mmol, 1.5 eq). The purification of the crude product using silica flash column chromatography, eluting with 1:1 petroleum ether: ethyl acetate solution, afforded the carboxamide product **BPCAR-89** as a white solid. Yield: 38%, ^{1}H NMR (300 MHz, Acetone-d_6) δ (ppm): 8.41 (1H, brs, $NHCH_2$), 7.82 (1H, s, C2′-H), 7.70 (1H, d, J = 12.00 Hz, C4′-H),7.23–7.40 (7H, m, 5H:OCH_2-C_6H_5; 2H: C5′-H and C6′-H), 7.18 (1H, d, J = 12.00 Hz, C5″-H), 6.28 (1H, s, C5-H), 5.30 (2H, s, OCH_2-C_6H_5), 4.50 (2H, d, J = 6.00 Hz, $NHCH_2$-C_6H_4), 2.40 (3H, s, CH_3), 2.24 (3H, s, CH_3).

N-(3-(1H-Pyrrol-1-yl)benzyl)-3-(benzyloxy)-6-methyl-4-oxo-4H-pyran-2-carboxamide (BPCAR-142)

Carboxamide derivative **BPCAR-142** was prepared according to the general procedure, using amine compound **AM-3** (98.2 mg, 0.57 mmol, 1.5 eq). The purification of the crude product using silica flash column chromatography, eluting with 1:1 petroleum ether: ethyl acetate solution, afforded the carboxamide product **BPCAR-142** as a white solid. Yield: 48%, ^{1}H NMR (300 MHz, $CDCl_3$) δ (ppm): 8.12 (1H, t, J = 8.00 Hz, $NHCH_2$), 7.16–7.38 (8H, m, 5H: $OCH_2C_6H_5$; 3H: C2′-H, C4′-H and C5′-H), 7.01–7.08 (3H, m, 2H: C2″-H, C5″-H; 1H: C6′-H), 6.36 (2H, t, J = 3.00 Hz, C3″-H, C4″-H), 6.25 (1H, S, C5-H), 5.32 (2H, s, $OCH_2C_6H_5$), 4.46 (2H, d, J = 8.30 Hz, $NHCH_2C_6H_4$), 2.35 (3H, s, 6-CH_3).

General Procedure for the Synthesis of 3-hydroxy-6-methyl-N-(substituted benzyl)-4-oxo-4H-pyran-2-carboxamide derivatives, HPCAR

40 mg of each of the desired BPCAR derivatives was dissolved in dry dichloromethane (3 mL) and flushed with nitrogen. Then, the reaction mixture was cooled to the temperature between 0 and −5°C in salty ice bath and the 1 M solution of boron tribromide in dichloromethane (3 eq) was slowly added drop-wise via a syringe. The reaction mixture was allowed to stir at room temperature and the reaction progress was monitored by TLC. The reaction was completed after almost 3 h. The excess BBr_3 was eliminated at the end of the reaction by the addition of cold methanol (5 mL) to the reaction mixture at 0°C and left to stir for half an hour. The mixture was concentrated to dryness in vacuum and the residue was dissolved several times in methanol and evaporated. This residue was purified by flash column chromatography to afford the final pure product (Ma and Hider, 2015; Sirous et al., 2019).

N-(3-Fluoro-5-(pyridin-2-yl)benzyl)-3-hydroxy-6-methyl-4-oxo-4H-pyran-2-carboxamide (HPCAR-28)

Compound **HPCAR-28** was prepared according to the general debenzylation procedure, starting from compound **BPCAR-28** (40 mg, 0.09 mmol, 1 eq) and 1 M solution of boron tribromide in CH_2Cl_2 (46 μL, 0.27 mmol, 3 eq). Purification using flash column chromatography (eluent: dichloromethane: methanol; 80:20 v/v) afforded a white solid as final product **HPCAR-28**. Yield: 71%, ^{1}H NMR (300 MHz, DMSO-d_6) δ (ppm): 8.60 (1H, d, J = 5.5 Hz, C6′-H), 8.12 (1H, brs, $NHCH_2$), 7.74 (1H, d, J = 5.5 Hz, Ar: C4-H), 7.62 (2H, s, Ar: C2-H and C6-H), 7.12–7.34 (1H, br, C4′-H), 7.00–7.13 (2H, m, C3′-H and C5′-H), 6.22 (1H, s, C5-H), 4.34 (2H, d, J = 8.00 Hz, $NHCH_2$-C_6H_4), 2.34 (3H, s, 6-CH_3). ^{13}C NMR (DMSO-d6) δ (ppm): 173.55 (4-C=O), 164.84 (CONH), 162.72 (C-3), 162.48 (Ar: $C_{3'}$-F, d, $^{1}J_{C-F}$: 220.4 Hz), 152.15 (Ar), 147.39 (Ar), 144.05 (C-2), 143.86 (Ar), 136.14 (C-6), 132.32 (Ar), 132.12 (Ar), 124.00 (Ar), 123.09 (Ar), 122.28 (Ar), 116.60 (Ar), 114.11 (Ar), 108.63 (C-5), 42.04 ($NHCH_2$), 19.31 (6-CH_3). ESI-MS (+) m/z (%): 355.3 $[M+H]^+$ (100).

3-Hydroxy-6-methyl-N-(3-(2-methyl-1H-imidazol-4-yl)benzyl)-4-oxo-4H-pyran-2 carboxamide (HPCAR-89)

Compound **HPCAR-89** was prepared according to the general procedure described above, starting from compound **BPCAR-89** (40 mg, 0.09 mmol, 1 eq) and 1 M solution of boron tribromide in CH_2Cl_2 (46 μL, 0.27 mmol, 3 eq). Purification using flash column chromatography (eluent: dichloromethane: methanol; 80:20 v/v) afforded a white solid as final product **HPCAR-89**. Yield: 82%, ^{1}H NMR (300 MHz, DMSO-d_6) δ (ppm): 11.80 (1H, brs, NH of imidazole ring), 10.63 (1H, brs, $NHCH_2$),7.60 (1H, s, C2′-H), 7.58 (1H, d, J = 12.00 Hz, C4′-H), 7.38 (1H, s, C5"-H), 7.20 (1H, t, J = 12.00 Hz, C5′-H), 7.05 (1H, d, J = 12.00 Hz, C6′-H), 6.20 (1H, s, C5-H), 4.40 (2H, d, J = 6.00 Hz, $NHCH_2$-C_6H_4), 2.24 (6H, s, CH_3-a and CH_3-b). ^{13}C NMR (DMSO-d6) δ (ppm): 173.53 (4-C=O), 164.78 (CONH), 162.72 (C-3), 156.60 ($C_3H_4N_2$: C2), 151.02 ($C_3H_4N_2$: C5), 147.44 (C-2), 142.54 (Ar), 136.14 (C-6), 134.64 (Ar), 129.47 (Ar), 128.30 (Ar), 125.52 (Ar), 123.14 ($C_3H_4N_2$: C4), 117.21 (Ar), 112.65 (C-5), 41.53 ($NHCH_2$), 19.30 (6-CH_3), 16.60 (CH_3-$C_3H_4N_2$). ESI-MS (+) m/z (%): 340.1 $[M+H]^+$ (100).

N-(3-(1H-Pyrrol-1-yl)benzyl)-3-hydroxy-6-methyl-4-oxo-4H-pyran-2-carboxamide (HPCAR-142)

Compound **HPCAR-142** was prepared according to the general procedure, starting from compound **BPCAR-142** (40 mg, 0.096 mmol, 1 eq) and 1 M solution of boron tribromide in CH_2Cl_2 (49 μL, 0.288 mmol, 3 eq). Purification using flash column chromatography (eluent: dichloromethane: methanol; 80:20 v/v) afforded a white solid as final product **HPCAR-142**. Yield: 86%, ^{1}H NMR (300 MHz, DMSO-d_6) δ (ppm): 10.30 (1H, brs,

$NHCH_2$), 7.2–7.56 (4H, m, C2′-H, C4′-H, C5′-H, C6′-H), 7.0–7.20 (2H, m, C2″-H, C5″-H), 6.23 (2H, d, $J = 7.50$ Hz, C3″-H, C4″-H), 6.18 (1H, s, C5-H), 4.50 (2H, d, $J = 7.00$ Hz, $NHCH_2$), 2.30 (3H, s, 6-CH_3). ^{13}C NMR (DMSO-d6) δ (ppm): 173.55 (4-C=O), 164.79 (CONH), 162.72 (C-3), 147.51 (C-2), 142.52 (Ar), 136.19 (C-6), 135.31 (Ar), 128.90 (Ar), 124.37 (Ar), 120.05 (C_4H_4N: C2, C5), 119.30 (Ar), 117.43 (Ar), 112.67 (C-5), 108.77 (C_4H_4N: C3, C4), 41.96 ($NHCH_2$), 20.65 (6-CH_3). ESI-MS (+) m/z (%): 324.9 $[M+H]^+$ (30), 346.7 $[M+Na]^+$ (100).

Biological Evaluation

Integrase Assays

The enzymatic integration reactions were carried out as previously described with minor modifications (Debyser et al., 2001; Christ et al., 2011). To determine the susceptibility of the HIV-1 IN enzyme to different compounds, an enzyme-linked immunosorbent assay (ELISA) adapted from Hwang et al. was used (Hwang et al., 2000). The overall integration assay uses an oligonucleotide substrate for which one oligonucleotide (5′-ACTGCTAGAGATTTTCCACACTGACTAAAAGGGTC-3′) is labeled with biotin at the 3′ end and the other oligonucleotide (5′-GACCCTTTTAGTCAGTGTGGAAAATCTCTAGCAGT-3′) is labeled with digoxigenin at the 5′ end. For the strand transfer assay, a pre-cleaved oligonucleotide substrate (the second oligonucleotide lacks GT [underlined] at the 3′ end) was used. The IN enzyme was diluted in 750 mM NaCl, 10 mM Tris (pH: 7.6), 10% glycerol, and 1 mM β-mercaptoethanol. To perform the reaction, 4 μL of diluted IN (corresponding to a concentration of 1.6 μM) and 4 μL of annealed oligonucleotides (7 nM) were added in a final reaction volume of 40 μL containing 10 mM $MgCl_2$, 5 mM dithiothreitol, 20 mM HEPES (pH 7.5), 5% polyethylene glycol, and 15% dimethyl sulfoxide. As such, the final concentration of IN in this assay was 160 nM. The reaction was carried out for 1 h at 37°C. Reaction products were denatured with 30 mM NaOH and detected by ELISA on avidin-coated plates. For determining the effect of compounds on the 3′-processing activity a classical cleavage assay with detection of products by denaturing gel electrophoresis was performed as described previously (Debyser et al., 2001; Christ et al., 2011). Briefly, 0.2 pmol of the radioactive labeled oligonucleotide substrate (INT1, ^{32}P-5′ TGTGGAAAATCTCTAGCAGT3′; INT2, 5′ACTGCTAGAGATTTTCCACA 3′) and 10 nmol IN in a final volume of 10 μL was incubated for 1 h at 37°C. The final reaction mixture contained 20 mM HEPES (pH 7.5), 5 mM dithiothreitol (DTT), 10 mM $MgCl_2$, 0.5% (v/v) polyethylene glycol 8000, 15% DMSO. IN was diluted previously in 750 mM NaCl, 10 mM Tris (pH 7.6), 10% glycerol and 1 mM β-mercaptoethanol. The reactions were stopped by the addition of formamide loading buffer (95% formamide, 0.1% xylene cyanol, 0.1% xylene cyanol, 0.1% bromophenol blue, and 0.1% sodium dodecyl sulfate). Samples were loaded on a 15% denaturing polyacrylamide/ureum gel. The extent of 3′-processing or DNA strand transfer was based on measuring the respective amounts of −2 bands or strand transfer products relative to the intensity of the total radioactivity present in the lane. These data were determined using the OptiQuant Acquisition and Analysis software (Perkin Elmer Corporate, Fremont, CA).

In vitro Anti-HIV and Drug Susceptibility Assays

The inhibitory effect of antiviral drugs on the HIV-induced cytopathic effect (CPE) in human lymphocyte MT-4 cell culture was determined by the MT-4/MTT-assay (Pauwels et al., 1988). This assay is based on the reduction of the yellow colored 3-(4,5-dimethylthiazol-2-yl)-2,5-diphenyltetrazolium bromide (MTT) by mitochondrial dehydrogenase of metabolically active cells to a blue formazan derivative, which can be measured spectrophotometrically. The 50% cell culture infective dose of the HIV strains was determined by titration of the virus stock using MT-4 cells. For the drug susceptibility assays, MT-4 cells were infected with 100–300 50% cell culture infective doses of the HIV strains in the presence of 5-fold serial dilutions of the antiviral drugs. The concentration of the compound achieving 50% protection against the CPE of HIV, which is defined as the 50% effective concentration (EC_{50}), was determined. In parallel, the concentration of the compound destroying 50% of the MT-4 cells, which is defined as the 50% cytotoxic concentration (CC_{50}), was determined as well.

RESULTS AND DISCUSSION

The main purpose of the present study is to identify novel chemical entities derived from HPCARs scaffold as new and useful hit compounds as HIV-1 INIs. Accordingly, an integrated computational protocol based on combinatorial library design protocol, physico-chemical properties prediction, molecular docking calculations, and MD simulation was developed in a stepwise filtering approach (**Figure 3**). The identified hit compounds were synthesized and submitted to biological evaluation in order to validate the proposed *in silico* strategy.

Generation of Combinatorial Hits Using CombiGlide

As the first step of the developed *in silico* protocol, HPCAR derivatives with $n = 1$ or 2 (**Figures 2, 3**) were submitted to CombiGlide software as a combinatorial docking tool. In each case, combinatorial virtual screening was applied in order to replace the aromatic groups of the original core, applying side-chain hopping method. The prepared sets of amine fragments, available in the library of reagents, were used to replace the original substituents at each defined attachment point (**Figure 3**). Variation in aromatic group resulted in the generation of a combinatorial library of more than 37,000 hit compounds for each studied core-containing molecule. The compounds from each new combinatorial library were sorted by GlideScore values. Only derivatives with score values lower than −6.0 kcal/mol were considered. The selected molecules were further analyzed by visual inspection to find compounds with an appropriate binding mode according to the key interactions found for HIV-1 INIs. From this first filter, 1,803 combinatorial compounds were chosen for the next step.

Molecular Properties Prediction

One of the major goals in drug discovery is the identification of innovative small molecular scaffolds exhibiting high efficacy and selectivity against the desired target along with a satisfactory ADME-T profile. Thus, the second filter in the screening workflow consisted in the prediction of the ADME-T properties and drug-like behavior of the above-mentioned 1,803 compounds using QikProp software. This step was performed to select molecules possessing satisfactory predicted membrane permeability (QPPCaco-2 and QPPMDCK models > 100), appropriate lipophilicity (QPlogP) including capability to cross the blood brain barrier and drug-likeness properties in accordance with Lipinski's rule of five. The potential interaction with *h*ERG K^+ channel (QPlog-HERG) was another key parameter considered in this step of filtering. 146 out of 1,803 compounds were predicted to have pharmacokinetic properties in the appropriate range. Moreover, the resulting compounds were filtered for behaving as PAINS using FAF-Drugs4 tool. Among 146 compounds, only two molecules contain sub-structural features that marked them as "frequent hitters" in high throughput screens. Finally, 144 candidates passed this step of screening and were chosen for the next step. A list of these top candidates with improved ADMET properties was provided in the **Table S1**.

Quantum Polarized Ligand Docking Simulation

The resulting 144 potential hit molecules were further computationally analyzed using QPLD calculations for guaranteeing a better prediction of their binding mode into HIV-1 IN active site. This docking protocol could provide a more accurate treatment of electronic interactions especially within metalloproteins active site, leading to the improvement of the accuracy of the docking results (Cho et al., 2005; Illingworth et al., 2008; Paolino et al., 2018). In this step, the potential inhibitors were selected based on their lower XP GlideScore and on the ability to engage in critical interactions in the HIV-1 IN active site. At the end, a total of 76 hit candidates with the favorable XP GlideScore values were identified (**Table S2**). As reported in **Table S2**, the 76 selected hit molecules showed XP GlideScore values < −6 kcal/mol (the values of the cut-off filters for the *in silico* studies were chosen taking into consideration the values found for the reference compounds **RLT**, **EVG**, and **DTG**). The detailed analysis of QPLD results indicated that these compounds adopt a reasonable interfacial binding mode similar to that found for the approved HIV-1 INIs, namely **RLT**, **EVG**, and **DTG** (Rostami et al., 2015; Sirous et al., 2015, 2019). Consistent with docking models of HP derivatives previously reported (Sirous et al., 2019), the same interaction pattern was found for the best docked pose of all the selected hit molecules within HIV-1 IN active site. In this context, combinatorial hits perfectly occupied the DNA/IN interface with donor oxygen triad of MBG interacting with both Mg^{2+} ions through a bis-bidentate mode of chelation. This orientation enables the aromatic side chain of the molecule to sit in a hydrophobic pocket close to the active site generated by the displacement of the terminal adenosine on the 3′-end of the viral DNA. As a result, the terminal aromatic moiety of ligands participates in π-π stacking interactions with the viral DNA nucleosides, DC_{16} and DG_4, and favorable hydrophobic contacts with the amino acids residues of the catalytic loop, Pro_{145}, Gln_{146}, and Gly_{149}. Particularly, Pro_{145} and Gln_{146} are directly involved in separation of the viral DNA strands upon the ST reaction. This can reduce the catalytic loop mobility and thus physically hamper the binding of the host DNA (Dirac and Kjems, 2001; Dolan et al., 2009). In some cases, further stabilization of the ligand in the active site was mediated by H-bonds with Asn_{117}, Pro_{145}, Gln_{146}, and Glu_{152} as well as nucleoside residues DG_4, DC_{16}, and DA_{17}. For example, **HPCAR-40** was involved in hydrogen bond interactions with Asn_{117} and Glu_{152} and **HPCAR-144** formed hydrogen bonds with Gln_{146} and Glu_{152}. Furthermore, in most of the docking models, the position of 4-pyran core of ligands was suitably located to establish strong hydrophobic interactions such as a π-π stacking with 3′-deoxyadenosine A_{17} (**Table S2**).

Prioritization of Hit Compounds Based on Relative Ligand Binding Energy

Although it is well established that docking calculations are highly successful in offering reliable ligand poses within the protein binding site, they often fail to rank compounds with respect to their binding affinities. This poor correlation may be due to severe approximations and simplifications employed by scoring functions of various docking tools. The scoring functions like GlideScore do not consider some essential thermodynamics factors in the ligand binding energy calculations such as protein and ligand solvation energy terms (Pearlman and Charifson, 2001; Taylor et al., 2002). Thus in the subsequent step of our computational workflow, relative ligand binding energy calculations using MM-GBSA rescoring method were carried out on the best docked pose of the ligands obtained from the previously described docking simulation. This approach may offer more reliable measuring criteria to prioritize screened HIV-1 INIs hits for chemical synthesis and biological evaluations as HIV-1 INIs (Huang et al., 2006). Rescoring using MM-GBSA leads to minor changes of the ligand conformations within receptor site. These changes result from minimization of the ligand in receptor's environment and consequent stabilization of receptor-ligand complex. The estimated binding energy values < −25 kcal/mol were considered to retrieve final set of combinatorial hits. Final ranking of the ligands in this step of screening workflow resulted in the identification of 40 top hit compounds as novel HIV-1 INIs, possessing relevant binding affinities for HIV-1 IN active site. The structures of these compounds are shown in **Table 2**. The calculated ΔG_{bind} of the final selected hits along with their contributions to total binding energy from various energy components are provided in **Table S3**.

Since the screened hit molecules share the same MBG, the main differences in ligand binding energies values between these inhibitors could be directly attributed to the hydrophobic aromatic moieties characterized by significant chemical diversity, including bicyclic and tricyclic structures. Inspection of energy

TABLE 2 | Chemical structures of 40 top combinatorial hits identified at the end of computational screening workflow applied in the present study.

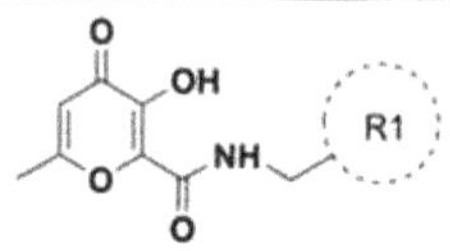

Cmpd	R_1	Cmpd	R_1	Cmpd	R_1
HPCAR-1	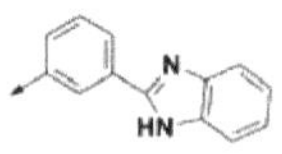	**HPCAR-33**	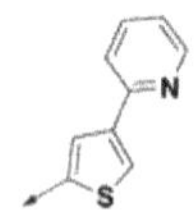	**HPCAR-89**	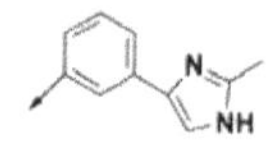
HPCAR-2	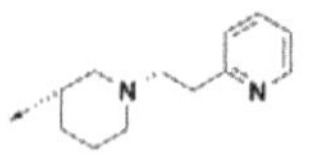	**HPCAR-35**	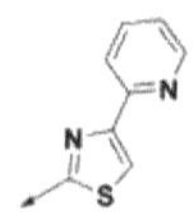	**HPCAR-90**	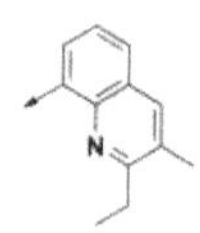
HPCAR-6	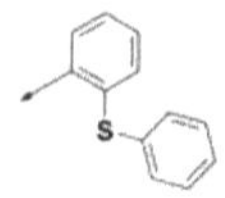	**HPCAR-37**	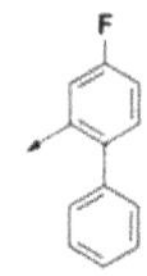	**HPCAR-91**	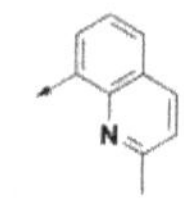
HPCAR-7	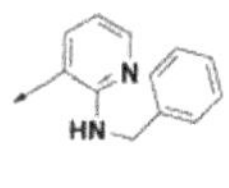	**HPCAR-41**	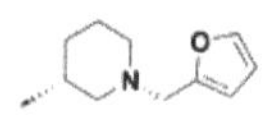	**HPCAR-92**	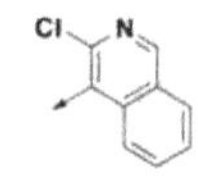
HPCAR-8	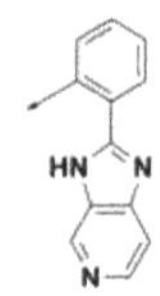	**HPCAR-44**	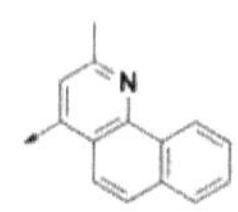	**HPCAR-108**	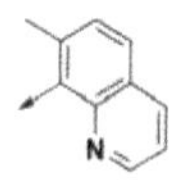
HPCAR-14	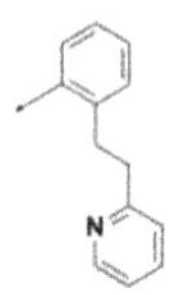	**HPCAR-45**	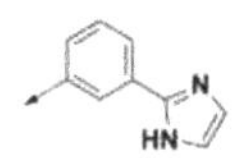	**HPCAR-111**	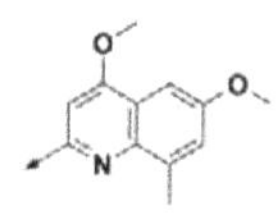
HPCAR-15	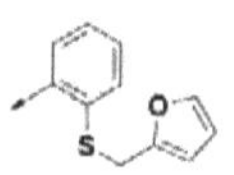	**HPCAR-46**	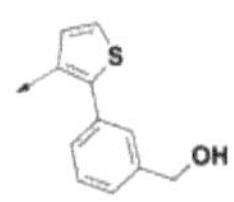	**HPCAR-114**	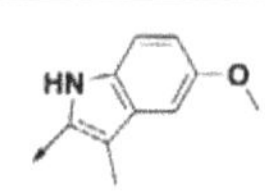
HPCAR-22	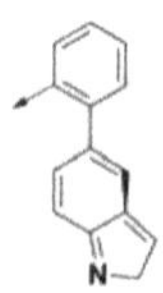	**HPCAR-52**	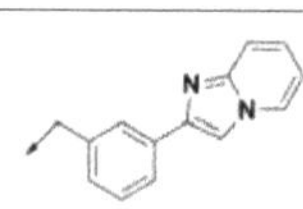	**HPCAR-123**	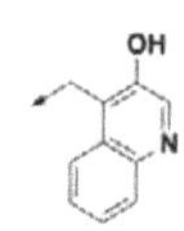
HPCAR-23	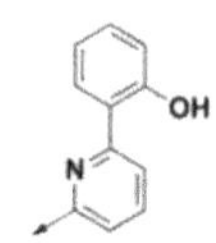	**HPCAR-54**	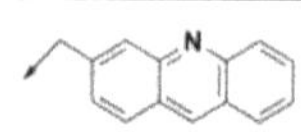	**HPCAR-126**	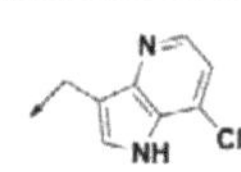
HPCAR-25	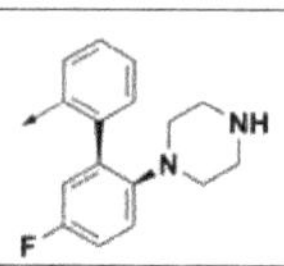	**HPCAR-55**	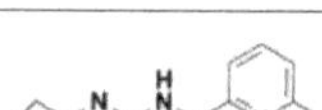	**HPCAR-130**	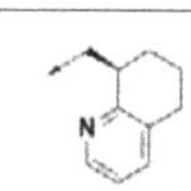

(Continued)

TABLE 2 | Continued

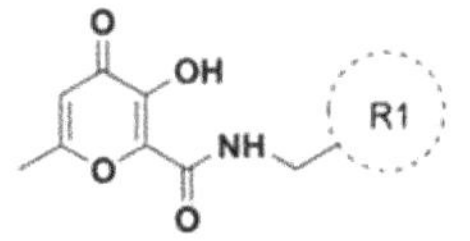

Cmpd	R_1	Cmpd	R_1	Cmpd	R_1
HPCAR-26	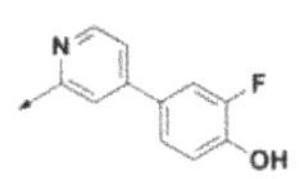	**HPCAR-56**	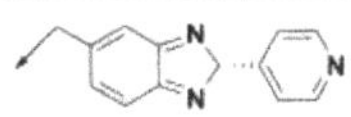	**HPCAR-140**	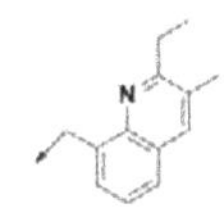
HPCAR-28	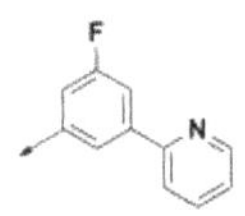	**HPCAR-66**	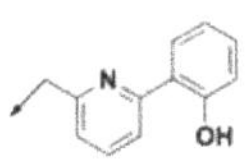	**HPCAR-142**	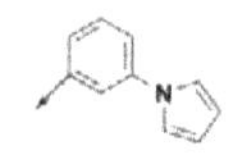
HPCAR-29	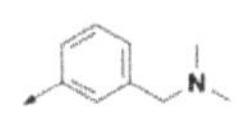	**HPCAR-69**	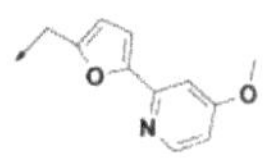	**HPCAR-144**	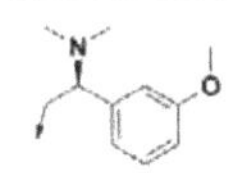
HPCAR-30	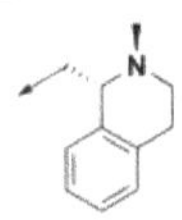				

*Three hit compounds (**HPCAR-28, HPCAR-89** and **HPCAR-142**) were selected from this final set for synthesis and biological assessment.*

terms in **Table S3** revealed that all selected ligands showed high values of van der Waals interaction energy ($\Delta G_{bindVdW}$ values), contributing to the ligand binding energy which emphasizes critical importance of hydrophobic interactions in the stability of the ligand-protein complexes.

Validation of Computational Screening Workflow

In order to validate the developed computational protocol, three compounds (**HPCAR-28**, **HPCAR-89**, and **HPCAR-142** in **Table 2**) from final set of 40 hit candidates were selected and synthesized. The selection was performed considering the favorable computational scores, the binding modes, the structural differences and synthetic accessibility. The best docked poses along with the detailed interaction into the HIV-1 IN active site of these representative compounds are depicted in **Figure 4**.

The compounds were able to establish a bis-bidentate chelation of the Mg^{2+} ions, strong hydrophobic interactions (π-π stackings) with the nucleotide DC_{16} and Pro_{145}. Interestingly, compounds **HPCAR-28** and **HPCAR-89** were able to form H-bonds with DG_4 that can further stabilize the binding mode compared to **HPCAR-142**. Moreover, the fluorine atom of **HPCAR-28** can guarantee additional interactions within the binding site with Pro_{145} and the sidechains of Glu_{152}. This slightly different pattern of interactions is also highlighted by the differences in docking scores and ΔG_{bind} values (**HPCAR-28** GlideScore −7.980 kcal/mol and ΔG_{bind} −34.102 kcal/mol; **HPCAR-89** GlideScore −6.648 kcal/mol and ΔG_{bind} −26.777 kcal/mol; **HPCAR-142** −6.622 kcal/mol and ΔG_{bind} −25.759 kcal/mol; as reported in **Tables S2**, **S3**). Overall, the *in silico* analysis showed that **HPCAR-28** and **HPCAR-89** can better interact with the active site of HIV IN with respect to **HPCAR-142**.

Regarding the investigation of the binding modes of our derivatives, in our previous study (Sirous et al., 2019), we discussed about the mutation of Tyr_{143} that confers resistance to **RLT**. In particular, **RLT** established interactions with Tyr_{143} by its oxadiazole moiety in both binary PFV-IN and modeled HIV-1 IN complexes. Interestingly, our most promising derivatives do not possess a moiety that can establish interactions with this residue (i.e., oxadiazole in **RLT**). Furthermore, in this study we investigated also two additional mutations that could confer resistance to drugs including **RLT** and **DTG**, $Gln_{148}His$ and $Gly_{140}Ser$. The *in silico* analysis reported in **Figure S1** showed the superposition of the binding mode of **RLT**, **DTG**, and **HPCAR-28** into HIV-1 IN active site. Notably, the only binding mode that can be strongly influenced by these residues (Tyr_{143}, Gln_{148}, and Gly_{140}) is the one of **RLT**. **DTG** can marginally interact with the mentioned residues, while **HPCAR-28** is largely distant from the residues that are responsible of the resistance (distance from Me of **HPCAR-28** to Tyr_{143} over 5 Å, to Gln_{148} over 9 Å, to Gly_{140} over 10 Å; measured by the measurement tool available in PyMOL). Remarkably, our HPCAR derivatives (**HPCAR-28** and **HPCAR-89**) can additionally target the nucleotide DC16 and DG4 (**Figure 4**). This analysis is in perfect agreement with the experimental data showing a dramatic decrease of affinity of **RLT** for mutant HIV-1 IN and a lower decrease of affinity of **DTG**. Consequently, it was assumed that the possible mutations

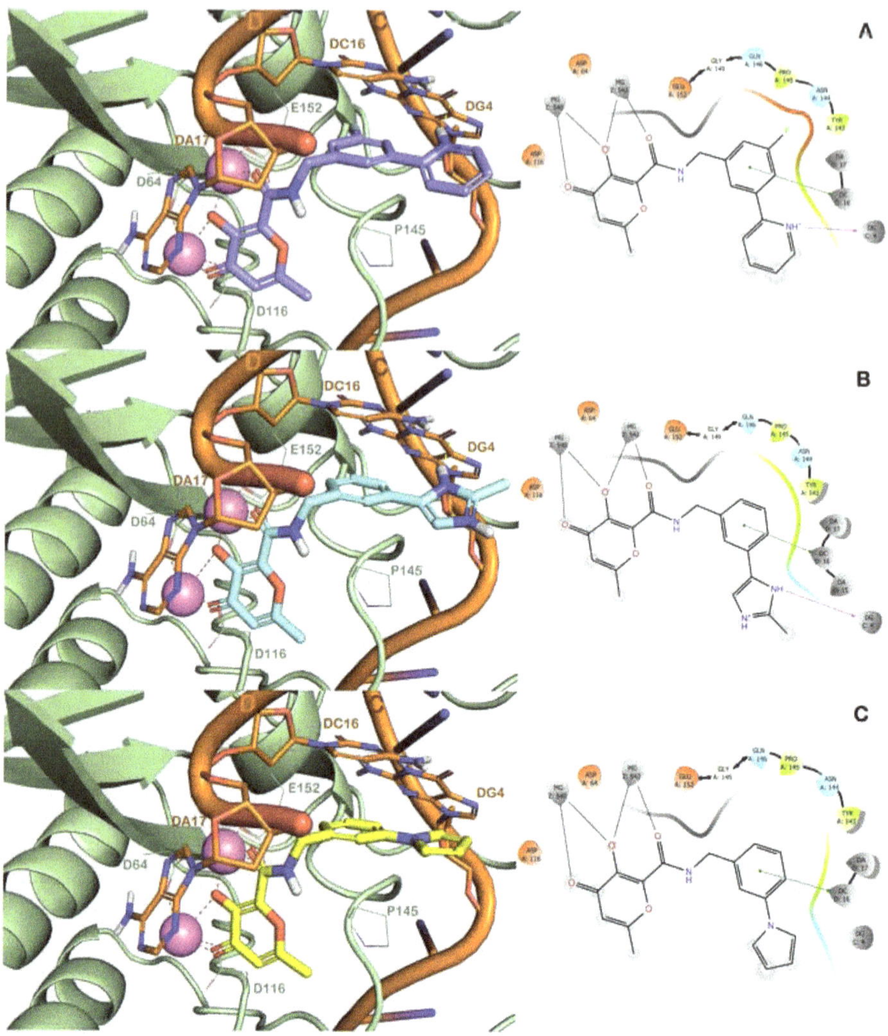

FIGURE 4 | (Left) Binding modes of **HPCAR-28** (purple sticks, **A**), **HPCAR-89** (cyan sticks, **B**), and **HPCAR-142** (yellow sticks, **C**) in the active site of the modeled HIV-1 IN, as found by QPLD method. The solid ribbon model shows the backbone of the modeled HIV-IN, and the key amino acids of the binding site are shown as lines. Two Mg^{2+} ions are displayed as violet spheres, while the viral DNA strands are depicted in orange. Hydrogen and metal coordination bonds are represented by dashed lines. These figures were prepared using PyMOL. (Right) Ligand interaction diagrams for the selected compounds. These figures were prepared using Maestro.

of residues Tyr_{143}, Gln_{148}, and Gly_{140} could not influence the binding of the HPCAR derivatives to IN.

Molecular Dynamics Simulation Studies

In order to better understand the behavior of the representative compounds into HIV-IN enzyme for providing more reliable results about the interactions of **HPCAR-28**, **HPCAR-89**, and **HPCAR-142** with HIV-IN, we performed MD simulations starting from the docked poses reported in **Figure 5** (see Experimental Section for further details).

The three INIs reached an overall stability about after 20 ns. We observed that the pattern of interaction indicated by the docking calculations are generally maintained during the MD, confirming **HPCAR-28** and **HPCAR-89** as more potent potential INIs with respect to the compound **HPCAR-142**. Accordingly, the three compounds maintained the coordination bond with the Mg^{2+} ions during the simulation as well as the hydrophobic interactions with DC_{16} and DA_{17}. We also observed that **HPCAR-28** and **HPCAR-89** were able to establish and maintain further contacts into the binding site with respect to the compound **HPCAR-142**. In fact, the presence of a nitrogen in the R_1 group as in of **HPCAR-28** and **HPCAR-89** allowed to the molecules to stabilize their binding mode by forming further H-bonds with DNA during the simulations. Briefly, the analysis of the computational studies allowed to propose **HPCAR-28** and **HPCAR-89** as more potent INIs with respect to the compound **HPCAR-142**.

In summary, combining different computational techniques for evaluating the affinity of the compounds for HIV IN binding site we provided a more comprehensive *in silico* protocol improving the probability to identify and select compounds with relevant affinity for the selected binding site (Brogi et al.,

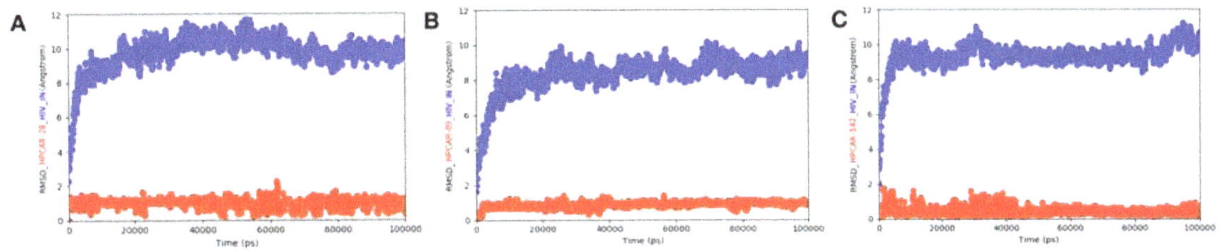

FIGURE 5 | RMSD of the complexes **HPCAR-28**/HIV IN **(A)**, **HPCAR-89**/HIV IN **(B)**, **HPCAR-142**/HIV IN **(C)** (RMSD of the protein in a line formed by blue circles; RMSD of the ligand in a line formed by red circles). RMSD were calculated between the final conformation and the starting conformation through the 100 ns of the MD simulation.

2009). Accordingly, the presented screening workflow allowed to select novel potential HIV-1 INIs based on HPCAR scaffold with improved predicted pharmacological profile. Taking into account also the synthetic feasibility three representative hit candidates were then chosen for the synthesis and then biologically evaluated for validating the applied computational approach.

Chemistry

In this study, 3-(benzyloxy)-6-methyl-4-oxo-4*H*-pyran-2-carboxylic acid, **BPCA** was used as a key intermediate material for the preparation of the three selected hit compounds. Thus, this intermediate was first synthesized starting from commercially available Kojic acid according to a synthetic procedure previously employed in our laboratory (Sirous et al., 2019). On the other hand, three different synthetic routes were developed for the preparation of the amine fragments needed for appending desired hydrophobic backbone to **BPCA**. The methodologies adopted for the synthesis of amine compounds **AM-(1-3)** are outlined in **Figures 6–9**, respectively.

As described in **Figure 6**, the synthesis of the amine fragment **AM-1** started using an efficient Suzuki–Miyaura cross-coupling (SMC) (Tan et al., 2014) by reacting 2-bromopyridine **1** with phenyl-boronic acid derivative **2** in the presence of tetrakis (triphenylphosphine) palladium (0) as the catalyst, affording the phenyl-pyridine derivative **3**. Subsequently the nitrile group of resulting compound **3** was reduced to the corresponding primary amine **AM-1** by treatment with sodium borohydride and dry nickel (II) chloride (Khurana and Gogia, 1997; Khurana and Kukreja, 2002; Caddick et al., 2003).

A four-step synthetic procedure was employed for the synthesis of the amine fragment **AM-2** starting from 2-methylimidazole **4** (**Figure 7**). The first step of the protocol consisted of the double bromination of the imidazole ring which afforded the dibromo-imidazole derivative **5** in a moderate yield. The selective debromination of the vicinal dibromide **5** employing sodium sulfite as the reducing agent in aqueous ethanol at reflux temperature effectively provided product **6** (yield: 75%) (Khurana and Gogia, 1997; Alonso-Alija et al., 2003). Bromo-imidazole **6** underwent a classical SM coupling reaction with phenyl-boronic acid **7**, providing phenyl-imidazole derivative **8**. Amine fragment **AM-2** was finally obtained by reduction of phenyl-imidazole derivative **8** using sodium borohydride and dry nickel (II) chloride as described for **AM-1** (Caddick et al., 2003).

The amine fragment **AM-3** was prepared from commercially available 3-aminobenzonitrile **9**, following **Figure 8**. A Clauson–Kaas reaction of 3-aminobenzonitrile **9** with dimethoxytetrahydrofuran **10** catalyzed by hydrochloric acid afforded the corresponding 1-phenylpyrrole derivative **11** in a good yield (82%) (Chatzopoulou et al., 2013). The nitrile functionality of the resulting product was then reduced in the presence of sodium borohydride and dry nickel (II) chloride to furnish the desired amine compound **AM-3** (Caddick et al., 2003).

Finally, the representative hit compounds were prepared by introduction of amine backbones to the benzyl-protected pyranone **BPCA** under standard amide coupling conditions (Sheehan et al., 1965; Sirous et al., 2019). The general procedure employed for the synthesis of the final compounds is summarized in **Figure 9**. The activation of carboxylic acid group of **BPCA** as the corresponding derivative **12** using EDCI and NHS as coupling reagents followed by treatment with the desired amines led to 2-amido substituted pyranone analogs **BPCAR**. The removal of the benzyl protecting group of the obtained amide derivatives was then accomplished by reaction with boron tribromide in dichloromethane at room temperature to obtain three final target products, **HPCAR-28, HPCAR-89**, and **HPCAR-142**, in 71–86% yield (Kosak et al., 2015; Sirous et al., 2019).

Biological Activity Evaluation

For validating the computational protocol herein presented, three representative compounds (**HPCAR-28**, **HPCAR-89**, and **HPCAR-142**) were synthesized and biologically assessed for HIV-1 IN catalytic inhibitory activity based on an *in vitro* enzymatic assay. Given that most HIV-1 INIs such as RLT target the ST step of the integration reaction, the inhibition of the ST activity of HIV-1 IN was examined in these assays in addition to overall HIV-1 IN inhibition. Moreover, assessment of the anti-HIV-1 potential in MT-4 cells was performed in a multiple round cell-based antiviral assay. Cytotoxicity of the selected compounds for the target host cell was also evaluated and their therapeutic indices were calculated. In these experiments, **RLT** was employed as a reference HIV-1 INI. The results for biological activities of these hits were summarized in **Table 3**.

As reported in **Table 3**, biological evaluation confirmed the favorable anti-HIV profile for the three newly synthesized

protocol. Gratifyingly, the results of pharmacological studies showed that the representative hit compounds inhibited HIV-1 IN in the low micromolar range. Among them, compound **HPCAR-28** showed the best inhibitory activity against HIV-1 IN as well as the best inhibitory activity against HIV-1 replication and HIV-1 IN strand transfer process along with a notable therapeutic index and no appreciable cell toxicity.

These promising and encouraging results provide further solid support for the potential exploitation of HPCAR scaffold in the development of anti-retroviral drugs, paving the way to the discovery of a new class of drugs against HIV-1 IN for treating HIV infection.

AUTHOR CONTRIBUTIONS

HS carried out the computational experiments and the synthesis of the selected compounds, contributing in writing the manuscript. GCh carried out the computational experiments and performed the acquisition, analysis, interpretation of data, contributing in writing, and revising the manuscript. SG and SBu advised in the synthesis of the compounds, contributing in revising the manuscript. ZD and FC performed the biological evaluation of the selected compounds. LS advised in the synthesis of the compounds. SBr conceived, designed, and performed the computational experiments, supervised the overall work, wrote and revised the manuscript. AF advised in the synthesis of the compounds and in the computational experiments, contributing in revising the manuscript. GCa supervised the overall work and contributing in revising the manuscript. MB conceived the synthetic strategy for the synthesis of the compounds and supervised the synthesis of them, contributing in revising the manuscript.

ACKNOWLEDGMENTS

The authors wish to thank the Department of Biotechnology Chemistry and Pharmacy at University of Siena for hosting HS during her Ph.D. training.

REFERENCES

Alonso-Alija, C., Micheles, M., Schirok, H., Schlemmer, K. H., Dodd, S., Fitgerald, M., et al. (2003). *Imidazopyridinones as p38 Map Kinase Inhibitors.* WO2003008413 A1. Available online at: https://patentscope.wipo.int/search/en/detail.jsf?docId=WO2003008413

Baell, J. B., and Holloway, G. A. (2010). New substructure filters for removal of pan assay interference compounds (PAINS) from screening libraries and for their exclusion in bioassays. *J. Med. Chem.* 53, 2719–2740. doi: 10.1021/jm901137j

Brindisi, M., Gemma, S., Kunjir, S., Di Cerbo, L., Brogi, S., Parapini, S., et al. (2015). Synthetic spirocyclic endoperoxides: new antimalarial scaffolds. *Medchemcomm* 6, 357–362. doi: 10.1039/C4MD00454J

Brindisi, M., Maramai, S., Brogi, S., Fanigliulo, E., Butini, S., Guarino, E., et al. (2016). Development of novel cyclic peptides as pro-apoptotic agents. *Eur. J. Med. Chem.* 117, 301–320. doi: 10.1016/j.ejmech.2016.04.001

Brindisi, M., Ulivieri, C., Alfano, G., Gemma, S., de Asis Balaguer, F., Khan, T., et al. (2019). Structure-activity relationships, biological evaluation and structural studies of novel pyrrolonaphthoxazepines as antitumor agents. *Eur. J. Med. Chem.* 162, 290–320. doi: 10.1016/j.ejmech.2018.11.004

Brogi, S., Brindisi, M., Butini, S., Kshirsagar, G. U., Maramai, S., Chemi, G., et al. (2018). (S)-2-Amino-3-(5-methyl-3-hydroxyisoxazol-4-yl)propanoic Acid (AMPA) and kainate receptor ligands: further exploration of bioisosteric replacements and structural and biological investigation. *J. Med. Chem.* 61, 2124–2130. doi: 10.1021/acs.jmedchem.8b00099

Brogi, S., Fiorillo, A., Chemi, G., Butini, S., Lalle, M., Ilari, A., et al. (2017a). Structural characterization of Giardia duodenalis thioredoxin reductase (gTrxR) and computational analysis of its interaction with NBDHEX. *Eur. J. Med. Chem.* 135, 479–490. doi: 10.1016/j.ejmech.2017.04.057

Brogi, S., Kladi, M., Vagias, C., Papazafiri, P., Roussis, V., and Tafi, A. (2009). Pharmacophore modeling for qualitative prediction of antiestrogenic activity. *J. Chem. Inf. Model.* 49, 2489–2497. doi: 10.1021/ci900254b

Brogi, S., Ramunno, A., Savi, L., Chemi, G., Alfano, G., Pecorelli, A., et al. (2017b). First dual AK/GSK-3beta inhibitors endowed with antioxidant properties as multifunctional, potential neuroprotective agents. *Eur. J. Med. Chem.* 138, 438–457. doi: 10.1016/j.ejmech.2017.06.017

Caddick, S., Judd, D. B., Lewis, A. K. D., Reich, M. T., and Williams, M. R. V. (2003). A generic approach for the catalytic reduction of nitriles. *Tetrahedron* 59, 5417–5423. doi: 10.1016/S0040-4020(03)00858-5

Cappelli, A., Manini, M., Valenti, S., Castriconi, F., Giuliani, G., Anzini, M., et al. (2013). Synthesis and structure-activity relationship studies in serotonin 5-HT(1A) receptor agonists based on fused pyrrolidone scaffolds. *Eur. J. Med. Chem.* 63, 85–94. doi: 10.1016/j.ejmech.2013.01.044

Chatzopoulou, M., Kotsampasakou, E., and Demopoulos, V. J. (2013). Clauson-kaas-type synthesis of pyrrolyl-phenols, from the hydrochlorides of aminophenols, in the presence of nicotinamide. *Synth. Commun.* 43, 2949–2954. doi: 10.1080/00397911.2012.753460

Chiu, T. K., and Davies, D. R. (2004). Structure and function of HIV-1 integrase. *Curr. Top. Med. Chem.* 4, 965–977. doi: 10.2174/1568026043388547

Cho, A. E., Guallar, V., Berne, B. J., and Friesner, R. (2005). Importance of accurate charges in molecular docking: quantum mechanical/molecular mechanical (QM/MM) approach. *J. Comput. Chem.* 26, 915–931. doi: 10.1002/jcc.20222

Christ, F., Busschots, K., Hendrix, J., Engelborghs, Y., and Debyser, Z. (2011). "Assays for the evaluation of HIV-1 integrase enzymatic activity, DNA-binding and co-factor interaction," in *HIV-1 Integrase*, ed N. Neamati (John Wiley & Sons, Inc), 151–163. doi: 10.1002/9781118015377

Debyser, Z., Cherepanov, P., Pluymers, W., and De Clercq, E. (2001). Assays for the evaluation of HIV-1 integrase inhibitors. *Methods Mol. Biol.* 160, 139–155. doi: 10.1385/1-59259-233-3:139

Debyser, Z., Cherepanov, P., Van Maele, B., De Clercq, E., and Witvrouw, M. (2002). In search of authentic inhibitors of HIV-1 integration. *Antivir. Chem. Chemother.* 13, 1–15. doi: 10.1177/095632020201300101

Delelis, O., Carayon, K., Saib, A., Deprez, E., and Mouscadet, J. F. (2008). Integrase and integration: biochemical activities of HIV-1 integrase. *Retrovirology* 5:114. doi: 10.1186/1742-4690-5-114

Di Santo, R. (2014). Inhibiting the HIV integration process: past, present, and the future. *J. Med. Chem.* 57, 539–566. doi: 10.1021/jm400674a

Dirac, A. M., and Kjems, J. (2001). Mapping DNA-binding sites of HIV-1 integrase by protein footprinting. *Eur. J. Biochem.* 268, 743–751. doi: 10.1046/j.1432-1327.2001.01932.x

Dolan, J., Chen, A., Weber, I. T., Harrison, R. W., and Leis, J. (2009). Defining the DNA substrate binding sites on HIV-1 integrase. *J. Mol. Biol.* 385, 568–579. doi: 10.1016/j.jmb.2008.10.083

Dyda, F., Hickman, A. B., Jenkins, T. M., Engelman, A., Craigie, R., and Davies, D. R. (1994). Crystal structure of the catalytic domain of HIV-1 integrase: similarity to other polynucleotidyl transferases. *Science* 266, 1981–1986. doi: 10.1126/science.7801124

Friesner, R. A., Banks, J. L., Murphy, R. B., Halgren, T. A., Klicic, J. J., Mainz, D. T., et al. (2004). Glide: a new approach for rapid, accurate docking and scoring. 1. Method and assessment of docking accuracy. *J. Med. Chem.* 47, 1739–1749. doi: 10.1021/jm0306430

Gasser, A., Brogi, S., Urayama, K., Nishi, T., Kurose, H., Tafi, A., et al. (2015). Discovery and cardioprotective effects of the first non-peptide agonists of the G protein-coupled prokineticin receptor-1. *PLoS ONE* 10:e0121027. doi: 10.1371/journal.pone.0121027

Hoover, W. G. (1985). Canonical dynamics - equilibrium phase-space distributions. *Physical Rev. A* 31, 1695–1697. doi: 10.1103/PhysRevA.31.1695

Huang, N., Kalyanaraman, C., Irwin, J. J., and Jacobson, M. P. (2006). Physics-based scoring of protein-ligand complexes: enrichment of known inhibitors in large-scale virtual screening. *J. Chem. Inf. Model.* 46, 243–253. doi: 10.1021/ci0502855

Humphreys, D. D., Friesner, R. A., and Berne, B. J. (1994). A multiple-time-step molecular-dynamics algorithm for macromolecules. *J. Phys. Chem.* 98, 6885–6892. doi: 10.1021/j100078a035

Hwang, Y., Rhodes, D., and Bushman, F. (2000). Rapid microtiter assays for poxvirus topoisomerase, mammalian type IB topoisomerase and HIV-1 integrase: application to inhibitor isolation. *Nucleic Acids Res.* 28, 4884–4892. doi: 10.1093/nar/28.24.4884

Illingworth, C. J., Morris, G. M., Parkes, K. E., Snell, C. R., and Reynolds, C. A. (2008). Assessing the role of polarization in docking. *J. Phys. Chem. A* 112, 12157–12163. doi: 10.1021/jp710169m

Irwin, J. J., and Shoichet, B. K. (2005). ZINC–a free database of commercially available compounds for virtual screening. *J. Chem. Inf. Model.* 45, 177–182. doi: 10.1021/ci049714+

Irwin, J. J., Sterling, T., Mysinger, M. M., Bolstad, E. S., and Coleman, R. G. (2012). ZINC: a free tool to discover chemistry for biology. *J. Chem. Inf. Model.* 52, 1757–1768. doi: 10.1021/ci3001277

Johns, B. A., and Svolto, A. C. (2008). Advances in two-metal chelation inhibitors of HIV integrase. *Expert. Opin. Ther. Pat.* 18, 1225–1237. doi: 10.1517/13543776.18.11.1225

Jorgensen, W. L., Maxwell, D. S., and TiradoRives, J. (1996). Development and testing of the OPLS all-atom force field on conformational energetics and properties of organic liquids. *J. Am. Chem. Soc.* 118, 11225–11236. doi: 10.1021/ja9621760

Kaminski, G. A., Friesner, R. A., Tirado-Rives, J., and Jorgensen, W. L. (2001). Evaluation and reparametrization of the OPLS-AA force field for proteins via comparison with accurate quantum chemical calculations on peptides. *J. Phys. Chem. B* 105, 6474–6487. doi: 10.1021/jp003919d

Katlama, C., and Murphy, R. (2012). Dolutegravir for the treatment of HIV. *Expert. Opin. Investig. Drugs* 21, 523–530. doi: 10.1517/13543784.2012.661713

Kawasuji, T., Fuji, M., Yoshinaga, T., Sato, A., Fujiwara, T., and Kiyama, R. (2006a). A platform for designing HIV integrase inhibitors. Part 2: a two-metal binding model as a potential mechanism of HIV integrase inhibitors. *Bioorg. Med. Chem.* 14, 8420–8429. doi: 10.1016/j.bmc.2006.08.043

Kawasuji, T., Yoshinaga, T., Sato, A., Yodo, M., Fujiwara, T., and Kiyama, R. (2006b). A platform for designing HIV integrase inhibitors. Part 1: 2-hydroxy-3-heteroaryl acrylic acid derivatives as novel HIV integrase inhibitor and modeling of hydrophilic and hydrophobic pharmacophores. *Bioorg. Med. Chem.* 14, 8430–8445. doi: 10.1016/j.bmc.2006.08.044

Khurana, J. M., and Gogia, A. (1997). Synthetically useful reactions with Nickle boride. A review. *Org. Prep. Proced. Int.* 29, 1–32. doi: 10.1080/00304949709355171

Khurana, J. M., and Kukreja, G. (2002). Rapid reduction of nitriles to primary amines with nickel boride at ambient temperature. *Synth. Commun.* 32, 1265–1269. doi: 10.1081/SCC-120003619

Kosak, T. M., Conrad, H. A., Korich, A. L., and Lord, R. L. (2015). Ether cleavage re-investigated: elucidating the mechanism of BBr3-facilitated demethylation of aryl methyl ethers. *Eur. J. Org. Chem.* 2015, 7460–7467. doi: 10.1002/ejoc.201501042

Lagorce, D., Maupetit, J., Baell, J., Sperandio, O., Tuffery, P., Miteva, M. A., et al. (2011). The FAF-Drugs2 server: a multistep engine to prepare electronic chemical compound collections. *Bioinformatics* 27, 2018–2020. doi: 10.1093/bioinformatics/btr333

Lagorce, D., Sperandio, O., Galons, H., Miteva, M. A., and Villoutreix, B. O. (2008). FAF-Drugs2: free ADME/tox filtering tool to assist drug discovery and chemical biology projects. *BMC Bioinformatics* 9:396. doi: 10.1186/1471-2105-9-396

Liao, C., Marchand, C., Burke, T. R. Jr., Pommier, Y., and Nicklaus, M. C. (2010). Authentic HIV-1 integrase inhibitors. *Future Med. Chem.* 2, 1107–1122. doi: 10.4155/fmc.10.199

Lipinski, C. A., Lombardo, F., Dominy, B. W., and Feeney, P. J. (2001). Experimental and computational approaches to estimate solubility and permeability in drug discovery and development settings. *Adv. Drug. Deliv. Rev.* 46, 3–26. doi: 10.1016/S0169-409X(00)00129-0

Ma, Y., and Hider, R. C. (2015). Novel synthetic approach to fluoro- and amido-disubstituted 3-hydroxypyridin-4-ones. *J. Fluor. Chem.* 173, 29–34. doi: 10.1016/j.jfluchem.2015.02.005

Maquiaveli, C. C., Lucon-Junior, J. F., Brogi, S., Campiani, G., Gemma, S., Vieira, P. C., et al. (2016). Verbascoside inhibits promastigote growth and arginase activity of *Leishmania amazonensis*. *J. Nat. Prod.* 79, 1459–1463. doi: 10.1021/acs.jnatprod.5b00875

Martyna, G. J., Tobias, D. J., and Klein, M. L. (1994). constant-pressure molecular-dynamics algorithms. *J. Chem. Phys.* 101, 4177–4189. doi: 10.1063/1.467468

Neamati, N., Lin, Z., Karki, R. G., Orr, A., Cowansage, K., Strumberg, D., et al. (2002). Metal-dependent inhibition of HIV-1 integrase. *J. Med. Chem.* 45, 5661–5670. doi: 10.1021/jm0201417

Nickolls, J., Buck, I., Garland, M., and Skadron, K. (2008). Scalable parallel programming with CUDA. *Queue* 6, 40–53. doi: 10.1145/1365490.1365500

Paolino, M., Brindisi, M., Vallone, A., Butini, S., Campiani, G., Nannicini, C., et al. (2018). Development of potent inhibitors of the *Mycobacterium tuberculosis* virulence factor Zmp1 and evaluation of their effect on mycobacterial survival inside macrophages. *ChemMedChem* 13, 422–430. doi: 10.1002/cmdc.201700759

Pauwels, R., Balzarini, J., Baba, M., Snoeck, R., Schols, D., Herdewijn, P., et al. (1988). Rapid and automated tetrazolium-based colorimetric assay for the detection of anti-HIV compounds. *J. Virol. Methods* 20, 309–321. doi: 10.1016/0166-0934(88)90134-6

Pearlman, D. A., and Charifson, P. S. (2001). Are free energy calculations useful in practice? A comparison with rapid scoring functions for the p38 MAP kinase protein system. *J. Med. Chem.* 44, 3417–3423. doi: 10.1021/jm0100279

Pommier, Y., Johnson, A. A., and Marchand, C. (2005). Integrase inhibitors to treat HIV/AIDS. *Nat. Rev. Drug. Discov.* 4, 236–248. doi: 10.1038/nrd1660

Rogolino, D., Carcelli, M., Sechi, M., and Neamati, N. (2012). Viral enzymes containing magnesium: metal binding as a successful strategy in drug design. *Coord. Chem. Rev.* 256, 3063–3086. doi: 10.1016/j.ccr.2012.07.006

Rostami, M., Sirous, H., Zabihollahi, R., Aghasadeghi, M. R., Sadat, S. M., Namazi, R., et al. (2015). Design, synthesis and anti-HIV-1 evaluation of a series of 5-hydroxypyridine-4-one derivatives as possible integrase inhibitors. *Med. Chem. Res.* 24, 4113–4127. doi: 10.1007/s00044-015-1443-4

Rowley, M. (2008). The discovery of raltegravir, an integrase inhibitor for the treatment of HIV infection. *Prog. Med. Chem.* 46, 1–28. doi: 10.1016/S0079-6468(07)00001-X

Santos, M. A., Marques, S. M., and Chaves, S. (2012). Hydroxypyridinones as "privileged" chelating structures for the design of medicinal drugs. *Coord. Chem. Rev.* 256, 240–259. doi: 10.1016/j.ccr.2011.08.008

Sato, M., Kawakami, H., Motomura, T., Aramaki, H., Matsuda, T., Yamashita, M., et al. (2009). Quinolone carboxylic acids as a novel monoketo acid class of human immunodeficiency virus type 1 integrase inhibitors. *J. Med. Chem.* 52, 4869–4882. doi: 10.1021/jm900460z

Sheehan, J. C., Preston, J., and Cruickshank, P. A. (1965). A rapid synthesis of oligopeptide derivatives without isolation of intermediates. *J. Am. Chem. Soc.* 87, 2492–2493. doi: 10.1021/ja01089a034

Sirous, H., Fassihi, A., Brogi, S., Campiani, G., Christ, F., Debyser, Z., et al. (2019). Synthesis, molecular modelling and biological studies of 3-hydroxy-pyrane-4-one and 3-hydroxy-pyridine-4-one derivatives as HIV-1 integrase inhibitors. *Med. Chem.* doi: 10.2174/1573406415666181219113225. [Epub ahead of print].

Sirous, H., Zabihollahi, R., Aghasadeghi, M. R., Sadat, S. M., Saghaie, L., and Fassihi, A. (2015). Docking studies of some 5-hydroxypyridine-4-one derivatives: evaluation of integrase and ribonuclease H domain of reverse transcriptase as possible targets for anti-HIV-1 activity. *Med. Chem. Res.* 24, 2195–2212. doi: 10.1007/s00044-014-1289-1

Still, W. C., Tempczyk, A., Hawley, R. C., and Hendrickson, T. (1990). Semianalytical treatment of solvation for molecular mechanics and dynamics. *J. Am. Chem. Soc.* 112, 6127–6129. doi: 10.1021/ja00172a038

Tan, J., Chen, Y., Li, H., and Yasuda, N. (2014). Suzuki-Miyaura cross-coupling reactions of unprotected haloimidazoles. *J. Org. Chem.* 79, 8871–8876. doi: 10.1021/jo501326r

Taylor, R. D., Jewsbury, P. J., and Essex, J. W. (2002). A review of protein-small molecule docking methods. *J. Comput. Aided Mol. Des.* 16, 151–166. doi: 10.1023/A:1020155510718

Vallone, A., D'Alessandro, S., Brogi, S., Brindisi, M., Chemi, G., Alfano, G., et al. (2018). Antimalarial agents against both sexual and asexual parasites stages: structure-activity relationships and biological studies of the Malaria Box compound 1-[5-(4-bromo-2-chlorophenyl)furan-2-yl]-N-[(piperidin-4-yl)methyl]methanamine (MMV019918) and analogues. *Eur. J. Med Chem.* 150, 698–718. doi: 10.1016/j.ejmech.2018.03.024

Zaccagnini, L., Brogi, S., Brindisi, M., Gemma, S., Chemi, G., Legname, G., et al. (2017). Identification of novel fluorescent probes preventing PrP(Sc) replication in prion diseases. *Eur. J. Med. Chem.* 127, 859–873. doi: 10.1016/j.ejmech.2016.10.064

12

Integrating Ligand and Target-Driven Based Virtual Screening Approaches with *in vitro* Human Cell Line Models and Time-Resolved Fluorescence Resonance Energy Transfer Assay to Identify Novel Hit Compounds Against BCL-2

Gurbet Tutumlu [1], *Berna Dogan* [1*], *Timucin Avsar* [2,3,4*], *Muge Didem Orhan* [3,4], *Seyma Calis* [4,5] and *Serdar Durdagi* [1,3*]

[1] Computational Biology and Molecular Simulations Laboratory, Department of Biophysics, School of Medicine, Bahcesehir University, Istanbul, Turkey, [2] Department of Medical Biology, Bahcesehir University, School of Medicine, Istanbul, Turkey, [3] Neuroscience Program, Health Sciences Institute, Bahcesehir University, Istanbul, Turkey, [4] Neuroscience Laboratory, Health Sciences Institute, Bahcesehir University, Istanbul, Turkey, [5] Molecular Biology, Genetics and Biotechnology Graduate Program, Istanbul Technical University, Istanbul, Turkey

***Correspondence:**
Berna Dogan
berna.dogan@med.bau.edu.tr
Timucin Avsar
timucin.avsar@med.bau.edu.tr
Serdar Durdagi
serdar.durdagi@med.bau.edu.tr

Antiapoptotic members of *B-cell leukemia/lymphoma*-2 (BCL-2) family proteins are one of the overexpressed proteins in cancer cells that are oncogenic targets. As such, targeting of BCL-2 family proteins raises hopes for new therapeutic discoveries. Thus, we used multistep screening and filtering approaches that combine structure and ligand-based drug design to identify new, effective BCL-2 inhibitors from a small molecule database (Specs SC), which includes more than 210,000 compounds. This database is first filtered based on binary *"cancer-QSAR"* model constructed with 886 training and 167 test set compounds and common 26 toxicity quantitative structure-activity relationships (QSAR) models. Predicted non-toxic compounds are considered for target-driven studies. Here, we applied two different approaches to filter and select hit compounds for further *in vitro* biological assays and human cell line experiments. In the first approach, a molecular docking and filtering approach is used to rank compounds based on their docking scores and only a few top-ranked molecules are selected for further long (100-ns) molecular dynamics (MD) simulations and *in vitro* tests. While docking algorithms are promising in predicting binding poses, they can be less prone to precisely predict ranking of compounds leading to decrease in the success rate of *in silico* studies. Hence, in the second approach, top-docking poses of each compound filtered through QSAR studies are subjected to initially short (1 ns) MD simulations and their binding energies are calculated via molecular mechanics generalized Born surface area (MM/GBSA) method. Then, the compounds are ranked based on their average MM/GBSA energy values to select hit molecules for further long MD simulations and *in vitro* studies. Additionally, we have applied text-mining approaches to identify molecules that contain *"indol"* phrase as many of the approved drugs contain indole and indol derivatives. Around 2700 compounds are filtered based on *"cancer-QSAR"* model and are then docked into BCL-2. Short MD simulations are performed for the top-docking poses for each compound in complex with BCL-2. The complexes are again ranked based on their MM/GBSA values to select hit molecules for further long MD simulations and *in vitro* studies. In total, seven molecules are subjected to biological activity tests in various human cancer cell lines as well as Time-Resolved Fluorescence Resonance Energy Transfer (TR-FRET) assay. Inhibitory concentrations are evaluated, and biological activities and apoptotic potentials are assessed by cell culture studies. Four molecules are found to be limiting the proliferation capacity of cancer cells while increasing the apoptotic cell fractions.

Keywords: BCL-2, molecular docking, MD simulations, virtual screening, text mining, *in vitro* human cell line models, TR-FRET assay, binary QSAR models

INTRODUCTION

Finding a cure for cancer is still a challenging task, despite the understanding of molecular mechanisms and causal relationships participating in the pathology of cancer since the mid-1980s (Fesik, 2005). As stated by Hanahan and Weinberg, multistage development of tumors consists of six biological features widely known as hallmarks of cancer: (i) maintaining proliferative signaling, (ii) avoiding growth suppressors, (iii) triggering invasion and metastasis, (iv) empowering replicative perpetuity, (v) inducing angiogenesis, and (vi) resisting cell death (Hanahan and Weinberg, 2000, 2011). The ability of cancer cells to escape from programmed cell death, namely, apoptosis, remains a critical feature of these six indicators (Mohamad Rosdi et al., 2018). Apoptosis is a molecular pathway that results with self-destruction of the cell, either following termination of physiological function or after a crucial damage to genetic material (Igney and Krammer, 2002; Reed, 2002; Verma et al., 2015). The well-defined basic apoptosis pathways, extrinsic and the intrinsic pathways, are variously stimulated, and they use determined signaling elements (Kollek et al., 2016). The extrinsic pathway is activated by outer stimulation of death receptors. Death receptors are members of the tumor necrosis factor (TNF) receptor family, which has an intracellular death domain that is able to accumulate and trigger caspase-8 followed by operation of effector caspases including caspase-3, -6, or -7 (Youle and Strasser, 2008; Eimon and Ashkenazi, 2010; Wu et al., 2018). The intrinsic pathway, also called mitochondrial pathway, is initiated by a variety of cytotoxic damages or growth signals, some of which are genetic instability, inadequate developmental stimulation, and invasion by viral pathogens. *B-cell leukemia/lymphoma*-2 (BCL-2) family proteins tightly regulate this process and subsequently leads to the activation of caspase-9 (Cory et al., 2003; Youle and Strasser, 2008; Eimon and Ashkenazi, 2010).

All members of BCL-2 protein family have retained sequence patterns regarded as the BCL-2 homology (BH) domains and could be divided into three main classes. The first class of proteins are made up of the proapoptotic activator BH domain 3 (BH3) only proteins such as BIM, BID, and PUMA. Immediately upon their activation, they serve as molecular guardians that connect outer spurs to the mitochondrial pathway. The following group contains the proapoptotic effectors, which are multidomain proteins, such as BAX and BAK, and each of them has three BH domains. These proteins distort the integrity of mitochondrial outer membrane, which leads to free movement of cytochrome C to cytoplasm, initiates downstream caspase activity, and ultimately to trigger the termination of cells. The last class of BCL-2 family are the antiapoptotic protein, BCL-XL, BCL-2, MCL-1, etc. All of these members consist of four BH domains and keeps cells safe by segregating their proapoptotic peers. The most important point in promoting apoptosis is to increase the amount of BH3-only proteins or switch off one of its antiapoptotic BCL-2 counterparts (Fesik, 2005; Dewson and Kluck, 2010; Chung, 2018; Mohamad Rosdi et al., 2018). The idea of BH3 mimetics as promising anticancer drugs is inspired by the conclusion that a great deal of cancers rely on BCL-2 family proteins and that the interaction between these proteins occurs through specific BH domains (Oltersdorf et al., 2005; Soderquist and Eastman, 2016). A genuine BH3 mimetic is expected to imitate the BH3 domain of a proapoptotic BCL-2 protein, thus deactivating the antiapoptotic family members by filling up their BH3-binding pockets.

Apoptotic cell death is an innate hurdle to growth of tumor cells; hence, one of the fundamental hallmarks of cancer cells is the avoidance of apoptosis, which comprises a crucial process in resistance to chemotherapeutics. This phenomenon led to peculiar approaches in anticancer therapies focusing on apoptosis such as suppression of survival factors that are detected to be overexpressed in numerous malignancies. In the group of survival factors, BCL-2 proteins are one of the families that step forward for drug discovery studies (Lessene et al., 2008; Hanahan and Weinberg, 2011; Billard, 2013). For example, a small molecule, named ABT-737, was issued as a potential inhibitor of BCL-2 and BCL-XL, which occupies their BH3-binding domain and further triggers apoptosis in diversified cancer types (Tse et al., 2008; Soderquist and Eastman, 2016). Ensuing pharmaceutical trials guided to clinical studies with ABT-263 (navitoclax), which had boosted bioavailability and indicated efficacy in leukemia and a few other neoplasias. However, they also manifested toxicities such as neutropenia and thrombocytopenia, leading to dose limitations (Tse et al., 2008; Gandhi et al., 2011). The thrombocytopenia was connected to the blockage of BCL-XL, as BCL-XL is essential for survival of platelets (Zhang et al., 2007). More recently, ABT-199 (venetoclax) was designed as a selective BCL-2 inhibitor and it evades the issue of thrombocytopenia (Souers et al., 2013). However, it also carries some side effects such as diarrhea, nausea, low white blood cell counts, high K^+ ion concentrations in the blood, headache, etc. Thus, novel BCL-2 inhibitors with better pharmacodynamic as well as pharmacokinetic profiles are needed.

It is well-established, especially in the last years, that taking a new drug into the market is both a time consuming and costly process. As a result, computer-aided drug design techniques have become prominent in drug development process (Lionta et al., 2014; Yoshino et al., 2015, 2017; Chiba et al., 2017; Halim et al., 2017; Durdagi et al., 2018a, 2019; Fu et al., 2018; Is et al., 2018; Mirza et al., 2018; Erol et al., 2019; Zaka et al., 2019). Different strategies depending on the availability of target molecules have been developed; structure-based drug design in which the target structure is known and ligand-based drug design that could be applied in cases that target structure is not known. It is also possible to combine both approaches to increase the possibility of "hit molecule" discovery as has been done in our previous studies (Durdagi et al., 2018a,b; Zaka et al., 2018; Kanan et al., 2019; Mollica et al., 2019). The most widely used technique in target-driven-based drug design is the molecular docking, and there are various docking programs as well as many different scoring functions to rank binding poses. Large molecule libraries can be screened using high throughput virtual screening, and lead compounds can be identified for further studies, quickly. By the use of more sophisticated docking algorithms and scoring functions, binding modes of compounds to target can also be determined. However, as expected, each of the docking algorithms and scoring functions have their own strengths and weaknesses. Numerous studies have been conducted to evaluate the comparative assessment of the docking and scoring functions (Bissantz et al., 2000; Bursulaya et al., 2003; Chen et al., 2006; Warren et al., 2006; Cross et al., 2009; Li et al., 2014). The latest evaluation study was conducted by Li et al. for 20 scoring functions on a diverse set of protein–ligand complexes (Li et al., 2014). Their comparison of scoring functions was based on four aspects: "scoring power" (binding affinity prediction), "ranking power" (relative ranking prediction), "docking power" (binding pose prediction), and "screening power" (discrimination of true binders from random molecules). Their results showed that scoring functions were generally more promising in docking and screening power tests than scoring and ranking power tests. In addition, scoring functions that were among top-ranked in docking power test were also more successful in screening power test but poor in other two power tests. This study, which shows that every scoring function has its own weaknesses, has represented that the ordering of compounds only by their docking scores may not accomplish the correct ranking of compounds; hence, if the molecules will only be selected according to their top docking scores for further studies such as *in vitro* tests, this may lead to false positive results (Rastelli et al., 2009; Rastelli and Pinzi, 2019). Therefore, in this study, we use another approach in ranking compounds that is based on molecular dynamics (MD) simulations and molecular mechanics generalized Born surface area (MM/GBSA) calculations after initial pose prediction by molecular docking.

In the present study, in order to identify novel BCL-2 inhibitors, ligand- and target-driven-based techniques were integrated with text mining approach, and novel hit molecules were identified with the virtual screening of small molecules library (Specs SC) that includes more than 212,000 compounds. In the identification of hits, two different approaches were considered: (i) Compounds were ranked by their docking scores, and MD simulations for 100 ns were carried out for the selected compounds and average MM/GBSA energies were calculated; (ii) Short (1-ns) MD simulations were applied for top-docking poses of all selected 342 compounds from binary quantitative structure-activity relationships (QSAR) models, and average MM/GBSA scores from short MD simulations were calculated. The average MM/GBSA scores were considered in the selection of compounds for longer MD simulations (100 ns) followed by MM/GBSA calculations. Additionally, it is known that many currently used Food and Drug Administration (FDA)-approved chemotherapeutics include indole fragment. To increase the probability of discovering hit molecules with potential anticancer properties, we screened Specs-SC database to identify molecules that contain *"indol"* groups by using text mining. Around 2700 compounds were screened against BCL-2, and novel hits that includes *"indol"* fingerprints were identified.

MATERIALS AND METHODS

Binary QSAR Models

MetaCore/MetaDrug (MC/MD) platform from Clarivate Analytics provides a comprehensive tool to analyze the pharmacodynamic and pharmacokinetic profiles for screening molecules. Using MC/MD, it is possible to calculate "therapeutic activity values (TAV)" of molecules for 25 common diseases including cancer by binary QSAR disease models. Additionally, toxicities of compounds could also be predicted in 26 different toxicity QSAR models using MC/MD. The *Tanimoto Prioritization (TP)* feature was applied to detect similarity between compounds and training and test set molecules analyzed in QSAR models based on fragments within the structure. QSAR models in the platform were constructed using various compounds based on experimental evidence of their activity/function on a particular protein of interest and then tested with validation sets. Estimated QSAR values (normalized between 0 and 1) >0.5 indicate potential therapeutic activity. The details about QSAR models could be found in the following reference (Kanan et al., 2019). In the current study, we used *"cancer-QSAR"* model, which has the following parameters: Training set $N = 886$, Test set $N = 167$, Sensitivity $= 0.89$, Specificity $= 0.83$, Accuracy $= 0.86$, MCC $= 0.72$.

Ligand Preparation and Protein Preparation

The compounds screened in this study (212, 520 molecules) were downloaded from Specs SC database (https://www.specs.net/index.php). 2D structures were used in binary QSAR models both for therapeutic activity prediction and toxicity prediction. After the target-driven screening and toxicity tests, 250 compounds were filtered and these molecules were prepared with the OPLS2005 forcefield using LigPrep module (Schrödinger Release 2015-2, 2015) of Maestro program (Banks et al., 2005). The possible ionization states at neutral pH 7.4 was determined by Epik module (Shelley et al., 2007). All possible tautomers as well as stereoisomers (if any) were generated. At the end, 342 structures were obtained and used in further docking and MD simulations. Two structures of BCl-2 solved by X-ray diffraction [Protein Data Bank (PDB) IDs, 4LXD (Souers et al., 2013), and 6GL8 (Casara et al., 2018)] along with two structures solved by NMR spectroscopy were retrieved from the PDB [1YSW (Oltersdorf et al., 2005) and 2O2F (Bruncko et al., 2007)]. Here, it should be mentioned that BCL-2 has a region predicted to adopt an unstructured and flexible loop, which caused the protein to be insoluble (Petros et al., 2001; Bruncko et al., 2007). Hence, in NMR studies, as first suggested by Petros et al., residues 35–91 were replaced with residues 35–50 from BCL-XL, and the C-terminal end (residues 208–219) was truncated (Petros et al., 2001). The resulting chimeric protein was very soluble, while still retaining its biological activity. Moreover, a 3D structure of BCL-2 with an intact loop region would be obtained. For crystal structures, although chimeric protein was used, the unstructured loop region could not be resolved due to low electron density and the fact that the loop region was not connected. As this could cause problems during MD simulations, we took the loop conformation from the NMR structure (PDB, 1YSW) for our modeling studies. The numbering of residues was based on the crystal structure with PDB code 4LXD. The missing atoms of proteins were added, and the ions, small molecules used to aid in crystallization, and water molecules not near the cocrystallized ligand (>5 Å) were removed using the Protein Preparation module of Maestro (Sastry et al., 2013). PROPKA (Bas et al., 2008) was employed to adjust protonation states of amino acids at pH of 7.4, and finally, in order to relax the proteins, the target protein was minimized employing the OPLS2005 forcefield parameters (Banks et al., 2005). The binding pocket of BCL-2 was classified based on cocrystallized ligands, and the residues in these regions, together with water molecules, were considered in the construction of grid lattice boxes in molecular docking.

Molecular Docking Simulations

The docking algorithms used in this study include standard precision (SP) module of Glide (Friesner et al., 2004; Halgren et al., 2004) and Induced Fit Docking (IFD) module of Maestro (Sherman et al., 2006a,b) with flexible ligand sampling. The IFD method consists of three consequent phases, including (i) docking of the compounds while the receptor is rigid; (ii) refining the complex residues within 5 Å of the ligand using Prime module (Jacobson et al., 2004); and finally, (iii) redocking of the compounds at the refined binding pocket.

Molecular Dynamics (MD) Simulations and Molecular Mechanics/Generalized Born Surface Area (MM/GBSA) Calculations

We performed MD simulations for apo form of BCL-2 and complexes of BCL-2 with hit compounds using Desmond program (Bowers et al., 2006). Protein–ligand complexes were placed in the cubic boxes with explicit TIP3P water models that have 10.0 Å thickness from surfaces of protein. All systems are neutralized by adding counter ions (Na^+ or Cl^- depending on the charge of the systems), and salt solution of 0.15 M NaCl was also used to adjust the concentration of the systems. The long-range electrostatic interactions were calculated by the particle mesh Ewald method (Essmann et al., 1995). A cut-off radius of 9.0 Å was used for both van der Waals and Coulombic interactions. The temperature was set as 310 K initially, and Nose–Hoover thermostat was used for adjustment (Nosé, 1984; Hoover, 1985). Martyna–Tobias–Klein protocol was employed to control the pressure, which was set at 1.01325 bar (Martyna et al., 1994). The time-step was assigned as 2.0 fs. The default values were used for minimization and equilibration steps, and finally 1-ns (for short MD simulations) and 100-ns (for long MD simulations) production run was performed for each simulation. Other details of the simulation protocols were described in our previous studies (Durdagi et al., 2016; Salmas et al., 2017; Rodrigues et al., 2018). The Prime module of Schrodinger (Jacobson et al., 2004) was used in binding free energy calculations of complexes by MM/GBSA approach (Bashford and Case, 2000). 100 trajectory frames from all MD simulation times were considered for short MD simulations. For longer MD simulations, on the other hand, 100 trajectory frames from the last half of the simulations were used for MM/GBSA calculations. OPLS3 forcefield (Banks et al., 2005) and VSGB 2.0 solvation model (Shan et al., 2011) were utilized during MM/GBSA calculations. All applied procedures for virtual screening in this study have been summarized in **Figure 1**.

Time Resolved Fluorescence Resonance Energy Transfer (TR-FRET)

The BCL-2 TR-FRET Assay (CISBio, Cat. No: 79601) was used to measure the inhibition of BCL-2 to bind its ligand in the presence of BCL-2 inhibitory molecules in a homogeneous 384 well-reaction format. The assay protocol for TR-FRET analysis was performed based on the suggestions of the manufacturer. Briefly, a sample containing terbium-labeled donor, dye-labeled acceptor, BCL-2 protein, peptide ligand, and each inhibitor were incubated for 2 h. All samples and controls were studied in triplicate. Tested concentrations for the molecules were 1 nM, 10 nM, 100 nM, 1 μM, and 10 μM. The fluorescence intensity was measured using a fluorescence reader (Varioskan LUXTM, Thermo Fischer). Two sequential measurements were conducted. First, terbium-donor emission was measured at 620 nm followed by dye-acceptor emission at 665 nm; each fluorescent read was excited at 344 nm. Data analysis was performed using the TR- FRET ratio (665 nm emission/620 nm emission) value. The percent inhibitory activity of tested molecules was calculated by:

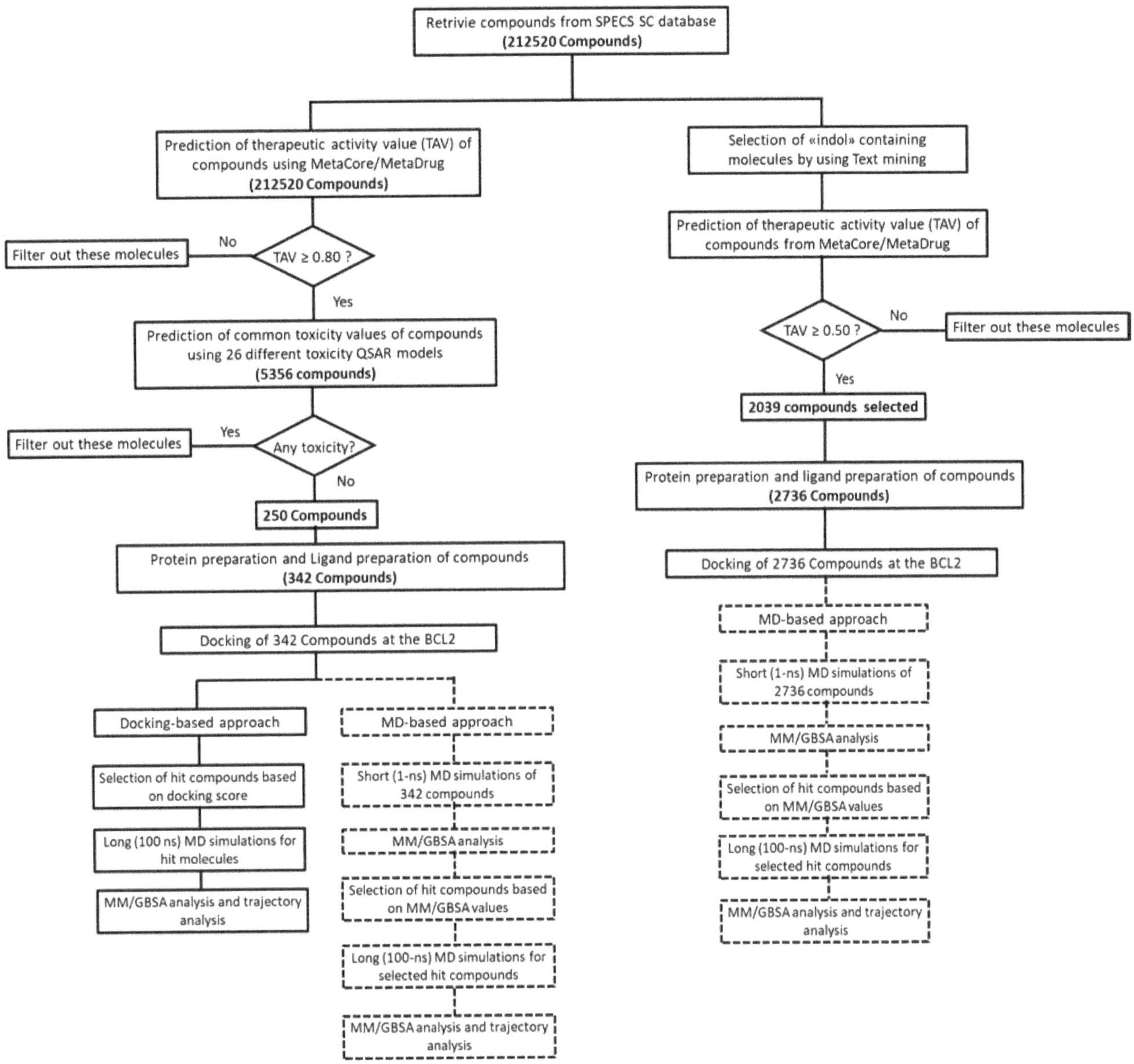

FIGURE 1 | The virtual screening workflow applied with two different approaches.

$$\%Activity = \frac{FRETs - FRETneg}{FRETp - FRETneg} x100\%$$

where *FRETs*, *FRETneg*, and *FRETp* are sample FRET, negative control FRET, and positive control FRET, respectively.

Cell Culture Experiments and 3-(4 5-dimethylthiazol-2-yl)-2 5-diphenyltetrazolium bromide (MTT) Analysis

Various cancer cell lines, such as HCT-116 colon cancer, U87-MG glial tumor, and MCF7 breast cancer cell lines, were used for cell culture experiments. Cells were seeded with high glucose *Dulbecco's* Modified Eagle Medium (DMEM) medium (Biosera) supplemented with 10% fetal bovine serum (FBS) (Gibco) and 1X penicillin/streptomycin (Multicell). Twenty-four hours prior to molecule treatment, 10,000 cells were seeded into each well of 24-well-cell culture plates. Molecules were used by preparing 4 mM stock solution in dimethyl sulfoxide (DMSO) (Amresco). For molecule treatment, molecule stock solutions were diluted in DMEM with 10% FBS and added onto cells in each corresponding well. Final concentration of vehicle DMSO was 2% at maximum. Therefore, the vehicle group in experiments only included a maximum of 2% DMSO concentration. We determined the number of cells to be seeded to make sure that none of the cells reaches more than 60% confluency during the treatment period, as higher plate confluency levels would slow down cell proliferation independently from the molecule treatment.

Values of half-maximal inhibitory concentration were (IC_{50}) determined by MTT cell proliferation assays. Different concentrations of molecules ranging between 10^{-9} and 10^{-4} M were tested on used cell lines with single treatment. Five hundred seventy nanometer absorbance values were recorded, and IC_{50} values were calculated by dose–response inhibition curves and non-linear regression analysis on GraphPad Prism 8 software. For cell proliferation assays, we performed 5-day experiments and repeated experiments at least three times with all cell lines. Survival rates did not change significantly after third day of treatment. Therefore, 3 days results were presented. MTT analysis was performed on 24-well plates with initially 1×10^4 cells/well, grown overnight, and then treated with the selected molecules with different concentrations for at least 3 days. Following the initial incubation day, molecules were added, and, after incubation with MTT at 37°C for 4 h, formazan was solubilized with DMSO (Sigma-Aldrich, St. Louis, USA) and absorbance was measured at 570 nm.

RESULTS

In this work, a small molecule library (Specs-SC) that has 212,520 available drug-like compounds as well as small molecules extracted from available literature were screened initially in MC/MD platform. The molecules were filtered based on their TAV against "cancer" disease model predicted by cancer-QSAR model of MetaCore. The cancer-QSAR model was constructed with 1,053 known compounds from literature, and obtained statistical results were found as follows: Sensitivity: 0.89; Specificity: 0.83; Accuracy: 0.86; MCC: 0.72. Thus, as it can be seen, statistical results validate the constructed cancer-QSAR model. Moreover, we have selected 30 compounds that have high ($IC_{50} \leq 10\,\mu M$) inhibitory activity against BCL-2 based on biological and cell line assays to further validate used QSAR model as suggested in various previous studies (Kumar Yadav et al., 2013, 2014a,b). These molecules are also subjected to cancer-QSAR model to predict their TAV against "cancer." Results showed that 23 out of 30 known inhibitors (more than 75% of the known inhibitors) have potential therapeutic activity (i.e., TAV $\geq$ 0.5) against cancer. Although the predicted QSAR values higher than 0.5 could potentially indicate therapeutic activity, in this study, we considered a higher threshold/cut-off value ($\geq$0.8). By this way, we only considered the molecules that would be predicted as highly therapeutically active in "Cancer-QSAR" model of MC/MD. 5356 molecules had the predicted cancer therapeutic activity values equal or higher than 0.8. Compounds may show high binding affinity, but if they carry undesired side effects, they cannot be considered for future clinical studies. Therefore, their toxicity and pharmacokinetic profiles must be investigated. In our study, we used 26 different toxicity QSAR models and these diverse toxicity models cover most of the commonly observed toxicities such as cardiotoxicity, nephrotoxicity, neurotoxicity, cytotoxicity, kidney necrosis, liver necrosis, etc. Out of 5,356 identified molecules, only 250 molecules showed no toxicities in all these 26 different toxicity QSAR models. These 250 compounds were then prepared with ligand preparation module of Maestro, and, at the end, 342 structures in total, with the possible tautomeric and protonation states, were obtained. All these molecules were then used in molecular docking studies for target protein BCL-2 along with two reference molecules venetoclax and S55746 (bcl201). For S55746, the crystal structure was available; hence, after the preparation of the complex as explained in Materials and Methods section, it was subjected to MD simulations. There was no available crystal structure of BCL-2 that was cocrystallized with venetoclax when this study was conducted, though its analogs were available. Hence, venetoclax was also prepared with LigPrep and molecular docking was used to obtain complex BCL-2/venetoclax.

The common weaknesses of docking algorithms were established by the comparative evaluation study of Li et al. (2014) as mentioned above. Molecular docking method sometimes could lead to elimination of true binders and/or false positive compounds since only top-ranked molecules would be considered as selected candidates for *in vitro* tests. Protein structure being considered as mainly rigid during docking is one of the major weaknesses. As such, here we have applied two different approaches: (i) an induced fit docking in which residues in binding pocket were considered as flexible; (ii) short MD simulations in which protein–ligand complex was relaxed to dispose clashes between protein and ligand. **Figure 1** shows the workflow applied in this study. It can be seen that we have also identified compounds that contain "*indol*" phrases using text mining to be considered for ligand- and structure-based studies of BCL-2 inhibitors.

Docking-Based Approach for Selection of Hit Molecules

The top-docking scores of five molecules and their 2D structures as well as corresponding data for reference molecules venetoclax and S55746 could be found in **Table S1**. To test the validity and reliability of docking approach as performed in previous studies (Chen et al., 2006), we have also redocked the cocrystallized ligand found in the crystal structure of BCL-2 (PDB ID, 4LXD). We have seen that the docking pose obtained with our protocol was able to reproduce the crystal pose with a root mean square deviation (RMSD) of 0.65 Å (i.e., after alignment between docked pose and cocrystallized pose, RMSD was 0.65 Å). As it can be seen from **Table S1**, venetoclax has the highest docking score (−15.46 kcal/mol) at BCL-2 cavity. However, venetoclax is a very large molecule [molecular weight (MW), 868 g/mol] that contains 61 non-hydrogen atoms, which could lead to high docking score, and in fact its ligand efficiency score (i.e., docking score per number of non-hydrogen atoms) was lower than the suggested compounds (**Table S1**). The molecules with the top-docking scores were smaller than venetoclax and S55746. However, they have high ligand efficiency scores, which could indicate that they could be lead compounds for further studies. For that reason, we performed MD simulations (100 ns) for these compounds in complex with BCL-2 protein starting from IFD docking poses. Although we carried out MD simulations for all five complexes as well as for two reference molecules in complex with BCL-2, we will only discuss the results for three compounds: **43** (Specs ID: AO-081/41887762); compound **58** (Specs ID: AJ-292/12931005); and compound **243** (Specs ID: AN-698/40780701), as they were chosen for *in vitro* studies.

MD-Based Approach for the Selection of Hit Molecules

The top-scoring docking poses for all 342 compounds were subjected to 1-ns short MD simulations, and the average binding free energies were calculated for MD trajectory frames using MM/GBSA approach. An in-house script was used for the preparation of simulation boxes as well as for the analysis of MD simulations. Compounds were then ranked based on average MM/GBSA scores, and, as shown in **Figure S1**, the normal distribution of MM/GBSA scores of studied 342 compounds and Z-scores of the distribution curves were plotted. Then, we selected compounds that have average MM/GBSA values above $Z \leq -2$, i.e., 12 molecules were chosen. The complexes of these compounds with BCL-2 were subjected to longer (100 ns) MD simulations. The structures and average MM/GBSA values of all these selected compounds could be found in **Table S2**. Although we have performed longer MD simulations for all 12 compounds in complex with the target protein, we selected only three of the compounds for *in vitro* tests, **258** (Specs ID: AK-968/12163470), **292** (Specs ID: AK-968/11842328), and **243** (Specs ID: AN-698/40780701). It should be noted that compound **243** was also found as a hit compound and selected based on docking approach.

Text Mining Approach for Selection of Hit Compounds

Since many currently used FDA-approved chemotherapeutics include indole derivatives, Specs-SC database that includes only *"indol"* groups (i.e., indoles, indolons, bisindoles, etc.) were also screened at the binding pocket of the BCL-2. Thus, *"indol"* keyword was searched as text within the 212,000 compounds and around 2700 compounds were identified. These *"indol"* phrase containing molecules were subjected to binary QSAR tests using MC/MD platform and specifically the "cancer-QSAR" model was chosen as before. Since indole derivatives are known to have high therapeutic activity potential, here we initially used a lower TAV threshold (0.5) to begin screening with a large number of molecules that include the *"indol"* phrase. Molecules that showed higher TAV values than 0.5 were docked at the binding pocket of BCL-2 using Glide/SP. Top-docking poses of these compounds were then used in MD simulations. 2700 individual MD simulations boxes were prepared with an in-house script, and 1-ns MD simulations were conducted and the average MM/GBSA scores were calculated. The normal distribution of MM/GBSA values as well as Z-scores of the distribution showed that there were 83 compounds with Z-scores lower than −2 (see **Figure 2**). As performing 100-ns MD simulation for all 83 complexes would require considerable computer time and power, we instead chose to perform 10-ns MD simulations for these compounds in complex with BCL-2 and again used MM/GBSA approach to calculate their average binding free energies. After 10-ns MD simulations, top-10 MM/GBSA-scored *"indol"* phrase containing molecules were forwarded for 100-ns MD simulations and their average MM/GBSA scores were calculated. **Table S3** shows the 2D structures and average MM/GBSA scores for these 10 compounds. We have selected two of them for *in vitro* studies: **ind-199** (AG-205/12549135) **and ind-435** (AN-329/13484046).

Analysis of Selected Compounds and Their Interactions With BCL-2

Although molecular docking studies could give an initial insight into protein–ligand interactions, it is always crucial to understand the maintenance of these interactions and perform dynamical studies as MD simulations for complexes. Hence, we performed MD simulations and analyzed the interactions observed during the simulations between protein and ligands. While we conducted 100-ns MD simulations for 29 compounds in total (including the reference molecules) in complex with BCL-2, we selected seven of them for *in vitro* studies based on their docking scores, MM/GBSA values, and their interactions with the target protein. Here, we will focus our analysis and discussion on these seven compounds that could be lead compounds as BCL-2 inhibitors. Before analyzing the ligand–protein interactions, the trajectories obtained from the simulations were firstly analyzed to examine the protein and ligand structure stability. RMSD and the root mean square fluctuations (RMSF) were used to measure the displacements of atoms for each frame with respect to the initial frame/structure and to categorize the local changes along protein structures, respectively (**Figures S2, S3**). Here, we have only plotted the RMSD graphs of studied proteins based on alpha carbons (C_α). As it can be seen from the figure, for compounds other than *"indol"* phrase containing ones, the RMSD plots do not change significantly after 50-ns and they reach a plateau. However, mainly in indol-containing molecules, RMSD values did not stabilize and conformational changes were observed during MD simulations (**Figure S4**). It can be seen that it was the unstructured loop region 31–89, not alpha-helix regions, that had higher displacement (**Figures S3, S4**). For **ind-199**, some unexpected helix formation is observed for this region, though the helix could not be conserved. The RMSF plot for protein targets in complex with selected compounds also confirmed that it was the loop region for which highest displacements were observed (**Figure S3**). Additionally, we checked the RMSD of the ligand molecules by considering two different fitting modes: "fit on protein/profit" and "fit on ligand/ligfit." While the first mode indicates the structural stability of ligand with respect to protein, i.e., its translational motion, the second mode shows the internal fluctuations of the ligand atoms in its binding pocket, i.e., its rotational motion. As can been seen from **Figure 3**, the profit RMSD plot shows that after initial 50 ns, most of the compounds did not move away from the binding pocket. However, compound **58** had a very high RMSD value (around 7.0 Å), which showed that it has high mobility in the binding pocket. In fact, **Figure S4** shows that the compound **58** completely changed its initial binding pose in the hydrophobic groove just after initial 20 ns, but then it did not have high mobility and stayed in the pocket as can be seen by lower

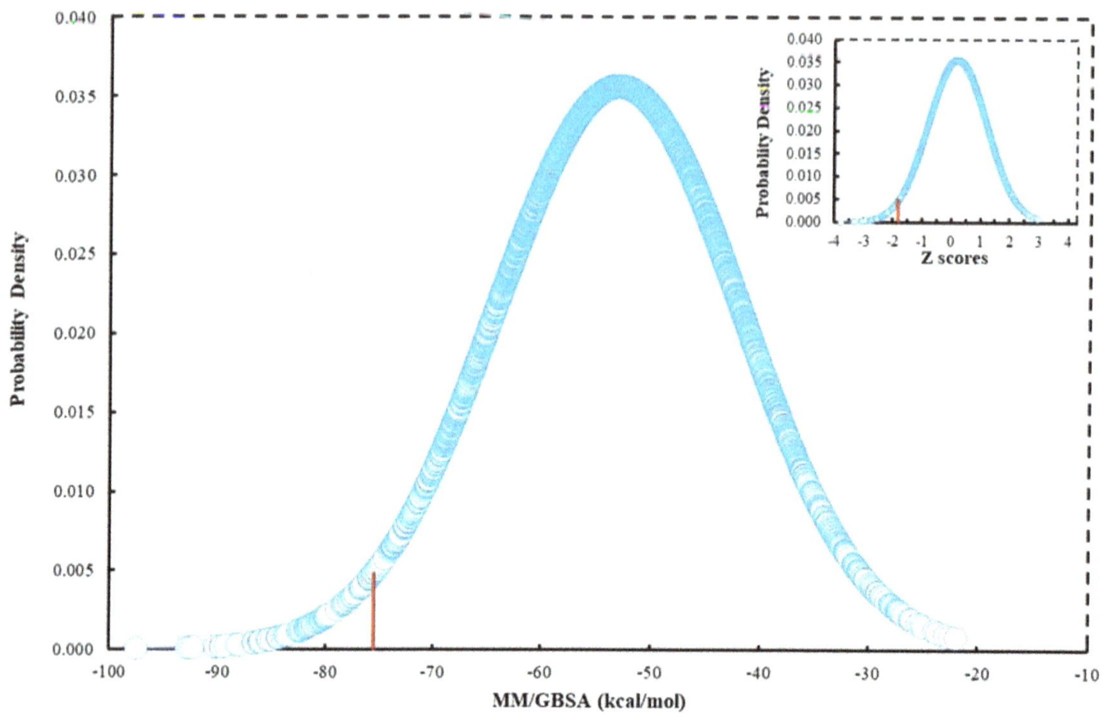

FIGURE 2 | MM/GBSA scores of around 2700 molecules that include "indol" phrases.

RMSD values and also small conformational changes. Indol-containing molecule **ind-435** also displayed high mobility in the binding pocket as can be observed in **Figure 3** and **Figure S4**. The RMSD for this compound did not really reach a plateau value. The size of this compound was actually considerably bigger than other molecules and has flexible regions. Hence, it extended from its initial binding pocket to the one next to it (e.g., hydrophobic grooves P1 to P4). Compound **243** has also higher profit RMSD values especially after 80 ns, and careful analysis of MD trajectories showed that it was mostly the phenyl ring that was attached thiazolidine group moving in pocket P1. The rotational movements (ligfit RMSDs) of the selected compounds could be seen in **Figure 4**. We observed that venetoclax did not also obtain a stable RMSD plot, though the values themselves were not higher than 3.0 Å for ligfit mode. As a large molecule, these rotational movements were not surprising. It was also not unexpected for **ind-435** as a large molecule with flexible alkyl chain to have high rotational RMSD values as seen in **Figure 4**. Compound **58** was found with higher RMSD values for ligfit mode; however, after 50 ns, the changes in RMSD values were smaller. All of the compounds at the end reached a kind of plateau value for rotational RMSD of ligands.

BCL-2 protein interacts with BH3-only proteins via hydrophobic groove on its surface, which contains four pockets: P1, P2, P3, and P4 pockets. To prevent the interaction of proapoptotic proteins such as BAX and BAK with BCL-2, which is an antiapoptotic protein, these pockets need to be filled by either small molecules or BH3-mimetics. It is important for these molecules to interact with key residues that mediate interaction between BCL-2 and BH3-only proteins. Based on the literature data, some of these crucial residues are as follows (numbering based on PDB code 4LXD): Asp100, Phe101, Arg104, Tyr105, Asp108, Phe109, Tyr199, Asn140, Gly142, Arg143, and Ala146. Additionally, we have analyzed the MD simulations of reference compounds venetoclax and S55746 in complex with BCL-2. The protein surfaces as well as 2D and 3D ligand interactions between protein and molecules were represented for venetoclax and S55746 in **Figure 5** and **Figure S5**, respectively. Consistent with the previously published data, S55746 bind and fill the pockets P1 to P2, while venetoclax could fill all four pockets on the surface from P1 to P4 (Birkinshaw et al., 2019). When this project was initiated, there was no cocrystallized venetoclax-bound form of the BCL-2. Here, we also checked the binding pose of venetoclax as the crystal structure of BCL-2 bound to venetoclax recently became available (Birkinshaw et al., 2019). A slight difference in binding pose of venetoclax was in the more flexible region of oxane fragment; however, with the rest of the compound, similar amino acid moieties interact by the identical parts of venetoclax in both poses. Based on the trajectory analysis of venetoclax, it was seen that venetoclax preserved its interactions with Asp100 and Phe101 more than 50% of the simulation time (**Figure S5**). Gly142 and Arg104 were also seen as interacting residues. Interaction with the backbone carbonyl oxygen atom of Ala143 was the most conserved interaction during MD simulations for S55746 (99%, **Figure 5**). Also, Arg143 and Phe101 formed π-cation and π-π stacking interactions with S55746, respectively. Based on these results, we analyzed the complexes of BCL-2 protein with selected hit

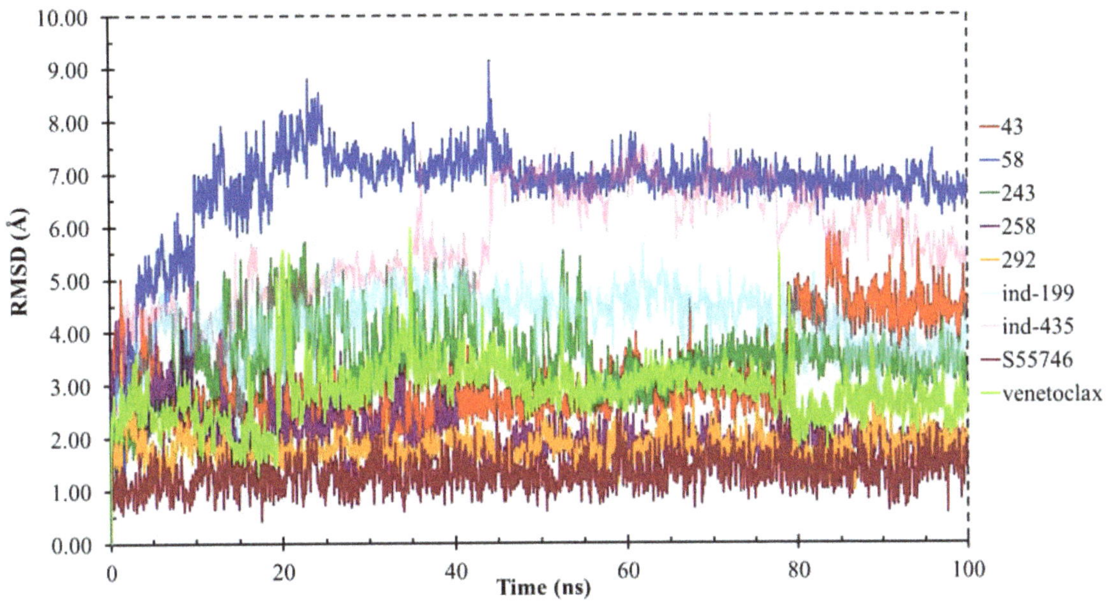

FIGURE 3 | ProFit RMSD graphs for the hit and reference compounds.

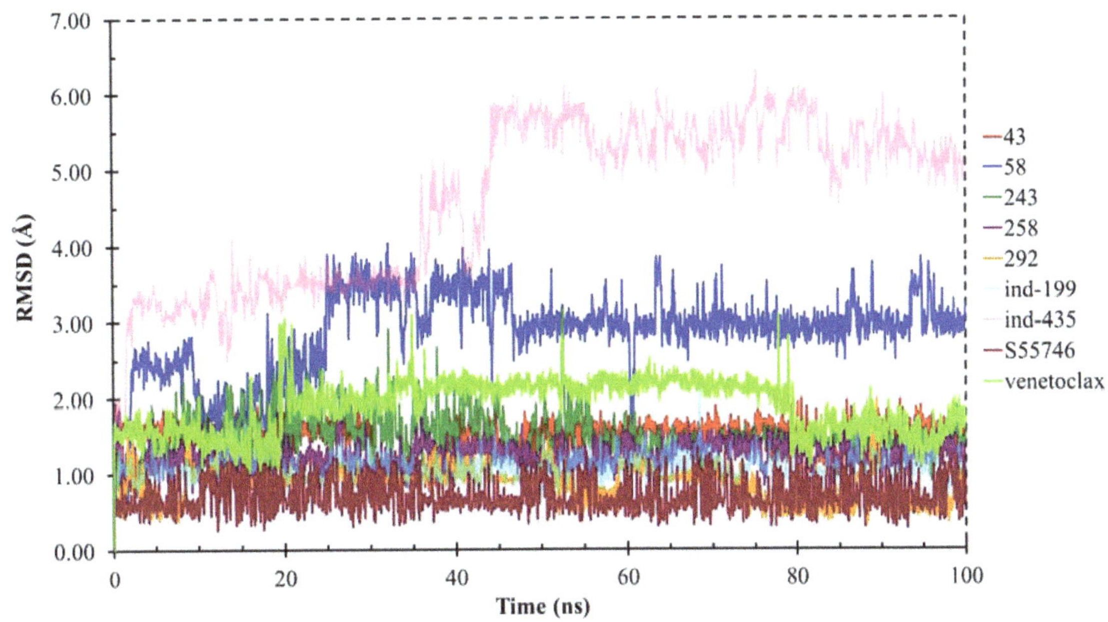

FIGURE 4 | LigFit RMSD graphs for the hit and reference compounds.

compounds as well as examined their ability to fill the pockets P1 to P4. Compound **43,** which can mainly bind BCL-2 via P2 and P3 pockets, consistently formed hydrogen bonds with Asp137 (96%) and π-π stacking interactions with residues Phe101 and Tyr105 of P2 pocket, although these later interactions were not preserved (16 and 24% of MD time, **Figure S6**). Compound **58** can mainly fill the pockets P1 to P3 of BCL-2 similar to S55746. It formed stable hydrogen bonding interactions with two key residues Asp108 and Asn140 (64 and 67%, respectively, **Figure 6**). Compound **243,** on the other hand, interacted with the residues of pockets P1 to P4. A π-π stacking interaction with Phe101 of P1 pocket was observed for 49% of MD simulation time, while its interactions with other key residues such as Tyr105, Asn140, and Arg143 were less conserved (**Figure S7**). Compound **258** was mainly found in pockets P2 to P4, and its most conserved interaction was observed to be with Tyr105.

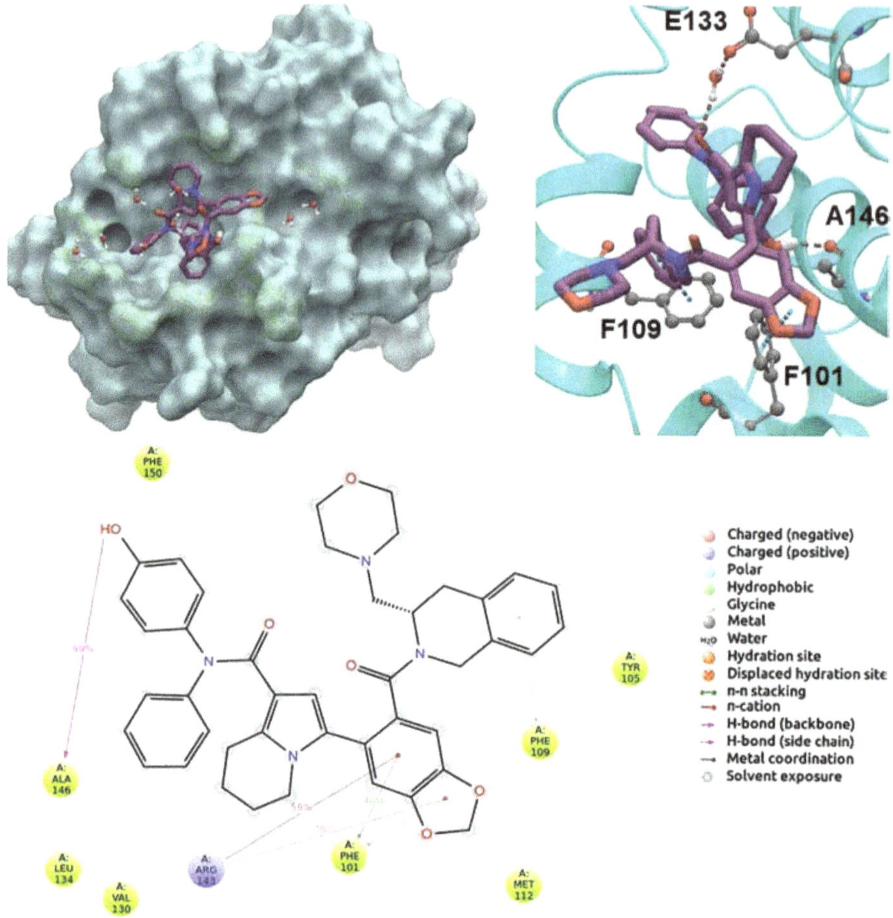

FIGURE 5 | 2D and 3D ligand interactions diagrams of selected positive control molecule S55746 at the binding pocket of BCL-2. Surface and ribbon representation are displayed for representative structure obtained from MD simulations, while 2D interaction diagram shows the systematic details of protein-ligand interactions observed during MD.

Not only did it form hydrogen bonds with Tyr105 but it also formed π-π stacking interactions, albeit they were not persistent interactions (17%, **Figure S8**). Compound **292** was an analog of compound **258;** as such, similar binding poses were expected, but their binding modes were quite different. Compound **292** formed persistent hydrogen bonding interactions with Asp108 (73%, **Figure S9**). H-bond and π-cation interactions with Arg143 were also observed for compound **292.** The chosen *"indol"* containing molecules were larger molecules compared to other five selected molecules; as such, they are able to fill the pockets P1 to P4. Compound **ind-199** formed a stable hydrogen bond with Asn140 (70%), π-cation, and salt bridge interactions with Arg104 (**Figure S10**). Although it also formed π-π stacking interactions with Phe109 and Phe150, these interactions were not persistent (13 and 22%, respectively). Compound **ind-435** not only filled all four pockets but also moved closer to carbonyl terminal part of BCL-2. A persistent hydrogen bond with Asp100 (55% of MD time) was observed, and additionally it interacts and with residues Phe100 and Arg143 (**Figure S11**).

We have also calculated the binding free energies for selected compounds as well as reference molecules in complex with BCL-2 using MM/GBSA approach after 100 ns MD simulations. In **Figure 7**, the MM/GBSA energies calculated for the trajectory frames observed during MD were plotted. It can be seen that venetoclax had lower MM/GBSA values compared to selected compounds. However, some of the selected compounds such as compound **243**, **ind-435,** and **ind-199** have considerable MM/GBSA values to other reference molecule S55746.

TR-FRET Analysis Confirms the Inhibitory Activity of Identified Hit Molecules on BCL2

TR-FRET analysis revealed that four of seven tested molecules compete with BCL2 ligand in binding. In presence of inhibitory molecules, BCL2 binding to its ligand was suppressed in a concentration- dependent manner. Compounds **58**, **ind-199**, **243**, and **292** showed the maximum inhibitory effect in ranging between 60 and 100% in 10 μM concentrations

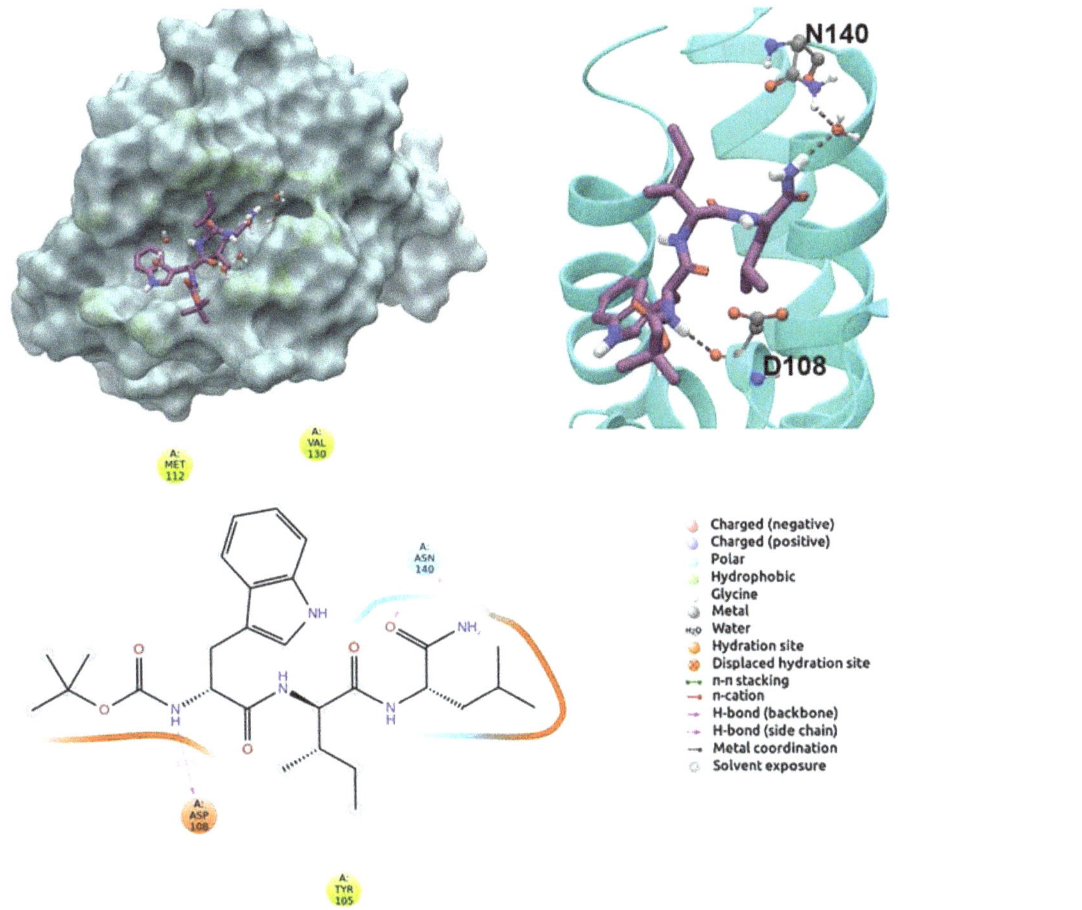

FIGURE 6 | 2D and 3D ligand interactions diagrams of selected hit molecule **58** at the binding pocket of BCL-2. Surface and ribbon representation are displayed for representative structure obtained from MD simulations, while 2D interaction diagram shows the systematic details of protein-ligand interactions observed during MD.

(**Figure 8**). However, three of selected molecules showed minimal inhibitory activity on BCL2 ranging from 10 to 40% with concentration-independent manner. We suppose that activity is correlated with solubility of the molecules since inactive molecules were found among partially soluble molecules.

Cell Proliferation Was Restricted by Using BCL2 Inhibitory Molecules

Together with TR-FRET analysis, selected hit compounds were also evaluated in various cancer cell lines, such as HCT-116 colon cancer, U87-MG glial tumor, MCF7 breast cancer cell lines, and IC_{50} values of selected molecules were calculated (**Table 1**). Of seven selected hits, five of them showed micromolar level of inhibitory concentrations, which is an acceptable range in cell culture experiments. Compound **258** did not show inhibitory activity on any of the tested cell-line assays.

To test whether BCL-2 inhibitory molecules had any effect on biological activity, we conducted cell proliferation assays and also evaluated apoptosis by observing cell structure and counting apoptotic cells. All molecules were tested on three different cancer cell lines, and all molecules showed similar effects on different cell types. The dose–response curves for all cell lines were shown in **Figures S12–S14**. Of seven molecules, four showed biological activity on MTT experiments. Molecules **58**, **ind-199**, **43,** and **243** with 100 μM concentration significantly limited the cell proliferation capacity of cancer cells. Four biologically active molecules showed their efficacy starting from the first hour of treatment by decreasing the number of proliferating cells. At the first day of treatment, only 60–70% of cells survived, while the number of proliferating cells decreased to <40% at the end of third day (**Figure 9**). MTT assay results for cell lines U87-MG and MCF7 were displayed in **Figures S15, S16**, respectively. Compared to untreated and DMSO only treated (vehicle) group, these four hit molecules showed significant activity. Lack of activity of other three compounds might be due to their low/moderate solubilities. Furthermore, the activity of the molecules was more dominant at cancer cells. We also tested these molecules on non-cancerous HUVEC cells, and none of the molecules showed significant reduction in cell viability (**Figure S17**). When we observed the cells under a microscope for the inactive molecules, we saw precipitates of molecules. Further, despite all efforts for

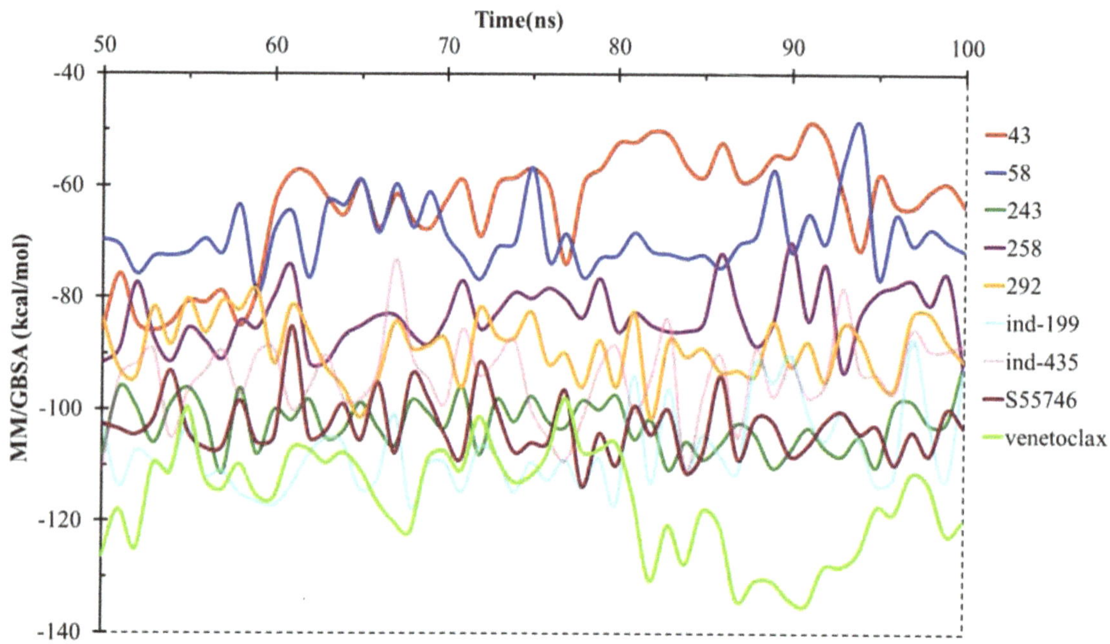

FIGURE 7 | MM/GBSA free energy analysis for the studied molecules at the binding pocket of BCL-2 throughout the last half of the MD simulations.

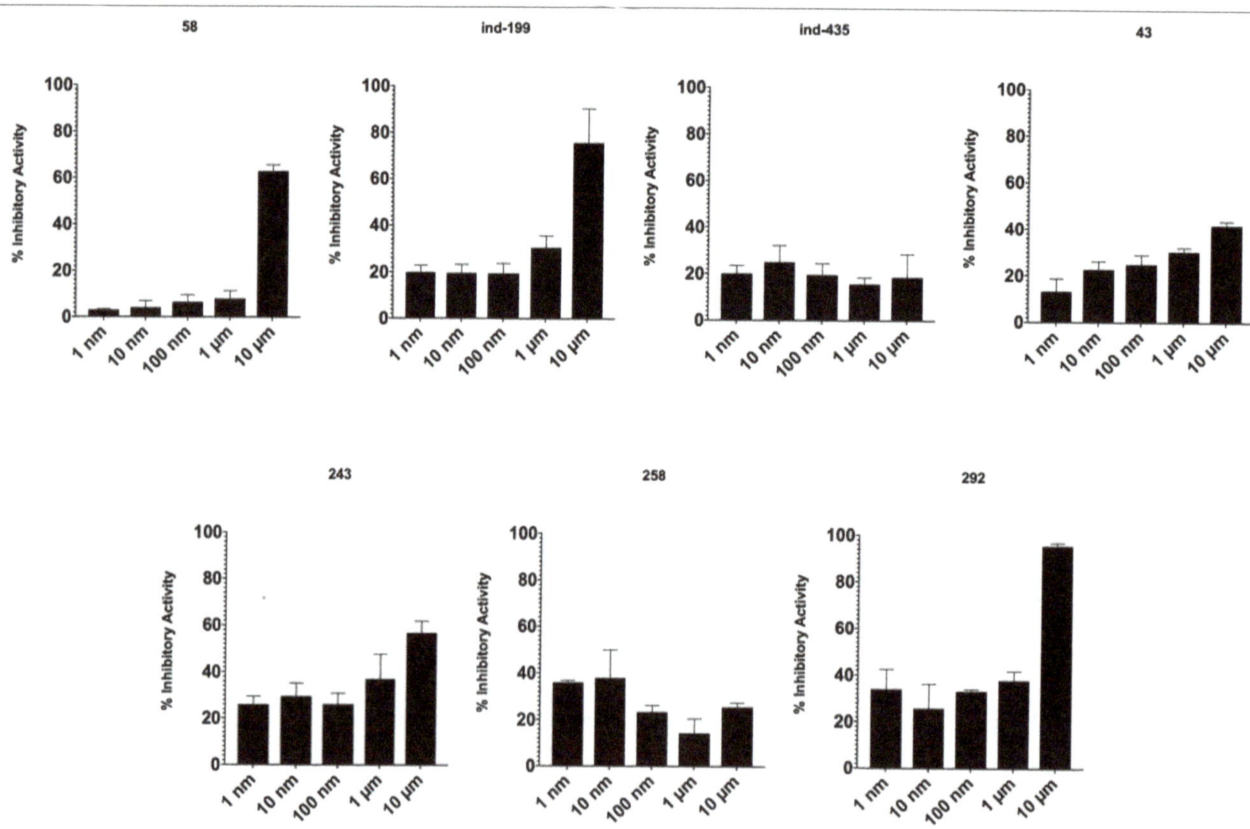

FIGURE 8 | Inhibitory activity of tested molecules. Activity of the molecules was assessed by the formula given in Materials and Methods section.

TABLE 1 | The specs ID, 2D structure, average MM/GBSA values, and maximal % inhibitory activity at 10μM concentrations, as well as IC_{50} values of selected hit compounds and reference molecules.

Compounds (specs ID)	2D structure	MM/GBSA (kcal/mol)	% inhibitory activity at 10 μM	IC_{50} (μM) for HTC116 cells	IC_{50} (μM) for U87-MG cells	IC_{50} (μM) for MCF7 cells
43 (AO-081/41887762)	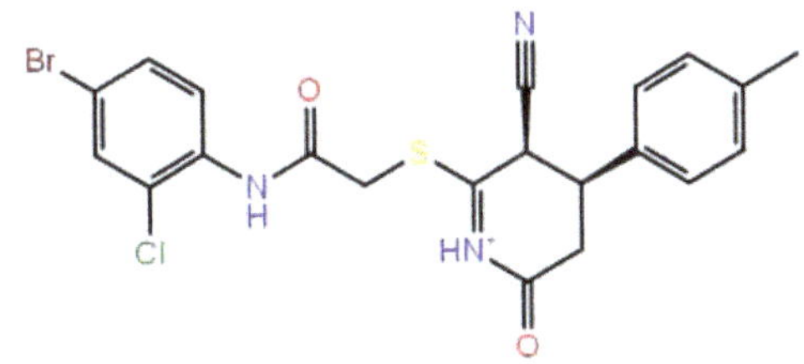	−64.15 ± 10.37	41.78 ± 1.76	24 ± 2.53	26 ± 1.73	30 ± 8.27
58 (AJ-292/12931005)	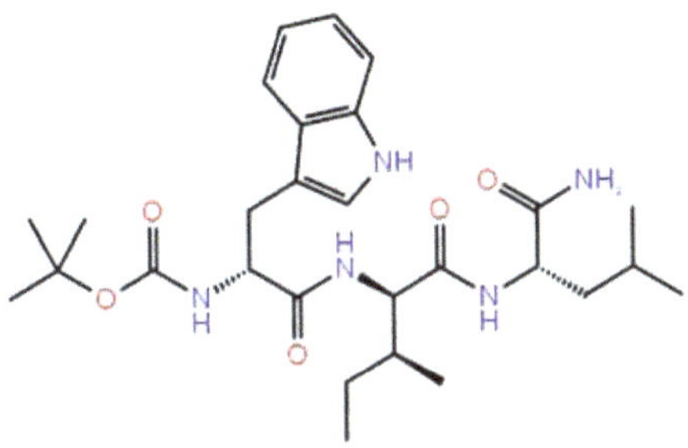	−68.84 ± 6.03	62.84 ± 2.73	17 ± 1.59	18 ± 2.29	21 ± 3.34
243 (AN-698/40780701)	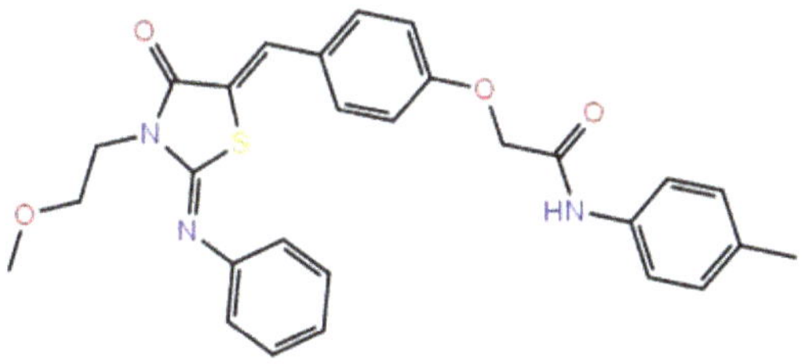	−102.65 ± 4.56	56.78 ± 5.02	25 ± 1.77	29 ± 2.55	31 ± 3.96
258 (AK-968/12163470)	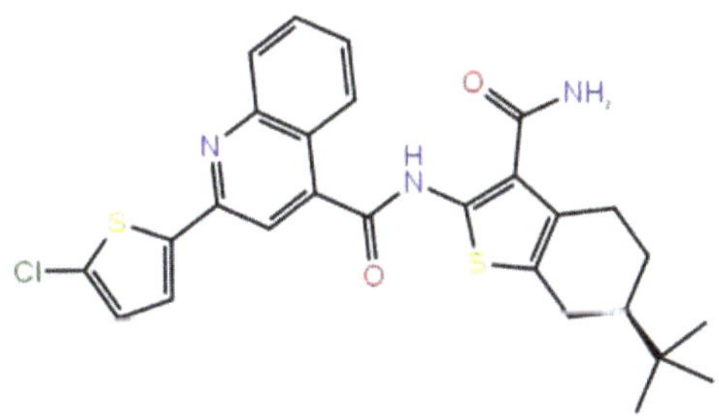	−83.50 ± 5.46	25.60 ± 1.84	NA[†]	NA[†]	NA[†]
292 (AK-968/11842328)	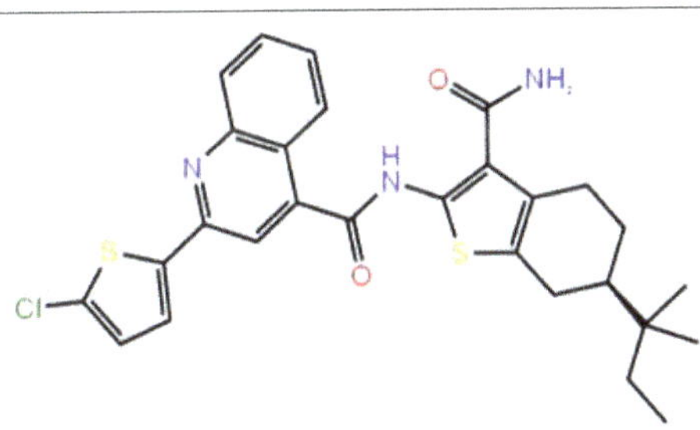	−88.93 ± 5.46	95.63 ± 1.27	130 ± 25.59	122 ± 33.21	150 ± 33.50

(Continued)

TABLE 1 | Continued

Compounds (specs ID)	2D structure	MM/GBSA (kcal/mol)	% inhibitory activity at 10 μM	IC_{50} (μM) for HTC116 cells	IC_{50} (μM) for U87-MG cells	IC_{50} (μM) for MCF7 cells
ind-199 **(AG-205/12549135)**	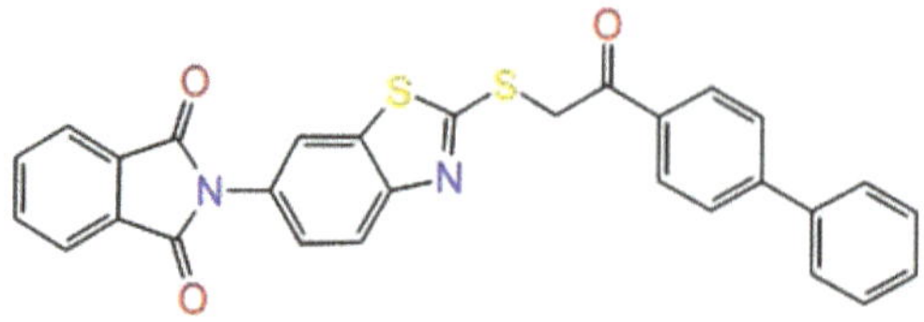	−107.41 ± 7.49	75.64 ± 14.65	22 ± 3.41	28 ± 4.46	26 ± 4.89
ind-435 (AN-329/13484046)	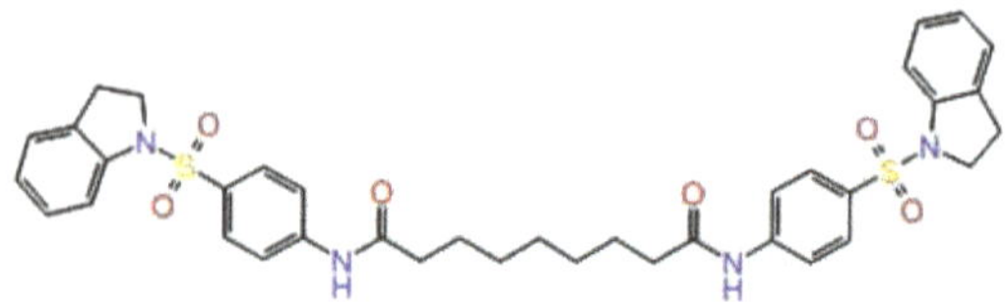	−94.17 ± 7.28	18.51 ± 9.91	NA†	NA†	NA†
venetoclax	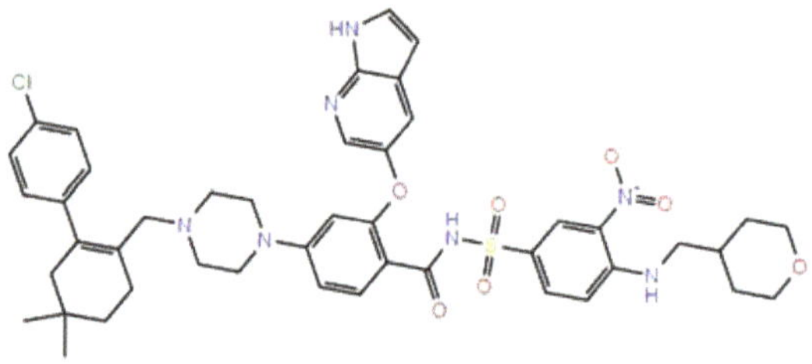	−116.31 ± 9.20	NA†	3.5*	22.9*	24.7*
S55746 (CHEMBL3958369)	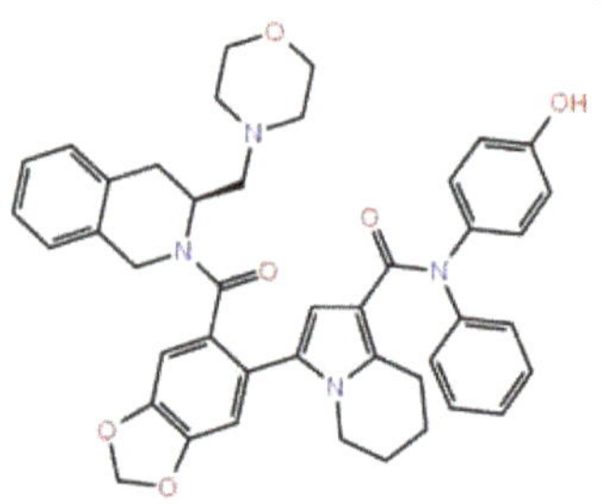	−101.43 ± 4.20	NA†	NA†	NA†	NA†

*†Not applied. *Taken from The Genomics of Drug Sensitivity in Cancer (GDSC) database (www.cancerRxgene.org) for HTC-116 cell line.*

increasing the solubility levels of these inactive compounds in DMSO, it failed to obtain a pure solubilized form of the molecules.

We also observed massive cell detachment and dying cells in cell culture plates (**Figure 10**), and formation of apoptotic cell bodies having circular structure rather than normal. Especially for the compound **58**, apoptotic cell bodies were abundant, and it immediately affected the cells upon the first hour of treatment. However, for the compounds **43** and **243**, despite apoptotic cell bodies having formed, there were still some unaffected cell residues that survived and proliferated. Cell detachment, cell death, and apoptotic bodies indicate apoptotic cell death. Our data altogether suggest that at 100 μM, concentrations of compounds **58, ind-199, 43,** and **243** induce apoptotic cell death.

Inhibition of antiapoptotic protein BCL-2 that is overexpressed in cancer cells is one of the most studied approaches in cancer research. Currently, venetoclax is the only approved drug by the FDA for the treatment of chronic lymphocytic leukemia (CLL), and it is a selective BCL-2 protein inhibitor. Although it has a very high affinity for BCL-2 as shown in various studies performed on different cancer cell lines (Yang et al., 2012) (www.cancerrxgene.org), resistance to this drug has already been observed (Birkinshaw et al., 2019). Hence, it is necessary to suggest new compounds and scaffolds as BCL-2 inhibitors that could be more efficient against mutations on the target structure and have no side effects. As such, in this study, we performed combined ligand- and structure-based approaches as well as text mining to propose new inhibitors against BCL-2 target protein. We selected seven hit compounds of which two are "*indol*"-based molecules. These compounds were considered in cancer cell line assays, and their IC_{50} values are calculated (**Table 1**). Based on the experimental findings, compound **58,** which has an IC_{50} value of 17 μM, was found to promote apoptosis, and it was the most effective of the seven compounds. Some of the selected hit molecules (compounds **258** and **292**) for *in vitro* analysis could only be partially solubilized in DMSO; therefore, solubility issue may restrict the activity of the compounds.

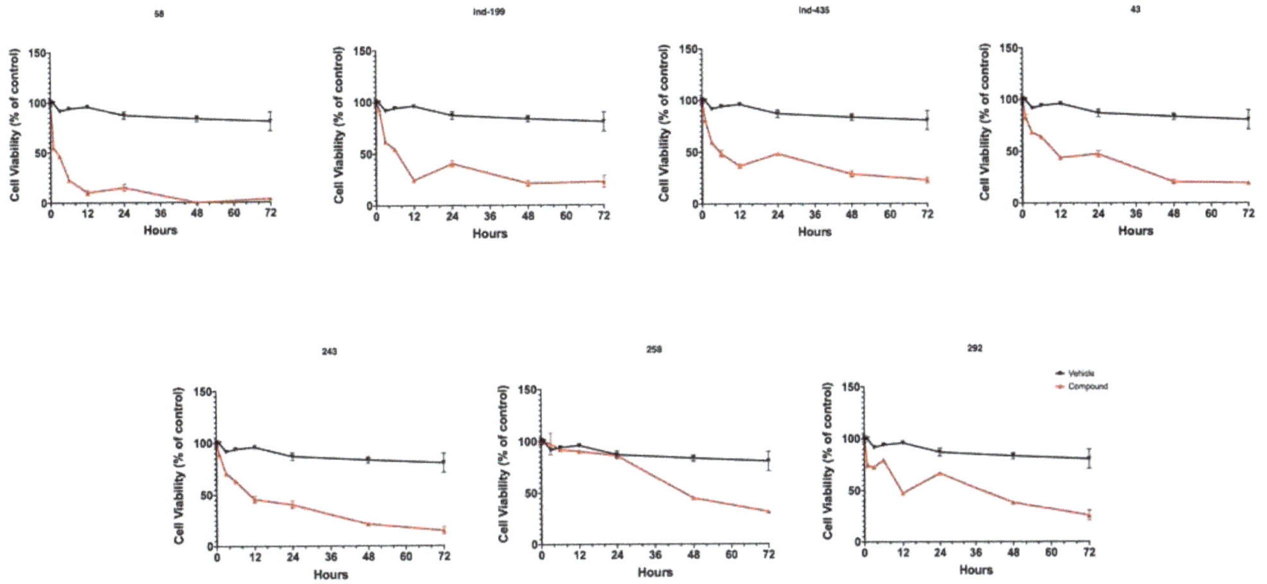

FIGURE 9 | MTT cell proliferation assay. Molecules having inhibitory activity were shown. Tested concentration for each drug was 100 μM. Statistical significance in graphs was determined by comparing each treatment group with DMSO control using ANOVA testing, and significance is considered as $p < 0.001$. Error bars show standard deviation.

When we have considered and compared the structures of selected hit molecules, specifically compounds that inhibited the proliferation of cancer cells such as compounds **58**, **ind-199**, **43**, and **243**, we have observed that all except compound **58** contains sulfur-containing groups such as sulfanyl or thiazole derivatives. All four molecules contain aromatic rings as well as amide groups in their structures, which are also groups observed in FDA-approved drug venetoclax and under development compound S55746. It must be noted that together with identified two indol-based compounds, **58** also involves an indole ring in its structure; thus, it validates the importance of indoles or indole derivatives in the scaffolds of potent BCL2 inhibitors. It must also be noted that the proposed hit molecules have lower molecular weights (MW) (between 490 and 529 g/mol) than the known BCL-2 inhibitors venetoclax (MW, 868 g/mol) and S55746 (MW, 710 g/mol) which indicate that the suggested compounds could be used as lead compounds for further optimization studies by small modifications. See .sdf file for structures of hit compounds along with their properties such as TAV, docking score, toxicity values, etc. in Data Sheet 1 in the **Supplementary Material**.

Overall, our results surprisingly show that docking-initiated screening has a better success rate compared to MD-initiated screening. However, this surprising result may be due to unexpected partial solubilities of some of the tested compounds that showed limited activity on cells.

CONCLUSIONS

In this work, a molecular library (Specs-SC) composed of 212,520 molecules was first filtered for their therapeutic effect against cancer, and then obtained molecules again filtered to remove toxic compounds using MC/MD from Clarivate Analytics. Identified 342 non-toxic and potent compounds using MC/MD were then screened based on target-driven approaches using available BCL-2 structures. In order to compare the both structural and energetic results, known BCL-2 inhibitors were used as positive control molecules and same computational protocols were applied for these compounds. Identified hit molecules from both docking and short (i.e., 1-ns) MM/GBSA calculations that have similar/better binding energies were compared to known inhibitors, then subjected to longer (i.e., 100-ns) MD simulations. In the virtual screening, two different strategies were considered and compared in the selection of hit compounds: (i) Compounds were ranked by their docking scores and long (100-ns) MD simulations were performed for the selected compounds and average MM/GBSA energies were calculated; (ii) Short (1-ns) MD simulations were performed for top-docking poses of all 342 compounds and average MM/GBSA scores were considered for the selection of molecules in long (100-ns) MD simulations of small molecules database. At the end, seven molecules were suggested as new scaffolds for inhibition of BCL-2. Compounds **58** (AJ-292/12931005), **ind-199** (AG-205/12549135), **43** (AO-081/41887762), and **243** (AN-698/40780701) with 100 μM concentration significantly limited the cell proliferation capacity of cancer cells. Four biologically active molecules showed their efficacy starting from the first hour of treatment by decreasing the number of proliferating cells. At the first day of treatment, only 60–70% of cells survived, while the number of proliferating cells decreased to <40% at the end of third day. TR-FRET analysis revealed that hit compounds **58**, **ind-199**, **243**, and **292** showed the maximum inhibitory effect ranging between 60 and 100% in 10 μM concentration. Thus, most of the active compounds found in the cell line tests

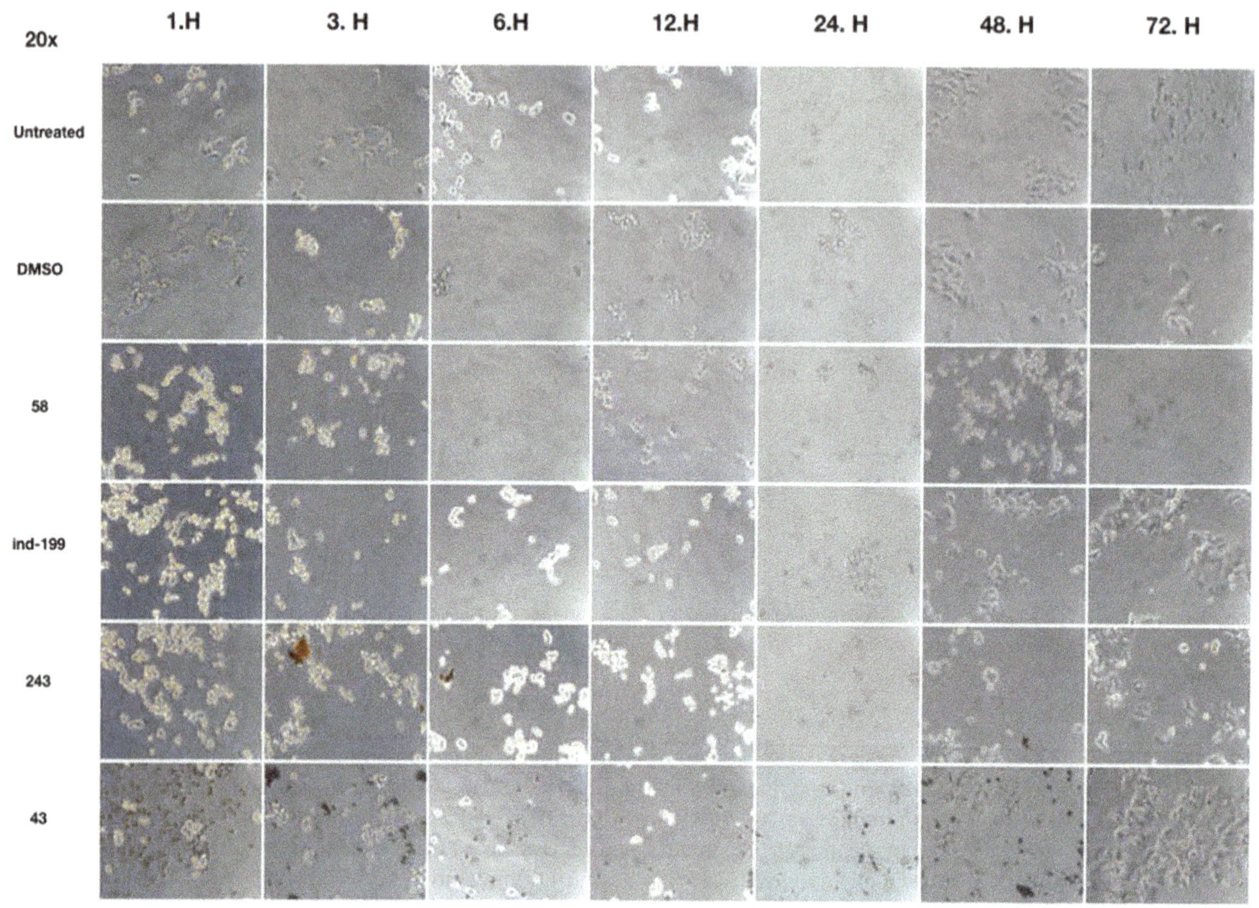

FIGURE 10 | Microscopic evaluation of HCT-116 cells for compounds **58** (AJ-292/12931005), **ind-199** (AG-205/12549135), **43** (AO-081/41887762), and **243** (AN-698/40780701). Cells were photographed and observed under microscope for 3 days. Vehicle group showed neat proliferation of cells as untreated group did, whereas molecule-treated groups reduced proliferation and showed apoptotic cell structures. Compound **58** (AJ-292/12931005) showed clear apoptotic activity from the first day, whereas other molecules showed limited activity. At 48 and 72 h of treatment in other groups, resistant cells are visible together with the unresolved molecule precipitates. However, there are no resistant cells and all cells seemed to be affected by the molecule **58** on treated group for all 3 days.

were also found potent in enzymatic assays. Results showed that compounds identified via integrated text-mining and docking initiated MM/GBSA-scores based approach has higher success rate. Thus, the results of this study may open new avenues for the designing of new BCL-2 inhibitor scaffolds.

AUTHOR CONTRIBUTIONS

BD and SD constructed the methodology and wrote the manuscript. SD also guided the studies, revised the paper, and managed laboratory resources and research funding. GT and BD performed molecular modeling studies. MO, SC, and TA conducted the experimental studies and wrote the manuscript.

FUNDING

BD has been supported by The Scientific and Technological Research Council of Turkey (TUBITAK) under the program of TUBITAK-2218. This work has been supported by Bahcesehir University, Project Code: BAP.2019-02.10. The numerical calculations reported in this paper were partially performed at TUBITAK ULAKBIM, High Performance and Grid Computing Center (TRUBA resources).

ACKNOWLEDGMENTS

We would like to thank Ismail Erol, Umit Yilmaz, and Canberk Ozbaykus for a helpful discussion.

REFERENCES

Banks, J. L., Beard, H. S., Cao, Y., Cho, A. E., Damm, W., Farid, R., et al. (2005). Integrated modeling program, applied chemical theory (IMPACT). *J. Comput. Chem.* 26, 1752–1780. doi: 10.1002/jcc.20292

Bas, D. C., Rogers, D. M., and Jensen, J. H. (2008). Very fast prediction and rationalization of pKa values for protein–ligand complexes. *Proteins* 73, 765–783. doi: 10.1002/prot.22102

Bashford, D., and Case, D. A. (2000). Generalized born models of macromolecular solvation effects. *Annu. Rev. Phys. Chem.* 51, 129–152. doi: 10.1146/annurev.physchem.51.1.129

Billard, C. (2013). BH3 mimetics: status of the field and new developments. *Mol. Cancer Ther.* 12, 1691–1700. doi: 10.1158/1535-7163.MCT-13-0058

Birkinshaw, R. W., Gong, J. N., Luo, C. S., Lio, D., White, C. A., Anderson, M. A., et al. (2019). Structures of BCL-2 in complex with venetoclax reveal the molecular basis of resistance mutations. *Nat. Commun.* 10:2385. doi: 10.1038/s41467-019-10363-1

Bissantz, C., Folkers, G., and Rognan, D. (2000). Protein-based virtual screening of chemical databases. 1. Evaluation of different docking/scoring combinations. *J. Med. Chem.* 43, 4759–4767. doi: 10.1021/jm001044l

Bowers, K. J., Chow, D. E., Xu, H., Dror, R. O., Eastwood, M. P., Gregersen, B. A., et al. (2006). "Scalable algorithms for molecular dynamics simulations on commodity clusters," *Paper Presented at the SC'06: Proceedings of the 2006 ACM/IEEE Conference on Supercomputing* (Tampa, FL). doi: 10.1145/1188455.1188544

Bruncko, M., Oost, T. K., Belli, B. A., Ding, H., Joseph, M. K., Kunzer, A., et al. (2007). Studies leading to potent, dual inhibitors of Bcl-2 and Bcl-xL. *J. Med. Chem.* 50, 641–662. doi: 10.1021/jm061152t

Bursulaya, B. D., Totrov, M., Abagyan, R., and Brooks, C. L. (2003). Comparative study of several algorithms for flexible ligand docking. *J. Comput. Aided Mol. Des.* 17, 755–763. doi: 10.1023/B:JCAM.0000017496.76572.6f

Casara, P., Davidson, J., Claperon, A., Le Toumelin-Braizat, G., Vogler, M., Bruno, A., et al. (2018). S55746 is a novel orally active BCL-2 selective and potent inhibitor that impairs hematological tumor growth. *Oncotarget* 9, 20075–20088. doi: 10.18632/oncotarget.24744

Chen, H., Lyne, P. D., Giordanetto, F., Lovell, T., and Li, J. (2006). On evaluating molecular-docking methods for pose prediction and enrichment factors. *J. Chem. Inf. Model* 46, 401–415. doi: 10.1021/ci0503255

Chiba, S., Ishida, T., Ikeda, K., Mochizuki, M., Teramoto, R., Taguchi, Y. H., et al. (2017). An iterative compound screening contest method for identifying target protein inhibitors using the tyrosine-protein kinase yes. *Sci. Rep.* 7:12038. doi: 10.1038/s41598-017-10275-4

Chung, C. (2018). Restoring the switch for cancer cell death: targeting the apoptosis signaling pathway. *Am. J. Health Syst. Pharm.* 75, 945–952. doi: 10.2146/ajhp170607

Cory, S., Huang, D. C., and Adams, J. M. (2003). The Bcl-2 family: roles in cell survival and oncogenesis. *Oncogene* 22, 8590–8607. doi: 10.1038/sj.onc.1207102

Cross, J. B., Thompson, D. C., Rai, B. K., Baber, J. C., Fan, K. Y., Hu, Y., et al. (2009). Comparison of several molecular docking programs: pose prediction and virtual screening accuracy. *J. Chem. Inf. Model.* 49, 1455–1474. doi: 10.1021/ci900056c

Dewson, G., and Kluck, R. (2010). Bcl-2 family-regulated apoptosis in health and disease. *Cell Health Cytoskeleton* 2, 9–22. doi: 10.2147/CHC.S6228

Durdagi, S., Aksoydan, B., Erol, I., Kantarcioglu, I., Ergun, Y., Bulut, G., et al. (2018a). Integration of multi-scale molecular modeling approaches with experiments for the *in silico* guided design and discovery of novel herg-neutral antihypertensive oxazalone and imidazolone derivatives and analysis of their potential restrictive effects on cell proliferation. *Eur. J. Med. Chem.* 145, 273–290. doi: 10.1016/j.ejmech.2017.12.021

Durdagi, S., Dogan, B., Erol, I., Kayik, G., and Aksoydan, B. (2019). Current status of multiscale simulations on GPCRs. *Curr. Opin. Struct. Biol.* 55, 93–103. doi: 10.1016/j.sbi.2019.02.013

Durdagi, S., Salmas, R. E., Stein, M., Yurtsever, M., and Seeman, P. (2016). Binding interactions of dopamine and apomorphine in D2High and D2Low states of human dopamine D2 receptor using computational and experimental techniques. *ACS Chem. Neurosci.* 7, 185–195. doi: 10.1021/acschemneuro.5b00271

Durdagi, S., Tahirul Qamar, M., Salmas, R. E., Tariq, Q., Anwar, F., and Ashfaq, U. A. (2018b). Investigating the molecular mechanism of staphylococcal DNA gyrase inhibitors: a combined ligand-based and structure-based resources pipeline. *J. Mol. Graph. Modell.* 85, 122–129. doi: 10.1016/j.jmgm.2018.07.010

Eimon, P. M., and Ashkenazi, A. (2010). The zebrafish as a model organism for the study of apoptosis. *Apoptosis* 15, 331–349. doi: 10.1007/s10495-009-0432-9

Erol, I., Cosut, B., and Durdagi, S. (2019). Toward understanding the impact of dimerization interfaces in angiotensin II type 1 receptor. *J. Chem. Inf. Model.* 59, 4314–4327. doi: 10.1021/acs.jcim.9b00294

Essmann, U., Perera, L., Berkowitz, M. L., Darden, T., Lee, H., and Pedersen, L. G. (1995). A smooth particle mesh Ewald method. *J. Chem. Phys.* 103, 8577–8593. doi: 10.1063/1.470117

Fesik, S. W. (2005). Promoting apoptosis as a strategy for cancer drug discovery. *Nat. Rev. Cancer* 5, 876–885. doi: 10.1038/nrc1736

Friesner, R. A., Banks, J. L., Murphy, R. B., Halgren, T. A., Klicic, J. J., Mainz, D. T., et al. (2004). Glide: a new approach for rapid, accurate docking and scoring. 1. Method and assessment of docking accuracy. *J. Med. Chem.* 47, 1739–1749. doi: 10.1021/jm0306430

Fu, Y., Sun, Y.-N., Yi, K.-H., Li, M.-Q., Cao, H.-F., Li, J.-Z., et al. (2018). Combination of virtual screening protocol by *in silico* toward the discovery of novel 4-hydroxyphenylpyruvate dioxygenase inhibitors. *Front. Chem.* 6:14. doi: 10.3389/fchem.2018.00014

Gandhi, L., Camidge, D. R., De Oliveira, M. R., Bonomi, P., Gandara, D., Khaira, D., et al. (2011). Phase I study of navitoclax (ABT-263), a novel Bcl-2 family inhibitor, in patients with small-cell lung cancer and other solid tumors. *J. Clin. Oncol.* 29, 909–916. doi: 10.1200/JCO.2010.31.6208

Halgren, T. A., Murphy, R. B., Friesner, R. A., Beard, H. S., Frye, L. L., Pollard, W. T., et al. (2004). Glide: a new approach for rapid, accurate docking and scoring. 2. Enrichment factors in database screening. *J. Med. Chem.* 47, 1750–1759. doi: 10.1021/jm030644s

Halim, S. A., Khan, S., Khan, A., Wadood, A., Mabood, F., Hussain, J., et al. (2017). Targeting dengue virus NS-3 helicase by ligand based pharmacophore modeling and structure based virtual screening. *Front. Chem.* 5:88. doi: 10.3389/fchem.2017.00088

Hanahan, D., and Weinberg, R. A. (2000). The hallmarks of cancer. *Cell* 100, 57–70. doi: 10.1016/S0092-8674(00)81683-9

Hanahan, D., and Weinberg, R. A. (2011). Hallmarks of cancer: the next generation. *Cell* 144, 646–674. doi: 10.1016/j.cell.2011.02.013

Hoover, W. G. (1985). Canonical dynamics: equilibrium phase-space distributions. *Phys. Rev. A* 31:1695. doi: 10.1103/PhysRevA.31.1695

Igney, F. H., and Krammer, P. H. (2002). Death and anti-death: tumour resistance to apoptosis. *Nat. Rev. Cancer* 2, 277–288. doi: 10.1038/nrc776

Is, Y. S., Durdagi, S., Aksoydan, B., and Yurtsever, M. (2018). Proposing novel MAO-B hit inhibitors using multidimensional molecular modeling approaches and application of binary QSAR models for prediction of their therapeutic activity, pharmacokinetic and toxicity properties. *ACS Chem. Neurosci.* 9, 1768–1782. doi: 10.1021/acschemneuro.8b00095

Jacobson, M. P., Pincus, D. L., Rapp, C. S., Day, T. J., Honig, B., Shaw, D. E., et al. (2004). A hierarchical approach to all-atom protein loop prediction. *Proteins* 55, 351–367. doi: 10.1002/prot.10613

Kanan, T., Kanan, D., Erol, I., Yazdi, S., Stein, M., and Durdagi, S. (2019). Targeting the NF-κB/IκBα complex via fragment-based E-Pharmacophore virtual screening and binary QSAR models. *J. Mol. Graph. Modell.* 86, 264–277. doi: 10.1016/j.jmgm.2018.09.014

Kollek, M., Müller, A., Egle, A., and Erlacher, M. (2016). Bcl-2 proteins in development, health, and disease of the hematopoietic system. *FEBS J.* 283, 2779–2810. doi: 10.1111/febs.13683

Kumar Yadav, D., Dhawan, S., Chauhan, A., Qidwai, T., Sharma, P., Singh Bhakuni, R., et al. (2014a). QSAR and docking based semi-synthesis and *in vivo* evaluation of artemisinin derivatives for antimalarial activity. *Curr. Drug Targets* 15, 753–761. doi: 10.2174/1389450115666140630102711

Kumar Yadav, D., Kalani, K., Singh, A. K., Khan, F., Srivastava, S. K., and Pant, A. B. (2014b). Design, synthesis and *in vitro* evaluation of 18β-glycyrrhetinic acid derivatives for anticancer activity against human breast cancer cell line MCF-7. *Curr. Med. Chem.* 21, 1160–1170. doi: 10.2174/09298673113206660330

Kumar Yadav, D., Kalani, K., Khan, F., and Kumar Srivastava, S. (2013). QSAR and docking based semi-synthesis and *in vitro* evaluation of 18 β-glycyrrhetinic acid derivatives against human lung cancer cell line A-549. *Med. Chem.* 9, 1073–1084. doi: 10.2174/1573406411309080009

Lessene, G., Czabotar, P. E., and Colman, P. M. (2008). BCL-2 family antagonists for cancer therapy. *Nat. Rev. Drug Discov.* 7, 989–1000. doi: 10.1038/nrd2658

Li, Y., Han, L., Liu, Z., and Wang, R. (2014). Comparative assessment of scoring functions on an updated benchmark: 2. Evaluation methods and general results. *J. Chem. Inf. Model.* 54, 1717–1736. doi: 10.1021/ci500081m

Lionta, E., Spyrou, G., K., Vassilatis, D., and Cournia, Z. (2014). Structure-based virtual screening for drug discovery: principles, applications and recent advances. *Curr. Top. Med. Chem.* 14, 1923–1938. doi: 10.2174/1568026614666140929124445

Martyna, G. J., Tobias, D. J., and Klein, M. L. (1994). Constant pressure molecular dynamics algorithms. *J. Chem. Phys.* 101, 4177–4189. doi: 10.1063/1.467468

Mirza, S. B., Lee, R. C. H., Chu, J. J. H., Salmas, R. E., Mavromoustakos, T., and Durdagi, S. (2018). Discovery of selective dengue virus inhibitors using combination of molecular fingerprint-based virtual screening protocols, structure-based pharmacophore model development, molecular dynamics simulations and *in vitro* studies. *J. Mol. Graph. Modell.* 79, 88–102. doi: 10.1016/j.jmgm.2017.10.010

Mohamad Rosdi, M. N., Mohd Arif, S., Abu Bakar, M. H., Razali, S. A., Mohamed Zulkifli, R., and Ya'akob, H. (2018). Molecular docking studies of bioactive compounds from Annona muricata Linn as potential inhibitors for Bcl-2, Bcl-w and Mcl-1 antiapoptotic proteins. *Apoptosis* 23, 27–40. doi: 10.1007/s10495-017-1434-7

Mollica, A., Zengin, G., Durdagi, S., Ekhteiari Salmas, R., Macedonio, G., Stefanucci, A., et al. (2019). Combinatorial peptide library screening for discovery of diverse α-glucosidase inhibitors using molecular dynamics simulations and binary QSAR models. *J. Biomol. Struct. Dyn.* 37, 726–740. doi: 10.1080/07391102.2018.1439403

Nosé, S. (1984). A unified formulation of the constant temperature molecular dynamics methods. *J. Chem. Phys.* 81, 511–519. doi: 10.1063/1.447334

Oltersdorf, T., Elmore, S. W., Shoemaker, A. R., Armstrong, R. C., Augeri, D. J., Belli, B. A., et al. (2005). An inhibitor of Bcl-2 family proteins induces regression of solid tumours. *Nature* 435, 677–681. doi: 10.1038/nature03579

Petros, A. M., Medek, A., Nettesheim, D. G., Kim, D. H., Yoon, H. S., Swift, K., et al. (2001). Solution structure of the antiapoptotic protein bcl-2. *Proc. Natl Acad. Sci. U.S.A.* 98, 3012–3017. doi: 10.1073/pnas.041619798

Rastelli, G., Degliesposti, G., Del Rio, A., and Sgobba, M. (2009). Binding estimation after refinement, a new automated procedure for the refinement and rescoring of docked ligands in virtual screening. *Chem. Biol. Drug Des.* 73:283–86. doi: 10.1111/j.1747-0285.2009.00780.x

Rastelli, G., and Pinzi, L. (2019). Refinement and rescoring of virtual screening results. *Front. Chem.* 7:498. doi: 10.3389/fchem.2019.00498

Reed, J. C. (2002). Apoptosis-based therapies. *Nat. Rev. Drug Discov.* 1, 111–121. doi: 10.1038/nrd726

Rodrigues, M. J., Slusarczyk, S., Pecio, Ł., Matkowski, A., Salmas, R. E., Durdagi, S., et al. (2018). *In vitro* and *in silico* approaches to appraise *Polygonum maritimum* L. as a source of innovative products with anti-ageing potential. *Indust. Crops Products* 111, 391–399. doi: 10.1016/j.indcrop.2017.10.046

Salmas, R. E., Seeman, P., Aksoydan, B., Erol, I., Kantarcioglu, I., Stein, M., et al. (2017). Analysis of the glutamate agonist LY404,039 binding to nonstatic dopamine receptor D2 dimer structures and consensus docking. *ACS Chem. Neurosci.* 8, 1404–1415. doi: 10.1021/acschemneuro.7b00070

Sastry, G. M., Adzhigirey, M., Day, T., Annabhimoju, R., and Sherman, W. (2013). Protein and ligand preparation: parameters, protocols, and influence on virtual screening enrichments. *J. Comput. Aided Mol. Des.* 27, 221–234. doi: 10.1007/s10822-013-9644-8

Schrödinger Release 2015-2 (2015) *LigPrep*. New York, NY: Schrödinger, LLC.

Shan, Y., Kim, E. T., Eastwood, M. P., Dror, R. O., Seeliger, M. A., and Shaw, D. E. (2011). How does a drug molecule find its target binding site? *JACS* 133, 9181–9183. doi: 10.1021/ja202726y

Shelley, J. C., Cholleti, A., Frye, L. L., Greenwood, J. R., Timlin, M. R., and Uchimaya, M. (2007). Epik: a software program for pK a prediction and protonation state generation for drug-like molecules. *J. Comput. Aided Mol. Des* 21, 681–691. doi: 10.1007/s10822-007-9133-z

Sherman, W., Beard, H. S., and Farid, R. (2006a). Use of an induced fit receptor structure in virtual screening. *Chem. Biol. Drug Des.* 67, 83–84. doi: 10.1111/j.1747-0285.2005.00327.x

Sherman, W., Day, T., Jacobson, M. P., Friesner, R. A., and Farid, R. (2006b). Novel procedure for modeling ligand/receptor induced fit effects. *J. Med. Chem.* 49, 534–553. doi: 10.1021/jm050540c

Soderquist, R. S., and Eastman, A. (2016). BCL2 inhibitors as anticancer drugs: a plethora of misleading BH3 mimetics. *Mol. Cancer Ther.* 15, 2011–2017. doi: 10.1158/1535-7163.MCT-16-0031

Souers, A. J., Leverson, J. D., Boghaert, E. R., Ackler, S. L., Catron, N. D., Chen, J., et al. (2013). ABT-199, a potent and selective BCL-2 inhibitor, achieves antitumor activity while sparing platelets. *Nat. Med* 19, 202–208. doi: 10.1038/nm.3048

Tse, C., Shoemaker, A. R., Adickes, J., Anderson, M. G., Chen, J., Jin, S., et al. (2008). ABT-263: a potent and orally bioavailable Bcl-2 family inhibitor. *Cancer Res.* 68, 3421–3428. doi: 10.1158/0008-5472.CAN-07-5836

Verma, S., Singh, A., and Mishra, A. (2015). Complex disruption effect of natural polyphenols on Bcl-2-Bax: molecular dynamics simulation and essential dynamics study. *J. Biomol. Struct. Dyn.* 33, 1094–1106. doi: 10.1080/07391102.2014.931823

Warren, G. L., Andrews, C. W., Capelli, A.-M., Clarke, B., LaLonde, J., Lambert, M. H., et al. (2006). A critical assessment of docking programs and scoring functions. *J. Med. Chem.* 49, 5912–5931. doi: 10.1021/jm050362n

Wu, H., Medeiros, L. J., and Young, K. H. (2018). Apoptosis signaling and BCL-2 pathways provide opportunities for novel targeted therapeutic strategies in hematologic malignances. *Blood Rev.* 32, 8–28. doi: 10.1016/j.blre.2017.08.004

Yang, W., Soares, J., Greninger, P., Edelman, E. J., Lightfoot, H., Forbes, S., et al. (2012). Genomics of Drug Sensitivity in Cancer (GDSC): a resource for therapeutic biomarker discovery in cancer cells. *Nucleic Acids Res.* 41, D955–D961. doi: 10.1093/nar/gks1111

Yoshino, R., Yasuo, N., Hagiwara, Y., Ishida, T., Inaoka, D. K., Amano, Y., et al. (2017). *In silico*, *in vitro*, X-ray crystallography, and integrated strategies for discovering spermidine synthase inhibitors for Chagas disease. *Sci. Rep.* 7:6666. doi: 10.1038/s41598-017-06411-9

Yoshino, R., Yasuo, N., Inaoka, D. K., Hagiwara, Y., Ohno, K., Orita, M., et al. (2015). Pharmacophore modeling for anti-chagas drug design using the fragment molecular orbital method. *PLoS ONE* 10:e0125829. doi: 10.1371/journal.pone.0125829

Youle, R. J., and Strasser, A. (2008). The BCL-2 protein family: opposing activities that mediate cell death. *Nat. Rev. Mol. Cell Biol.* 9, 47–59. doi: 10.1038/nrm2308

Zaka, M., Abbasi, B. H., and Durdagi, S. (2018). Proposing novel TNFα direct inhibitor Scaffolds using fragment-docking based e-pharmacophore modeling and binary QSAR-based virtual screening protocols pipeline. *J. Mol. Graph. Modell.* 85, 111–121. doi: 10.1016/j.jmgm.2018.07.007

Zaka, M., Abbasi, B. H., and Durdagi, S. (2019). Novel tumor necrosis factor-α (TNF-α) inhibitors from small molecule library screening for their therapeutic activity profiles against rheumatoid arthritis using target-driven approaches and binary QSAR models. *J. Biomol. Struct. Dyn.* 37, 2464–2476. doi: 10.1080/07391102.2018.1491423

Zhang, H., Nimmer, P., Tahir, S., Chen, J., Fryer, R., Hahn, K., et al. (2007). Bcl-2 family proteins are essential for platelet survival. *Cell Death Differ.* 14, 943–951. doi: 10.1038/sj.cdd.4402081

13

Novel Quinoline Compound Derivatives of NSC23925 as Potent Reversal Agents Against P-Glycoprotein-Mediated Multidrug Resistance

Xingping Quan[1†], *Hongzhi Du*[2†], *Jingjing Xu*[3†], *Xiaoying Hou*[1], *Xiaofeng Gong*[1], *Yao Wu*[1], *Yuqi Zhou*[1], *Jingwei Jiang*[1], *Ligong Lu*[4], *Shengtao Yuan*[1], *Xiangyu Yang*[4*], *Lei Shi*[3*] and *Li Sun*[1*]

[1] *Jiangsu Key Laboratory of Drug Screening, China Pharmaceutical University, Nanjing, China,* [2] *School of Pharmacy, Hubei University of Chinese Medicine, Wuhan, China,* [3] *Henan Key Laboratory of Organic Functional Molecules and Drug Innovation, School of Chemistry and Chemical Engineering, Henan Normal University, Xinxiang, China,* [4] *Zhuhai Interventional Medical Center, Zhuhai Precision Medical Center, Zhuhai People's Hospital, Zhuhai Hospital Affiliated with Jinan University, Zhuhai, China*

Correspondence:
Xiangyu Yang
yangxygdzhh@163.com
Lei Shi
shirlei@sina.com
Li Sun
sunli@cpu.edu.cn

† These authors have contributed equally to this work

Multidrug resistance is a serious problem and a common cause of cancer treatment failure, leading to patient death. Although numerous reversal resistance inhibitors have been evaluated in preclinical or clinical trials, efficient and low-toxicity reversal agents have not been identified. In this study, a series of novel quinoline compound derivatives from NSC23925 were designed to inhibit P-glycoprotein (P-gp). Among them, YS-7a showed a stronger inhibitory effect against P-gp than verapamil, as a positive control, when co-incubated with chemotherapy drugs at minimally cytotoxic concentrations. YS-7a suppressed the P-gp transport function without affecting the expression of P-gp but stimulated the ATPase activity of P-gp in a dose-dependent manner. Next, molecular docking was used to predict the six most probable binding sites, namely, SER270, VAL273, VAL274, ILE354, VAL357, and PHE390. Moreover, YS-7a had no effect on cytochrome P450 3A4 activity and showed little toxicity to normal cells. In addition, combined treatment of YS-7a with vincristine showed a better inhibitory effect than the positive control verapamil *in vivo* without a negative effect on mouse weight. Overall, our results showed that YS-7a could reverse cancer multidrug resistance through the inhibition of P-gp transport function *in vitro* and *in vivo*, suggesting that YS-7a may be a novel therapeutic agent.

Keywords: molecular docking, multidrug resistance (MDR), P-glycoprotein (P-gp), quinoline, reversal cancer resistance

INTRODUCTION

Cancer multidrug resistance (MDR) is a major cause of chemotherapy failure leading to patient death. MDR cancer cells often show pleiotropic cross-resistance to a wide range of chemotherapy drugs. Mechanisms of MDR can be classified into non-cellular-based and cellular-based resistance mechanisms (Krishna and Mayer, 2000). Numerous potential mechanisms of MDR have been reported involving the ABC transporter family, DNA damage and repair, cancer stem cell regulation, microRNA regulation, and epigenetic regulation (Wu et al., 2014). Among these, the ABC transporter families play an important role in cellular-based resistance mechanisms by facilitating exocytosis of chemotherapy drugs (Choi and Yu, 2014; Wu et al., 2014). These transporters are universally expressed across MDR cancer cells, especially P-glycoprotein (P-gp; encoded by MDR1), which is functionally equivalent to an efflux pump that translocate substrates or chemotherapy drugs from the intracellular to the extracellular environment (Fojo et al., 1987; Konstantinos, 2015). Studies have confirmed that P-gp is highly expressed or overactivated in a large number of patients with failed chemotherapy (Alfarouk et al., 2015). Therefore, P-gp is a potential target for reversing drug resistance.

P-gp inhibitors, also known as MDR modulators, have been used to reverse MDR and block P-gp function in combination with chemotherapy drugs (Coley, 2010; Kumar and Jaitak, 2019). Several pharmacological P-gp inhibitors have been developed, including verapamil (VP), PSC-833, and tariquidar. VP was the first to be identified, and is commonly used as a P-gp inhibitor for its low affinity and other pharmacological activities, but has many side effects (Bellamy et al., 1988; Yusa and Tsuruo, 1989). Dexverapamil (Pirker et al., 1995; Thürlimann et al., 1995) and PSC-833 (Boesch et al., 1991; Kusunoki et al., 2010) lack the pharmacological activities of VP and cyclosporin A, but inhibit cytochrome P450 (CYP) 3A4 activity. This leads to complicated drug–drug interactions and limits their application (Chico et al., 2001; Labrie et al., 2006). Meanwhile, tariquidar (XR9576) (Federica et al., 2004; Fox and Bates, 2007), LY335979 (Dantzig et al., 1999; Shepard et al., 2003), and HM30181 (Cha et al., 2013; Köhler and Wiese, 2015) show more specific affinities to P-gp with fewer side effects. Several clinical trials are underway that are expected to address clinical drug resistance. Oraxol, the oral preparation consisting of paclitaxel and HM30181A, showed a strong trend in progression-free survival (p = 0.077), favoring oral paclitaxel over *intravenous* paclitaxel and a strong trend in overall survival (p = 0.11) (https://ir.athenex.com/, ClinicalTrials.gov Identifier: NCT02594371). However, improved novel inhibitors are required to make P-gp a reliable target for reversing resistance.

NSC23925 was identified from 2,000 small molecule compounds using a high-throughput cell-based screening assay, and can specifically inhibit P-gp and reverse MDR with no effect on P-gp expression (Duan et al., 2009). NSC23925 was shown to prevent the emergence of MDR in ovarian cancer both *in vitro* and *in vivo* (Yang et al., 2015) and in osteosarcoma (Yang et al., 2014) without affecting P-gp expression. NSC23925 also reversed MDR in cancer cells (Duan et al., 2012).

In this study, we designed and synthesized a series of NSC23925 analogs with improved potency through two mechanisms (**Figures 1B,C**). Owing to their new structure and superior activity, these compounds were granted a patent (CN 108017615A, CN 107973781A). Among the synthesized compounds, YS-7a and YS-7b showed better P-gp inhibition than the positive control VP and the parent compound NSC23925. Our findings demonstrated that substituting -OH with -OMe increased the intracellular accumulation of Rhodamine 123 (Rho123); therefore, YS-7a was selected for further evaluation of its potent reversal effect. Next, the target of YS-7a was confirmed using small interfering (si)RNA. YS-7a had no effect on mRNA and protein expression of P-gp but inhibited its efflux pumping effect and stimulating P-gp ATPase instead, supporting its direct effect on P-gp. The binding sites were predicted through molecular docking. There was no significant effect on CYP3A4 activity and almost no toxicity toward normal cells. Finally, YS-7a improved the anti-tumor effect of chemotherapy drugs, showing better reversal of drug resistance than VP when combined with vincristine (VCR) *in vivo*. Overall, our study showed that YS-7a inhibited P-gp with high efficiency and low toxicity both *in vitro* and *in vivo*. Therefore, YS-7a is a novel P-gp inhibitor that may be used for the treatment of MDR cancers.

MATERIALS AND METHODS

General Chemistry

All the reagents were obtained from commercial sources and used without further purification unless otherwise indicated. All organic solvents were dried and freshly distilled before use by standard methods. The reactions were monitored by thin layer chromatography (TLC) on GF254 silica gel coated plates and visualized by UV light (254 and 365 nm). Purification by column and flash chromatography was carried out using silica gel (200–300 mesh). Melting points were taken on a X-4B melting-point apparatus and were uncorrected. ^{1}H and ^{13}C NMR spectra were recorded in DMSO-d6 or $CDCl_3$ on a Bruker Avance/600 (^{1}H: 600 MHz, ^{13}C: 150 MHz at 25°C) or Bruker Avance/400 (^{1}H: 400 MHz, ^{13}C: 100 MHz at 25°C, Bruker Instruments, Inc., Billerica, MA, USA) Chemical shifts are expressed in values (ppm) relative to tetramethylsilane as an internal standard, and coupling constants (J values) were given in hertz (Hz). Abbreviations are represented as follows: br, broad; s, singlet; d, doublet; dd, double doublet; t, triplet; q, quartet; m, multiplet. HRMS analysis was performed on a mass spectrometer using electrospray ionization (ESI-oa-TOF), and the purity of all samples used for HRMS (>95%) was confirmed by ^{1}H and ^{13}C NMR spectroscopic analyses. HPLC was performed on Agilent Technologies 1200 LC Column 250 × 4.6 nm and using H_2O (95–5%)/MeOH (5–95%) during 22 min as the mobile phase. Flow rate was1.0 mL/min (all solvents were HPLC grade). The HPLC system was monitored at 254 nm.

Biology

Cell Lines and Cell Culture

Human leukemia cell line K562, human oral squamous carcinoma KB cells, human hepatocellular carcinoma cell line HepG2 and Human umbilical vein endothelial cells (HUVEC) were obtained from the Cell Bank of the Institute of Biochemistry and Cell Biology, Chinese Academy of Sciences (Shanghai, China).The MDR1-overexpressed cell lines, 3 μM adriamycin (ADR)-selected (Dalian Meilun Biotech Co., Ltd., China) multidrug resistance cell K562/ADR and 0.1 μM vincristine (VCR)-selected (Lingnan Pharmaceutical Co., China) multidrug resistance cell KB/VCR were obtained from Nanjing Shenghe Pharmaceutical Ltd (Nanjing, China). All the cells were cultured in RPMI-1640 medium (Gibco) supplemented with 10% (v/v)

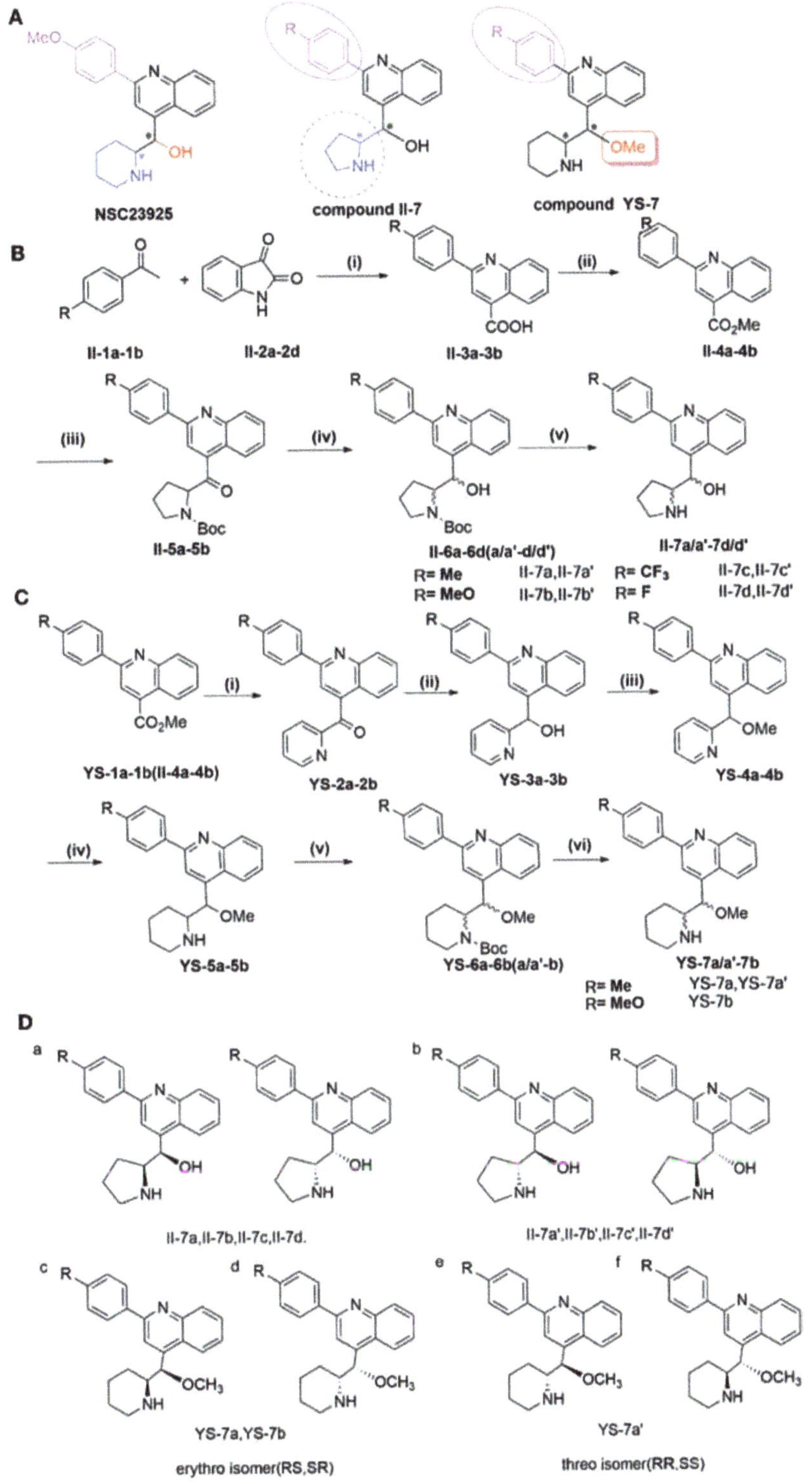

FIGURE 1 | (A) Synthesis of compounds II-7a, II-7a′, II-7b, II-7b′, II-7c, II-7c′, II-7d, and II-7d′; **(B)** synthesis of compounds YS-7a, YS-7a′, and YS-7b. Reagents and conditions **(A)**: (i) 1-(4-3-methoxyphenyl)ethanone, KOH, EtOH, 85°C, 24 h; (ii) concentrated H_2SO_4, MeOH, 65°C reflux overnight; (iii) 1-Boc-pyrrole (1 equiv), sec-BuLi (1.3 equiv) tetramethylethylenediamine 1.7 mL, −78°C, 2 h, dropping compound, stirring 2 h at room temperature, dry tetrahydrofuran; (iv) $NaBH_4$ (9 equiv), EtOH, 0°C, 0.75–1 h. (v) 2 M HCl, 30°C, 48 h. **(B)**: (i) 2-bromopyridine, n-BuLi, Et_2O/tetrahydrofuran, −78°C, 2 h; (ii) 7 $NaBH_4$, EtOH, 0°C, 1 h; (iii) dry N,N-dimethylformamide, NaCl, N_2, 0°C, 10 min, methyl iodide, stirring 1 h at 25°C; (iv) platinum dioxide, HCl, MeOH, H_2; (v) triethylamine, di-tert-butyl decarbonate dissolved in tetrahydrofuran at 0°C, stirring at room temperature overnight; (vi) 2 M HCl, 30°C, 48 h. **(C)** Design of target compounds. **(D)** Structure of compounds II-7a, II-7a′, II-7b, II-7b′, II-7c, II-7c′, II-7d, II-7d′, YS-7a, YS-7a′, and YS-7b (a–d).

heat-inactivated fetal bovine serum (FBS, HyClone) at 37°C and 5% CO_2.

Antibodies and Reagents

The antibodies and reagents included β-actin (AC026, ABclonal), MDR1 (22336-1-AP, proteintech), Anti-rabbit IgG (H+L) (Biotinylated Antibody #14708, Cell Signaling Technology), Anti-mouse IgG (H+L) (Biotinylated Antibody #14709, Cell Signaling Technology).

Rhodamine-123 (Rho-123) Accumulation

Intracellular fluorescence intensity was measured by Flow Cytometry (Wang et al., 2000). Cells in the exponential growth phase were seeded in 12-well plates, with about 10^4 cells per well. After a 24 h incubation at 37°C in a 5% CO_2, cells were treated with various concentrations of candidate compounds and verapamil (VP) for 4 h. Then 1 μg/mL Rhodamine-123 (Rho-123) was added directly to the cells. Additional incubation for 1 h at 37°C protected from light, the cells were harvested and immediately detected by flow cytometric (BD) at an excitation wavelength of 488 nm and emission wavelength of 530 nm. The results were calculated by GraphPad Prism 6.0 software.

Cell Proliferation Assays *in vitro*

The inhibition of the compounds on the growth of cancer cells KB/VCR and KB or human leukemia cell line K562/ADR and K562 cells were estimated by the 3-(4,5-dimethyl-2-thiazolyl)-2,5-diphenyl-2-H-tetrazolium bromide (MTT). Cells were plated in 96-well-plates, with about 1–2 × 10^3 cells per well. After 24 h, cells were incubated with various concentrations of compounds and verapamil (VP) for 72 h. MTT was added directly to the cells, and incubated for a further 4 h at 37°C protected from light. Finally, the absorbance at 490 nm was read on a microplate reader (Thermo Fisher Scientific). Experiments were conducted in triplicate at least and repeated three times independently. The inhibition rate was calculated as follows (Wei et al., 2019): inhibition rate (%) = (1− absorbance of the treated group/absorbance of the control group) × 100%. The reversing tumor resistance fold (RF) in resistance cancer cells = IC_{50} (concentration at half-maximum inhibition) of single chemotherapeutic drug/IC_{50} of chemotherapeutic drug combined with YS-7a.

siRNA Treatment

All siRNA fragments were synthesized by GenePharma (Shanghai, China). Cells in the logarithmic growth phase were seeded in 6-well-plates, with about 5–6 × 10^5 cells per well. Once the cells attached (often 8 h later), the medium with 10% FBS was replaced by fresh serum-free medium containing different siRNA for 6–8 h. The sequence of siRNA are as follows:

Negative Control	5′-UUCUCCGAACGUGUCACGUTT-3′
	5′-ACGUGACACGUUCGGAGAATT-3′
MDR1-homo-824	5′-GACCAGGUAUGCCUAUUAUTT-3′
	5′-AUAAUAGGCAUACCUGGUCTT-3′
MDR1-homo-2187	5′-GCGAAGCAGUGGUUCAGGUTT-3′
	5′-ACCUGAACCACUGCUUCGCTT-3′
MDR1-homo-3323	5′-CACCCAGGCAAUGAUGUAUTT-3′
	5′-AUACAUCAUUGCCUGGGUGTT-3′.

The medium should then be changed to fresh medium with 10% FBS for a further 24 h. Cells were used to evaluate the effectiveness of knockdown and the cytotoxicity effects; methods were the same as cell proliferation assays *in vitro*. The reversing tumor resistance fold (RF) in P-gp knockdown cancer cells = IC_{50} of single chemotherapeutic drug in P-gp knockdown cancer cells/IC_{50} of chemotherapeutic drug combined with YS-7a in P-gp knockdown cancer cells.

RT-qPCR Assays

The expression of the relative genes of cells was detected by RT-qPCR as reported (Hou et al., 2018b). The total RNA was isolated with the TRIzol® Reagent (Vazyme) and then reverse transcribed with the HiScript™ QRT SuperMix for qPCR (Vazyme). The mRNA level was measured using the SYBR Green master mix (Vazyme). The β-actin mRNA served as the control. Primer sequences used for qRT-PCR were as follows:

β-actin	5′-GGACTTCGAGCAAGAGATGG-3′ (forward)
	5′- AGCACTGTGTTGGCGTACAG-3′ (reverse)
MDR1	5′-GGAGCCTACTTGGTGGCACATAA-3′(forward)
	5′-TGGCATAGTCAGGAGCAAATGAAC-3′ (reverse).

Western Blot

The expression of the MDR1 protein was analyzed by Western Blot assays. After being treated with compounds, cells were harvested and lysed, the total protein concentrations were consistent according to the BCA kit (Beyotime Biotechnology, China). Protein lysates (20–30 μg protein per lane) were separated by 8% SDS-PAGE, and then the PVDF membranes were incubated with primary antibodies and second antibodies. The results were quantified by image analyzer (Bio-Rad, USA). The expression of β-actin was used as the control.

P-gp ATPase Activity Assays

The P-gp ATPase activity was tested by Pgp-Glo™ Assay Systems (Promega). The impact of candidate compounds on P-gp ATPase activity were examined by comparing untreated samples and samples treated with Na_3VO_4 (sodium orthovanadate). The compounds could be assessed as stimulating, inhibiting, or having no effect on basal P-gp ATPase activity.

Molecular Docking

Schrödinger was used for the molecular modeling studies as we have used before (Hou et al., 2018a). The crystal structure of the P-gp (PDB ID: 3WME) was prepared using Protein Preparation Wizard. The structure of compounds YS-7a were prepared using ChemBioDraw Ultra 13.0. The calculation was performed based on the force field OPLS (optimized potentials for liquid simulations) 2005 selecting water as the solvent. The following structure was obtained from the result of 1,000 calculation cycles.

CYP3A4 Activity Assays

The effect of the candidate compounds against CYP3A4 activity was performed by P450-Glo™ CYP3A4 Assay (Luciferin-IPA) Cell-Based/Biochemical Assay (Promega). The expression of the CYP3A4 gene of HepG2 cells could be induced by 25 μM rifampicin. Cells were typically exposed for 24–72 h. The cells were then treated with various concentrations of test compounds for 72 h. Ketoconazole was used as the positive group. Finally, the P450-Glo™ CYP3A4 Assay (Luciferin-IPA) Cell-Based/Biochemical Assay (Promega) was added to pyrolysis, the treated HepG2 cells, and the fluorescence was detected by SoftMax Pro 6.1 (Beckman counter). The relative CYP3A4 activity was estimated as the formula: (the fluorescence of YS-7a treated/YS-7a treated HepG2 cells)/(the fluorescence of control/control HepG2 cells).

In vivo Experiments

Female BALB/c mice aged 4–6 weeks and weighing 18–20 g were purchased by the Model Animal Research Center of Nanjing University (Nanjing, China). KB/VCR cells (2×10^6) were transplanted to establish the subcutaneous xenograft model. Intraperitoneal administration once the tumor volume (TV) reached 100 mm^3, all the mice could be divided into six groups: the normal group (saline, 0.2 ml/kg), single chemotherapy drug group (VCR 0.5 mg/kg), positive drug single group (VP 10 mg/kg), single YS-7a group (YS-7a 10 mg/kg), positive drug group (VP 10 mg/kg+ VCR 0.5 mg/kg), and the combination YS-7a group (YS-7a 10 mg/kg + VCR 0.5 mg/kg). All the drugs were given by intraperitoneal injection every 3 days. After 24 days, all the animals were sacrificed and the final tumor obtained to calculate the relative tumor volume (RTV). TV and RTV were calculated as follows: TV (mm^3) = $½ \times A \times B^2$, where A represents the longest diameter of tumor, B represents the shortest diameter. RTV = V_{24}/V_0, V_{24} represents the TV of day 24, and V_0 represents the TV of day 0. Additionally, all of the final tumors were weighted, and the weight loss ratio counted. The weight loss ratio (%) = $M_{24(drugtreated)}/M24^*_{(control)}100\%$. In this study, animal administration was guided by the Animal Care and Control Committee of the China Pharmaceutical University.

Statistical Analysis

All results are shown as the mean ± S.D of triplicate experiments. One-way ANOVA or the student's *t*-test was performed for the statistical analysis using the GraphPad Prism 5.0 software as previously reported (Du et al., 2018). All comparisons are made relative to the untreated controls. $^*P < 0.05$ was considered statistically significant; $^{**}P < 0.01$ and $^{***}P < 0.001$ was considered very statistically significant.

RESULTS

Design Novel Derivatives With Potent Reversal Activity

The natural compound NSC23925 contains a quinoline structure with one benzene ring and two chiral carbons in the side chain (**Figure 1A**). Based on the structural mode, we designed and obtained some derivatives **II-7a-a′**, **II-7b-b′**, **II-7c-c′**, **II-7d-d′**, **YS-7a-a′**, and **YS-7b** by changing the substituent on benzene ring in the side chain and replacing piperidine with tetrahydropyrrole (**compound II-7**) or replacing -OH with -OMe (**compound YS-7**) (**Figure 1A**). Each compound was purified by column chromatography and the purity of compounds was evaluated using high-performance liquid chromatography (HPLC) (**Table S1, Figures S1–S11**).

The general procedure for the synthesis of the compounds shown in **Figures 1B,C** is as follows: 2-(4-R-Phenyl)quinoline-4-carboxylic acid (**II-3**) was prepared from 4-R-1-phenyl ethenone (**II-1**) and indoline-2,3-dione (**II-2**) (yield: 80–82%), and was then esterified to afford methyl-2-(4-R-phenyl)quinoline-4-carboxylate (**II-4** or **YS-1**) (yield: 80–88%). Using n-BuLi as a base, 2-bromopyrrole or 2-bromopyridine was reacted with (**II-4** or **YS-1**) to give (2-(4-R-phenyl)quinolin-4-yl)(pyrrole-2-yl)-methanone (**II-5**) (yield: 20–25%) and (2-(4-R-phenyl)quinolin-4-yl)(pyridin-2-yl)-methanone (**YS-2**) (yield: 80–85%). Subsequent reduction of **II-5** or **YS-2** by $NaBH_4$ afforded 2-(4-R-phenyl) (quinolin-4-yl)(pyridin-2-yl)methanol (**II-6**) (yield: 87–96%) and 2-(4-R-phenyl) (quinolin-4-yl)(pyridin-2-yl)methanol (**YS-3**) (yield: 90–98%). **II-6** was separated by column chromatography to obtain a pair of diastereomers **II-6** (**a, a′-d, d′**) that could be separated based on polarity; the less polar compound was named **II-6 (a-d)** and the more polar was named **II-6 (a′-d′)**. Methyl iodide was used as a methyl donor to produce methyl-2-(4-R-phenyl) (quinolin-4-yl)(pyridin-2-yl)methyl ether (**YS-4**) (yield: 85%). We then performed a reduction reaction of **YS-4** by hydrogen to produce 2-(hydroxy(2-(4-R-phenyl) quinolin-4-yl) methyl) piperidine-1-carboxylic acid tert-butyl ester (**YS-5**) (yield: 95%). A triethylamine and di-tert-butyl decarbonate reaction with **YS-5** was used to produce **YS-6**, after which **YS-6** was separated by column chromatography to obtain a pair of diastereomers that could be separated based on polarity; the less polar compound was named **YS-6** (**a** or **b**) and the more polar was named **YS-6** (**a′** or **b′**) (yield: 75%). The deprotection reaction of **II-6** or **YS-6** was performed and finally solid washed with dichloromethane to yield the corresponding diastereomer **II-7** (**a, a′-d, d′**) and **YS-7** (**a, a′** or **b**).

Based on a previous study of the Erythro/Threo configuration of phenyl 2-piperidylcarbinols by NMR, after knowing its absolute configuration (Lapidus and Fauley, 1971; Solladié-Cavallo et al., 2003), the ^{3}J-erythro and ^{3}J-threo in the CH(OH)-CH(NH) systems were different, always showing ^{3}J-erythro(RS, SR) $<^3$J-threo(RR, SS). Therefore, ^{1}H NMR was applied to determine the structure of these compounds. By analyzing these data, we found that the low polarity compounds (II-7a,7b,7c) could belong to etythro (RS, SR) isomer, and the highly polar compounds (II-7a',7b',7c') belong to threo (RR, SS) isomer. Therefore, we inferred that YS-7a and YS-7b (the lower polarity) belongs to etythro (RS, SR) isomer compounds, and YS-7a' belongs to the threo (RR, SS) isomer compound (**Figure 1D**). All NMR spectra of these compounds are provided in **Figures S12–S55**. After obtaining these 11 compounds, the reversal activities were measured.

Screening of Novel P-gp Inhibitors in MDR Cells

We evaluated the cancer MDR reversal activities of the candidate compounds. First, quantitative reverse transcription PCR and

Western blotting were performed to characterize the resistance of the KB/VCR and K562/ADR cell lines (**Figures 2A–F**). P-gp expression was increased at both the mRNA and protein levels. MDR of KB/VCR and K562/ADR cells was detected based on the half-maximal inhibitory concentration (IC_{50}) using the MTT assay. KB/VCR cells (IC_{50} = 0.8294 ± 0.241 μM) showed a 46.8-fold greater resistance to VCR than KB cells (IC_{50} = 0.01770 ± 0.094 μM), whereas K562/ADR cells (IC_{50} = 6.919 ± 0.01992 μM) showed a 347.3-fold greater resistance to adriamycin (ADR) than K562 cells (IC_{50} = 0.01992 ± 0.008 μM). Because the resistance of cancer cells decreased in the absence of chemotherapy drugs, compounds at a dose below the 20% inhibition concentration (0.1 μM VCR in KB/VCR cells; 3 μM ADR in K562/ADR cells) were co-incubated during the entire process. These findings supported the use of KB/VCR and K562/ADR cells for subsequent experimentation.

After confirming the overexpression of P-gp in MDR cancer cells, we detected the intracellular accumulation of Rho123 to screen for potential novel P-gp inhibitors and to assess P-gp inhibition. Rho123 was added to KB and KB/VCR cells at a final concentration of 5 μM for 1 h; 10 μM VP in KB/VCR cells were used as the positive control. The intracellular concentration of Rho123 decreased significantly in KB/VCR cells, which was reversed by VP (**Figure 2G**). Subsequently, II-7a, II-7a′, II-7b, II-7b′, II-7c, II-7c′, II-7d, II-7d′, YS-7a, YS-7a′, and YS-7b were evaluated by flow cytometry for their capacity to inhibit Rho123 efflux. Among the candidate compounds, the low-polarity compounds YS-7a (fold change = 82.19 ± 17.79) and YS-7b (65.85 ± 10.04) showed the greatest degree of Rho123 efflux inhibition, compared to VP (9.79 ± 0.70) and NSC23925 (40.53 ± 0.49) (**Figure 2H**), suggesting that they can potently reverse MDR. Further characterization was performed to measure their reversal efficiency *in vitro*.

Structure–Activity Relationship

Next, we investigated the structure–activity relationship (SAR) of the candidate compounds (**Table 1**). The low-polarity compound **II-7b**, which substituted piperidine for tetrahydropyrrole, showed significantly decreased activity compared to the parent compound. Changing the substituent on the benzene ring in the side chain with an electron-donating or electron-withdrawing group resulted in compounds **II-7a-a′** (R_1: -Me), **II-7c-c′** (R_1: -CF_3), and **II-7d-d′** (R_1: -F); these compounds did not improve the efflux of intracellular Rho123. Among these eight compounds (i.e., **II-7a-a′ to d-d′**), higher polarity damaged the activity.

Based on these results, we focused on the replacement of -OH with -OMe in the chiral carbons. The addition of a methoxy group in chiral carbons (**YS-7b**) promoted the activity, suggesting that reducing the polarity of the molecule and hydrogen bonding are beneficial to its activity. Interestingly, **YS-7a**, with an electron-donating methyl substitution, was more potent (fold change = 82.19 ± 17.79) than NSC23925, whereas the high-polarity compound **YS-7a′** (38.42 ± 25.09) showed no obvious improvement in activity. Considering the bioactivity and polarity of the compounds, we selected compounds **YS-7a** and **YS-7b** for further characterization.

In vitro Drug Resistance Reversal Effects of YS-7a and YS-7b

As potential P-gp inhibitors, YS-7a and YS-7b may reverse the resistance to chemotherapy drugs. Before testing YS-7a and YS-7b in combination with chemotherapy drugs, the antiproliferation effects of YS-7a and YS-7b were measured using the MTT assay. A concentration with low antiproliferation effects (<20% inhibition) was used to evaluate their MDR reversal effects (**Figures 3A,B**). In both KB/VCR and K562/ADR cells, 10 μM YS-7a, 2.5 μM YS-7b, and 2.5 μM VP were selected as the low-toxicity dose.

The drug resistance reversal effects of YS-7a and YS-7b were measured in combination with chemotherapy drugs based on cytotoxicity. Series concentrations of the chemotherapy drugs VCR and doxorubicin (ADR) were applied individually to explore the reversal effects of YS-7a and YS-7b. YS-7a exerted powerful reversal activity compared to the classical P-gp inhibitor VP in both KB/VCR and K562/ADR cells (**Figures 3C,D**). The IC_{50} values of the combined YS-7a + chemotherapy drug in drug-resistant KB/VCR and K562/ADR cells were 0.0376 ± 0.0116 μM and 0.268 ± 0.053 μM, respectively, whereas the IC_{50} values of the chemotherapy drugs in drug-sensitive KB and K562 cells were 0.435 ± 0.286 μM and 6.571 ± 1.758 μM, respectively; therefore, YS-7a showed a 10.11 ± 3.51 and 30.59 ± 5.83 reversal of drug resistance in KB/VCR and K562/ADR cells, respectively. Meanwhile, the IC_{50} values of the combined YS-7b + chemotherapy drug in drug-resistant KB/VCR and K562/ADR cells were 0.0561 ± 0.0390 μM and 0.616 ± 0.185 μM, respectively, whereas the IC_{50} values of the chemotherapy drugs in drug-sensitive KB and K562 cells were 0.375 ± 0.246 μM and 6.571 ± 1.758 μM, respectively; therefore, YS-7b showed a 6.92 ± 0.55 and 10.79 ± 0.87 reversal of drug resistance in KB/VCR and K562/ADR cells, respectively. Overall, YS-7a showed a significantly better drug resistance reversal effect in MDR cells and was selected for further experimentation of its reversal capabilities.

P-gp May Be a Target of YS-7a

Although YS-7a was screened for its potent reversal effect in MDR cancer cells, it remained unclear whether it targeted P-gp. To clarify this, knockdown of P-gp was implemented by three siMDR1 fragments. siMDR1-2 and siMDR1-3 were chosen for further experiments, both of which downregulated P-gp mRNA and protein levels in KB/VCR and K562/ADR cells (**Figures 4A–D**). Knockdown by siMDR1-2 and siMDR1-3 decreased P-gp transporter function (**Figures 4E,F**). After knockdown of P-gp, the drug resistance reversal potency of YS-7a decreased from 16.12- to 1.57-fold (siMDR1-2) and 1.63-fold (siMDR1-3) in KB/VCR cells, whereas that of VP decreased from 6.26- to 1.56-fold (siMDR1-2) and 1.63-fold (siMDR1-3) (**Figure 4G**). In other words, the reversal effect of YS-7a almost entirely disappeared after P-gp knockdown. Altogether, these results show that the drug resistance reversal effect of YS-7a relies on P-gp.

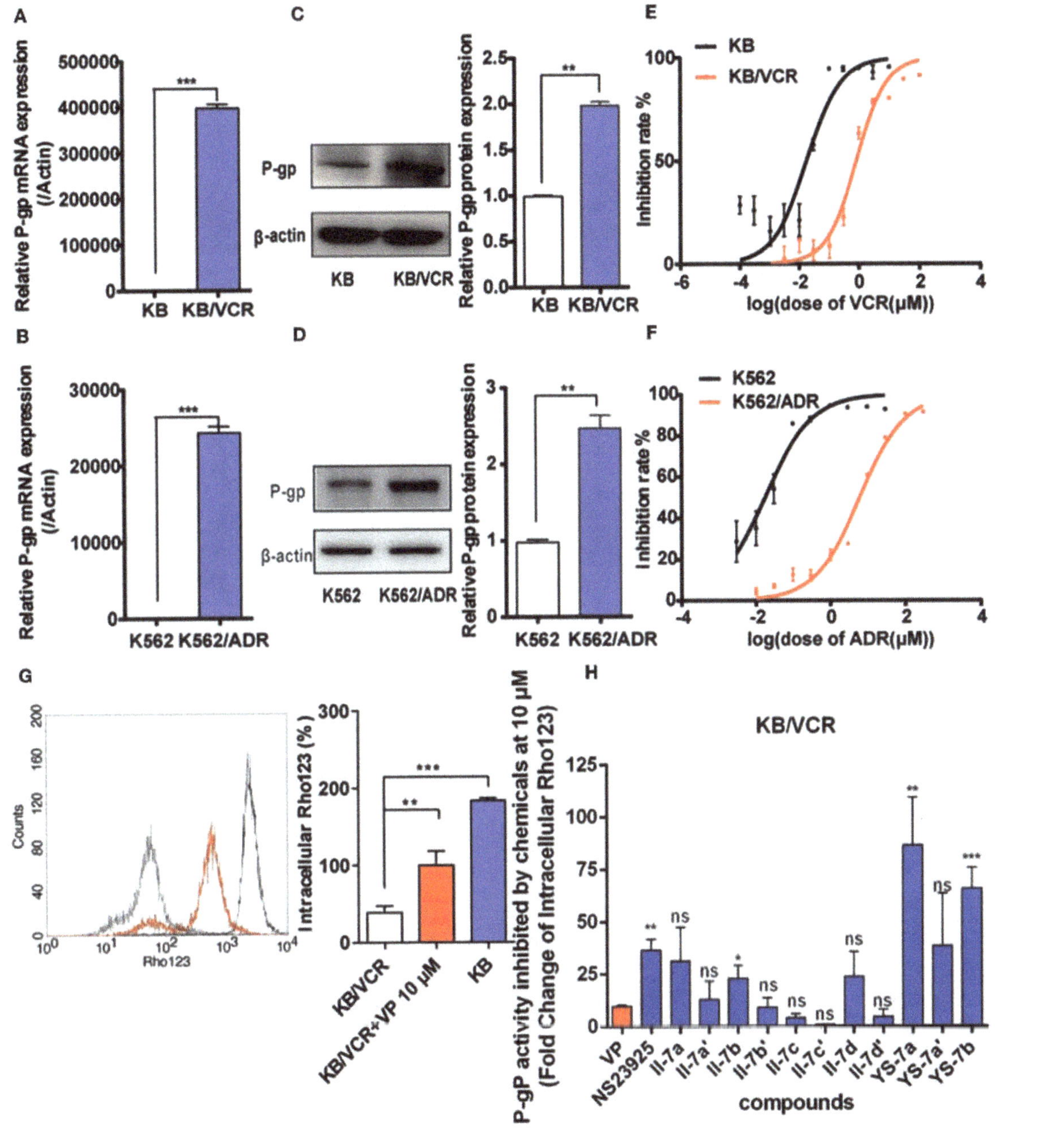

FIGURE 2 | Drug resistance of the KB/VCR and K562/ADR cell lines and screening for novel P-gp inhibitors. **(A,B)** Expression of P-gp mRNA in KB, KB/VCR, K562, and K562/ADR cells. **(C,D)** Expression of P-gp protein in KB, KB/VCR, K562, and K562/ADR cells. **(E,F)** The IC_{50} was determined after exposure to a series concentration of chemotherapy drugs (VCR or ADR) in KB, KB/VCR, K562, and K562/ADR cells for 72 h, and were measured using the MTT assay. **(G)** Intracellular content of Rho123 in KB cells, KB/VCR cells, and KB/VCR cells exposed to 10 μM VP for 4 h. **(H)** Flow cytometry was used to screen compounds that exhibited strong P-gp inhibition after incubation for 4 h; YS-7a and YS-7b resulted in more than 50 times accumulation of Rho123, and were chosen for further study. All experiments were repeated at least three times. $^{**}P < 0.01$ and $^{***}P < 0.001$.

YS-7a Does Not Affect P-gp Expression but Directly Inhibits Transport Function

MDR cells often exhibit overactivated or overexpressed P-gp and abnormal P-gp ATPase activity. To explore the specific mechanisms of YS-7a, flow cytometry was performed to monitor the function of P-gp transporters *via* Rho123 efflux. Treatment of KB/VCR cells with 10 μM YS-7a resulted in a significant increase compared to the group treated with 2.5 μM VP (positive control) (**Figure 5A**). Consistent results were obtained in K562/ADR cells (**Figure 5B**). However, YS-7a did not affect P-gp mRNA and protein levels in KB/VCR and K562/ADR cells (**Figures 5C–E**). These results showed that YS-7a inhibited P-gp function, but

TABLE 1 | SAR study of novel quinoline compounds

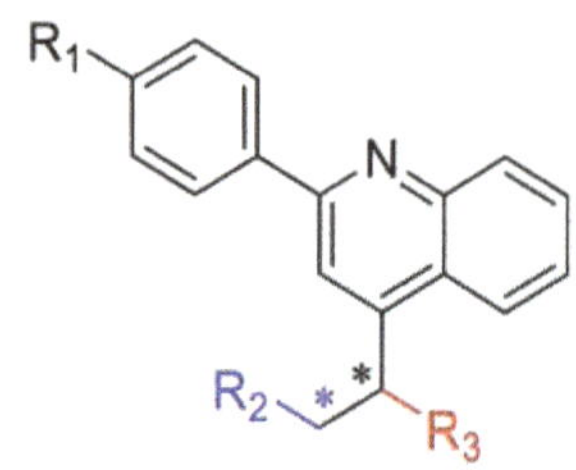

Compound	-R_1	-R_2	-R_3	Structure	tR(min) /HPLC	Fold change of intracellular Rho123 (FC)
NSC23925	-OMe	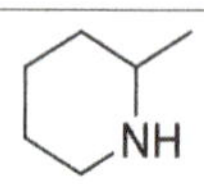	-OH			36.50 ± 5.20
II-7a	-Me	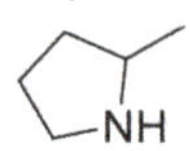	-OH	Etythro (RS, SR) isomer	tR = 19.23 min 96.61%	31.35 ± 16.05
II-7a′				Threo (RR, SS) isomer	tR = 19.718 min 95.66%	12.94 ± 8.72
II-7b	-OMe			Etythro (RS, SR) isomer	tR = 19.068 min 96.17%	23 ± 6.13
II-7b′				Threo (RR, SS) isomer	tR = 19.488 min 95.10%	9.16 ± 4.66
II-7c	-CF_3			Etythro (RS, SR) isomer	tR = 10.917 min 97.35%	4.15 ± 1.96
II-7c′				Threo (RR, SS) isomer	tR = 13.772 min 95.03%	1.04 ± 0.01
II-7d	-F			Etythro (RS, SR) isomer	tR = 9.931 min 95.70%	23.79 ± 11.86
II-7d′				Threo (RR, SS) isomer	tR = 12.429 min 95.00%	4.63 ± 3.57
YS-7a	-Me	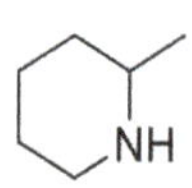	-OMe	Etythro (RS, SR) isomer	tR = 18.222 min 96.33%	86.43 ± 22.92
YS-7-a′				Threo (RR, SS) isomer	tR = 19.923 min 96.93%	38.42 ± 25.09
YS-7b	-OMe			Etythro (RS, SR) isomer	tR = 19.409 min 97.22%	65.85 ± 10.04

not expression. We further measured P-gp ATPase activity in the presence of YS-7a using the Pgp-Glo™ Assay Systems Kit (Promega; Madison, WI, USA), and found that YS-7a stimulated P-gp ATPase activity in a dose-dependent manner (**Figure 5F**). These results demonstrate that YS-7a may inhibit the P-gp substrate binding site in a similar manner as VP.

To explore the involvement of P-gp as a therapeutic target of YS-7a, we performed molecular docking experiments of YS-7a with P-gp (PDB: 3WME). The binding energies for all YS-7a poses were −11.3 kcal/mol, indicating that YS-7a could strongly bind to P-gp. Our results also showed that YS-7a formed six hydrophobic interactions with residues SER270, VAL273, VAL274, ILE354, VAL357, and PHE390 (**Figure 5G**). Based on these observations, YS-7a can directly bind to the functional domains of P-gp. Altogether, YS-7a may suppress the P-gp transport function without affecting its expression, by stimulating the ATPase activity of P-gp by directly binding to the six probable sites instead.

YS-7a Has No Effect on CYP3A4 Activity and Little Toxicity Toward Normal Cells

P-gp inhibitors, such as PSC-833 (Boesch et al., 1991; Kusunoki et al., 2010), can inhibit CYP3A4 activity, resulting in complicated drug–drug interactions and unexpected side effects; the ensuing toxicity can lead to failure of the final inhibitor clinical trial. To explore the potential for drug–drug interactions, we measured CYP3A4 activity after treatment with YS-7a. The results showed that YS-7a had no effect on CYP3A4 activity, even

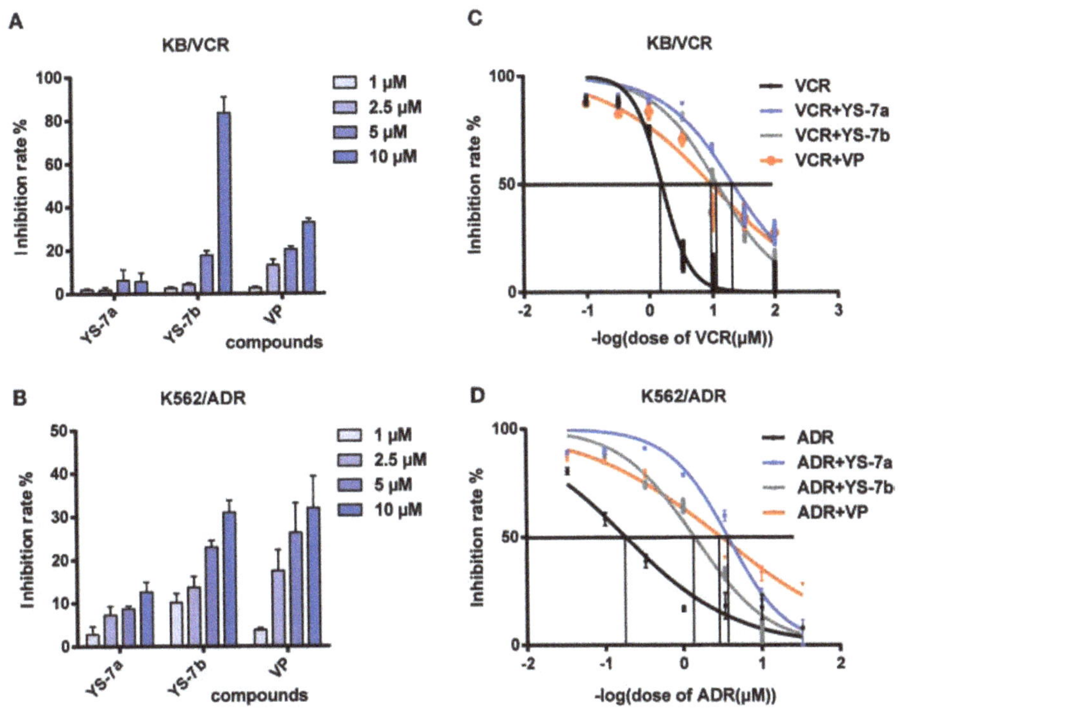

FIGURE 3 | Cytotoxicity and reversal effect of the candidate compounds YS-7a and YS-7b in KB/VCR and K562/ADR cells. The compounds were diluted to four concentrations, 1, 2.5, 5, and 10 μM, and cytotoxicity was evaluated after 72 h using the MTT assay in **(A)** KB/VCR and **(B)** K562/ADR cells. **(C)** Combined treatment of 10 μM YS-7a and 2.5 μM YS-7b with a series of VCR concentrations in KB/VCR cells for 72 h. **(D)** Combined treatment of 10 μM YS-7a and 2.5 μM YS-7b with a series of ADR concentrations in K562/ADR cells for 72 h. The data shown represent the mean ± SD of three independent experiments.

at high doses (100 μM) (**Figure 6A**). Thus, YS-7a may not have drug metabolism interactions.

Drugs can also show toxicity to vascular endothelial cells after entering the blood circulation (Cao et al., 2017). Thus, we evaluated the potential toxicity of YS-7a in human umbilical vein endothelial cells (HUVECs). The IC_{50} of YS-7a in HUVECs was 45.33 ± 2.55 μM (**Figure 6B**), suggesting that YS-7a (10 μM) has low potential for toxicity at concentrations used to reverse drug resistance. These results support the application of YS-7a as a novel potent P-gp inhibitor that can inhibit its transporter functions without undesirable side effects on CYP3A4 activity or endothelial cell toxicity.

In vivo Drug Resistance Reversal Effect of YS-7a

The mechanism and potential toxicity of YS-7a was confirmed *in vitro*. However, whether YS-7a reverses MDR *in vivo* remained unclear. Thus, we performed an *in vivo* xenograft experiment to evaluate the reversal effect of YS-7a (**Figure 7**). When combined with 0.5 mg/kg VCR, YS-7a at a dose of 10 mg/kg showed tumor growth inhibition of approximately 50.11%, while the single 10 mg/kg YS-7a group and single VCR group showed poor inhibition rates. Simultaneously, no YS-7a groups showed a decrease in mouse weight, indicating that YS-7a may have minimal toxicity *in vivo*. These findings indicate that YS-7a can reverse MDR *in vivo* with minimal potential toxicity.

DISCUSSION

To combat MDR cancer, the development of novel P-gp inhibitors is important, and most P-gp inhibitors are in preclinical or clinical trials. In this study, we synthesized 11 novel quinoline compounds, which could be divided into low-polarity (II-7a, II-7b, II-7c, II-7d, YS-7a, and YS-7b) and high-polarity (II-7a′, II-7b′, II-7c′, II-7d′, and YS-7a′) groups based on HPLC. Among these, YS-7a had the best MDR reversal effect *in vitro*, showing a reversal effect of over 10-fold in KB/VCR cells and over 30-fold in K562/ADR cells at low-toxicity concentrations.

We confirmed that YS-7a directly inhibited the transporter function of P-gp without affecting its expression, stimulating P-gp ATPase activity in a dose-dependent manner instead. Furthermore, YS-7a did not inhibit CYP3A4 activity and showed little cytotoxicity toward HUVECs at a concentration of 10 μM. In the KB/VCR xenograft model, 10 mg/kg YS-7a combined with 0.5 mg/kg VCR showed significant differences in tumor volumes compared to the control, with an average tumor growth inhibition exceeding 50%. These findings support YS-7a as a novel P-gp inhibitor, and can provide a reference for the design and development of additional P-gp inhibitors.

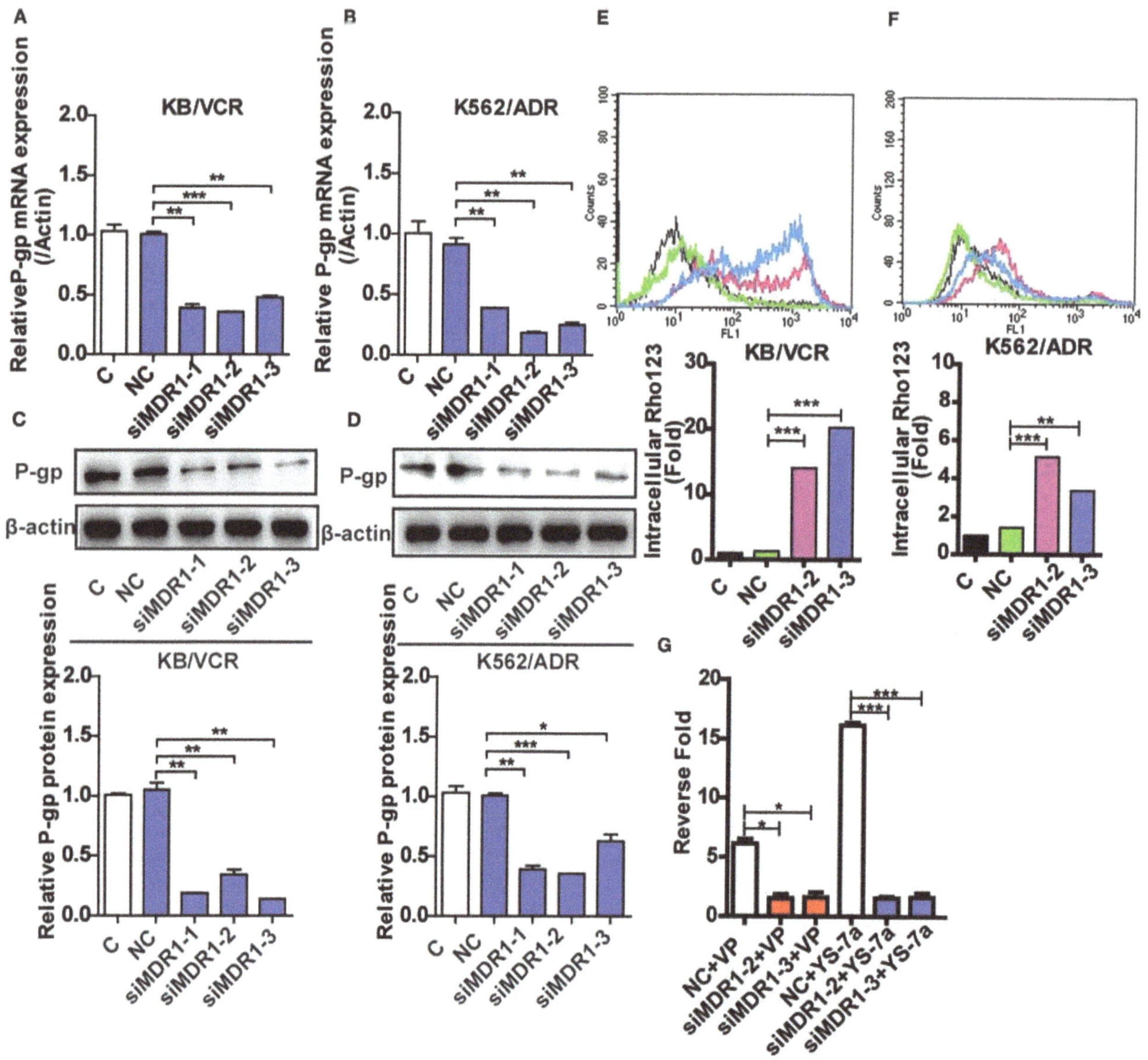

FIGURE 4 | Confirmation of the target of YS-7a in MDR cells. The expression of P-45 gp mRNA and protein in *MDR1* knockdown **(A,C)** KB/VCR cells and **(B,D)** K562/ADR cells. Changes in P-gp transporter function in *MDR1* knockdown **(E)** KB/VCR cells and **(F)** K562/ADR cells. **(G)** The target of YS-7a was verified through the fold change in drug resistance reversal in KB/VCR cells using the MTT assay after *MDR1* knockdown. All results were repeated at least three times. $^{*}P < 0.05$, $^{**}P < 0.01$, and $^{***}P < 0.001$.

P-gp inhibitors are generally classified based on their inhibition mechanism: inhibiting the substrate binding site, interfering with ATP hydrolysis, or altering the integrity or fluidity of cell membrane lipids, which inhibits P-gp structural transformation (Shapiro and Ling, 1997; Varma et al., 2003; Drori et al., 2010). Most P-gp inhibitors inhibit the substrate binding site. Based on these reports, we screened P-gp inhibitors by performing Rho123 efflux experiments (**Figure 3**). Furthermore, MDR cancer cells show overexpression or excessive activation of P-gp, and P-gp inhibitors may inhibit the expression or function of P-gp (Silva et al., 2015). Therefore, the effects of YS-7a on P-gp function and expression were measured (**Figure 5**). Our results showed that YS-7a suppressed P-gp transport function without affecting its expression. In addition, P-gp ATPase activity is affected by various drug resistance regulators, such as VP (Sharom et al., 1995). The YS-7a inhibition effect of P-gp ATPase was reflected by ATP consumption measurement using the P-gp-Glo™ Assay Systems Kit (**Figure 5F**). Our results suggest that YS-7a inhibits the P-gp substrate binding site, similar to VP; however, further studies are required to verify its mechanism of action.

P-gp and CYP3A4 play important roles in reducing intracellular concentrations of xenobiotics and drug absorption through their respective roles in xenobiotic excretion and

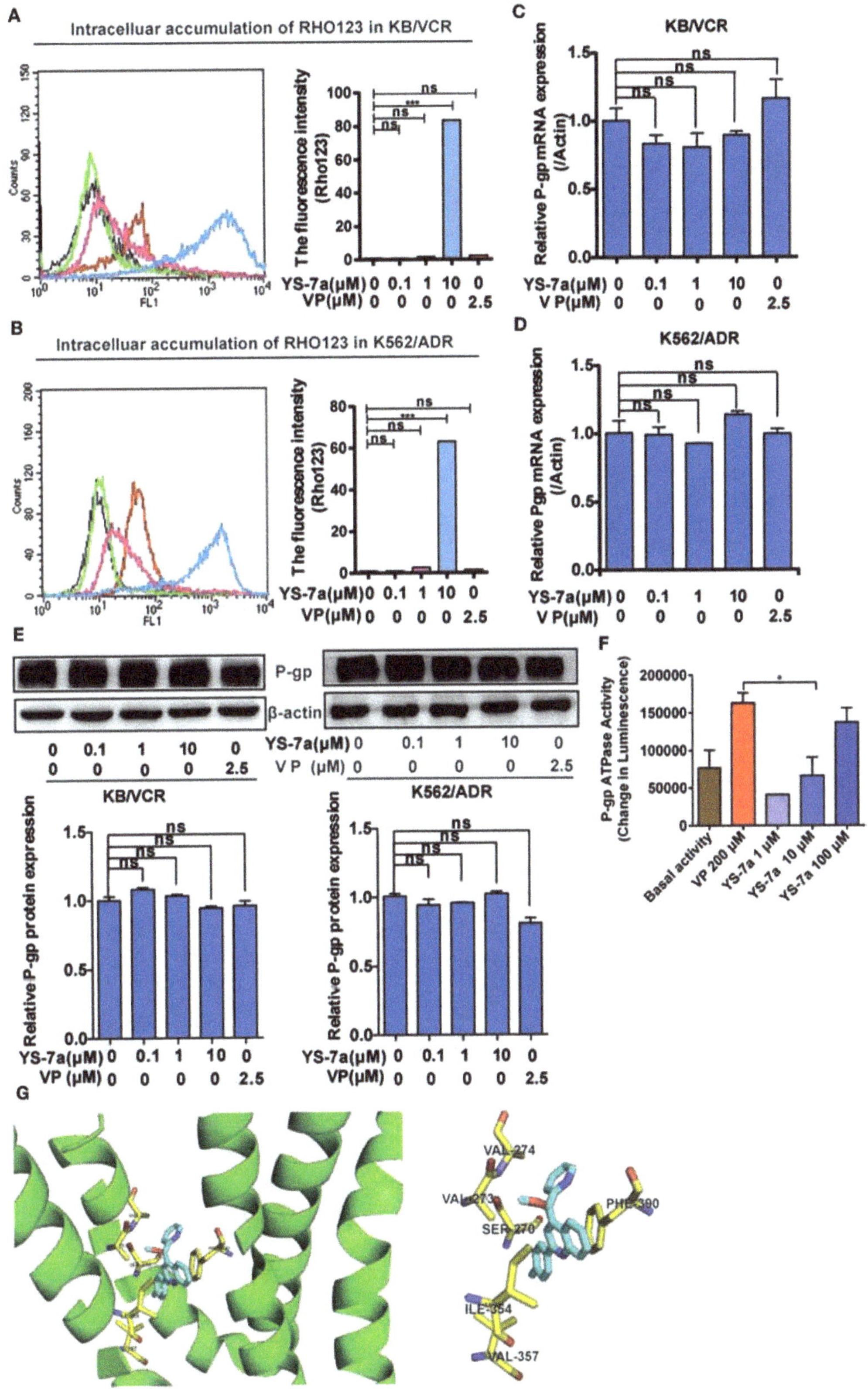

FIGURE 5 | Mechanism of P-gp inhibition by YS-7a. Intracellular accumulation of Rho123 in **(A)** KB/VCR and **(B)** K562/ADR cells after exposure to YS-7a. Effect of YS-7a on the expression of P-gp **(C,D)** mRNA and **(E)** protein in KB/VCR and K562/ADR cells. **(F)** Effect of YS-7a on P-gp ATPase activity after different drug concentrations were incubated with recombinant P-gp protein; VP was used as the positive control and basal activity as the negative control. **(G)** Molecular docking of YS-7a with P-gp (3WME); the yellow amino acid residues represent a distance of 1 angstrom or less, $^{***}P < 0.001$.

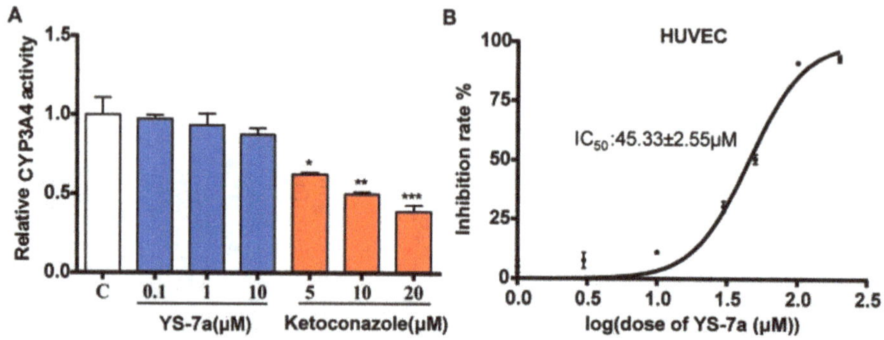

FIGURE 6 | Potential toxicity of YS-7a *in vitro*. **(A)** Effect of different concentrations of YS-7a on CYP3A4 activity. **(B)** The 72-h cytotoxicity of YS-7a in HUVECs measured using the MTT assay. All experiments were repeated at least three times. $^{*}P < 0.05$, $^{**}P < 0.01$, and $^{***}P < 0.001$.

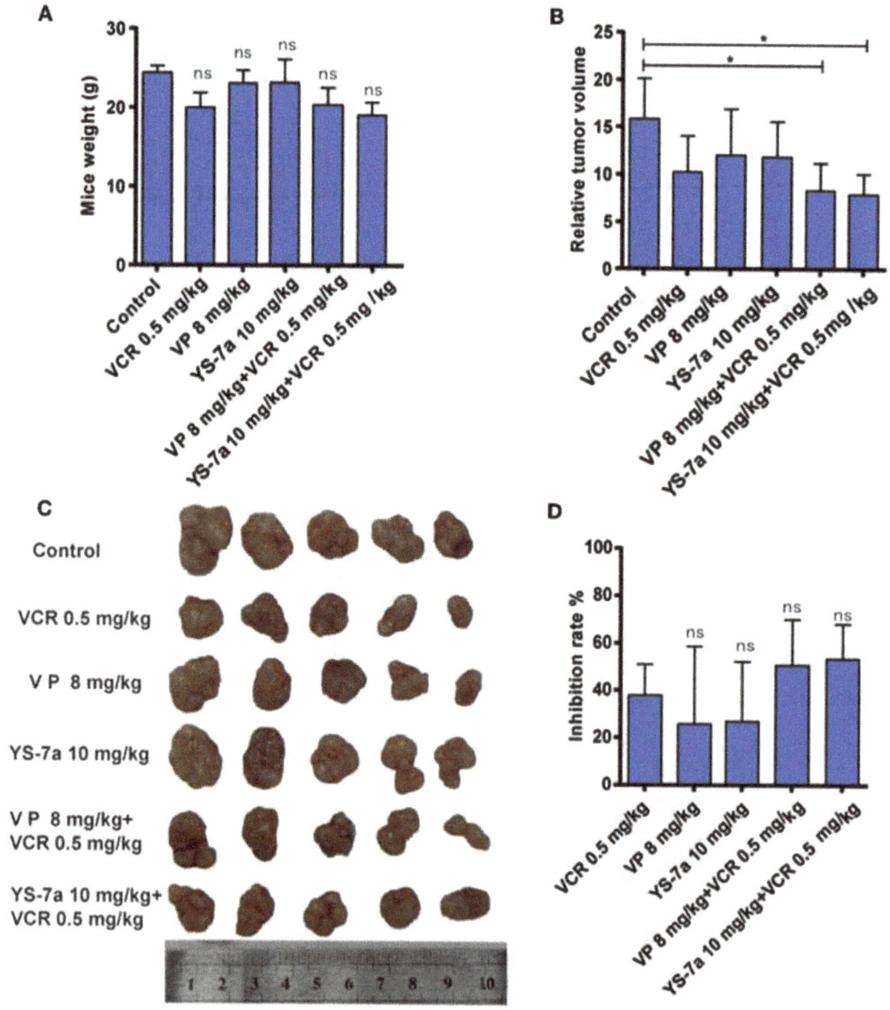

FIGURE 7 | *In vivo* drug resistance reversal effect of YS-7a in KB/VCR xenograft nude mice. **(A)** The weight of KB/VCR xenograft nude mice in all groups after treatment for 24 days. **(B)** The relative tumor volume of KB/VCR xenograft nude mice in all treatment groups after 24 days. **(C)** Images of tumors from the KB/VCR xenograft nude mice in every treatment group. **(D)** Tumor inhibition rate in every treatment group after 24 days, $^{*}P < 0.05$.

metabolism. P-gp and CYP3A4 work in coordination, given their co-localization in intestinal epithelial tissue and similarly overlapping substrates (Watkins, 1997; Katoh et al., 2001; Oliver et al., 2004). Several studies have reported that P-gp inhibitors inhibit CYP3A4, leading to unexpected toxicity (Wacher et al., 1998; Mathias et al., 2015). To predict potential drug–drug interactions, we measured the inhibitory effects of YS-7a on CYP3A4 activity (**Figure 6**). Our results suggested that YS-7a did not inhibit CYP3A4 activity. Therefore, YS-7a may have fewer side effects than PSC-833 and dexverapamil.

As shown *in vitro* (**Figures 3–6**), the novel P-gp inhibitor YS-7a showed superior reversal effects compared to VP by binding directly to P-gp. However, confirming whether YS-7a binds at the sites predicted by molecular docking, requires further study. Various methods, such as mutating the corresponding sites or radioisotope tracing (Hrycyna et al., 1999; Tsujimura et al., 2008), could be applied. *In vivo*, the drug resistance reversal effect of YS-7a was relatively low (about 50%). However, YS-7a at a dose of 10 mg/kg did not significantly decrease mouse body weight, suggestive of little-to-no toxicity or side effects. Thus, YS-7a may exhibit better reversal effects at higher doses. Many reports (Krepler et al., 2016; Vaidhyanathan et al., 2016) have shown that the patient-derived xenograft (PDX) model is ideal to evaluate the efficiency and toxicity of small-molecule inhibitors *in vivo*. Therefore, future studies should apply the PDX model to confirm the drug resistance reversal effect of YS-7a. Moreover, the pharmacokinetics of YS-7a should be explored to investigate its potential therapeutic mechanism in future studies.

CONCLUSIONS

We obtained a novel potent quinoline P-gp inhibitor derived from NSC23925, which showed a cancer MDR reversal effect both *in vitro* and *in vivo*. First, 11 novel quinoline compounds were synthesized, and potential P-gp inhibitors were screened using the classic screening model. YS-7a showed a significant inhibition effect against cellular Rho123 efflux. The MDR reversal effect and potential mechanisms of YS-7a were verified *in vitro*. YS-7a suppressed the P-gp transport function without affecting its expression, by stimulating the ATPase activity of P-gp in a dose-dependent manner instead. In addition, potential binding sites were predicted based on molecular docking. Finally, *in vitro* experiments support the low toxicity of YS-7a and the MDR reversal effect of YS-7a was verified in a KB/VCR cancer xenograft model with minimal toxicity. Overall, these results suggest that YS-7a may be a potential candidate compound for the development for new agents to reverse cancer MDR.

AUTHOR CONTRIBUTIONS

XQ, HD, JX, XY, LSh, and LSu defined the research subject and its aims, conceived, and designed the experiments. XQ, HD, JX, XH, XG, YZ, LSh, and YW conducted the experiments. XQ, HD, JJ, LL, and SY analyzed the data and wrote the paper.

FUNDING

This work was supported by National Key Research and Development Program of China (No. 2017YFA0205200), the National Natural Science Foundation of China (No. 21702051, 81773766, and 81903845), the Double First-Class University Project (No. CPU2018GY38), the Natural Science Foundation of Jiangsu Province (BK20181330) and the Key Scientific Research Project of Henan Province (No. 18A150009 and 17A350006).

REFERENCES

Alfarouk, K. O., Stock, C. M., Taylor, S., Walsh, M., Muddathir, A. K., Verduzco, D., et al. (2015). Resistance to cancer chemotherapy: failure in drug response from ADME to P-gp. *Cancer Cell Int.* 15:71. doi: 10.1186/s12935-015-0221-1

Bellamy, W. T., Dalton, W. S., Kailey, J. M., Gleason, M. C., Mccloskey, T. M., Dorr, R. T., et al. (1988). Verapamil reversal of doxorubicin resistance in multidrug-resistant human myeloma cells and association with drug accumulation and DNA damage. *Cancer Res.* 48, 6365–6370.

Boesch, D., Muller, K., Pourtiermanzanedo, A., and Loor, F. (1991). Restoration of daunomycin retention in multidrug-resistant P388 cells by submicromolar concentrations of SDZ PSC 833, a nonimmunosuppressive cyclosporin derivative. *Exp. Cell Res.* 196, 26–32. doi: 10.1016/0014-4827(91)90452-Z

Cao, Y., Gong, Y., Liu, L., Zhou, Y., Fang, X., Zhang, C., et al. (2017). The use of human umbilical vein endothelial cells (HUVECs) as an *in vitro* model to assess the toxicity of nanoparticles to endothelium: a review. *J. Appl. Toxicol.* 37, 1359–1369. doi: 10.1002/jat.3470

Cha, Y. J., Lee, H., Gu, N., Kim, T. E., Lim, K. S., Yoon, S. H., et al. (2013). Sustained increase in the oral bioavailability of loperamide after a single oral dose of HM30181, a P-glycoprotein Inhibitor, in healthy male participants. *Basic Clin. Pharmacol. Toxicol.* 113, 419–424. doi: 10.1111/bcpt.12108

Chico, I., Kang, M. H., Bergan, R., Abraham, J., Bakke, S., Meadows, B., et al. (2001). Phase I study of infusional paclitaxel in combination with the P-glycoprotein antagonist PSC 833. *J. Clin. Oncol.* 19, 832–842. doi: 10.1200/JCO.2001.19.3.832

Choi, Y. H., and Yu, A. M. (2014). ABC transporters in multidrug resistance and pharmacokinetics, and strategies for drug development. *Curr. Pharm. Des.* 20, 793–807. doi: 10.2174/138161282005140214165212

Coley, H. M. (2010). Overcoming multidrug resistance in cancer: clinical studies of p-glycoprotein inhibitors. *Methods Mol. Biol.* 596, 341–358. doi: 10.1007/978-1-60761-416-6_15

Dantzig, A. H., Shepard, R. L., Law, K. L., Tabas, L., Pratt, S., Gillespie, J. S., et al. (1999). Selectivity of the multidrug resistance modulator, LY335979, for P-glycoprotein and effect on cytochrome P-450 activities. *J. Pharmacol. Exp. Ther.* 290, 854–862.

Drori, S., Eytan, G. D., and Assaraf, Y. G. (2010). Potentiation of anticancer-drug cytotoxicity by multidrug-resistance chemosensitizers involves alterations in membrane fluidity leading to increased membrane permeability. *FEBS J.* 228, 1020–1029. doi: 10.1111/j.1432-1033.1995.tb20352.x

Du, H., Huang, Y., Hou, X., Quan, X., Jiang, J., Wei, X., et al. (2018). Two novel camptothecin derivatives inhibit colorectal cancer proliferation via induction of cell cycle arrest and apoptosis *in vitro* and *in vivo*. *Eur. J. Pharm. Sci.* 123, 546–559. doi: 10.1016/j.ejps.2018.08.018

Duan, Z., Choy, E., and Hornicek, F. J. (2009). NSC23925, identified in a high-throughput cell-based screen, reverses multidrug resistance. *PLoS ONE* 4:e7415. doi: 10.1371/journal.pone.0007415

Duan, Z., Li, X., Huang, H., Yuan, W., Zheng, S.-L., Liu, X., et al. (2012). Synthesis and evaluation of (2-(4-Methoxyphenyl)-4-quinolinyl)(2-piperidinyl)methanol (NSC23925) isomers to reverse multidrug resistance in cancer. *J. Med. Chem.* 55, 3113–3121. doi: 10.1021/jm300117u

Federica, D. N., Knight, L. A., Sharon, G., Whitehouse, P. A., Mercer, S. J., Sanjay, S., et al. (2004). *Ex vivo* reversal of chemoresistance by tariquidar (XR9576). *Anticancer. Drugs* 15, 861–869. doi: 10.1097/00001813-200410000-00006

Fojo, A. T., Ueda, K., Slamon, D. J., Poplack, D. G., Gottesman, M. M., and Pastan, I. (1987). Expression of a multidrug-resistance gene in human tumors and tissues. *Proc. Natl. Acad. Sci. U.S.A.* 84, 265–269. doi: 10.1073/pnas.84.1.265

Fox, E., and Bates, S. E. (2007). Tariquidar (XR9576): a P-glycoprotein drug efflux pump inhibitor. *Expert Rev. Anticancer Ther.* 7, 447–459. doi: 10.1586/14737140.7.4.447

Hou, X., Du, H., Quan, X., Shi, L., Zhang, Q., Wu, Y., et al. (2018a). Silibinin inhibits NSCLC metastasis by targeting the EGFR/LOX pathway. *Front. Pharmacol.* 9:21. doi: 10.3389/fphar.2018.00021

Hou, X., Du, H., Yang, R., Qi, J., Huang, Y., Feng, S., et al. (2018b). The antitumor activity screening of chemical constituents from Camellia nitidissima Chi. *Int. J. Mol. Med.* 41, 2793–2801. doi: 10.3892/ijmm.2018.3502

Hrycyna, C. A., Ramachandra, M., Germann, U. A., Cheng, P. W., Pastan, I., and Gottesman, M. M. (1999). Both ATP sites of human P-glycoprotein are essential but not symmetric. *Biochemistry* 38, 13887–13899. doi: 10.1021/bi991115m

Katoh, M., Nakajima, M., Yamazaki, H., and Yokoi, T. (2001). Inhibitory effects of CYP3A4 substrates and their metabolites on P-glycoprotein-mediated transport. *Eur. J. Pharm. Sci.* 12, 505–513. doi: 10.1016/S0928-0987(00)00215-3

Köhler, S. C., and Wiese, M. (2015). HM30181 derivatives as novel potent and selective inhibitors of the breast cancer resistance protein (BCRP/ABCG2). *J. Med. Chem.* 58, 3910–3921. doi: 10.1021/acs.jmedchem.5b00188

Konstantinos, B. (2015). Structural basis for the mechanism of ABC transporters. *Biochem. Soc. Trans.* 43, 889–893. doi: 10.1042/BST20150047

Krepler, C., Xiao, M., Katrin, S., Brafford, P., Shannan, B., Beqiri, M., et al. and Herlyn, M. (2016). Personalized pre-clinical trials in BRAF inhibitor resistant patient derived xenograft models of melanoma identify c-Met as an effective second line combination therapy target. *Clin. Cancer Res.* 75, 1592–1602. doi: 10.1158/1078-0432.CCR-15-1762

Krishna, R., and Mayer, L. D. (2000). Multidrug resistance (MDR) in cancer-mechanisms, reversal using modulators of MDR and the role of MDR modulators in influencing the pharmacokinetics of anticancer drugs. *Eur. J. Pharm. Sci.* 11, 265–283. doi: 10.1016/S0928-0987(00)00114-7

Kumar, A., and Jaitak, V. (2019). Natural products as multidrug resistance modulators in cancer. *Eur. J. Med. Chem.* 176, 268–291. doi: 10.1016/j.ejmech.2019.05.027

Kusunoki, N., Takara, K., Tanigawara, Y., Yamauchi, A., Ueda, K., Komada, F., et al. (2010). Inhibitory effects of a cyclosporin derivative, SDZ PSC 833, on transport of doxorubicin and vinblastine via human P-glycoprotein. *Cancer Sci.* 89, 1220–1228. doi: 10.1111/j.1349-7006.1998.tb00518.x

Labrie, P., Maddaford, S. P., Lacroix, J., Catalano, C., Lee, D. K. H., Rakhit, S., et al. (2006). *In vitro* activity of novel dual action MDR anthranilamide modulators with inhibitory activity at CYP-450. *Bioorg. Med. Chem.* 14, 7972–7987. doi: 10.1016/j.bmc.2006.07.055

Lapidus, J. B., and Fauley, J. J. (1971). Absolute configuration of the phenyl 2-piperidylcarbinols. *J. Organic Chem.* 36, 3065–3067. doi: 10.1021/jo00819a045

Mathias, T. J., Natarajan, K., Shukla, S., Doshi, K. A., Singh, Z. N., Ambudkar, S. V., et al. (2015). The FLT3 and PDGFR inhibitor crenolanib is a substrate of the multidrug resistance protein ABCB1 but does not inhibit transport function at pharmacologically relevant concentrations. *Invest. New Drugs* 33, 300–309. doi: 10.1007/s10637-015-0205-y

Oliver, V. R., Oliver, B., Fromm, M. F., Thon, K. P., Michel, E., and Kivistö, K. T. (2004). Cytochrome P450 3A4 and P-glycoprotein expression in human small intestinal enterocytes and hepatocytes: a comparative analysis in paired tissue specimens. *Clin. Pharm. Ther.* 75, 172–183. doi: 10.1016/j.clpt.2003.10.008

Pirker, R., Zöchbauer, S., Kupper, H., Laßmann, A., Gsur, A., Frass, M., et al. (1995). Dexverapamil as resistance modifier in acute myeloid leukaemia. *J. Cancer Res. Clin. Oncol.* 3, 21–24. doi: 10.1007/BF02351067

Shapiro, A. B., and Ling, V. (1997). Effect of quercetin on Hoechst 33342 transport by purified and reconstituted P-glycoprotein. *Biochem. Pharmacol.* 53, 587–596. doi: 10.1016/S0006-2952(96)00826-X

Sharom, F. J., Yu, X., Chu, J. W., and Doige, C. A. (1995). Characterization of the ATPase activity of P-glycoprotein from multidrug-resistant Chinese hamster ovary cells. *Biochem. J.* 308(Pt 2), 381–390. doi: 10.1042/bj3080381

Shepard, R. L., Cao, J., Starling, J. J., and Dantzig, A. H. (2003). Modulation of P-glycoprotein but not MRP1- or BCRP-mediated drug resistance by LY335979. *Int. J. Cancer* 103, 121–125. doi: 10.1002/ijc.10792

Silva, R., Vilas-Boas, V., Carmo, H., Dinis-Oliveira, R. J., Carvalho, F., De Lourdes Bastos, M., et al. (2015). Modulation of P-glycoprotein efflux pump: induction and activation as a therapeutic strategy. *Pharmacol. Ther.* 149, 1–123. doi: 10.1016/j.pharmthera.2014.11.013

Solladié-Cavallo, A., Marsol, C., Yaakoub, M., Azyat, K., Klein, A., Roje, M., et al. (2003). erythro-1-Naphthyl-1-(2-piperidyl)methanol: synthesis, resolution, NMR relative configuration, and VCD absolute configuration. *J. Org. Chem.* 68, 7308–7315. doi: 10.1021/jo0345502

Thürlimann, B., Kröger, N., Greiner, J., Mross, K., Schüller, J., Schernhammer, E., et al. (1995). Dexverapamil to overcome epirubicin resistance in advanced breast cancer. *J. Cancer Res. Clin. Oncol.* 121, R3–R6. doi: 10.1007/BF02351063

Tsujimura, S., Saito, K., Nawata, M., Nakayamada, S., and Tanaka, Y. (2008). Overcoming drug resistance induced by P-glycoprotein on lymphocytes in patients with refractory rheumatoid arthritis. *Ann. Rheum. Dis.* 67, 380–388. doi: 10.1136/ard.2007.070821

Vaidhyanathan, S., Wilken-Resman, B., Ma, D. J., Parrish, K. E., Mittapalli, R. K., Carlson, B. L., et al. (2016). Factors influencing the central nervous system distribution of a novel phosphoinositide 3-kinase/mammalian target of rapamycin inhibitor GSK2126458: implications for overcoming resistance with combination therapy for melanoma brain metastases. *J. Pharmacol. Exp. Ther.* 356, 251–259. doi: 10.1124/jpet.115.229393

Varma, M. V., Ashokraj, Y., Dey, C. S., and Panchagnula, R. (2003). P-glycoprotein inhibitors and their screening: a perspective from bioavailability enhancement. *Pharmacol. Res.* 48, 347–359. doi: 10.1016/S1043-6618(03)00158-0

Wacher, V. J., Silverman, J. A., Zhang, Y., and Benet, L. Z. (1998). Role of P-glycoprotein and cytochrome P450 3A in limiting oral absorption of peptides and peptidomimetics. *J. Pharm. Sci.* 87, 1322–1330. doi: 10.1021/js980082d

Wang, E., Casciano, C. N., Clement, R. P., and Johnson, W. W. (2000). *In vitro* flow cytometry method to quantitatively assess inhibitors of P-glycoprotein. *Drug Metab. Dispos.* 28, 522–528.

Watkins, P. B. (1997). The barrier function of CYP3A4 and P-glycoprotein in the small bowel. *Adv. Drug Deliv. Rev.* 27, 161. doi: 10.1016/S0169-409X(97)00041-0

Wei, X., Mao, T., Li, S., He, J., Hou, X., Li, H., et al. (2019). DT-13 inhibited the proliferation of colorectal cancer via glycolytic metabolism and AMPK/mTOR signaling pathway. *Phytomedicine* 54, 120–131. doi: 10.1016/j.phymed.2018.09.003

Wu, Q., Yang, Z., Nie, Y., Shi, Y., and Fan, D. (2014). Multi-drug resistance in cancer chemotherapeutics: Mechanisms and lab approaches. *Cancer Lett.* 347, 159–166. doi: 10.1016/j.canlet.2014.03.013

Yang, X., Feng, Y., Gao, Y., Shen, J., Choy, E., Cote, G., et al. (2015). NSC23925 prevents the emergence of multidrug resistance in ovarian cancer *in vitro* and *in vivo*. *Gynecol. Oncol.* 137, 134–142. doi: 10.1016/j.ygyno.2015.02.002

Yang, X., Yang, P., Shen, J., Osaka, E., Choy, E., Cote, G., et al. (2014). Prevention of multidrug resistance (MDR) in osteosarcoma by NSC23925. *Br. J. Cancer* 110, 2896–2904. doi: 10.1038/bjc.2014.254

Yusa, K., and Tsuruo, T. (1989). Reversal mechanism of multidrug resistance by verapamil: direct binding of verapamil to P-glycoprotein on specific sites and transport of verapamil outward across the plasma membrane of K562/ADM cells. *Cancer Res.* 49, 5002–5006.

14

Exploring the Use of Compound-Induced Transcriptomic Data Generated from Cell Lines to Predict Compound Activity Toward Molecular Targets

Benoît Baillif[1], *Joerg Wichard*[2], *Oscar Méndez-Lucio*[1,3†] and *David Rouquié*[1*†]

[1] Bayer SAS, Bayer CropScience, Sophia Antipolis, France, [2] Department of Genetic Toxicology, Bayer AG, Berlin, Germany, [3] Bloomoon, Villeurbanne, France

Correspondence:
David Rouquié
david.rouquie@bayer.com

† These authors jointly supervised this work

Pharmaceutical or phytopharmaceutical molecules rely on the interaction with one or more specific molecular targets to induce their anticipated biological responses. Nonetheless, these compounds are also prone to interact with many other non-intended biological targets, also known as off-targets. Unfortunately, off-target identification is difficult and expensive. Consequently, QSAR models predicting the activity on a target have gained importance in drug discovery or in the de-risking of chemicals. However, a restricted number of targets are well characterized and hold enough data to build such *in silico* models. A good alternative to individual target evaluations is to use integrative evaluations such as transcriptomics obtained from compound-induced gene expression measurements derived from cell cultures. The advantage of these particular experiments is to capture the consequences of the interaction of compounds on many possible molecular targets and biological pathways, without having any constraints concerning the chemical space. In this work, we assessed the value of a large public dataset of compound-induced transcriptomic data, to predict compound activity on a selection of 69 molecular targets. We compared such descriptors with other QSAR descriptors, namely the Morgan fingerprints (similar to extended-connectivity fingerprints). Depending on the target, active compounds could show similar signatures in one or multiple cell lines, whether these active compounds shared similar or different chemical structures. Random forest models using gene expression signatures were able to perform similarly or better than counterpart models built with Morgan fingerprints for 25% of the target prediction tasks. These performances occurred mostly using signatures produced in cell lines showing similar signatures for active compounds toward the considered target. We show that compound-induced transcriptomic data could represent a great opportunity for target prediction, allowing to overcome the chemical space limitation of QSAR models.

Keywords: target prediction, compound-induced transcriptomic data, QSAR, machine learning, cellular context

INTRODUCTION

Biologically active molecules rely on the interaction with one or more molecular targets (Hughes et al., 2000). In the context of hit discovery both in pharmaceutical or in phytopharmaceutical industries, a major objective is to be able to screen molecule candidates for their activity toward a target of interest, and assessing compound activity toward off-targets, that can cause adverse effects *in vivo* (Rouquié et al., 2015). Testing activity of every candidate on a battery of targets represent a complex task that requires major R&D costs. A potential solution to predict candidate's activity with a lower cost is to perform computational methods using more general measured or calculated descriptors (Chen et al., 2016; Vamathevan et al., 2019).

A commonly used technique is to compute descriptors from chemical structures, like the extended-connectivity fingerprints (ECFPs) and use them for prediction, relying on the quantitative structure-activity relationship (QSAR) principle, i.e., molecules sharing a similar structure may share a similar activity profile (Rogers and Hahn, 2010; Cherkasov et al., 2014). However, such molecule descriptors show limitations: they do not perform well for all target prediction tasks depending on the quantity and quality of available activity data, prediction is limited to the applicability domain (depending on the training set used), and a small change in chemical structure can lead to a large change in biological response (activity cliffs) (Cruz-Monteagudo et al., 2014).

Additional descriptors have been proposed to circumvent such QSAR drawbacks, such as measurements from large scale biological assays (Petrone et al., 2012; Laufkötter et al., 2019). Results from high throughput screening (HTS) assays, such as bioactivity experiments, can be used as fingerprints (HTSFPs) in predictive models for specific targets. Petrone et al. (2012) showed that models using HTSFPs were outperforming models using ECFPs for certain targets, and that HTSFP models' predictions were covering a large structural diversity. The main limiting factor of such models is the sparsity of available activity data. Besides bioactivity data, more integrative large-scale biological measurements, like transcriptomics or cell morphology readouts can be used for target prediction (Aliper et al., 2016; Pabon et al., 2018; Scheeder et al., 2018; Simm et al., 2018; Hofmarcher et al., 2019; Kuthuru et al., 2019; Lapins and Spjuth, 2019).

Compound-induced gene expression data are gathered from biological experiments reflecting how the compound acted on one or multiple targets in a specific biological context. Cancer cell lines, being easily cultured, are a commonly used model to generate gene expression data. Hughes et al. (2000) proved that enough data allows to use pattern-matching algorithms to study similarity between signatures coming from drug induction (Hughes et al., 2000). Lamb et al. (2006) invented the concept of Connectivity Map (CMAP), creating relationships between small molecules, genes and diseases (Lamb et al., 2006). Since then, transcriptomics data have been shown to be useful to identify new molecules with biological activity (Hieronymus et al., 2006; Wei et al., 2006). Recently, a large public CMAP L1000 dataset was released representing more than 300,000 Gene Expression Signatures (GESs) of cell line responses to so-called perturbagens (Subramanian et al., 2017). GESs were produced for more than 20,000 compounds in 80 human cancer cell lines, tested at various concentration and exposition time. The large scale of this dataset allows the use of GESs in machine learning models for target prediction or drug repurposing (Lee et al., 2016; De Wolf et al., 2018).

In the current work, we investigated whether we could predict compound activity toward a larger number of molecular targets based on their GESs extracted from the CMAP L1000 dataset. In addition, we were interested to reveal how machine learning models using GESs perform compared to models using more traditional QSAR descriptors, such as the Morgan fingerprints.

We show that random forest models built using compound-induced GES were able to effectively predict targets, especially if they were produced from a cell line showing similar GESs between active compounds on the evaluated target. For 25% of the target prediction tasks, GESs models had similar or higher performances than models using Morgan fingerprints, offering an opportunity to escape from the chemical space limitation associated with QSAR approaches.

MATERIALS AND METHODS

Gene Expression Signatures (GESs) Acquisition

The CMAP L1000 dataset was obtained from two GEO repositories: GSE92742, corresponding to the first phase of L1000 (pilot, 2012–2015) and GSE70138, which is the second phase (production, on-going). GESs generation was described by Subramanian et al. (2017).

For this study, we only used Level 5 GESs meaning that each GES is represented by an instance, that is a combination of a perturbagen (chemical or gene deletion), cell line, concentration and time point, and is composed by the plate-normalized expression z-scores of the whole genome, inferred from 978 landmark genes (measured gene that can be used for whole transcriptome inference). We focused on landmark signatures of compound perturbagens, which comprises 333,273 GESs for 21,300 unique compounds. GESs obtained in the exact same condition were averaged, to have one signature per condition.

Among all obtained GESs, the ones generated at a 10 μM and 24 h time point were selected (as shown in **Figure 1**), as this condition was the most represented in the dataset and facilitate the comparison of results. GESs from the 8 most profiled cell lines were used; cell line and number of GESs are presented in **Table 1**. Also, only GESs generated by compounds with known structure were selected. In total, the working dataset contains 39,544 GESs obtained from 9,035 compounds.

Activity Data Acquisition

Annotations about activity or inactivity was retrieved from the PubChem BioAssay database, using available CIDs documented in the L1000 signature metadata, excepted for TUBB actives, that were extracted from the Drug Repurposing Hub of the LINCS (Wang et al., 2014; Corsello et al., 2017). Activity data were compiled in a binary activity matrix (1 for active, 0 for

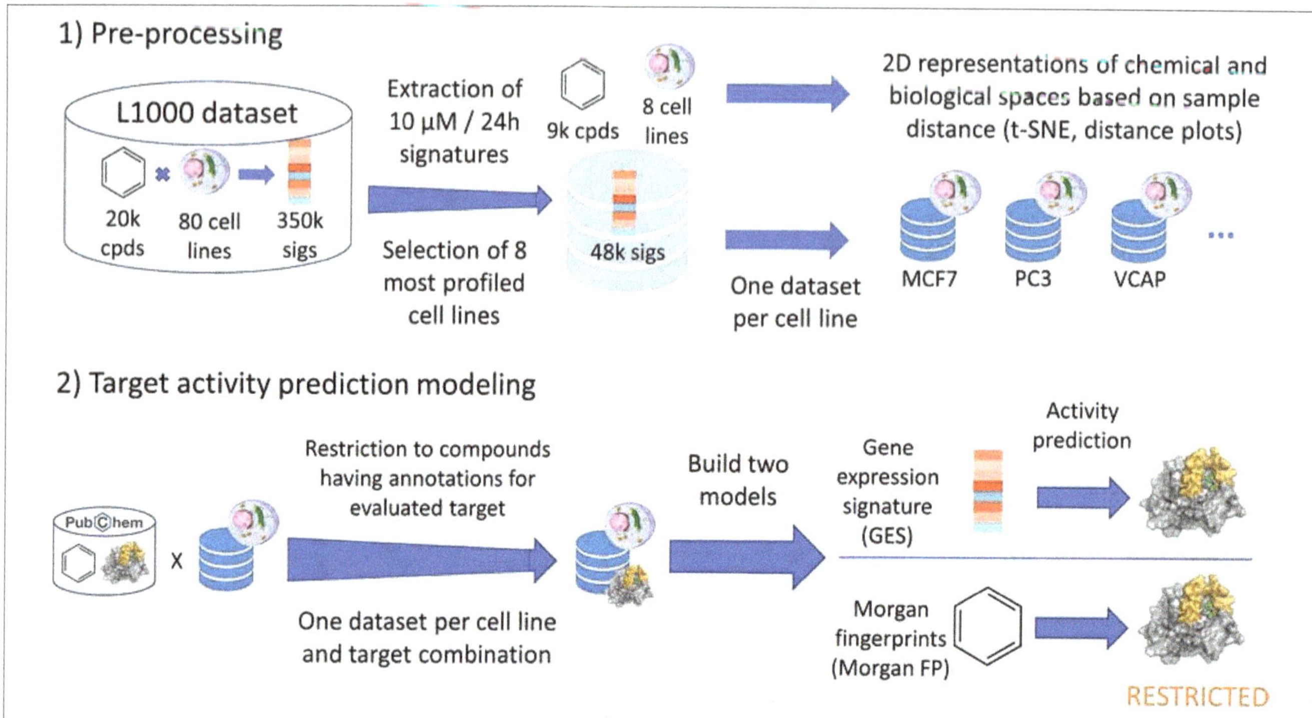

FIGURE 1 | Data analysis pipeline performed in current work. Starting from the CMAP L1000 dataset, signatures produced at 10 µM and 24 h from 8 cell lines were extracted and used in t-SNE and distance plots. One dataset was built per cell line (GES and corresponding compound structure), and each of these datasets were restricted to compounds having known annotations (active or inactive) for the evaluated target. For each target—cell line dataset, a first model was built using the gene expression signatures (GES model). Alongside, a second counterpart model was built using the Morgan fingerprints of compounds whose signatures were used in the first model (Morgan FP model).

TABLE 1 | The 8 core cell lines used in this work, with their corresponding number of GESs for compounds with known structure tested at 10 µM/24 h.

Cell line	Primary site	Subtype	Number of 10 µM–24 h signatures
A375	Skin	Malignant melanoma	3,525
A549	Lung	Non small cell lung cancer| carcinoma	5,267
HA1E	Kidney	Normal kidney	3,646
HCC515	Lung	Carcinoma	1,932
HT29	Large intestine	Colorectal adenocarcinoma	3,192
MCF7	Breast	Adenocarcinoma	7,546
PC3	Prostate	Adenocarcinoma	8,071
VCAP	Prostate	Carcinoma	6,365

inactive, empty if unknown). At least one annotation among 1,388 targets was found for 7,804 of the 9,035 compounds (512,406 annotations were found, representing 4.8% of the full activity matrix).

Representation of Chemical and Biological Spaces

For each compound, binary Morgan fingerprints were computed. The Morgan fingerprints were employed as input of a t-SNE (t-distributed stochastic neighbor embedding) algorithm (using the sklearn implementation) using Dice distance as metric, to reduce the data to a two-dimensional output that can be plotted to represent the chemical space (Van Der Maaten and Hinton, 2008; Pedregosa et al., 2011). Information of the number of targets per compound was included as color-code using a blue gradient in the plot.

The whole extracted 10 µM/24 h signature dataset was used as input for a second t-SNE using the cosine distance metric, representing the overall biological (response) space wherein each cell line was color-coded in the plot. For every cell line, a t-SNE using the cosine distance metric was performed using all GESs profiled in the cell line, generating 2D biological space.

Machine Learning Modeling

Targets for which we know at least 50 active compounds (representing between 1 and 63% of active per target) were selected for machine learning modeling in order to have a minimum number of actives in test sets to evaluate the model performances, and for computational time purposes. Complete information on the number of active and inactive compounds for these selected targets is listed in **Table 2**.

Subsequently, for each cell line GES dataset, we created a target—cell line GES dataset, restricting to compounds for which target activity was known as shown in **Figure 1** (this step caused the number of possible models to drop from 1,104 to 990). Datasets for each target prediction task were split into a training set (67% of the data) and a test set (remaining 33% of the data). Two models for target activity prediction were trained using

TABLE 2 | Molecular targets used in this work, with number of active and inactive compounds in total, and in each cell line GES dataset.

Gene name	Total inactive	Total active	Description	A375		A549		HA1E		HCC515		HT29		MCF7		PC3		VCAP	
				Inactive	Active	Inactive	Active	Inactive	Active	Inactive	Active	Inactive	Active	Inactive	Active	Inactive	Active	Inactive	Active
ABCB1	801	96	ATP binding cassette subfamily B member 1 [HGNC:40]	331	42	545	60	424	50	211	32	317	32	770	95	772	95	608	68
ABHD5	2,458	57	Abhydrolase domain containing 5 [HGNC:21396]	908	22	1,533	47	-	-	-	-	-	-	2,030	57	2,045	57	1,730	52
ALOX15	1,136	101	Arachidonate 15-lipoxygenase [HGNC:433]	508	27	764	92	808	52	496	33	498	27	1,062	97	1,066	96	804	91
AR	1,085	103	Androgen receptor [HGNC:644]	580	36	639	64	757	62	374	36	572	37	1,038	94	1,036	93	682	69
ATAD5	2,213	97	Atpase family, AAA domain containing 5 [HGNC:25,752]	1,007	43	1,466	70	1288	60	638	41	922	42	2,087	90	2,090	88	1,629	72
ATXN2	1,897	143	Ataxin 2 [HGNC:10555]	695	36	1,139	104	950	50	501	41	652	41	1556	123	1,558	129	1,243	102
BAZ2B	1,252	143	Bromodomain adjacent to zinc finger domain 2B [HGNC:963]	516	63	873	101	653	76	319	37	470	56	1,199	135	1,197	136	974	112
BRCA1	3,008	160	BRCA1, dna repair associated [HGNC:1100]	1,117	67	1945	116	1,519	63	800	33	1,014	50	2,537	148	2,549	150	2,134	131
CBX1	1,999	80	Chromobox 1 [HGNC:1551]	899	41	1,412	64	1,120	61	532	38	809	40	1,899	75	1,904	76	1,576	67
CHRM1	2,433	86	Cholinergic receptor muscarinic 1 [HGNC:1950]	906	49	1,544	62	1,055	59	460	39	791	48	2,036	84	2051	83	1,739	65
CHRM4	2,476	70	Cholinergic receptor muscarinic 4 [HGNC:1953]	908	45	1,552	54	1,057	55	460	40	793	45	2,049	68	2,064	67	1,751	54
CHRM5	2,478	62	Cholinergic receptor muscarinic 5 [HGNC:1954]	908	41	1,553	47	1,057	49	461	36	793	39	2,050	62	2,065	61	1,751	50
CYP1A2	307	526	Cytochrome P450 family 1 subfamily A member 2 [HGNC:2596]	145	265	183	399	219	428	136	277	144	261	299	505	294	505	183	410
CYP2C19	717	276	Cytochrome P450 family 2 subfamily C member 19 [HGNC:2621]	329	151	514	213	486	228	289	138	324	148	688	271	684	272	524	225
CYP2C9	708	270	Cytochrome P450 family 2 subfamily C member 9 [HGNC:2623]	310	157	510	197	476	222	285	126	305	154	679	264	674	263	517	207
CYP3A4	1,153	164	Cytochrome P450 family 3 subfamily A member 4 [HGNC:2637]	472	113	780	104	847	133	561	64	467	110	1,070	160	1069	161	802	118
DRD1	1,843	99	Dopamine receptor D1 [HGNC:3020]	807	54	1,295	71	1028	78	526	55	725	54	1,762	91	1,762	91	1,450	71
DRD2	2,262	95	Dopamine receptor D2 [HGNC:3023]	769	58	1,371	73	956	84	474	55	683	57	1,858	93	1873	93	1,541	74
DRD3	2,446	142	Dopamine receptor D3 [HGNC:3024]	877	76	1,432	110	1,129	114	551	78	823	75	2,004	139	2,017	139	1,569	111
EPAS1	2,443	70	Endothelial PAS domain protein 1 [HGNC:3374]	–	–	1,524	52	–	–	–	–	–	–	2,021	64	2,033	67	1,723	57
FEN1	2,100	53	Flap structure-specific endonuclease 1 [HGNC:3650]	961	23	1,496	29	1,213	28	–	–	866	21	1,990	46	1,999	46	1,669	32
GFER	1,589	89	Growth factor, augmenter of liver regeneration [HGNC:4236]	679	37	1,153	59	813	46	363	21	600	29	1,519	81	1,519	81	1,294	70

(Continued)

TABLE 2 | Continued

Gene name	Total inactive	Total active	Description	A375		A549		HA1E		HCC515		HT29		MCF7		PC3		VCAP	
				Inactive	Active	Inactive	Active	Inactive	Active	Inactive	Active	Inactive	Active	Inactive	Active	Inactive	Active	Inactive	Active
GLS	2,989	66	Glutaminase [HGNC:4331]	1,240	22	1,878	46	1,515	31	–	–	–	–	2,560	58	2,574	59	2,072	53
GMNN	2,079	161	Geminin, DNA replication inhibitor [HGNC:17493]	969	67	1,392	121	1,224	72	569	43	884	63	1,972	146	1,974	153	1,552	128
HPGD	1,464	92	15-Hydroxyprostaglandin dehydrogenase [HGNC:5154]	575	38	1,000	74	962	62	618	39	567	37	1363	89	1,363	86	1,060	71
HSD17B10	1,211	107	Hydroxysteroid 17-beta dehydrogenase 10 [HGNC:4800]	516	48	827	84	858	81	548	47	506	48	1,134	99	1,135	95	866	81
HSP90AA1	666	56	Heat shock protein 90 alpha family class A member 1 [HGNC:5253]	295	25	453	39	419	38	–	–	288	25	640	50	637	50	502	40
HSPB1	876	76	Heat shock protein family B (small) member 1 [HGNC:5246]	461	40	522	45	600	53	304	26	454	41	837	72	837	71	558	47
HTR1A	412	60	5-Hydroxytryptamine receptor 1A [HGNC:5286]	186	34	279	49	232	55	122	37	180	34	401	58	400	58	315	50
IL1B	1,773	206	Interleukin 1 beta [HGNC:5992]	589	54	1,005	165	768	78	382	54	541	54	1,385	190	1,391	196	1,122	163
JAK2	895	80	Janus kinase 2 [HGNC:6192]	378	39	663	58	478	43	248	29	364	40	867	71	867	74	723	55
JUN	842	97	Jun proto-oncogene, AP-1 transcription factor subunit [HGNC:6204]	442	49	491	67	570	72	279	41	435	49	801	91	799	91	523	70
KCNH2	363	190	Potassium voltage-gated channel subfamily H member 2 [HGNC:6251]	174	119	212	136	250	161	128	104	173	119	331	183	329	184	228	139
KDM4A	1,607	192	Lysine demethylase 4A [HGNC:22978]	693	76	1,130	125	834	87	379	42	603	69	1,529	173	1,536	175	1,286	140
KDM4E	1,389	124	Lysine demethylase 4E [HGNC:37098]	543	43	999	88	880	70	547	40	530	42	1,320	109	1,321	110	1,057	95
MITF	3,626	132	Melanogenesis associated transcription factor [HGNC:7105]	1,170	42	2,238	91	1,562	51	858	42	1,083	37	2,832	116	2,871	120	2,460	93
MLLT3	14,566	101	MLLT3, super elongation complex subunit [HGNC:7136]	–	–	2,244	26	–	–	–	–	–	–	3,002	33	3,461	50	3,095	46
MPHOSPH8	506	52	M-Phase phosphoprotein 8 [HGNC:29810]	278	21	365	39	403	41	253	29	278	21	490	48	485	50	382	43
MYC	2,069	121	MYC proto-oncogene, bHLH transcription factor [HGNC:7553]	–	–	1,067	113	–	–	–	–	–	–	1,230	114	1,249	117	1,151	115
NFE2L2	2,850	226	Nuclear factor, erythroid 2 like 2 [HGNC:7782]	1,142	94	1,816	148	1,355	153	620	83	1,013	95	2,425	204	2,439	204	2,023	152
NFKB1	2,875	107	Nuclear factor kappa B subunit 1 [HGNC:7794]	730	23	1,608	91	1,237	37	814	29	716	22	1,978	100	2,000	101	1,742	94
NOD1	1,056	51	Nucleotide binding oligomerization domain containing 1 [HGNC:16390]	–	–	754	43	–	–	–	–	409	21	1,010	47	1,010	49	844	40
NOD2	2,578	59	Nucleotide binding oligomerization domain containing 2 [HGNC:5331]	952	23	1,629	53	1,124	21	–	–	836	23	2,152	57	2,165	59	1,837	48
NPSR1	1,007	55	Neuropeptide S receptor 1 [HGNC:23631]	–	–	712	44	554	21	–	–	–	–	959	52	956	54	777	50

(Continued)

TABLE 2 | Continued

Gene name	Total inactive	Total active	Description	A375		A549		HA1E		HCC515		HT29		MCF7		PC3		VCAP	
				Inactive	Active	Inactive	Active	Inactive	Active	Inactive	Active	Inactive	Active	Inactive	Active	Inactive	Active	Inactive	Active
NR3C1	925	54	Nuclear receptor subfamily 3 group C member 1 [HGNC:7978]	–	–	636	38	692	34	451	25	–	–	896	54	890	54	659	47
NR5A1	419	69	Nuclear receptor subfamily 5 group A member 1 [HGNC:7983]	190	22	285	50	239	29	–	–	–	–	408	60	407	64	322	50
OPRK1	1,122	51	Opioid receptor kappa 1 [HGNC:8154]	455	29	805	41	564	34	–	–	428	29	1,068	51	1,070	50	895	41
PIP4K2A	1,898	88	Phosphatidylinositol-5-phosphate 4-kinase type 2 alpha [HGNC:8997]	609	31	1,082	66	812	34	–	–	566	23	1,486	84	1,501	83	1,206	72
PLA2G7	1,907	57	Phospholipase A2 group VII [HGNC:9040]	828	27	1,367	37	995	37	–	–	737	28	1,825	52	1,826	51	1,534	37
PLK1	1,935	108	Polo like kinase 1 [HGNC:9077]	631	45	1,125	82	836	39	431	23	590	36	1,531	100	1,542	102	1,241	88
POLB	1,166	53	DNA polymerase beta [HGNC:9174]	480	22	850	37	646	30	–	–	462	21	1,113	50	1,113	50	932	39
POLH	2,202	70	DNA polymerase eta [HGNC:9181]	858	26	1,342	44	1,015	37	–	–	749	23	1,827	61	1,838	64	1,532	48
POLI	1,726	79	DNA polymerase iota [HGNC:9182]	775	29	1,210	52	945	43	448	24	689	27	1,629	71	1,637	72	1,359	55
POLK	2,895	79	DNA polymerase kappa [HGNC:9183]	1,248	30	2,048	49	1,799	43	986	27	1,154	26	2,713	69	2,722	70	2,225	54
PRMT1	2,886	80	Protein arginine methyltransferase 1 [HGNC:5187]	1,114	28	1,704	59	1,073	23	–	–	–	–	2,394	74	2,415	74	2,081	68
RAD52	14,593	132	RAD52 homolog, DNA repair protein [HGNC:9824]	–	–	2,291	25	–	–	–	–	–	–	3,043	40	3,496	54	3,121	49
SIRT5	14,103	141	Sirtuin 5 [HGNC:14933]	–	–	2,086	30	–	–	–	–	–	–	2,769	40	3,211	44	2,844	42
SLC6A3	1,006	94	Solute carrier family 6 member 3 [HGNC:11049]	461	49	773	71	584	72	252	54	453	49	976	91	973	90	823	73
SMN2	1,633	53	Survival of motor neuron 2, centromeric [HGNC:11118]	–	–	1,136	44	1,059	28	–	–	–	–	1,520	49	1,521	49	1,209	45
STK33	3,358	423	Serine/threonine kinase 33 [HGNC:14568]	1,127	101	2,077	304	1,458	163	776	131	1,034	102	2,660	329	2,663	360	2,268	328
TARDBP	1,802	60	TAR DNA binding protein [HGNC:11571]	–	–	1,044	50	748	25	–	–	–	–	1,409	58	1,418	59	1,156	52
TNFRSF10B	2,429	80	TNF receptor superfamily member 10b [HGNC:11905]	–	–	1,510	66	1,056	26	–	–	786	27	2,008	73	2,021	75	1,718	58
TP53	2,310	198	Tumor protein p53 [HGNC:11998]	974	97	1,554	137	1,380	130	737	84	891	98	2,172	179	2,174	181	1,714	137
TSHR	2,259	70	Thyroid stimulating hormone receptor [HGNC:12373]	968	25	1,579	58	1,317	43	727	35	–	–	2,133	68	2,131	67	1,739	64
TUBB	697	51	Tubulin beta class I [HGNC:20773]	–	–	503	32	373	32	–	–	–	–	692	48	693	49	563	32
USP1	2,356	64	Ubiquitin specific peptidase 1 [HGNC:12607]	877	30	1,425	46	1,260	45	697	29	833	30	1,972	55	1,985	58	1,557	44
VDR	2,696	140	Vitamin D receptor [HGNC:12679]	1,161	44	1,901	101	1,673	80	915	50	1,076	43	2,530	127	2,536	128	2,059	107
YES1	138	101	YES proto-oncogene 1, Src family tyrosine kinase [HGNC:12841]	106	89	99	86	117	89	77	76	106	89	132	97	131	99	90	67

each subset: a first model used the 978-landmark GES as input (referred as GES models), and the second one used the Morgan fingerprints of corresponding compounds to fairly compare model performances (referred as Morgan FP models). Models were trained using random forest classifiers (Breiman, 2001).

The training was performed using a 4-fold cross-validation on training set to tune the maximum depth of tree, before assessing prediction performances on the test set. The number of trees per model was set to 200. Models were built in Python 2.7 using the sklearn package: to account for unbalanced dataset, the "class_weight" parameter was set to "balanced_subsample," to increase the weight of the under-represented class samples when training the trees (Pedregosa et al., 2011). A first step of feature selection was performed using an initial random forest classifier, computing the feature importance (Breiman, 2001). Sum of importance of all feature was 1, with each feature importance between 0 (non-important) and 1 (important). This step was performed 5 times, feature importance was averaged by feature, and only the 20 most important features were selected to be loaded into a final random forest model. This whole modeling pipeline, from train-test split to final model was performed 10 times per task, to account for variable performances depending on the dataset split.

Models were evaluated by counting the numbers of true positive (TP), true negative (TN), false positive (FP) and false negative (FN). These parameters were combined in the following metrics in order to compare model performances:

- $Sensitivity = TP/(TP + FN)$
- $Specificity = TN/(TN + FP)$
- Balanced accuracy (BA) : $BA = (Sensitivity + Specificity)/2$
- Matthews correlation coefficient (MCC) :

$$MCC = \frac{TP^*TN - FP^*FN}{\sqrt{(TP + FP)\,(TP + FN)\,(TN + FP)\,(TN + FN)}}$$

Balanced accuracy allows for a fair evaluation of model performances when using unbalanced datasets, by averaging accuracy for each class (here active and inactives).

Quadrant Plots

Between each possible pair of compounds active on the same target and in each cell line, Dice distance between Morgan fingerprints, and cosine distance between GESs in given cell line were computed. These 2 distances were plotted in a 2D plot (referred as distance plot), Dice distance on X-axis and cosine distance on Y-axis. These plots were theoretically split in 4 quadrants.

Quadrant I in the top-right corner contains active compound pairs having different structures (Morgan fingerprints Dice distance > 0.5) and presenting different GESs (cosine distance > 0.5); quadrant II in top-left corner contains active compound pairs having similar structures (Morgan fingerprints Dice distance < 0.5) and presenting different GESs (cosine distance > 0.5); quadrant III in bottom-left corner contains active compound pairs having similar structures (Morgan fingerprints Dice distance < 0.5) and presenting similar GESs (cosine distance < 0.5), quadrant IV in bottom-right corner contains active compound pairs having different structures (Morgan fingerprints Dice distance > 0.5) and presenting similar GESs (cosine distance < 0.5). Number of active compound pairs in each quadrant were counted for each distance plot. Similar calculations were made using not only active compounds, but all compounds having an annotation (active or inactive) for considered target and profiled in the same cell line.

RESULTS

In the present work, we investigated the link between compound structure information ($n = 9{,}035$) and their corresponding induced biological responses captured by GESs ($n = 39{,}544$) in human tumor cell lines and evaluated the potential of machine learning approaches to infer about molecular targets involved in the compound bioactivity. In addition, we compared these machine learning models using GESs with counterpart models using Morgan fingerprints.

Exploration of Chemical and Biological Spaces

As a first step, to observe the diversity of the 9,035 compounds profiled in the 10 μM/24 h L1000 signature dataset, the corresponding chemical space was visualized. **Figure 2A** is a 2-dimensional t-SNE representation of the chemical space, illustrating the variability in terms of Morgan fingerprints. The 9,035 compounds form a broad chemical space, with a mean Dice distance between compound pairs of 0.81 (ChEMBL has a mean pairwise Dice distance of 0.82). The center of the chemical space is mostly composed by small molecules having on average a molecular weight lower than 500 Da whereas the outer part is populated by clusters of compounds with higher molecular weights (>500 Da). Overall, we were able to retrieve, in the public domain, at least one activity information for 7,837 compounds, from which 4,872 were active in at least one target. The majority of those compounds were found active in a low number of targets, on average 6 per compound, with a median of 2. Not surprisingly, a set of 23 kinase inhibitors were found to be active in more than 100 targets.

Figure 2B shows a t-SNE plot created using all GESs induced by the 9,035 compounds in the different cell lines to examine the complete biological space. This t-SNE is color coded by the different cell lines used to generate the gene signatures. Each cell line is represented by a set of 4 to 5 main clusters of GESs differing in size and some overlap of the cluster indicates similar GESs derived from different cell lines. In order to better appreciated the differences and communalities in GESs obtained with the selected compounds, t-SNE plots were created highlighting the clusters derived for cell lines originating from the same tumor type namely prostate tumor (VCAP and PC3 in **Figure 2C**) and lung tumor (A549 and HCC515 in **Figure 2D**). GESs derived from cell lines coming

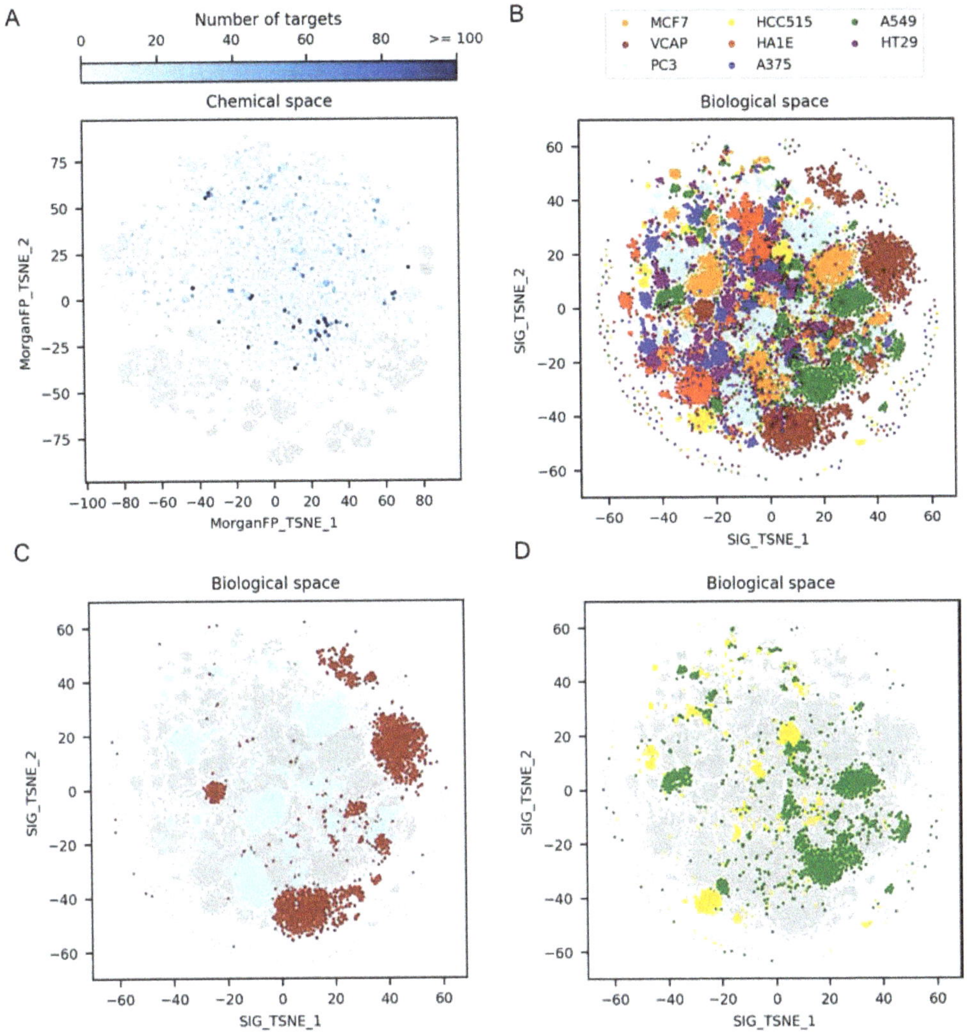

FIGURE 2 | Exploration of the 2D chemical space, along with the corresponding 2D biological space formed by all GES. **(A)** t-SNE on Morgan fingerprints from the 9,035 compounds in working dataset, representing the chemical space. Points corresponding to compounds for which there is no known target are represented by gray points ($n = 4,163$). Points corresponding to compounds for which there is at least one known target are in blue ($n = 4,872$), with darker blue depending on the increasing number of targets. **(B)** t-SNE on all GESs in the working dataset, representing the biological (transcriptomic response) space. Points corresponding to GESs are colored by cell line. **(C)** Biological space highlighting only PC3 and VCAP signatures, 2 cell lines originating from prostate cancer. **(D)** Biological space highlighting only A549 and HCC515 signatures, 2 cell lines originating from lung cancer.

from the same tissue present very little overlap as can be observed in **Figures 2C,D**.

These results illustrate the variability in the cellular modifications occurring during carcinogenesis (Hanahan and Weinberg, 2011) and show that each cell line represent a distinct biological space even if the cell lines are derived from the same tissue type. Interestingly, when comparing, for a set of compounds showing GESs in a single cluster in VCAP, GESs of these compounds in PC3 are spread across various clusters from the PC3 biological space (data not shown). This shows that each cell line explores different biological responses to compounds.

After having described the global variability of GESs in the different cell lines, we explored the chemical and biological spaces corresponding to active and inactive compounds on different targets. Since each compound-induced GES obtained in each cell line was shown to represent a unique biological space, t-SNE plots were computed per cell line in order to further explore the link between the different biological spaces and the corresponding chemical ones. For this, we decided to focus on three cell lines derived from different tissues and among the largest GES dataset generated that is to say A549 (lung cancer), MCF7 (breast cancer) and PC3 (prostate cancer). In addition, we selected 3 representative molecular targets showing different chemical and biological space profiles: compounds active on the glucocorticoid receptor (NR3C1) have similar structures, and similar GESs in some cell lines (**Figures 3A–D**); tubulin beta I (TUBB) actives have more diverse structures but show similar GESs in each cell line considered in this work (**Figures 4A–D**); and dopamine receptor D1 (DRD1) actives have diverse structure and GESs in every used cell line (**Figures 5A–D**).

NR3C1 actives compounds are mostly grouped together in the chemical space, as shown in **Figure 3A** ($n = 54$; mean Dice distance = 0.67). Most of NR3C1 active GESs are also grouped in a cluster in the A549 biological space ($n = 38$; mean cosine distance = 0.76), visible in **Figure 3B**, and remaining NR3C1 active GESs are spread across this biological space. Following the similarity principle, we could conjecture that other GESs that are close to this cluster are responses from other NR3C1 actives, especially in the PC3 biological space where the cluster contains compounds known to be active. The same phenomenon can be observed in the biological space of PC3 (**Figure 3D**), HCC515, HA1E and VCAP (data not shown). Surprisingly, the GES clusters populated by numerous known NR3C1 actives in the biological spaces of A549 and PC3 also contain some known inactive compounds. In the biological spaces of MCF7, A375 and HT29, there is no such clustering, like shown in **Figure 3C** representing the MCF7 biological space ($n = 54$; mean cosine distance = 0.92). Overall, these results show that compounds that are known to be active on the NR3C1 target can show a similar response in only certain cellular contexts.

TUBB actives compounds are spread in the chemical space (represented in **Figure 4A**), indicating that they have diverse chemical structures ($n = 51$; mean Dice distance = 0.76). Most importantly, in each cell lines used in this work, GESs induced by TUBB actives compounds were similar (as illustrated in **Figures 4B–D**), with a rather low mean cosine distance between active compounds ranging between 0.61 and 0.75 depending on the cell line dataset. Moreover, GESs of TUBB actives tend to be similar across all cell lines used in this work (highlighted in **Supplementary Figure 1**). This conserved pattern in GESs induced by tubulin binding compounds likely illustrate certainly the ubiquitous role of tubulin polymerization of the eukaryotic cytoskeleton (Chaaban and Brouhard, 2017).

Finally, DRD1 actives compounds, that are represented in the chemical space t-SNE, have diverse chemical structures ($n = 99$; mean Dice distance = 0.81), associated with diverse GESs for the 3 cell lines presented (mean cosine distance between 0.88 and 0.92 depending on the cell line), as illustrated in **Figures 5A–D**. Since GESs of active compounds in any cell lines are not similar, nor their chemical structures, actives cannot be easily discriminated from inactives using these two types of descriptors, as opposed to what was observed with NR3C1 actives that have similar structures, or TUBB actives having similar GESs in every cell line used in this study.

Model Performances: GES Vs. Morgan Fingerprints

Based on the observed GES similarity of compounds sharing target activity in appropriate cellular contexts, we tested building predictive machine learning models using GESs as descriptors and compare their performances with the ones of the models using Morgan fingerprints.

In order to avoid building models with too unbalanced datasets and to ensure a minimum of active compounds when testing model performances, we first pre selected targets having at least 50 active compounds in the total dataset (representing between 1 and 63% of active compounds per target). We obtained one dataset per cell line—target combination (restricted to compounds having signatures in the considered cell line, as shown in **Figure 1**) and carried out a second selection by performing prediction tasks using datasets containing at least 20 active compounds for the considered target (representing between 1 and 69% of active compounds per dataset). For each selected cell line—target dataset, one model using GESs (referred as GES model) was computed. In order to perform a fair comparison per task, one counterpart model using corresponding compound Morgan fingerprints (referred as Morgan FP model) was built using the same set of compounds as the one used in the corresponding GES models. Performances of models were evaluated using the balanced accuracy (BA) metric on a test set, to account for class imbalance in datasets. In total, 990 models were built for a total of 69 different targets. BAs of all built models are presented in **Table 3**. MCC of all built models are presented in **Supplementary Table 1**.

Overall, GES model performances appeared to be variable depending on the predicted target and on the cell line that was used to generate the GESs, with a BA ranging from 0.49 to 0.88. Counterpart models trained with Morgan fingerprints also had variable performances, with a BA ranging from 0.50 to 0.98. On average, Morgan FP models (mean BA = 0.65) yielded better performances for the target activity prediction than their counterpart GES models (mean BA = 0.58). On the 495 cell line—target combinations, BA of GES models was higher than BA of counterpart Morgan FP models for 124 combinations (25%).

On the 990 models, 208 models reached a BA higher than 0.7 (21%) for 40 targets (59 GES models for 18 targets; 138 Morgan FP models for 28 targets), and 33 models reached a BA higher than 0.8 (3%) for 10 targets (10 GES models for 4 targets; 21 Morgan FP models for 7 targets). For all 138 Morgan FP models reaching BA higher than 0.7, BA was superior to counterpart GES models, and for the 59 GES models reaching BA higher than 0.7, only 6 had counterpart Morgan FP model with higher BA.

For NR3C1 activity prediction, Morgan FP models yielded a BA between 0.93 and 0.98 depending on the cell line dataset. It is not surprising considering that that NR3C1 actives have similar structure as shown in **Figure 3A**. On the GES models, a BA of 0.77 was reached using the A549 signature dataset, correlating to similar GESs that were observed in the A549 biological space (**Figure 3B**), whereas a BA of 0.6 was obtained using the MCF7 signature dataset (no GES cluster in MCF7 biological space, shown in **Figure 3C**). A549 and MCF7 signature model performances cannot be fairly compared because they were built using different sets of compounds. In fact, performances of different GES models cannot be compared across cell lines nor across targets, performances can only be compared to observed similarity between active compounds in either chemical and biological space plots for a given target.

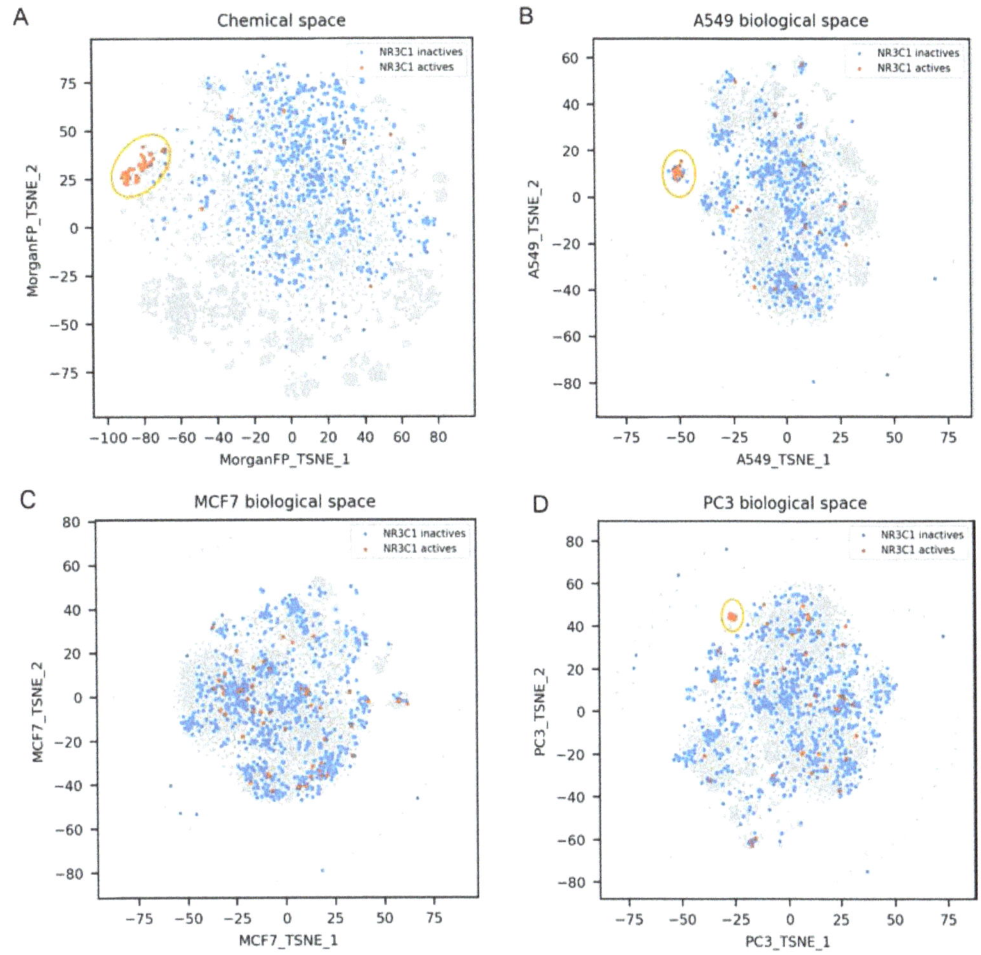

FIGURE 3 | NR3C1 active and inactives compounds in the chemical space and the different biological spaces formed by GES produced in a single cell line. **(A)** Chemical space; **(B)** t-SNE on all A549 signatures (A549 biological space); **(C)** t-SNE on all MCF7 signatures (MCF7 biological space); **(D)** t-SNE on all PC3 signatures (PC3 biological space). Points corresponding to NR3C1 actives are red ($n = 54$), NR3C1 inactives ($n = 925$) are blue, gray points have no available label concerning NR3C1 activity. Orange circles point out clustering of active compounds.

For TUBB activity prediction, GES models yielded BA between 0.81 and 0.88 depending on the cell line dataset, which was among the 10 best GES models. Interestingly, their counterpart Morgan FP models were not significantly underperforming (BA ranging from 0.78 to 0.82). Even though the TUBB active structures are diverse, the models still managed to identify structural fragments that could produce such predictive performance.

For DRD1 activity prediction, Morgan FP models yielded BA between 0.68 and 0.74 depending on the cell line dataset, and were always better than their counterpart GES model, with a BA ranging from 0.58 to 0.64.

Overall, we conclude that it was possible to build GES models with acceptable performances, performing similarly or better than their counterpart Morgan FP models in 25% of the target prediction tasks. Moreover, we see an important advantage in the GES models: they are theoretically performing independently of the chemical space considered, allowing target identification of new compounds even if their corresponding structural diversity is not represented in the training set.

Rationalizing Model Performances Using Distance Plots

To further describe and understand the reasons for the differences in performances between GES model and Morgan FP model, for every dataset used in each cell line—target combinations, Morgan fingerprints Dice distance was plotted against GES cosine distance between each pair of active compounds in the given dataset.

Generated distance plots were split in 4 quadrants separated by a 0.5 threshold for Dice distance (dotted vertical line) and a 0.5 threshold for cosine distance (dotted horizontal line). Data points in top right (Quadrant I) represent pairs of active compounds showing diverse structures and different GESs in the considered cell line and contains most of compound pairs (average of 95.1%). Data points in top left (Quadrant II) represent pairs of active

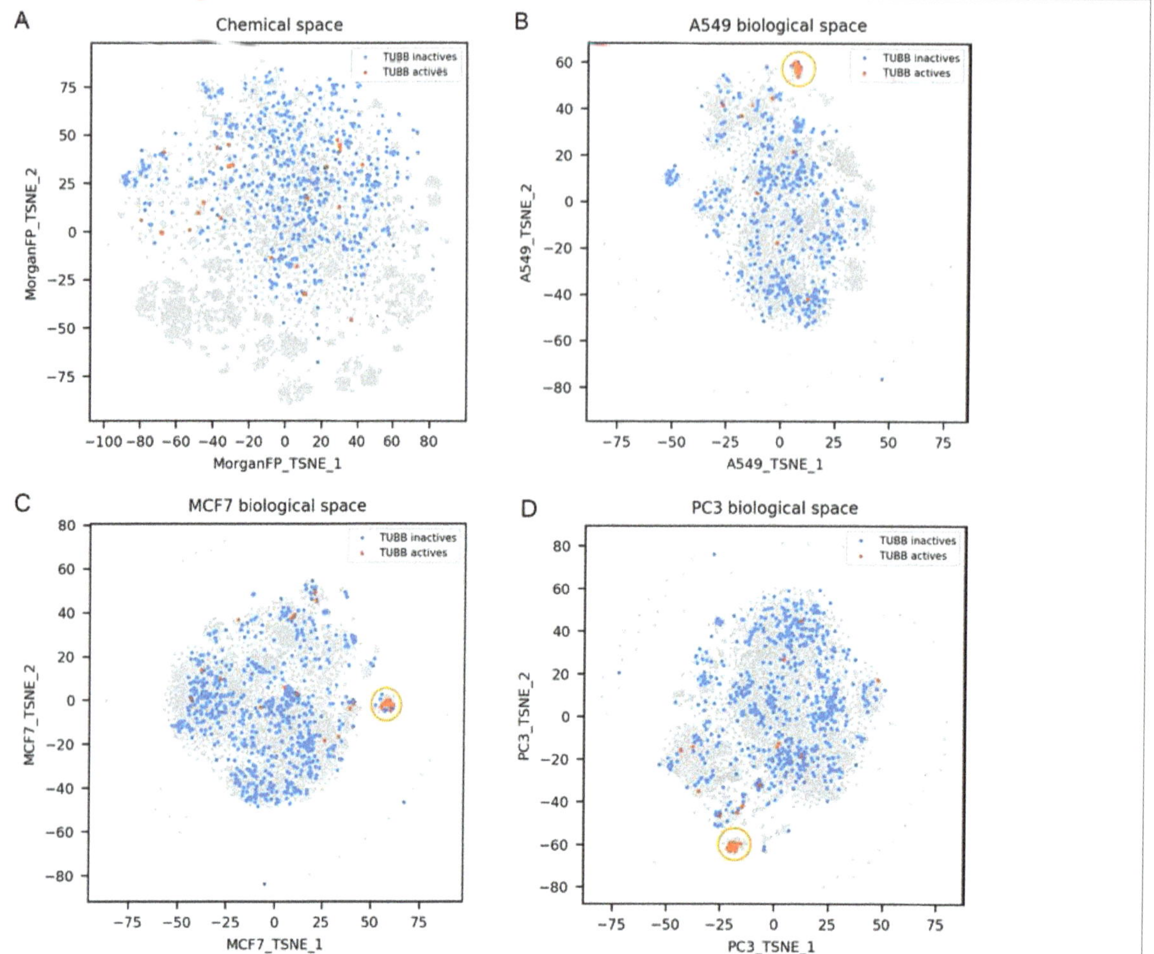

FIGURE 4 | TUBB active and inactives compounds in the chemical space and the different biological spaces formed by GES produced in a single cell line. **(A)** Chemical space; **(B)** A549 biological space; **(C)** MCF7 biological space; **(D)** PC3 biological space. Points corresponding to TUBB actives ($n = 51$) are red, TUBB inactives ($n = 697$) are blue, gray points have no available label concerning TUBB activity. Orange circles point out clustering of active compounds.

compounds showing similar structures while showing diverse GESs in the considered cell line (average of 1.9%). Data points in bottom left (Quadrant III) represents pairs of active compounds showing similar structures and similar GESs in the considered cell line and contains least compound pairs (average of 0.5%). Data points in bottom right (Quadrant IV) represents pairs of active compounds showing similar GESs while having different structures (average of 2.5%). Intuitively, we think that sample similarity within the same class (here: actives) is a good indicator to know if a machine learning model will be able to properly predict samples from this class.

Overall, the mean percentage of compound pairs (active and inactives) were 99.3, 0.3, 0.01 and 0.4% for quadrants I, II, III and IV respectively. Based on this dataset, compounds active toward a molecular target have on average more similar structures and GESs than the totality of the compounds.

We expected to reach good Morgan FP model prediction for combinations having a high proportion of points in quadrants II and III (similar structures), and good GES model prediction for combinations having a high proportion of points in quadrants III and IV (similar GESs). We evaluated the use of distance plots on the three targets and three cell lines used in previous space plots (**Figures 3, 5**). Similar work was performed using not only active compounds, but all compounds having at least one annotation for each of the three previously described targets, shown in **Supplementary Figure 2.**

For NR3C1 distance plots, there are approximately 10% of compound pairs in quadrants II and III of the 3 plots (**Figures 6A–C**), coherent with good Morgan FP model performances. However, depending on which cell line the GESs were generated from, there were different proportions of compound pairs in quadrants III and IV: there are 20% of pairs for A549, and only 1% of pairs in MCF7. This is in agreement with what was observed in model performances: performance of GES models using the A549 dataset (BA = 0.77) was much better than performances using MCF7 dataset (BA = 0.60). Surprisingly, prediction using GESs from the PC3 dataset showed good performances (BA = 0.73), even though the proportion

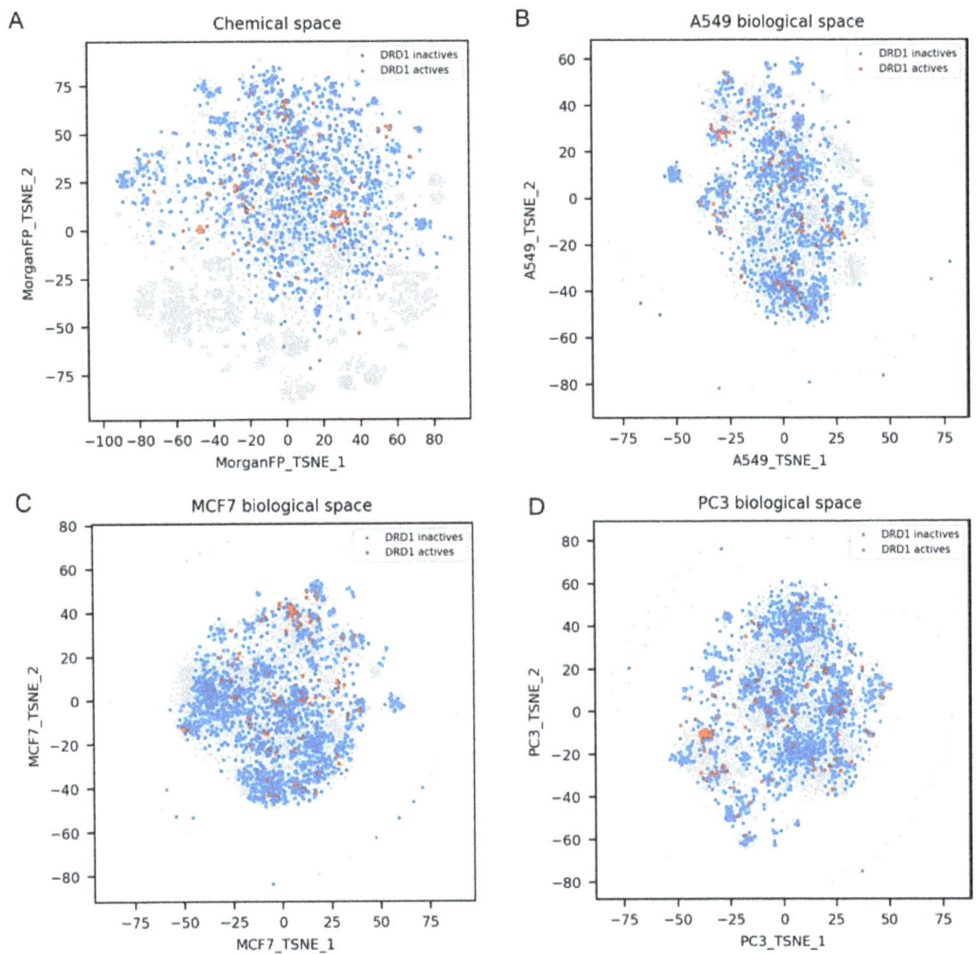

FIGURE 5 | DRD1 active and inactives compounds in the chemical space and the different biological spaces formed by GES produced in a single cell line. **(A)** Chemical space; **(B)** A549 biological space; **(C)** MCF7 biological space; **(D)** PC3 biological space. Points corresponding to DRD1 actives ($n = 99$) are red, DRD1 inactives ($n = 1843$) are blue, gray points have no available label concerning DRD1 activity.

of active compound pairs in quadrants III and IV was around 1% (similar to the proportion observed for the MCF7 dataset that showed worse performances). This suggests that the GES model built with PC3 was able to capture a subset of genes to discriminate active compounds from inactives, even with active compounds showing different GESs.

For TUBB distance plots (**Figures 6D–F**), between 7 and 10% of compound pairs was observed in quadrants II and III, matching the good Morgan FP model performances with the 3 cell line datasets (BA ranging from 0.80 to 0.82). Most importantly, there are between 26 and 40% of compound pairs in quadrants III and IV, echoing the better performances of the GES models in these cell lines (BA ranging from 0.81 to 0.88).

For DRD1 distance plots (**Figures 6G–I**), 98% of compound pairs are in quadrant I, leaving low number of active compound pairs in the other quadrants (with similar Morgan fingerprints and/or GESs). This is coherent with the average performances of GES (BA ranging from 0.68 to 0.74) and Morgan FP models (BA ranging from 0.58 to 0.64) built for this target.

Among the 50 best GES models, the mean percentage of active pairs in quadrants III and IV was 5.2% (vs. 2.3% in quadrants II and III). For the 50 best Morgan FP models, the mean percentage of active pairs in quadrants II and III was 4.0% (vs. 2.2% in quadrants III and IV). This suggests a positive relationship between sample similarity between active compounds using a given set of descriptors for active compounds and performances of models using these descriptors.

In the current work, GESs were shown to be effective descriptors to predict compound activity toward molecular targets. In 25% of target prediction tasks, GES models outperformed their counterpart Morgan FP models, especially when using GES produced in a cell line exhibiting similar GESs between compounds active toward the target of interest. Such GES models performs independently of the structural diversity of compounds that were used to produce GESs, offering a great opportunity to escape the classical chemical space limitations associated with QSAR models. In addition, t-SNE plots, along with 2D distance plots, can give insights to assess the predictive

TABLE 3 | Mean BAs of models (mean per condition).

Target class	Target name	Cell line	A375		A549		HA1E		HCC515		HT29		MCF7		PC3		VCAP	
		Target/ Descriptor	**GES**	**Morgan FP**	**GES**	**Morgan FP**	**GES**	**Morgan FP**	**GES**	**Morgan FP**	**GES**	**Morgan FP**	**GES**	**Morgan FP**	**GES**	**Morgan FP**	**GES**	**Morgan FP**
Enzyme	15-Hydroxyprostaglandin dehydrogenase	HPGD	0.5	0.65	0.51	0.7	0.52	0.67	0.5	0.72	0.51	0.68	0.5	0.71	0.52	0.67	0.52	0.64
	Arachidonate 15-lipoxygenase	ALOX15	0.54	0.74	0.57	0.75	0.54	0.67	0.5	0.63	0.5	0.73	0.56	0.74	0.65	0.75	0.53	0.75
	ATP binding cassette B1	ABCB1	0.54	0.62	0.51	0.61	0.5	0.54	0.5	0.5	0.51	0.5	0.56	0.62	0.59	0.63	0.51	0.63
	BRCA1, dna repair associated	BRCA1	0.74	0.69	0.69	0.62	0.67	0.57	0.6	0.52	0.71	0.6	0.78	0.64	0.75	0.64	0.67	0.65
	Cytochrome P450 1A2	CYP1A2	0.54	0.6	0.56	0.6	0.57	0.61	0.59	0.58	0.5	0.59	0.59	0.63	0.6	0.63	0.56	0.61
	Cytochrome P450 2C19	CYP2C19	0.52	0.57	0.55	0.59	0.5	0.55	0.52	0.55	0.51	0.57	0.56	0.58	0.56	0.59	0.53	0.58
	Cytochrome P450 2C9	CYP2C9	0.55	0.57	0.52	0.61	0.52	0.6	0.51	0.6	0.53	0.58	0.55	0.58	0.6	0.58	0.54	0.6
	Cytochrome P450 3A4	CYP3A4	0.51	0.55	0.52	0.59	0.52	0.58	0.49	0.6	0.51	0.54	0.52	0.6	0.54	0.6	0.53	0.57
	DNA polymerase beta	POLB	0.5	0.66	0.5	0.69	0.51	0.82	–	–	0.5	0.69	0.5	0.69	0.53	0.73	0.5	0.69
	DNA polymerase eta	POLH	0.55	0.71	0.51	0.74	0.66	0.82	–	–	0.5	0.76	0.51	0.73	0.55	0.72	0.52	0.69
	DNA polymerase iota	POLI	0.5	0.7	0.5	0.71	0.54	0.71	0.5	0.6	0.51	0.65	0.51	0.72	0.51	0.73	0.5	0.68
	DNA polymerase kappa	POLK	0.58	0.77	0.51	0.78	0.56	0.83	0.52	0.79	0.5	0.76	0.54	0.81	0.56	0.83	0.5	0.83
	Flap structure-specific endonuclease 1	FEN1	0.5	0.72	0.5	0.68	0.5	0.77	–	–	0.5	0.74	0.5	0.77	0.51	0.75	0.5	0.7
	Glutaminase	GLS	0.5	0.64	0.51	0.64	0.53	0.58	–	–	–	–	0.51	0.74	0.51	0.69	0.51	0.7
	Growth factor, augmenter of liver regeneration	GFER	0.51	0.72	0.5	0.72	0.59	0.74	0.5	0.71	0.5	0.72	0.52	0.72	0.56	0.71	0.5	0.7
	Hydroxysteroid 17-beta dehydrogenase 10	HSD17B10	0.51	0.57	0.54	0.62	0.55	0.63	0.51	0.63	0.49	0.58	0.54	0.65	0.53	0.64	0.5	0.62
	Janus kinase 2	JAK2	0.71	0.57	0.73	0.63	0.69	0.56	0.63	0.56	0.68	0.56	0.8	0.63	0.73	0.59	0.65	0.58
	MDM2 proto-oncogene	MDM2	0.77	0.69	0.71	0.61	0.7	0.62	0.76	0.53	0.67	0.59	0.83	0.65	0.81	0.64	0.76	0.66
	Phosphatidylinositol-5-phosphate 4-kinase type 2 alpha	PIP4K2A	0.51	0.69	0.54	0.75	0.53	0.66	–	–	0.5	0.58	0.53	0.76	0.5	0.76	0.52	0.74
	Phospholipase A2 group VII	PLA2G7	0.5	0.71	0.51	0.65	0.57	0.72	–	–	0.5	0.69	0.54	0.69	0.57	0.71	0.51	0.69
	Polo like kinase 1	PLK1	0.5	0.62	0.52	0.64	0.54	0.52	0.49	0.56	0.5	0.52	0.52	0.68	0.52	0.67	0.49	0.68
	Serine/threonine kinase 33	STK33	0.78	0.58	0.68	0.62	0.78	0.59	0.74	0.6	0.7	0.56	0.72	0.61	0.71	0.64	0.66	0.65
	Ubiquitin specific peptidase 1	USP1	0.5	0.54	0.51	0.58	0.51	0.53	0.51	0.53	0.5	0.55	0.52	0.57	0.57	0.59	0.5	0.57
	YES proto-oncogene 1, Src family tyrosine kinase	YES1	0.7	0.72	0.67	0.7	0.71	0.72	0.63	0.69	0.66	0.71	0.66	0.75	0.7	0.72	0.54	0.68
Epigenetic regulator	Bromodomain adjacent to zinc finger domain 2B	BAZ2B	0.6	0.66	0.54	0.68	0.63	0.69	0.52	0.6	0.5	0.65	0.55	0.67	0.6	0.66	0.53	0.68
	Chromobox 1	CBX1	0.56	0.57	0.55	0.62	0.6	0.6	0.57	0.61	0.54	0.55	0.61	0.6	0.57	0.62	0.55	0.61
	Lysine demethylase 4A	KDM4A	0.64	0.62	0.56	0.67	0.65	0.7	0.57	0.63	0.6	0.65	0.58	0.68	0.6	0.65	0.53	0.63
	Lysine demethylase 4E	KDM4E	0.59	0.76	0.52	0.75	0.61	0.75	0.53	0.75	0.5	0.72	0.53	0.73	0.57	0.74	0.52	0.72
	M-phase phosphoprotein 8	MPHOSPH8	0.52	0.53	0.52	0.64	0.54	0.64	0.51	0.65	0.5	0.54	0.63	0.63	0.54	0.64	0.51	0.65
	Protein arginine methyltransferase 1	PRMT1	0.5	0.65	0.51	0.71	0.5	0.54	–	–	–	–	0.52	0.7	0.51	0.71	0.51	0.72
	Sirtuin 5	SIRT5	–	–	0.51	0.65	–	–	–	–	–	–	0.51	0.62	0.5	0.61	0.5	0.6

(Continued)

TABLE 3 | Continued

Target class	Target name	Target/Descriptor	A375 GES	A375 Morgan FP	A549 GES	A549 Morgan FP	HA1E GES	HA1E Morgan FP	HCC515 GES	HCC515 Morgan FP	HT29 GES	HT29 Morgan FP	MCF7 GES	MCF7 Morgan FP	PC3 GES	PC3 Morgan FP	VCAP GES	VCAP Morgan FP
	Survival of motor neuron 2, centromeric	SMN2	–	–	0.5	0.62	0.51	0.56	–	–	–	–	0.52	0.63	0.52	0.6	0.5	0.62
Ion channel	Potassium voltage-gated channel H2	KCNH2	0.72	0.82	0.64	0.8	0.66	0.79	0.65	0.76	0.74	0.8	0.65	0.84	0.65	0.8	0.67	0.8
Membrane receptor	5-hydroxytryptamine receptor 1A	HTR1A	0.5	0.72	0.51	0.75	0.54	0.75	0.53	0.75	0.51	0.7	0.55	0.77	0.52	0.76	0.55	0.79
	Cholinergic receptor muscarinic 1	CHRM1	0.6	0.69	0.64	0.69	0.66	0.71	0.7	0.69	0.67	0.62	0.59	0.71	0.6	0.73	0.65	0.72
	Cholinergic receptor muscarinic 4	CHRM4	0.63	0.71	0.67	0.75	0.64	0.72	0.7	0.68	0.63	0.66	0.66	0.7	0.62	0.73	0.62	0.72
	Cholinergic receptor muscarinic 5	CHRM5	0.6	0.69	0.62	0.76	0.64	0.72	0.69	0.72	0.63	0.68	0.64	0.73	0.59	0.71	0.61	0.68
	Dopamine receptor D1	DRD1	0.64	0.68	0.6	0.73	0.63	0.7	0.58	0.72	0.62	0.69	0.62	0.74	0.61	0.72	0.59	0.74
	Dopamine receptor D2	DRD2	0.61	0.74	0.61	0.79	0.61	0.79	0.6	0.79	0.61	0.73	0.65	0.79	0.62	0.79	0.63	0.8
	Dopamine receptor D3	DRD3	0.6	0.66	0.58	0.72	0.56	0.71	0.58	0.71	0.58	0.66	0.63	0.72	0.57	0.72	0.58	0.73
	Neuropeptide S receptor 1	NPSR1	–	–	0.59	0.64	0.5	0.55	–	–	–	–	0.63	0.66	0.57	0.66	0.58	0.63
	Opioid receptor kappa 1	OPRK1	0.5	0.61	0.52	0.65	0.5	0.61	–	–	0.54	0.63	0.57	0.65	0.53	0.64	0.55	0.68
	Thyroid stimulating hormone receptor	TSHR	0.51	0.64	0.5	0.56	0.56	0.52	0.57	0.5	–	–	0.56	0.61	0.56	0.6	0.55	0.61
	TNF receptor superfamily member 10b	TNFRSF10B	–	–	0.69	0.61	0.56	0.52	–	–	0.7	0.56	0.71	0.61	0.78	0.58	0.65	0.56
Other cytosolic protein	Heat shock protein 90 alpha A1	HSP90AA1	0.53	0.65	0.5	0.67	0.59	0.73	–	–	0.53	0.67	0.55	0.67	0.59	0.65	0.51	0.64
	Heat shock protein family B1	HSPB1	0.58	0.58	0.54	0.53	0.63	0.58	0.54	0.51	0.5	0.55	0.66	0.59	0.66	0.61	0.55	0.57
Secreted protein	Interleukin 1 beta	IL1B	0.62	0.55	0.65	0.6	0.65	0.55	0.65	0.55	0.66	0.57	0.68	0.63	0.69	0.62	0.63	0.62
Structural protein	Tubulin beta class I	TUBB	–	–	0.81	0.8	0.82	0.78	–	–	–	–	0.88	0.82	0.84	0.8	0.82	0.8
Transcription factor	Androgen receptor	AR	0.51	0.63	0.58	0.75	0.55	0.71	0.53	0.75	0.51	0.62	0.61	0.77	0.55	0.74	0.67	0.76
	Jun proto-oncogene, AP-1 transcription factor subunit	JUN	0.6	0.69	0.54	0.63	0.58	0.65	0.56	0.61	0.59	0.67	0.6	0.65	0.57	0.67	0.6	0.63
	Melanogenesis associated transcription factor	MITF	0.81	0.64	0.7	0.61	0.73	0.57	0.73	0.56	0.68	0.57	0.82	0.65	0.79	0.68	0.69	0.61
	Nuclear factor kappa B1	NFKB1	0.51	0.51	0.5	0.66	0.51	0.5	0.5	0.51	0.55	0.5	0.5	0.63	0.51	0.64	0.51	0.63
	Nuclear receptor 3C1	NR3C1	–	–	0.77	0.96	0.67	0.94	0.76	0.98	–	–	0.6	0.93	0.73	0.95	0.69	0.95
	Nuclear receptor 5A1	NR5A1	0.55	0.53	0.65	0.56	0.64	0.57	–	–	–	–	0.72	0.62	0.73	0.62	0.65	0.6
	Tumor protein p53	TP53	0.72	0.57	0.62	0.55	0.65	0.55	0.7	0.57	0.62	0.58	0.71	0.58	0.7	0.57	0.6	0.56
	Vitamin D receptor	VDR	0.5	0.57	0.5	0.6	0.52	0.6	0.51	0.54	0.53	0.53	0.58	0.62	0.55	0.59	0.53	0.59
Transporter	Abhydrolase domain containing 5	ABHD5	0.51	0.57	0.51	0.66	–	–	–	–	–	–	0.55	0.68	0.54	0.68	0.53	0.69
	Solute carrier family 6 member 3	SLC6A3	0.64	0.65	0.62	0.66	0.65	0.65	0.67	0.62	0.61	0.65	0.66	0.66	0.66	0.67	0.64	0.68
Unclassified protein	Ataxin 2	ATXN2	0.78	0.5	0.7	0.62	0.74	0.52	0.7	0.53	0.69	0.58	0.72	0.62	0.72	0.61	0.7	0.61
	ATPase family, AAA domain containing 5	ATAD5	0.58	0.56	0.52	0.67	0.59	0.62	0.55	0.62	0.52	0.6	0.6	0.65	0.64	0.65	0.52	0.68

(Continued)

TABLE 3 | Continued

Target class	Target name	Cell line	A375		A549		HA1E		HCC515		HT29		MCF7		PC3		VCAP	
		Target/ Descriptor	GES	Morgan FP	GES	Morgan FP	GES	Morgan FP	GES	Morgan FP	GES	Morgan FP	GES	Morgan FP	GES	Morgan FP	GES	Morgan FP
	Endothelial PAS domain protein 1	EPAS1	–	–	0.63	0.62	–	–	–	–	–	–	0.73	0.68	0.76	0.65	0.69	0.67
	Geminin, DNA replication inhibitor	GMNN	0.7	0.59	0.71	0.58	0.69	0.55	0.65	0.59	0.67	0.55	0.76	0.62	0.75	0.59	0.68	0.6
	MLLT3, super elongation complex subunit	MLLT3	–	–	0.5	0.54	–	–	–	–	–	–	0.55	0.55	0.51	0.63	0.51	0.67
	MYC proto-oncogene, bHLH transcription factor	MYC	–	–	0.73	0.65	–	–	–	–	–	–	0.69	0.65	0.63	0.66	0.77	0.64
	Nuclear factor, erythroid 2 like 2	NFE2L2	0.57	0.51	0.57	0.6	0.55	0.58	0.57	0.59	0.58	0.53	0.56	0.61	0.61	0.6	0.59	0.6
	Nucleotide binding oligomerization domain containing 1	NOD1	–	–	0.58	0.66	–	–	–	–	0.6	0.58	0.66	0.69	0.65	0.68	0.56	0.7
	Nucleotide binding oligomerization domain containing 2	NOD2	0.5	0.53	0.53	0.61	0.56	0.54	–	–	0.52	0.53	0.58	0.68	0.61	0.68	0.56	0.64
	RAD52 homolog, DNA repair protein	RAD52	–	–	0.54	0.57	–	–	–	–	–	–	0.52	0.61	0.53	0.63	0.53	0.69
	TAR DNA binding protein	TARDBP	–	–	0.5	0.56	0.51	0.54	–	–	–	–	0.54	0.55	0.54	0.54	0.5	0.57

Target in lines, and cell line and used descriptor in columns. GES, model using gene expression signature. Morgan FP, model using chemical fingerprints from counterpart GES model dataset. Cells containing "-" corresponds to models that were not computed in cause of a too low number of actives (< 20) in the dataset to perform appropriate classification. Model presenting BA between 0.7 and 0.8 are highlighted in orange whereas those with BA > 0.8 are highlighted in red.

power of GESs and Morgan fingerprints for target prediction, based on a limited dataset depending on biological (GES and bioactivity assay) data availability.

DISCUSSION

Our results show that compound-induced transcriptomic responses derived from cell lines have the potential to support target prediction of unknown compounds with large structural diversity. Interestingly, we observed that compound induced biological responses are mostly cell line specific even when cell lines are derived from the same tissue. Nevertheless, machine learning models using GESs were shown to perform well as long as the appropriate cell line was used. Exploring biological spaces can help to overcome the limitations derived from a restricted chemical space when using traditional QSAR. To improve the predictivity of GES models, we have identified several limitations, and discuss possible improvements.

Data Acquisition

First limitations come from gene expression data preprocessing. Gene expression values were obtained through multiple preprocessing steps from the initial generated raw data. For instance, there is a first peak deconvolution step to determine the gene expression levels, that as well as the plate-normalized z-scoring to obtain the normalized ("Level 5") can still be improved as already stated by Li et al. (2017). Using GESs obtained with different preprocessing methods could potentially give more accurate normalized values leading to increased performances in machine learning models.

Secondly, the CMAP L1000 technology relies on the measurement of 978 landmark genes, representing about 5% of the human transcriptome (Pertea, 2012). The gene values of the remaining transcriptome can be inferred through different computational methods (Subramanian et al. (2017) method reached good prediction for 81% of inferred genes), that are still under improvement (Blasco et al., 2019). We decided to only use the 978 landmarks as input data for the machine models generated, to reflect real measured gene expression. Doing so, we might have missed some valuable information captured by a change of expression of the non-measured genes. Therefore, it would be interesting to explore the potential added value of expanding the number of descriptors by adding the inferred gene information to the target prediction models.

Data Restrictions

Another limitation is also coming with the activity dataset that was used. Since compound activity is a selective interaction, there is for each target a low number of active compounds compared to the number of inactive compounds. As a consequence, the training sets used for model building were highly unbalanced favorizing the prediction of the category inactive. Moreover, not every compound was tested for activity in all targets, leading to a sparse dataset (5% of total compound target interactions are known).

On top of this activity data limitation, not all available compounds were profiled in all the 8 cell lines used in this work.

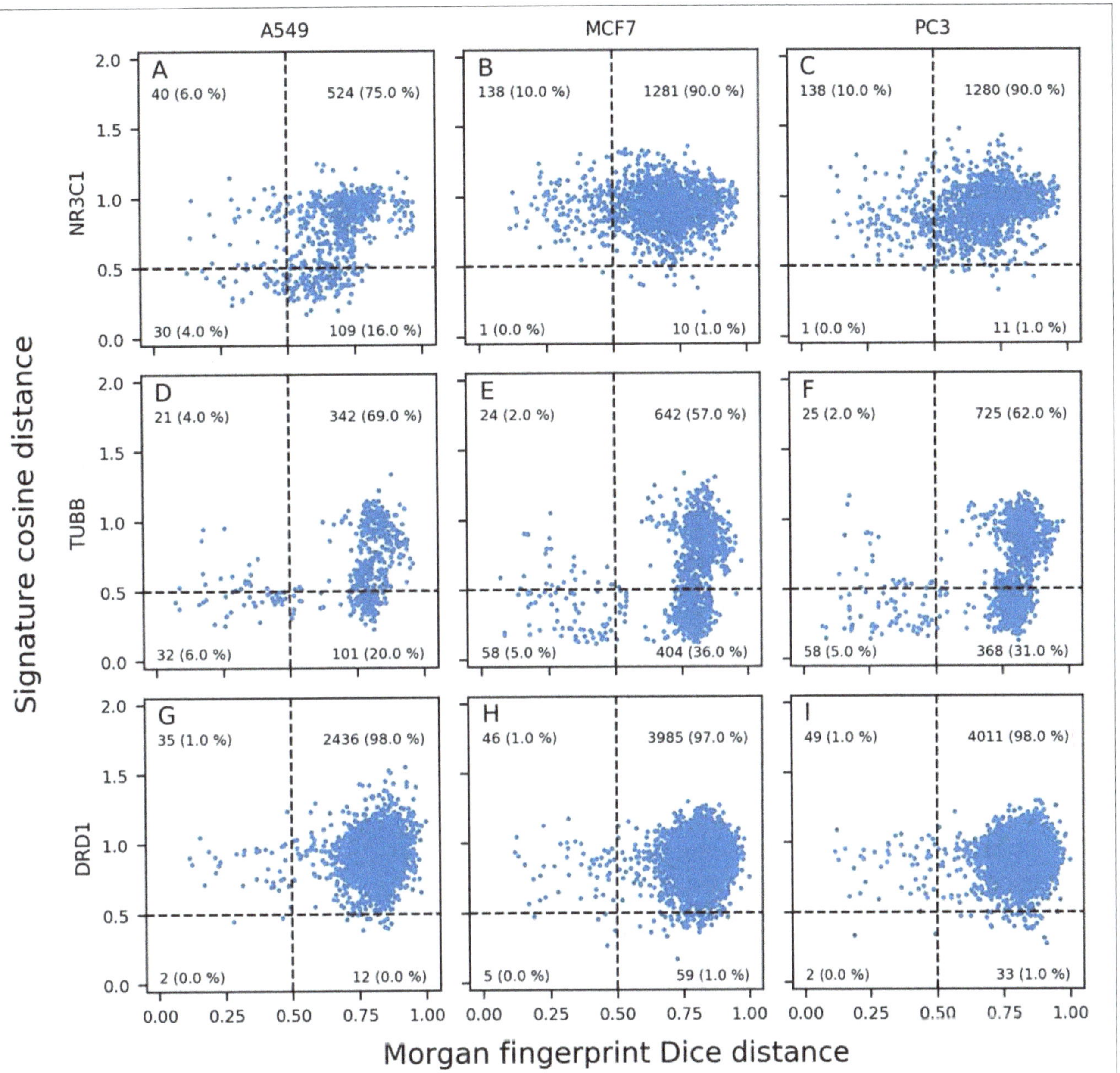

FIGURE 6 | Morgan fingerprints Dice distance vs. GES cosine distance (distance plots). Different panels show information for pairs of NR3C1 **(A–C)**, TUBB **(D–F)**, and DRD1 **(G–I)**; active compounds in A549 **(A,D,G)**, MCF7 **(B,E,H)**, and PC3 **(C,F,I)** cell lines.

There were only about 600 compounds profiled in all the cell lines, which is too limited to build predictive models, with regard to available activity data. Consequently, one dataset per cell line was created, formed by compounds profiled in this cell line and resulting GESs. For each target prediction, the cell line datasets were restricted to compounds having a known label for the target of interest. Since each task used a different dataset, performances of models across cell lines or targets the comparison across GES models was not possible. The difference in dataset sizes is explaining at least partly the variation of performances of GES models across targets, ranging from models close to a random predictor (BA = 0.50) to good GES models (BA = 0.88), as well as the variation of performances of counterpart Morgan FP models (BA ranging from 0.50 to 0.98).

Biological Response Constraints

Biologically, variation of GES model performances can also be caused by the difference in the pathway representation in the cell lines and consequently to compound induced signatures. Compounds active on a given target might show GESs with different degree of similarity or no similarity among the considered cell lines. as illustrated by the cases of NR3C1, TUBB and DRD1. Gene expression responses depend on the cellular context as shown in this work and elsewhere (Chen et al., 2013;

Yu et al., 2019). Thus, the biological system in which the GESs are generated is of utmost importance for target prediction.

Due to practical aspects (scalability, low price, etc.), biological systems such as *in vitro* immortalized cell cultures (like cancer cell lines used in this work) are widely used, but they come with some disadvantages: they show limited physiological representativity and have been shown to drift along passages (Hughes et al., 2007). Even within the same cell line, it was shown that strains show different responses to the same compounds, indicating a reduced reproducibility between generated GESs (Ben-David et al., 2018). Ideally, the GESs should be derived from biological systems mimicking as much as possible the biological responses observed in the corresponding target organ.

The advantage of transcriptomic evaluations over single endpoint assays is that in theory they have the potential to capture integrative responses from compound treatments, ranging from on target activity at high potency to off-target activities at lower potencies, depending on the tested concentrations. GESs responses are also known to be variable depending on time exposition (Aguayo-Orozco et al., 2018). That is the reason why we selected data sets originating from the same study design. GESs measured at a concentration of 10 μM after 24 h of treatment of the cell lines were extracted, as this is the most represented experimental condition (De Wolf et al., 2016; Lv et al., 2017).

GES Models Versus Morgan FP Models

We showed that using GES datasets produced by the Broad Institute with the CMAP L1000 technique (Subramanian et al., 2017), random forest models outperformed counterpart Morgan FP models for target prediction in 25% of the cases. Evidently, the outcome of this comparison is depending on the available data for the different targets to build the models as illustrated by the wide range of differences of BA between the two types of predictive models. Practically, both QSAR and transcriptomic descriptors represent good opportunities for target prediction, but each come with advantages and constraints that needs to be considered when building predictive models.

QSAR models for target prediction are widely used because of the wide dataset available, with existing databases like PubChem or ChEMBL. Most QSAR descriptors are discrete unambiguous values extracted from the chemical formula of compounds, thus easily computed. In the context of hit discovery, a major drawback of QSAR models is that they show significant error rate when trying to predict activity for compounds that are too structurally different from the training set (Cherkasov et al., 2014). Using a new set of descriptors, like compound bioactivity such as GESs extracted from *in vitro* experiments, can help in target prediction while escaping from the classical chemical space limitation observed in QSAR approaches.

On the other hand, GESs represents a number of changes on a certain number of genes (the 978 landmarks), capturing the effect of compounds. These data could be used to make inference about biology (i.e., finding targets or biomarkers). Each cell line shows a unique biological space that can be explored. However, these biological experiment data are prone to technical and biological variability like discussed earlier. Gene expression can be measured in different dose and time conditions, adding dimensions to explore in order to find the conditions reaching best performances in GES models. Finally, the gene expression measurements are more and more cost effective, making the use of such data at a large scale possible.

When exploring a new chemical class in hit discovery, evaluating chemical-induced biological responses in appropriate cell-lines using transcriptomic profiling can support chemical prioritization. This biologically-based approach present the advantage in a given biological space of being in principle chemical space independent as opposed to QSAR modeling that is constrained by the chemical space of the training set. Furthermore, during lead optimization, biological spaces inform about the direct activity of candidates, which can help fine-tuning their desired activity profile, by optimizing the on-target activity. It has been recently shown that this type of data can be used for *de novo* chemical design fulfilling a specific GES (Méndez-Lucio et al., 2020). In a chemical safety approach, it can be used to detect compound interaction with off-targets. However, a difference between these 2 applications would be the conditions in which the GESs are generated: on-target effects are observable at low concentrations (Kd often in the nanomolar range), while off-target effect are known to typically appear at higher concentration as illustrated by Li et al. (2019).

In conclusion, in this work, we evaluated the use of a large public dataset of compound-induced transcriptomic data, to predict compound activity on 69 molecular targets. We compared machine learning models built with transcriptomics data with counterpart models built using Morgan fingerprints. Active compounds on a given target could exhibit similar signatures in one or multiple cell lines, independent from the chemical structure similarity between these active compounds. For 25% of the tasks, random forest models using transcriptomics signatures performed similarly or better than counterpart models built with Morgan fingerprints, occurring mostly using signatures produced in cell lines that showed similar signatures for active compounds on a given target. Compound-induced transcriptomic data could offer a great opportunity for target prediction based on cell response similarity and allows to circumvent the applicability domain limitation of QSAR models.

AUTHOR CONTRIBUTIONS

BB, OM-L, and DR contributed to the conception of the work. BB performed the workflow with the help of OM-L. BB wrote the first draft of the manuscript. JW, OM-L, and DR provided guidance and helped with the manuscript preparation and contributed to manuscript revision, read and approved the submitted version. DR and OM-L wrote sections of the manuscript.

ACKNOWLEDGMENTS

Authors thank Karen Tilmant for proof reading the text and for her useful comments. We are also grateful to Arwa Al-Dilaimi, Djork-Arne Clevert and Angela Becker for supporting the project and for insightful discussions.

REFERENCES

Aguayo-Orozco, A., Bois, F. Y., Brunak, S., and Taboureau, O. (2018). Analysis of time-series gene expression data to explore mechanisms of chemical-induced hepatic steatosis toxicity. *Front. Genet.* 9:396. doi: 10.3389/fgene.2018.00396

Aliper, A., Plis, S., Artemov, A., Ulloa, A., Mamoshina, P., and Zhavoronkov, A. (2016). Deep learning applications for predicting pharmacological properties of drugs and drug repurposing using transcriptomic data. *Mol. Pharm.* 13, 2524–2530. doi: 10.1021/acs.molpharmaceut.6b00248

Ben-David, U., Siranosian, B., Ha, G., Tang, H., Oren, Y., Hinohara, K., et al. (2018). Genetic and transcriptional evolution alters cancer cell line drug response. *Nature* 560, 325–330. doi: 10.1038/s41586-018-0409-3

Blasco, A., Endres, M. G., Sergeev, R. A., Jonchhe, A., Macaluso, N. J. M., Narayan, R., et al. (2019). Advancing computational biology and bioinformatics research through open innovation competitions. *PLoS ONE* 14:e0222165. doi: 10.1371/journal.pone.0222165

Breiman, L. (2001). Randomforest2001. *Mach. Learn.* 45, 5–32. doi: 10.1017/CBO9781107415324.004

Chaaban, S., and Brouhard, G. J. (2017). A microtubule bestiary: structural diversity in tubulin polymers. *Mol. Biol. Cell* 28, 2924–2931. doi: 10.1091/mbc.E16-05-0271

Chen, M., Xiao, J., Zhang, Z., Liu, J., Wu, J., and Yu, J. (2013). Identification of human HK genes and gene expression regulation study in cancer from transcriptomics data analysis. *PLoS ONE* 8:e54082. doi: 10.1371/journal.pone.0054082

Chen, X., Yan, C. C., Zhang, X., Zhang, X., Dai, F., Yin, J., et al. (2016). Drug-target interaction prediction: databases, web servers and computational models. *Brief Bioinform.* 17, 696–712. doi: 10.1093/bib/bbv066

Cherkasov, A., Muratov, E. N., Fourches, D., Varnek, A., Baskin, I. I., Cronin, M., et al. (2014). QSAR modeling: where have you been? where are you going to?. *J. Med. Chem.* 57, 4977–5010. doi: 10.1021/jm4004285

Corsello, S. M., Bittker, J. A., Liu, Z., Gould, J., McCarren, P., Hirschman, J. E., et al. (2017). The drug repurposing hub: a next-generation drug library and information resource. *Nat. Med.* 23, 405–408. doi: 10.1038/nm.4306

Cruz-Monteagudo, M., Medina-Franco, J. L., Pérez-Castillo, Y., Nicolotti, O., Cordeiro, M. N. D. S., and Borges, F. (2014). Activity cliffs in drug discovery: Dr Jekyll or Mr Hyde? *Drug Discov. Today* 19, 109–1080. doi: 10.1016/j.drudis.2014.02.003

De Wolf, H., Cougnaud, L., Van Hoorde, K., De Bondt, A., Wegner, J. K., Ceulemans, H., et al. (2018). High-throughput gene expression profiles to define drug similarity and predict compound activity. *Assay Drug Dev. Technol.* 16, 162–176. doi: 10.1089/adt.2018.845

De Wolf, H., De Bondt, A., Turner, H., and Göhlmann, H. W. H. (2016). Transcriptional characterization of compounds: lessons learned from the public LINCS data. *Assay Drug Dev. Technol.* 14, 252–260. doi: 10.1089/adt.2016.715

Hanahan, D., and Weinberg, R. A. (2011). Hallmarks of cancer: the next generation. *Cell* 144, 646–674. doi: 10.1016/j.cell.2011.02.013

Hieronymus, H., Lamb, J., Ross, K. N., Peng, X. P., Clement, C., Rodina, A., et al. (2006). Gene expression signature-based chemical genomic prediction identifies a novel class of HSP90 pathway modulators. *Cancer Cell* 10, 321–330. doi: 10.1016/j.ccr.2006.09.005

Hofmarcher, M., Rumetshofer, E., Clevert, D. A., Hochreiter, S., and Klambauer, G. (2019). Accurate prediction of biological assays with high-throughput microscopy images and convolutional networks. *J. Chem. Inf. Model* 59, 1163–1171. doi: 10.1021/acs.jcim.8b00670

Hughes, P., Marshall, D., Reid, Y., Parkes, H., and Gelber, C. (2007). The costs of using unauthenticated, over-passaged cell lines: how much more data do we need? *BioTechniques.* 43, 575, 577–578, 581–582. doi: 10.2144/000112598

Hughes, T. R., Marton, M. J., Jones, A. R., Roberts, C. J., Stoughton, R., Armour, C. D., et al. (2000). Functional discovery via a compendium of expression profiles. *Cell* 102, 109–126. doi: 10.1016/S0092-8674(00)00015-5

Kuthuru, S., Szafran, A. T., Stossi, F., Mancini, M. A., and Rao, A. (2019). Leveraging image-derived phenotypic measurements for drug-target interaction predictions. *Cancer Inform.* 18:1176935119856595. doi: 10.1177/1176935119856595

Lamb, J., Crawford, E. D., Peck, D., Modell, J. W., Blat, I. C., Wrobel, M. J., et al. (2006). The connectivity map: using gene-expression signatures to connect small molecules, genes, and disease. *Science* 313, 1929–1935. doi: 10.1126/science.1132939

Lapins, M., and Spjuth, O. (2019). Evaluation of gene expression and phenotypic profiling data as quantitative descriptors for predicting drug targets and mechanisms of action. *Biorxiv.* doi: 10.1101/580654. [Epub ahead of print].

Laufkötter, O., Sturm, N., Bajorath, J., Chen, H., and Engkvist, O. (2019). Combining structural and bioactivity-based fingerprints improves prediction performance and scaffold hopping capability. *J. Cheminform.* 11:54. doi: 10.1186/s13321-019-0376-1

Lee, H., Kang, S., and Kim, W. (2016). Drug repositioning for cancer therapy based on large-scale drug-induced transcriptional signatures. *PLoS ONE* 11:e0150460. doi: 10.1371/journal.pone.0150460

Li, A., Lu, X., Natoli, T., Bittker, J., Sipes, N. S., Subramanian, A., et al. (2019). The carcinogenome project: *in vitro* gene expression profiling of chemical perturbations to predict long-term carcinogenicity. *Environ. Health Perspect.* 127:47002. doi: 10.1289/EHP3986

Li, Z., Li, J., and Yu, P. (2017). l1kdeconv: an R package for peak calling analysis with LINCS L1000 data. *BMC Bioinformatics* 18:356. doi: 10.1186/s12859-017-1767-9

Lv, C., Wu, X., Wang, X., Su, J., Zeng, H., Zhao, J., et al. (2017). The gene expression profiles in response to 102 traditional Chinese medicine (TCM) components: a general template for research on TCMs. *Sci. Rep.* 7:352. doi: 10.1038/s41598-017-00535-8

Méndez-Lucio, O., Baillif, B., Clevert, D. A., Rouquié, D., and Wichard, J. (2020). *De novo* generation of hit-like molecules from gene expression signatures using artificial intelligence. *Nat. Commun.* 11:10. doi: 10.1038/s41467-019-13807-w

Pabon, N. A., Xia, Y., Estabrooks, S. K., Ye, Z., Herbrand, A. K., Süß, E., et al. (2018). Predicting protein targets for drug-like compounds using transcriptomics. *PLoS Comput. Biol.* 14:e1006651. doi: 10.1371/journal.pcbi.1006651

Pedregosa, F., Varoquaux, G., Gramfort, A., Michel, V., Thirion, B., Grisel, O., et al. (2011). Scikit-learn: machine learning in python. *J. Mach. Learn. Res.* 12, 2825–2830. Available online at: http://jmlr.org/papers/v12/pedregosa11a.html

Pertea, M. (2012). The human transcriptome: an unfinished story. *Genes* 3, 344–360. doi: 10.3390/genes3030344

Petrone, P. M., Simms, B., Nigsch, F., Lounkine, E., Kutchukian, P., Cornett, A., et al. (2012). Rethinking molecular similarity: Comparing compounds on the basis of biological activity. *ACS Chem. Biol.* 7, 1399–1409. doi: 10.1021/cb3001028

Rogers, D., and Hahn, M. (2010). Extended-connectivity fingerprints. *J. Chem. Inf. Model.* 50, 742–754. doi: 10.1021/ci100050t

Rouquié, D., Heneweer, M., Botham, J., Ketelslegers, H., Markell, L., Pfister, T., et al. (2015). Contribution of new technologies to characterization and prediction of adverse effects. *Crit. Rev. Toxicol.* 45, 172–183. doi: 10.3109/10408444.2014.986054

Scheeder, C., Heigwer, F., and Boutros, M. (2018). Machine learning and image-based profiling in drug discovery. *Curr. Opin. Syst. Biol.* 10, 43–52. doi: 10.1016/j.coisb.2018.05.004

Simm, J., Klambauer, G., Arany, A., Steijaert, M., Wegner, J. K., Gustin, E., et al. (2018). Repurposing high-throughput image assays enables biological activity prediction for drug discovery. *Cell Chem. Biol.* 25, 611-618. doi: 10.1016/j.chembiol.2018.01.015

Subramanian, A., Narayan, R., Corsello, S. M., Peck, D. D., Natoli, T. E., Lu, X., et al. (2017). A Next Generation Connectivity Map: L1000 Platform and the First 1,000,000 Profiles. *Cell* 171, 1437–1452 e17. doi: 10.1016/j.cell.2017.10.049

Vamathevan, J., Clark, D., Czodrowski, P., Dunham, I., Ferran, E., Lee, G., et al. (2019). Applications of machine learning in drug discovery and development. *Nat. Rev. Drug Discov.* 18, 463–477. doi: 10.1038/s41573-019-0024-5

Van Der Maaten, L., and Hinton, G. (2008). Visualizing data using t-SNE. *J. Mach. Learn. Res.* 9, 2579–2605. Available online at: http://www.jmlr.org/papers/v9/vandermaaten08a.html

Wang, Y., Suzek, T., Zhang, J., Wang, J., He, S., Cheng, T., et al. (2014). PubChem Bioassay: 2014 update. *Nucleic Acids Res.* 1, D1075–D1082. doi: 10.1093/nar/gkt978

Wei, G., Twomey, D., Lamb, J., Schlis, K., Agarwal, J., Stam, R. W., et al. (2006). Gene expression-based chemical genomics identifies rapamycin as a modulator of MCL1 and glucocorticoid resistance. *Cancer Cell* 10, 331–342. doi: 10.1016/j.ccr.2006.09.006

Yu, K., Chen, B., Aran, D., Charalel, J., Yau, C., Wolf, D. M., et al. (2019). Comprehensive transcriptomic analysis of cell lines as models of primary tumors across 22 tumor types. *Nat. Commun.* 10:3574. doi: 10.1038/s41467-019-11415-2

15

GLORY: Generator of the Structures of Likely Cytochrome P450 Metabolites Based on Predicted Sites of Metabolism

Christina de Bruyn Kops[1†], Conrad Stork[1†], Martin Šícho[1,2†], Nikolay Kochev[3,4†], Daniel Svozil[2†], Nina Jeliazkova[3†] and Johannes Kirchmair[1,5,6]*

[1] Department of Computer Science, Center for Bioinformatics (ZBH), Faculty of Mathematics, Informatics and Natural Sciences, Universität Hamburg, Hamburg, Germany, [2] CZ-OPENSCREEN: National Infrastructure for Chemical Biology, Department of Informatics and Chemistry, Faculty of Chemical Technology, University of Chemistry and Technology Prague, Prague, Czechia, [3] Ideaconsult Ltd., Sofia, Bulgaria, [4] Department of Analytical Chemistry and Computer Chemistry, University of Plovdiv, Plovdiv, Bulgaria, [5] Department of Chemistry, University of Bergen, Bergen, Norway, [6] Computational Biology Unit (CBU), University of Bergen, Bergen, Norway

***Correspondence:**
Johannes Kirchmair
johannes.kirchmair@uib.no
orcid.org/0000-0003-2667-5877

†Christina de Bruyn Kops
orcid.org/0000-0001-8890-2137
Conrad Stork
orcid.org/0000-0002-5499-742X
Martin Šícho
orcid.org/0000-0002-8771-1731
Nikolay Kochev
orcid.org/0000-0001-6547-3675
Daniel Svozil
orcid.org/0000-0003-2577-5163
Nina Jeliazkova
orcid.org/0000-0002-4322-6179

Computational prediction of xenobiotic metabolism can provide valuable information to guide the development of drugs, cosmetics, agrochemicals, and other chemical entities. We have previously developed FAME 2, an effective tool for predicting sites of metabolism (SoMs). In this work, we focus on the prediction of the chemical structures of metabolites, in particular metabolites of xenobiotics. To this end, we have developed a new tool, GLORY, which combines SoM prediction with FAME 2 and a new collection of rules for metabolic reactions mediated by the cytochrome P450 enzyme family. GLORY has two modes: MaxEfficiency and MaxCoverage. For MaxEfficiency mode, the use of predicted SoMs to restrict the locations in the molecule at which the reaction rules could be applied was explored. For MaxCoverage mode, the predicted SoM probabilities were instead used to develop a new scoring approach for the predicted metabolites. With this scoring approach, GLORY achieves a recall of 0.83 and can predict at least one known metabolite within the top three ranked positions for 76% of the molecules of a new, manually curated test set. GLORY is freely available as a web server at https://acm.zbh.uni-hamburg.de/glory/, and the datasets and reaction rules are provided in the **Supplementary Material**.

Keywords: metabolism prediction, metabolite structure prediction, rule-based approach, sites of metabolism, xenobiotic metabolism, cytochrome P450, metabolites

INTRODUCTION

Metabolism is responsible for creating metabolites with different physicochemical and pharmacological properties compared to those of the original parent molecule. Xenobiotic metabolism in particular is directly relevant for humans, especially as it relates to, for example, the development of drugs, cosmetics, and agrochemicals. In fact, it is supposed that metabolism is the main clearance pathway for the vast majority of all xenobiotics (Kirchmair et al., 2015). However, metabolism can also result in pharmacologically active metabolites as well as toxic metabolites (Testa et al., 2012).

The cytochrome P450 (CYP) family of enzymes plays an important role in the metabolism of xenobiotics, especially in the formation of first-generation metabolites, of which roughly 60% are formed by CYPs (Testa et al., 2012). The importance of CYPs to drug discovery is clear from the observation that many drugs are metabolized by CYPs; common estimates range from 50% (Di, 2014) to 80% (Testa et al., 2012). A detailed meta-analysis of the metabolites of over 1,000 different xenobiotic substrates carried out by Testa et al., showed that 40% of all metabolites are formed by CYPs, including a substantial proportion of all toxic or highly reactive metabolites (Testa et al., 2012).

There are 57 known human CYP enzymes, the majority of which are primarily involved in endogenous metabolism. The CYP2 and CYP3 subfamilies are mainly responsible for metabolizing xenobiotics (Testa et al., 2012), and the key CYP isozymes for drug metabolism are CYP3A4, 3A5, 2D6, 2C8, 2C9, 2C19, 1A1, 2B6, and 2E1 (Di, 2014). Among the xenobiotic-metabolizing CYP isozymes, the binding pockets vary greatly; in some cases the binding pocket of a single isozyme is highly flexible and can accommodate a broad range of substrates with widely varying sizes (Kirchmair et al., 2015).

Computational methods can make a significant contribution to predicting xenobiotic metabolism, because they can be used to quickly make predictions that can focus the experimental aspects of the drug development process. Such a focusing effect is both cost-effective and time-effective (Kirchmair et al., 2015).

One relatively well-developed aspect of the computational prediction of xenobiotic metabolism is the identification of the metabolically labile atom positions, also known as sites of metabolism (SoMs) (Kirchmair et al., 2012). Being able to predict SoMs is important because knowing an atom position in a molecule at which a metabolizing reaction is likely to occur usually provides a chemist with a good idea of the ensuing metabolite structure. Besides a range of commercial offerings, several freely available tools, such as SMARTCyp (Olsen et al., 2019), SOMP (Rudik et al., 2015), Xenosite (Zaretzki et al., 2013), and FAME 2 (Šícho et al., 2017), are able to predict SoMs with high accuracy (Tyzack and Kirchmair, 2018). FAME 2, which is used in the present work for SoM prediction, is a machine learning-based tool developed recently in our group. The extra trees classifier models of FAME 2, which are based on a set of 2D circular descriptors, were developed specifically to predict SoMs of metabolic reactions catalyzed by the CYP family of enzymes in humans. FAME 2 is highly accurate, achieving, on an independent test set, a Matthews correlation coefficient of 0.57 and an area under the receiver operating characteristic curve (AUC) of 0.91.

In contrast to *in silico* SoM prediction, computational prediction of the structures of metabolites lags behind with respect to prediction accuracy. In general, existing methods for predicting metabolite structures for xenobiotics are dominated by rule-based approaches. There are a number of well-established commercial tools for metabolite structure prediction, including Meteor Nexus (Lhasa Ltd.), a rule-based metabolite prediction software (Marchant et al., 2008). Meteor Nexus offers three different reasoning methods to prioritize the plethora of generated metabolites. The current default reasoning method is SoM scoring, which compares the SoM identified by the reaction rule to experimental data in order to assign scores to the predicted metabolites[1]. Other rule-based computational tools include TIMES (LMC; Mekenyan et al., 2004), which uses a heuristic algorithm to generate possible metabolic maps, and MetabolExpert (CompuDrug; Darvas, 1987).

In addition to commercial metabolite structure prediction tools, there is an increasing number of freely available options. Again, many of the available options rely primarily on a set of reaction rules to generate structures of possible metabolites. One well-known approach that has been around for some time is SyGMa (Ridder and Wagener, 2008), which in this work is used as a reference method. SyGMa predicts metabolites using knowledge-based reaction rules, some of which were derived from common knowledge of metabolism reactions and some of which were developed using the Metabolite Database (MDL Metabolite Database, Elsevier, 2001), for a total of 144 reaction rules covering both phase I and phase II metabolism. The predicted metabolites are ranked by empirical probability scores calculated based on the fraction of predicted metabolites produced by the particular reaction rule that match reported metabolites in the database. Using all 144 phase I and phase II reaction rules in up to three successive reaction steps, SyGMa was able to predict 68% of all known metabolites in the test set. In terms of ranking, SyGMa ranked 45% of the known metabolites in the test set in the top 10. The authors additionally examined SyGMa's potential usefulness for predicting CYP-mediated metabolism by evaluating its performance on a set of 127 single-step CYP-mediated reactions. Using only the 118 phase I reaction rules, which include but are not specific to CYP-mediated reactions, SyMGa was able to predict 84% of all known CYP-formed metabolites and predict 66% of the known metabolites within the top three ranked predicted metabolites. However, the proprietary nature of the dataset that was used to derive SyGMa's reaction rules and validate the method, not to mention the current unavailability of the dataset, hinders the reproducibility of the results as well as further use of the models derived from the data.

A recent, free software designed to predict metabolites from multiple sources and enzyme families is BioTransformer (Djoumbou-Feunang et al., 2019), which in this work is used as the second reference method. BioTransformer is a comprehensive metabolite prediction tool that contains a CYP metabolite prediction module (in addition to four other metabolite prediction modules). BioTransformer predicts CYP-formed metabolites using a knowledge-based approach combined with built-in CYP selectivity prediction by CypReact (Tian et al., 2018), a machine learning-based tool, as a precursor to metabolite prediction. Aside from the initial CYP isoform-specificity prediction, the basis of BioTransformer's CYP450 metabolite prediction module is a rule-based method whose

Abbreviations: AUC, area under the receiver operating characteristic curve; CYP, cytochrome P450; ROC, receiver operating characteristic; SoM, site of metabolism.

[1] Meteor Reasoning Methodologies, Lhasa Limited, https://www.lhasalimited.org/products/meteor-reasoning-methodologies.htm

reaction rules are derived partly from the metabolic reactions in MetXBioDB (Djoumbou-Feunang et al., 2019), a freely available database of metabolism reactions that was established in the context of developing BioTransformer. In the current version of BioTransformer, the predicted metabolites are not ranked. BioTransformer also offers an option for identifying metabolites based on masses from mass spectrometry data. On a test dataset of 60 parent molecules with a total of 180 known metabolites, BioTransformer's CYP450 metabolite prediction module achieved a recall of 0.90 and a precision of 0.46.

Another freely available metabolite prediction tool is MetaTox (Rudik et al., 2017), which encompasses both phase I and phase II metabolism and combines the prediction of the reaction class and the reacting atom in order to predict metabolites. Additionally, the open-source software Toxtree (Patlewicz et al., 2008) contains a metabolism prediction module called "SMARTCyp—Cytochrome P450-Mediated Drug Metabolism" that predicts SoMs using SMARTCyp (Rydberg et al., 2010) and then applies a small set of reaction rules to the predicted SoMs in order to predict metabolites.

Common to all modern approaches for metabolite prediction is that they remain challenged by the combinatorial explosion of predictions, in particular when looking at several generations of metabolites (Judson, 2014). It is not unusual for metabolite structure predictors to produce several pages full of predicted metabolites, a fact which is often and not without reason criticized, particularly by experts in metabolism. The key to tackling this problem lies in the development of approaches for the accurate ranking of metabolites according to their relevance in terms of metabolic rates and biological properties. A number of methods attempt to get a handle on the immense number of predicted metabolites by ranking their predictions according to various approaches.

Another option, which has primarily been implemented in commercial tools to date, is to use SoM prediction as a preliminary step to reduce the number of generated metabolites. Commercial tools for metabolite prediction that incorporate SoM prediction include ADMET Predictor (SimulationsPlus)[2], which predicts SoMs and the corresponding metabolite structures for nine CYP isoforms, and StarDrop (Optibrium; Tyzack et al., 2016), whose "P450 metabolism" module predicts SoMs using quantum mechanical simulations and displays the structures of the metabolites corresponding to the predicted SoMs. In addition, META Ultra (MultiCASE Inc.; Klopman et al., 1994) predicts SoMs and metabolites, and MetaSite (Cruciani et al., 2005) was a SoM and CYP isoform selectivity prediction software that now also predicts metabolite structures[3].

Few freely available metabolite prediction methods combine information on predicted SoMs with a rule set. MetaTox predicts reaction classes and reacting atoms (i.e., SoMs, in principle) separately for each parent molecule, then combines the predictions to generate metabolites. The probability that the metabolite is formed is calculated based on the predicted probabilities of the reaction class and of the SoM predicted with the SOMP method (Rudik et al., 2015). However, the validation of MetaTox considers the performance of the reaction class prediction and the reacting atom prediction separately, without evaluating the prediction of the metabolite structures themselves, and it is unclear how exactly the reaction class and reacting atom predictions are combined to generate a metabolite structure (Rudik et al., 2017). On the other hand, it is clear that SoM prediction is used directly as a prefilter before applying reaction rules in the SMARTCyp Toxtree module. However, a validation of this method has not been published.

In terms of the availability of rule sets for metabolite structure prediction, there are a few existing freely available collections of reaction rules described in an easily accessible, computer-readable format such as SMIRKS[4], a reaction transform language within the Daylight system. One source of CYP reaction rules is the SMARTCyp Toxtree module, which uses 16 reaction rules and makes the SMIRKS freely available as part of the source code. A larger selection of reaction rules is provided in the freely available SyGMA Python package. The reaction rules are clearly separated into phase I and phase II rules; however, there is no indication of which of the 118 phase I reaction rules specifically describe CYP-mediated reactions. In addition, these rules were derived from a proprietary and no longer distributed dataset. BioTransformer offers a large number of CYP-specific biotransformation rules in SMIRKS format as well as additional constraint(s) for each rule as part of its Reaction Knowledgebase.

In this work, we present a multipronged approach to the prediction of metabolites formed by the CYP enzyme family in humans. In reference to FAME, we name this approach GLORY. One fundamental aspect of GLORY is a new, easily interpretable rule base for CYP metabolism that was developed solely from the scientific literature and basic chemistry knowledge, without relying on any dataset of metabolic reactions. In addition, we have examined the effect of using SoM prediction as a preliminary filter for the positions at which reaction rules are allowed to be applied and also as part of a new approach to ranking the predicted metabolites. GLORY therefore has two modes: MaxCoverage, which focuses solely on recall, and MaxEfficiency, which focuses more on precision. Further, we have validated GLORY on a new, high quality, manually curated dataset that is provided in the **Supplementary Material**.

RESULTS AND DISCUSSION

Two key aspects are at the core of GLORY, which aims to predict metabolites within the context of human, CYP-mediated metabolism: reaction rules and predicted SoMs. In terms of the rule-based aspect, GLORY uses reaction rules to convert parent molecules into their possible metabolites. To this end, we developed a collection of rules based entirely on the scientific literature to ensure that the rule set was not biased by any particular metabolism dataset. The information on the CYP-mediated reactions from the literature was combined with

[2]ADMET Predictor Metabolism Module, SimulationsPlus, https://www.simulations-plus.com/software/admetpredictor/metabolism/

[3]MetaSite, https://www.moldiscovery.com/software/metasite/

[4]SMIRKS—A Reaction Transform Language, Daylight, http://www.daylight.com/dayhtml/doc/theory/theory.smirks.html

basic chemistry knowledge to develop SMIRKS to describe each reaction type. In some cases, such as for O-dearylation, multiple SMIRKS were required for a single reaction type, resulting in a total of 73 SMIRKS for the 61 reaction types present in our collection (**Supplementary Table 1**). We additionally use a simple binary distinction between common and uncommon reaction types, which were thoroughly discussed and distinguished from each other in Guengerich (2001), and which distinction we were able to extrapolate to the CYP-mediated reactions found elsewhere in the literature (see Methods for details). We do not use occurrence ratios calculated based on a given dataset in order to rank the predicted metabolites, due to the limited size, quality, and accessibility of existing datasets. Out of our collection of 61 CYP reaction types, 22 have been designated as common.

The second key aspect of GLORY is its use of the SoM probabilities predicted by FAME 2 for each heavy atom in a molecule to (i) reduce the false-positive prediction rate while maintaining an acceptable recovery rate and (ii) augment the ranking of predicted metabolites. In order to reduce the false-positive prediction rate, the possibility of utilizing a hard cutoff based on SoM probabilities was explored. This cutoff was used to determine at which atom positions the rules were allowed to be applied. In the context of GLORY, we have called this approach, in which SoM prediction is used as a preliminary filter, MaxEfficiency mode. In contrast, we designate the approach in which SoM probabilities are used for ranking metabolites derived for all positions in a molecule regardless of SoM probability the MaxCoverage mode. The difference in workflow between the two modes is illustrated in **Figure 1**.

Datasets

To choose a SoM probability cutoff for the MaxEfficiency mode and develop a priority score to rank predicted metabolites, a large reference dataset was generated by combining the CYP metabolism data extracted from DrugBank (Wishart et al., 2018) and MetXBioDB. MetXBioDB is a recently published database of metabolic reactions, whose substrates are mainly comprised of xenobiotics and also include a few sterol lipids and mammalian primary metabolites, and whose reaction data came from the scientific literature as well as publicly available databases (Djoumbou-Feunang et al., 2019). In addition, a manually curated, high-quality dataset was compiled from the scientific literature for the validation of GLORY. This test dataset contains 29 parent molecules and a total of 81 metabolites, resulting in 2.79 metabolites per parent molecule on average. Importantly, any parent compounds that are in the test dataset were removed from the reference dataset before any analysis occurred. In total, the reference dataset contains 848 parent molecules and a total of 1,588 metabolites, for an average of 1.87 metabolites per parent molecule. Predictions could be made for 847 of 848 molecules in the reference dataset (one molecule could not be processed successfully with FAME 2; see Methods for details).

MaxEfficiency Mode: Selection of a Cutoff for Metabolite Structure Generation Based on SoM Probability

In order to determine the effect of a SoM prediction-based prefilter on predicting preferably only the most relevant metabolites and reducing the number of false positive predictions, we tried several different cutoffs for the SoM probability that must be achieved by at least one atom involved in the reaction (as defined by the reaction's SMIRKS). For each heavy atom in a molecule, FAME 2 reports a probability between 0 and 1, corresponding to the fraction of trees of the extra trees classifier that predict that a particular atom is a SoM. The decision threshold in FAME 2 for whether or not an atom is considered likely enough to be a SoM to be designated as such was determined by the trained model to be 0.4 (Šícho et al., 2017).

We examined the effect of different SoM probability cutoffs using the reference dataset and selected the cutoff to be used

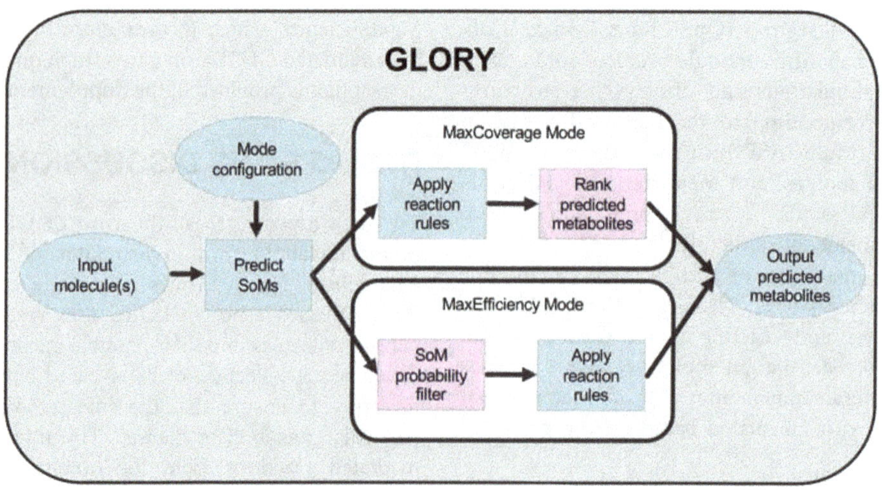

FIGURE 1 | Workflow for GLORY indicating the difference between MaxCoverage mode and MaxEfficiency mode.

in MaxEfficiency mode based on these results. In particular, we inspected the effect of the SoM probability cutoffs on precision and recall, which are defined as follows:

$$Recall = TP / (TP + FN)$$
$$Precision = TP / (TP + FP)$$

where TP is the number of true positive predictions, FP is the number of (putative) false positive predictions, and FN is the number of false negative predictions. In other words, recall measures the portion of known metabolites that were reproduced by the method and precision measures the fraction of all predicted metabolites that are represented in the dataset.

Here it is worth noting that the number of false positives, and the designation of a prediction as false positive, is especially dependent on the dataset that is being used for comparison. Many metabolites that are formed in humans have not yet been discovered, or their structures have not yet been exactly elucidated. Since even the highest-quality dataset is limited by the available experimental data, the reality is that the distinction between a real false positive prediction and the true positive prediction of an as yet unknown or unconformed metabolite may not be possible. Nevertheless, with this caveat, we evaluate our method based on the available data, including the putative false positives.

The purpose of the MaxEfficiency mode is to use the SoM probability cutoff to predict metabolites with increased precision compared to no cutoff (i.e., MaxCoverage mode). At the same time, however, we did not want to sacrifice too much in terms of recall, as it is still important to predict a molecule's actual metabolites even while reducing the number of putative false positive predictions.

For the purpose of metabolite prediction, we found that using FAME 2's decision threshold of 0.4 as the cutoff for SoM probability resulted in a relatively low recall of 0.65 (especially when compared to the recall of 0.83 achieved in MaxCoverage mode, as will be discussed later in this work). Hence, despite the increased precision afforded by a cutoff of 0.4, it was determined that this cutoff too greatly reduced the achieved recall. We therefore additionally tested lower SoM probability cutoffs (**Table 1**). Observing the trade-off between precision and recall with cutoffs ranging from 0.4 to 0.1 and comparing them to MaxCoverage mode, we determined that a SoM probability cutoff of 0.2, which resulted in a precision of 0.19 and a still-high recall of 0.75, offered the best compromise. A SoM probability cutoff of 0.2 for MaxEfficiency mode was therefore fixed based on the results shown in this section. Note that although all of the precision values shown in **Table 1** are quite low, the precision of GLORY using a SoM probability cutoff is comparable to the precision of existing methods for metabolite structure prediction (see below for the results on the test dataset).

TABLE 1 | Effect of different SoM probability cutoffs on precision and recall over the entire reference dataset.

SoM Probability Cutoff[a]	0.4	0.3	0.2	0.1	None
Precision	0.24	0.22	0.19	0.13	0.07
Recall	0.65	0.71	0.75	0.80	0.83

[a] *Note that 0.4 is the default decision threshold in FAME 2, a cutoff of none corresponds to MaxCoverage mode, and a cutoff of 0.2 was chosen for MaxEfficiency mode.*

Development of a Priority Score to Rank Predicted Metabolites for MaxCoverage Mode

In order to rank the predicted metabolites for a particular molecule, we developed a priority score for each predicted metabolite based on the SoM probability of the atoms involved in the transformation and whether the reaction type is common or not. Specifically, the SoM probability calculated by FAME 2 for all atoms in the parent molecule that are involved in a reaction as defined by the SMIRKS is considered, and the maximum SoM probability among these atoms is then incorporated into the score, as illustrated in **Figure 2**. The priority score was calculated using a simple formula:

$$score_{predictedmetabolite} = P \times F$$

where P is the maximum SoM probability out of the atoms in the parent molecule that were matched by the applied transformation and F is the factor according to whether the reaction type was designated as common or uncommon. In case the same predicted metabolite resulted from multiple transformations, the maximum priority score over all transformations leading to that prediction was used. A higher priority score is intended to indicate a higher likelihood of the prediction being true. For all uncommon reaction types, $F = 1$. The factor F for common reaction types affects the early enrichment of the predictions. Specifically, the early enrichment improves when common reaction types are given more weight in the score than uncommon reaction types, i.e. $F_{common} > 1$ (**Figure 3**). Based on an analysis of the receiver operating characteristic (ROC) curves and area under the ROC curves (AUC) for varying F_{common}, shown in **Figure 3**, a factor of 5, resulting in an AUC of 0.90, was chosen. All subsequent results based on ranking the predicted metabolites therefore used $F_{common} = 5$ in the calculation of the priority score, and the priority score can therefore range from 0 to 5.

Comparison of Performance on a New, Manually Curated Test Set

The performance of the MaxEfficiency and MaxCoverage modes of GLORY was evaluated on the curated test set of 29 parent molecules with a total of 81 metabolites. This evaluation includes a comparison with BioTransformer and SyGMa as well as an analysis of how well the scoring and ranking aspects of the different approaches work. Specifically, we employed the CYP450 module of BioTransformer and the phase I metabolism reactions of SyGMa (SyGMa does not feature a dedicated module for CYP metabolism, but phase I metabolism is carried out to a significant extent by CYP enzymes) for the comparison.

Analysis of MaxEfficiency Mode

GLORY's MaxEfficiency mode was designed to address the problem of low precision caused by a high number of putative

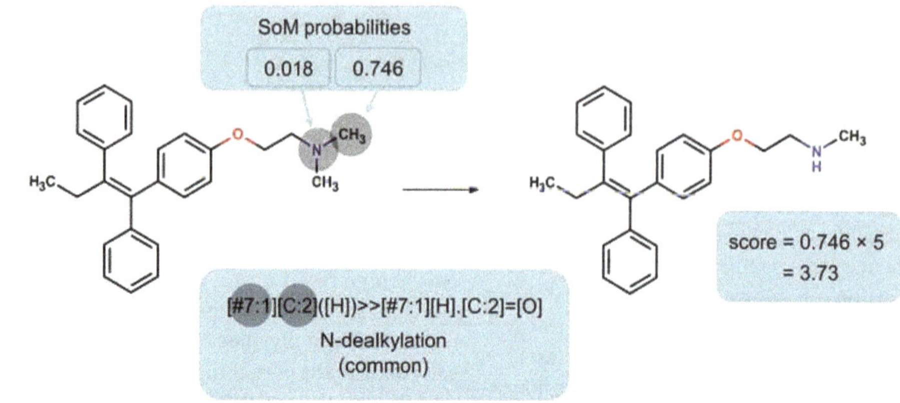

FIGURE 2 | Illustration of the determination of the maximum SoM probability of all heavy atoms in the parent molecule that are matched by the reaction rule, using the N-dealkylation reaction rule (common reaction type; factor $F = 5$) as an example. This maximum probability is used to calculate the priority score of the product.

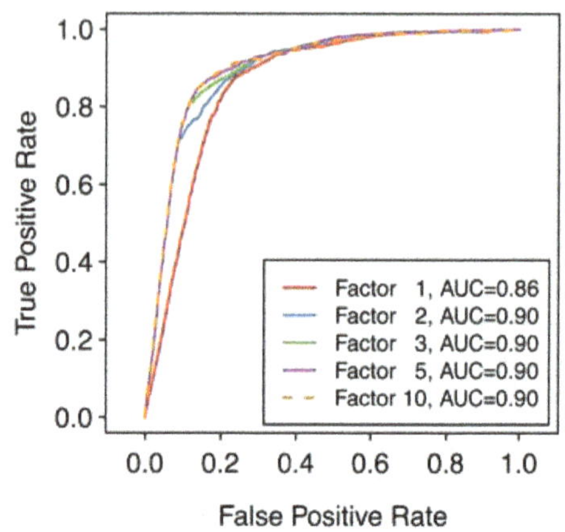

FIGURE 3 | Receiver operating characteristic (ROC) curves over the entire reference dataset of 848 compounds with 1,588 known metabolites, with varying values of the factor used for common reaction types when calculating the priority score for each metabolite. Note that a factor of 1 means that only the SoM probability (i.e., the maximum SoM probability for all atoms that are matched by the SMIRKS) affects the priority score of the predicted metabolite, regardless of the reaction type. Note also that a ROC curve can be calculated despite there being no "true negative" predictions overall (all predicted metabolites are "positive" predictions). To generate the ROC curve, the false positive rate (FPR) is calculated at each score threshold. At each point, predictions with scores below the threshold are considered "negative" predictions and predictions with scores above the threshold are considered "positive" predictions. Hence the number of "true negative" predictions and therefore the FPR can be calculated for each point of the ROC curve.

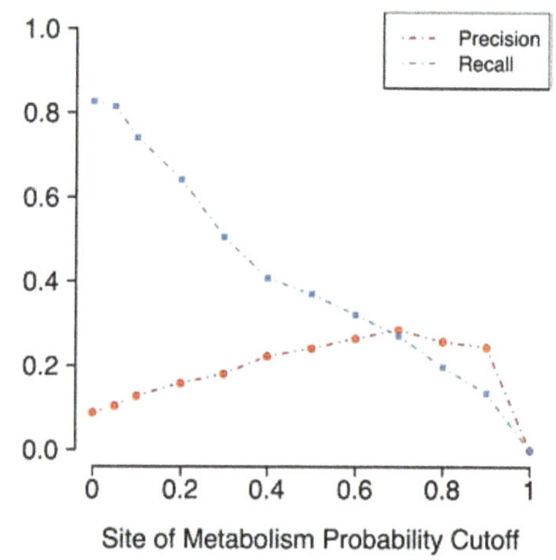

FIGURE 4 | Precision (portion of predictions that are true positives) and recall (portion of known metabolites that are predicted) vary according to the cutoff for FAME 2's predicted SoM probability. A SoM probability cutoff of 0.4 corresponds to the decision threshold used in FAME 2. The SoM probability cutoff chosen for the MaxEfficiency mode of GLORY was 0.2.

false positive metabolite predictions. This general problem of an excess of predictions is well-documented for metabolite prediction tools (Judson, 2014). However, as mentioned above, it is important to note that the designation of predictions as false positive is particularly dataset-dependent.

As described previously, the MaxEfficiency mode uses a cutoff based on the SoM probabilities that FAME 2 predicts for each heavy atom in order to restrict the locations in the molecule at which the reaction rules are allowed to be applied. This SoM probability cutoff was set to 0.2 based on the analysis on the reference dataset; however, we also examine the effect of different SoM probability cutoffs using the high-quality test dataset in order to get a more complete picture of how much can be gained by a cutoff-based approach.

As expected, using SoM predictions to confine the application of reaction rules to certain positions does involve a trade-off between precision and recall (**Figure 4**). Recall measures the portion of known metabolites that the method was able to reproduce, and precision measures the fraction of all predicted metabolites that are actually known metabolites (see previous section for definitions). The larger the SoM probability required to be present among the atoms involved in the transformation, the lower the recall but the higher the precision as measured across the entire test dataset. In addition, the larger the SoM probability cutoff, the more parent molecules there are for which

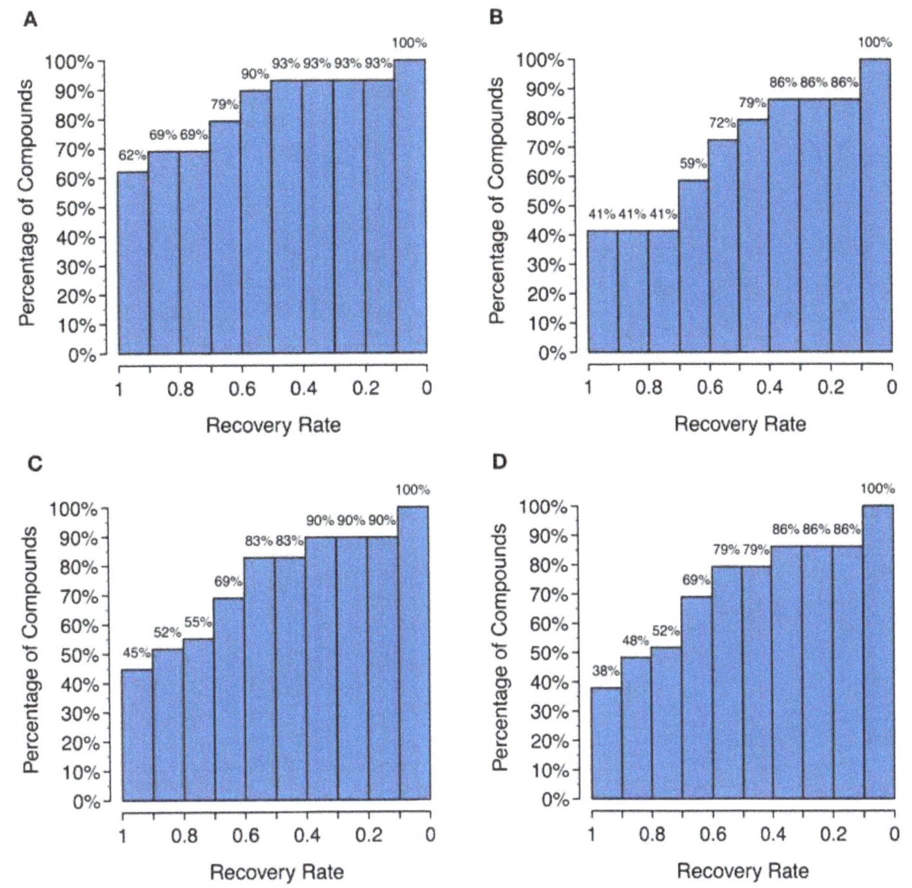

FIGURE 5 | Histograms of the recovery rate of known metabolites broken down by parent compound: **(A)** GLORY in MaxCoverage mode, **(B)** GLORY in MaxEfficiency mode, **(C)** SyGMa, **(D)** BioTransformer. For example, a recovery rate of 0.5 indicates that for x% of all parent molecules, at least half of all recorded metabolites from the test dataset were predicted.

no metabolite predictions can be made. Without any such cutoff and even up to a SoM probability cutoff of 0.2, metabolites can be predicted for all parent molecules in the test dataset. However, with a SoM probability cutoff of 0.3, no metabolites are predicted for two parent molecules, and this number increases to three for a cutoff of 0.4 (**Supplementary Table 2**). The number of molecules affected is small in this case, yet is approximately 10% of the size of the test dataset. Overall, as the cutoff increases, the total number of predicted metabolites decreases drastically (**Supplementary Table 2**).

Unfortunately, as **Figure 4** shows, there is a large decrease in recall for a small increase in precision when using SoM probability cutoffs of 0.1 or greater. Looking more closely at the recovery rates per parent molecule, we see that GLORY's MaxEfficiency mode (using the selected cutoff of 0.2 as described above) can predict at least half of the known metabolites for 72% of the parent molecules in the test dataset, as opposed to 83% for SyGMa and 79% for BioTransformer (**Figure 5**). GLORY's MaxEfficiency mode can predict all known metabolites for 41% of the parent molecules in the test dataset, as opposed to 45% for SyGMa and 38% for BioTransformer. On the other hand, the number of putative false positives per parent molecule is brought to within the same range as was measured for SyGMa and BioTransformer (**Figure 6**). Using MaxEfficiency mode, most parent molecules have fewer than 10 putative false positives, which is also the case for BioTransformer but not quite the case for SyGMa (however, as mentioned above, SyGMa's rule base also includes rules for non-CYP-mediated phase I reactions).

Based on these results, it appears that using FAME 2's predicted SoM probabilities as a hard cutoff for metabolite prediction may not be sufficient for many use cases. However, the SoM predictions are useful for more than just as a hard cutoff, namely to rank the predicted metabolites, as will be shown in the next section.

Comparison of MaxCoverage Mode to SyGMa and BioTransformer

Neither SyGMa nor BioTransformer uses regioselectivity prediction as a prefilter before applying reaction rules. The same is true of MaxCoverage mode, which only uses SoM prediction in order to score and rank the predicted metabolites. Hence, we compared SyGMa and BioTransformer to GLORY's

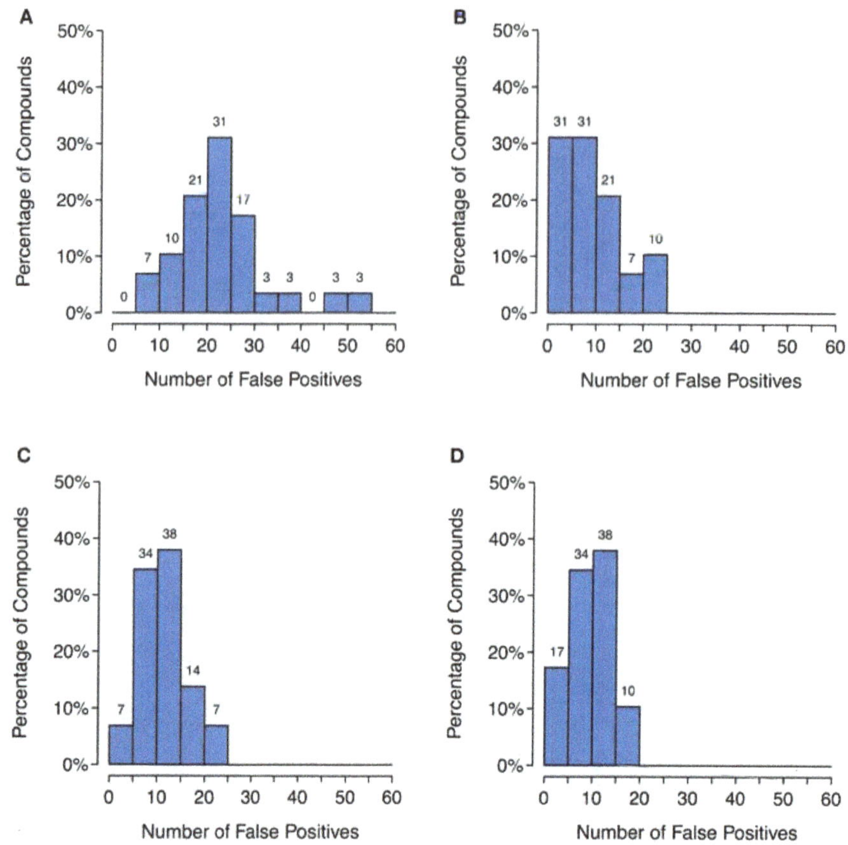

FIGURE 6 | Histograms of the number of putative false positive predictions: **(A)** GLORY in MaxCoverage mode, **(B)** GLORY in MaxEfficiency mode, **(C)** SyGMa, **(D)** BioTransformer. These histograms use right-closed intervals.

MaxCoverage mode in terms of recall, precision, and ability to rank the predicted metabolites.

A high recall is important for any use case of a metabolite structure predictor, but even more so for applications in which it is of utmost importance to not miss any physically existing metabolites, such as, for example, when attempting to identify metabolites based on MS data. GLORY's MaxCoverage mode performs well in terms of recall, with a recall of 0.83 compared to 0.74 and 0.72 for SyGMa and BioTransformer, respectively, across the entire test dataset (**Table 2**). A closer look at recall broken down to the level of the recovery rate of known metabolites for each parent molecule shows that GLORY is able to predict all known metabolites for 62% of the parent molecules, whereas SyGMa and BioTransformer achieve only 45% and 38%, respectively, in this regard (**Figure 5**). The number of parent molecules for which GLORY is able to predict at least half of the known metabolites is 90%, compared to 83% for SyGMa and 79% for BioTransformer (**Figure 5**).

Precision can be a useful metric for measuring how well a method is able to keep the number of putative false positive predictions under control. Precision was low across the board for metabolite prediction on the test dataset, with BioTransformer reaching the highest precision of the three tools at 0.17. SyGMa was close behind at 0.15, and GLORY's MaxCoverage mode lagged further behind at a precision of only 0.08 (**Table 2**). Again breaking this down to a slightly more detailed overview, we see that BioTransformer and SyGMa both always produce fewer than 25 putative false positives per parent molecule and, for the majority of parent molecules, fewer than 15 putative false positives or even, in the case of BioTransformer, fewer than 10 (**Figure 6**). GLORY in MaxCoverage mode, on the other hand, often produces so many predictions per parent molecule that there are up to 53 putative false positives per parent molecule in the test dataset and on average a relatively high number of putative false positive predictions compared to the other two tools (**Figure 6**).

In the case of the low precision observed for SyGMa, it is important to note that SyGMa's rule set is not specific to CYP-mediated metabolism but rather covers phase I metabolism in general. This could indicate that SyGMa might achieve higher precision if only the CYP-specific rules were used.

BioTransformer's CYP450 prediction module, which has the highest precision of all three methods, uses isoform prediction as a preliminary filter. Only the relevant reactions for the predicted metabolizing CYP isoform(s) are applied to the parent molecule, which could contribute to the observed precision.

Although the precision of MaxCoverage mode (as well as SyGMa and BioTransformer) was found to be low and high rates

TABLE 2 | Evaluation results for SyGMa, BioTransformer, and GLORY's MaxCoverage and MaxEfficiency modes on the manually curated test dataset.

	SyGMa	BioTransformer	GLORY, MaxCoverage mode	GLORY, MaxEfficiency mode[b]
Precision	0.15	0.17	0.08	0.16
Recall	0.74	0.72	0.83	0.64
Total number of predicted metabolites	406	344	793	327
Number of successfully predicted reported metabolites[a]	60	58	67	52
Top-1	0%	N/A	68.97%	68.97%
Top-2	48.28%	N/A	72.41%	72.41%
Top-3	68.97%	N/A	75.86%	75.86%

[a] *The total number of reported metabolites in the dataset was 81.*
[b] *The SoM probability cutoff used for MaxEfficiency mode is 0.2, chosen based on the results of the analysis on the reference dataset. Data on the performance of MaxEfficiency mode with different SoM probability cutoffs are reported in* ***Supplementary Table 2***.

of false positive predictions are problematic in general, in the case of metabolite structure predictors a low precision is only problematic if there is no way to distinguish between the true positive and putative false positive predicted metabolites. This distinction can be achieved with a well-working ranking of the predicted metabolites, which circumvents the need to reduce the total number of predicted metabolites. Hence it is important that a metabolite prediction tool can rank the predicted metabolites in terms of likelihood of occurrence.

GLORY scores its predicted metabolites based partly on the maximum SoM probability of all the atoms involved in the reaction and also takes the type of reaction into account (see above for a more detailed description of the priority score). SyGMa uses empirical probability scores calculated based on the percentage of all predictions for each reaction rule that are found in the training dataset. SyGMa's scoring system thereby relies entirely on the discontinued Metabolite dataset. The scores generated by GLORY or by SyGMa can be used to rank the predicted metabolites for a given parent compound in terms of their likelihood of occurring. The current version of BioTransformer, on the other hand, does not score or rank its predictions.

We compared the ranking capability of GLORY's MaxCoverage mode with that of SyGMa. SyGMa was able to predict a known metabolite within the top three ranked positions for 69% of the parent molecules in the test dataset, whereas GLORY's MaxCoverage mode predicted a known metabolite within the top three predictions for 76% of the parent molecules (**Table 2**).

To look at the overall quality of the scoring as well as the ranking ability of SyGMa compared to GLORY, we generated ROC curves for each method using the score of each predicted metabolite as well as the rank of each predicted metabolite for a given molecule. The rank-based analysis corresponds better to the actual use case, in which it is desired to prioritize the predicted metabolites for a particular parent molecule, as opposed to over an entire dataset [note that SyGMa was originally only evaluated in terms of ranking per parent molecule (Ridder and Wagener, 2008)]. However, we additionally used the score-based ROC curve to visualize the performance of GLORY's priority score across the whole test dataset. To better allow for comparison of the ROC curves, false negatives were included in the ROC curves and thereby in the calculated AUCs by adding those molecules to the set of data points and artificially assigning them a score of 0 or rank of 1,000, as applicable, for the purpose of this evaluation.

Though the AUC values are low, due in part to the inclusion of false negative data points in the ROC curves, the ROC curves show a much better earlier enrichment for GLORY than for SyGMa (**Figure 7**). SyGMa does not rank a known metabolite in the best-ranked position for any parent molecule in the test dataset (**Table 2**), which is reflected in the ROC curve. This decent early enrichment with GLORY, which is corroborated by the top-3 value, is a highly encouraging result indicating that the most likely predictions are closer to the top of the ranked list than the putative false positive predictions are.

One possible explanation for why SyGMa performs poorly in terms of scoring could be that its scoring scheme was derived from occurrence ratios in the Metabolite database and therefore optimized to predict the metabolites in that particular dataset. Although the Metabolite database was large, the authors of SyGMa report that the database was nevertheless biased toward compounds with one known metabolite and postulate that many of the metabolite profiles were incomplete (Ridder and Wagener, 2008). Our manually curated test dataset consists of parent molecules with metabolites that have been published since 2014, while SyGMa was developed using the 2001 version of Metabolite, so we assume that the overlap, if any, between SyGMa's training dataset and our test dataset is low. Without access to the dataset that was used to develop SyGMa's scoring methodology, it remains unclear how well the types of the reactions that lead to the metabolites in the test dataset were represented in their training dataset. Related to that, an additional downside of SyGMa's approach of basing their scoring approach on a database of metabolic reactions is that, since reaction rules can only be included if the database contains enough examples of a specific reaction type to calculate

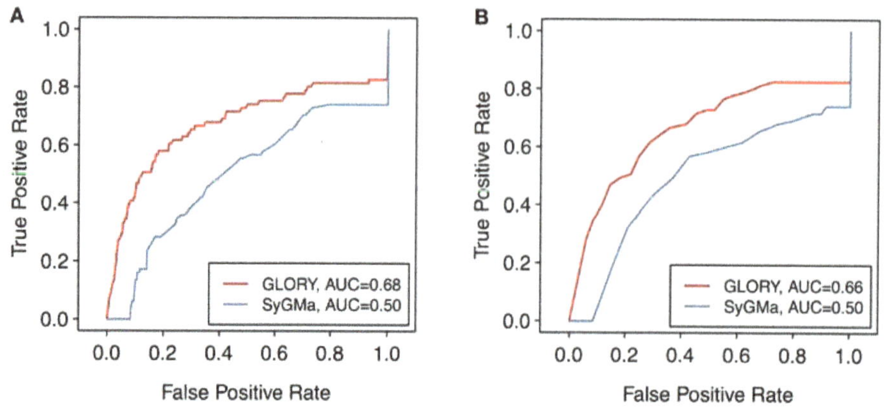

FIGURE 7 | ROC curves over the entire test dataset comparing the **(A)** scoring and **(B)** ranking approaches of SyGMa to GLORY's MaxCoverage mode. For a better comparison of the two methods, false negatives were included in the ROC curve by assigning those data points a score of 0 or rank of 1,000, as applicable.

a probability score, more unusual reaction types or reaction types that are for some reason not well enough represented in the database may be missing from SyGMa's rule base (Ridder and Wagener, 2008).

There are several other differences in methodology between GLORY and SyGMa that could contribute to the difference in performance. Firstly, SyGMa does not specifically predict CYP-mediated metabolism but rather phase I metabolism in general, meaning that it could predict other phase I metabolites that are simply not present in the test dataset because they are not formed by CYPs. Second, in the current Python package implementation that was used for this validation, SyGMa does not appear to require its predicted metabolites to have a certain minimum size. Unlike GLORY, which does not output a potential metabolite if it has fewer than three heavy atoms, SyGMa predicts a handful of metabolites (across the whole test dataset) with only one or two heavy atoms.

Computation Time

The run time for GLORY was measured on a workstation equipped with eight Intel(R) Core(TM) i7-4790 CPUs, 32 GB of main memory, and a Linux operating system. For the test dataset, the total run time (using eight cores) was 4.6 min in MaxCoverage mode and 4.3 min in MaxEfficiency mode (averaged over three runs). On average, the computation time per molecule required to predict metabolites was 10.9 s for MaxCoverage mode and 10.3 for MaxEfficiency mode (averaged over three runs).

METHODS

Development of a Collection of Transformations

A collection of transformations, defined by SMIRKS and representing reaction types, was assembled based on known CYP-mediated reactions found in the literature (see **Supplementary Material** for details). The SMIRKS were defined to be as general as possible while being restricted to reasonable reaction chemistry, as indicated by the literature and common chemical knowledge. Therefore, if a reaction was found in the literature but it was not clear how the reaction would apply to other molecules besides the provided example, the reaction was excluded from the collection. This was the case for most reactions involving large ring systems as well as ring fusions and ring contractions. Specifically, the following types of reactions were excluded from our collection: reactions that appeared to be singleton reactions, reactions involving more than two fused rings that are not part of a steroid backbone, ring fusions, ring contractions, reactions in which the substrate or product is a radical, and reactions specifically indicated to have been found only in the case of plant CYP isozymes.

A few of the SMIRKS used to describe the transformations were taken from the Toxtree SMARTCyp module[5]. Most of the SMIRKS, however, were newly developed specifically for GLORY. When developing the SMIRKS expressions, care was taken to include as few atoms as possible in the explicit mapping, since SoM probabilities were considered for all atoms in the mapping.

Each reaction type was designated as either "common" or "uncommon." Whenever possible, this label was assigned according to the reaction's classification by Guengerich in his 2001 review of CYP-mediated reactions (Guengerich, 2001), which explicitly divided the reactions into these two categories. If the reaction type was not described in that publication, a "common" or "uncommon" label was chosen based on extrapolation (on the basis of empirical similarity to reaction types present in the publication).

Our collection of CYP reaction rules consists of 61 reaction types. In some cases, multiple transformations were required to describe the same reaction type, leading to a total of 73 transformations in the collection of defined reactions. A full list of the reaction types and their SMIRKS can be found in **Supplementary Table 1**.

Metabolite Prediction Program

Predicting the structures of the metabolites involves applying the reaction rules at all relevant positions. The relevant positions

[5]Toxtree Module: SMARTCyp—Cytochrome P450-Mediated Drug Metabolism, http://toxtree.sourceforge.net/smartcyp.html

are determined by the reaction rule itself and, in the case of the MaxEfficiency mode, by the SoM probability predicted for each heavy atom. In MaxCoverage mode, the SoM probabilities are also used to score the predicted metabolites.

SoM Prediction With FAME 2

The SoM predictions were carried out using the FAME 2 software (Šícho et al., 2017), which included preprocessing of the molecules. The circCDK_ATF_6 trained model, which had the best average performance during the independent test set validation in Šícho et al. (2017), was used for the SoM prediction within GLORY.

Application of Transformations

The transformations of parent molecules into predicted metabolites based on the defined SMIRKS strings were performed using Ambit-SMIRKS [Kochev et al., 2018; Ambit-SMARTS Java Library, version 3.1.0. http://ambit.sourceforge.net/smirks.html (accessed Oct 4, 2017)]. Some transformations may result in multiple products. Products that contain fewer than three heavy atoms are not included in the set of predicted metabolites generated by GLORY.

When SoM prediction is used as a preliminary filter, a transformation rule is only applied at a particular location in the parent molecule if one of the heavy atoms involved is predicted to be a SoM with a probability over a certain threshold (see Results for more information on this threshold).

Scoring of Predicted Metabolites

The scoring of the predicted metabolites was based on SoM probability predictions and whether the reaction type was designated as common or uncommon. Each atom in the parent molecule was assigned a likelihood of being a SoM by FAME 2. When applying the transformations defined by SMIRKS, Ambit-SMIRKS maps the reactant portion of the defined transformation to any matching set of atoms in the parent molecule. Within this mapping, the maximum SoM probability was calculated and used to score the predicted metabolite that resulted from this particular transformation and mapping.

For each predicted metabolite, the priority score is calculated by multiplying the maximum SoM probability within the mapping with a factor F depending on whether the reaction type was classified as "common" or "uncommon." Priority scores for the predicted metabolites therefore range from 0 to F_{common}. The higher the score, the more likely the predicted metabolite is considered to be. See Results for further details on the selection of values for F.

If multiple transformations of a given parent molecule lead to the same metabolite structure, the priority score is calculated separately in each case and the highest score is retained. To calculate top-k values and rank-based ROC curves, it was necessary to rank the predicted metabolites for each parent molecule based on their priority scores. If different metabolites of the same parent compound have the same priority score, then they receive the same rank. In the case of a tie, one or more rank numbers, according to the number of tied predictions, following the tied rank are skipped. For example, if the highest score is 2.5 and two predicted metabolites both have this score, then both of these metabolites are assigned a rank of 1, no predicted metabolite is assigned a rank of 2, and the predicted metabolite(s) with the next highest score are assigned the rank of 3.

Program Output

The predicted metabolites are provided as an SD file with the following information for each predicted metabolite: rank (out of all predicted metabolites for a particular parent molecule), priority score, reaction name, and the InChI, SMILES, and ID of the parent molecule. If multiple transformations led to the same product, the highest priority score and the corresponding reaction name are reported. If the input consists of multiple molecules, the ID of a parent molecule is set to the molecule's position in the ordered list of input molecules (i.e., its position in the input file).

Creation of the Reference Dataset

The reference dataset was made by combining the CYP metabolism data from DrugBank and MetXBioDB. The total size of the combined reference dataset, not including any metabolism information for any of the parent molecules contained in the manually curated test dataset, is 848 parent molecules and 1588 metabolites (an average of 1.87 metabolites per parent molecule).

DrugBank Dataset

The DrugBank database (DrugBank, version 5.1.2. https://www.drugbank.ca/ [accessed Jan 14, 2019]) was downloaded from the website. In addition to the database in XML format, the structures of all of the molecules, both parents and metabolites, were downloaded in SD format from the website (drug group "All" for the parent molecules).

Any parent or metabolite molecule without an available structure was ignored. One parent compound (DrugBank ID: DB09327) was ignored because its SMILES had two components of which the main component could not be unambiguously identified. All available generations of metabolism reactions were considered, as long as the reaction was annotated as mediated by one or more CYP isozymes. The enzymes for the reactions listed in DrugBank do not have any apparent species information, so all were assumed to be human and thereby relevant for this dataset.

For all CYP-mediated reactions, the reactant was considered to be the parent molecule and the product was considered to be a first-generation metabolite of that particular parent molecule. Any metabolite with the same InChI, ignoring stereochemistry information, as its parent molecule was removed from the set of metabolites for that parent molecule. Only those parent molecules with at least one valid metabolite were included in the final dataset.

Finally, the six parent molecules that are also present in the manually curated test dataset were removed from the DrugBank dataset prior to any evaluation, along with their corresponding metabolism information. These parent compounds were bupropion, ticlopidine, imipramine, ifosfamide, bosentan, and olanzapine.

After preprocessing, including removal of the overlap with the manually curated test dataset, the DrugBank dataset contained

364 parent molecules and 702 metabolites in total, with an average of 1.93 metabolites per parent molecule in the dataset.

MetXBioDB Dataset

The human, CYP-mediated reactions were extracted from the MetXBioDB dataset (MetXBioDB, version 1.0. https://bitbucket.org/djoumbou/biotransformerjar/src/master/database/ [accessed Jan 11, 2019]). As the only structural information provided in the MetXBioDB is in the form of InChIs and InChIKeys, any substrate or product without a reported InChI could not be considered. A lacking InChI was only the case for one out of 1468 CYP-mediated, human reactions in MetXBioDB.

Stereochemistry information was removed by generating InChIs without a stereochemistry layer, resulting in 751 CYP, human parent compounds in total. Of these, 259 are also present in the DrugBank dataset. For these overlapping parent compounds, 512 of 569 DrugBank metabolites are also in MetXBioDB, and MetXBioDB has an additional 93 metabolites for these overlapping parent compounds.

Eight parent compounds (olanzapine, bupropion, metoclopramide, bosentan, imipramine, ticlopidine, ifosfamide, and atomoxetine) from the manually curated test dataset were also present in the MetXBioDB dataset, only two of which (metoclopramide and atomoxetine) were not also present in the DrugBank dataset. These parent compounds and the corresponding metabolism data were removed from the MetXBioDB dataset.

After preprocessing, including removal of the overlap with the manually curated test dataset, the MetXBioDB dataset contained 743 parent molecules and 1385 metabolites in total, with an average of 1.86 metabolites per parent molecule in the dataset.

Merger of the DrugBank and MetXBioDB Datasets

The DrugBank dataset and the MetXBioDB dataset were combined to form the reference dataset via a straightforward consolidation of the parent and metabolite information. All molecule comparisons occurred using InChIs generated without stereochemistry information. For any parent molecule that was present in both the DrugBank and the MetXBioDB datasets, which was the case for 259 parent molecules, the sets of metabolites from both datasets were combined, disregarding stereochemistry, to yield the final set of metabolites for that parent molecule in the reference dataset.

Creation of the Manually Curated Test Dataset

A new dataset for testing GLORY was manually assembled from the scientific literature. The data were extracted from publications on metabolism that were found in two journals: *Xenobiotica* and *Drug Metabolism and Disposition.* The time frame considered was from January 2014 to June 2018 for *Xenobiotica* and from January 2014 to June 2017 for *Drug Metabolism and Disposition.*

Publications were chosen and the metabolism information they contain included in the dataset if the following criteria were fulfilled:

1. The publication must contain a figure that depicts the metabolism scheme and includes the chemical structures of the parent compound and the first-generation metabolites.
2. The metabolism data must have been experimentally determined from a human source (i.e., either humans, human cells, or recombinant human CYP enzymes). If some but not all of the data were from humans, any non-human metabolites in the metabolism scheme were excluded from the dataset.
3. For at least 75% of all of the first-generation human metabolites depicted in the metabolism scheme (note that any metabolite that is depicted as merely being an intermediate is not considered), the following two criteria must be satisfied. First, the identity of the enzyme(s) responsible for the formation of the metabolite must be known. For this purpose, it is sufficient to know whether or not this metabolite is formed by CYPs. Second, the exact chemical structure, including the connectivity of all atoms, of the metabolite must be known. There is one exception to this rule: If the metabolite is known to not be CYP-formed, then the exact structure is not relevant and the metabolite is counted anyway.

Based on these criteria, 29 metabolism schemes containing at least one human, CYP-formed first-generation metabolite with a fully defined structure were found and included in the dataset. For these 29 parent molecules, there are 81 metabolites in total that fulfill the criteria (first-generation, human, CYP, fully defined structure) for inclusion in the dataset. Note that only first-generation metabolites are included in the dataset. Note also that intermediates, as depicted in the metabolism scheme, are not included in the dataset. Instead, the first non-intermediate metabolite in the pathway is used.

The SMILES for the metabolites were generated using ChemSpider (ChemSpider. http://www.chemspider.com/ [accessed Feb 13, 2019]). Consistency of stereochemistry information between parents and their metabolites was maintained.

Validation of Metabolite Structure Predictors

Predicted metabolites were compared to known metabolites from the reference and test datasets using their InChIs. The InChIs used for this comparison were generated without stereochemistry information using CDK (Willighagen et al., 2017; Chemistry Development Kit, version 2.0. https://cdk.github.io/ [accessed Nov 3, 2017]).

During the validation, a predicted aldehyde metabolite was considered equivalent to the corresponding carboxylic acid, because there is evidence that some percentage of an aldehyde metabolite acts as an intermediate that is further oxidized to a carboxylic acid without leaving the CYP enzyme active site (Bell-Parikh and Guengerich, 1999).

In the case of one parent molecule in the reference dataset, no predictions could be made because the parent molecule contains boron. FAME 2 is unable to make predictions for molecules containing boron because no boron-containing molecules were present in the dataset used to train the model.

The SyGMa predictions were carried out in Python using the SyGMa Python package (SyGMa, version 1.1.0), and RDKit (RDKit: Open-Source Cheminformatics, version 2017_03_01, 2017). Only the phase I reaction rule set was used and one reaction cycle was applied.

The BioTransformer predictions were performed using the CYP450 mode of the BioTransformer (BioTransformer, version 1.0.8. https://bitbucket.org/djoumbou/biotransformerjar/src/master/ [accessed Feb 5, 2019]) command line tool. BioTransformer was run individually for each parent compound using single SMILES input.

The ROC curves were generated using the ROCR R package (Sing et al., 2005; ROCR, version 1.0-7, 2015). When false negative data points were added to the curve, these data points were assigned a score of 0 or a rank of 1,000, respectively, depending on whether the ROC curve represented scores or ranks.

CONCLUSIONS

We have developed GLORY, a new tool for predicting the structures of human metabolites formed by CYPs. GLORY incorporates two key ideas: a literature-based collection of CYP-mediated reaction rules and SoM prediction, which was used particularly auspiciously to develop a new scoring approach for the predicted metabolites.

For GLORY, we developed a new collection of 73 reaction rules, describing 61 reaction types, for CYP-mediated metabolism. In developing this collection, we prioritized the reproducibility of our rule set and therefore based the rules on the scientific literature rather than on any dataset. In addition to the rules themselves, each reaction type was designated as either common or uncommon, again based on the scientific literature rather than on any dataset.

In addition, we have devised a priority score for predicted metabolites based on predicted SoM probabilities and the simple, literature-based distinction between common and uncommon reaction types. Hence neither our rule set nor our scoring approach is directly based on any dataset of metabolic reactions, setting our approach apart from other tools, for example SyGMa, which uses reaction rules and occurrence ratios derived from a proprietary dataset, and BioTransformer, whose rules were to some extent based on a freely available dataset.

GLORY has two modes: MaxEfficiency, which uses SoM prediction as a prefilter for the positions in a molecule at which reactions are allowed to occur, and MaxCoverage, which does not use a prefilter and instead focuses on high recall and an accurate ranking of the predicted metabolites. Using SoM prediction as a preliminary filter, i.e., in MaxEfficiency mode, does not work as well as might be expected in terms of reducing the number of putative false positive predictions while still keeping a high rate of recovery of reported metabolites. However, by developing a priority score for the predicted metabolites using SoM prediction combined with a simple binary distinction between common and uncommon reaction types, we are able to rank the metabolites predicted by MaxCoverage mode to the extent that GLORY can predict at least one known metabolite within the top three ranked positions for 76% of the molecules in the independent test set while achieving a recall of 0.83. GLORY's MaxCoverage mode outperforms both SyGMa and BioTransformer in terms of recall and outperforms SyGMa in terms of ranking (BioTransformer does not currently rank its metabolite predictions). One use case for the MaxCoverage mode could be, for example, identifying metabolites from mass spectrometry data.

Along with the collection of reaction rules, we provide a new, manually curated test dataset for free use as a benchmark dataset. In addition, GLORY is freely available as a web server at https://acm.zbh.uni-hamburg.de/glory/.

Importantly, the concept of GLORY is such that it can be extended to predict metabolites formed by enzymes not belonging to the CYP family. The enzymes that this approach can be expanded to is limited, in principle, only by the extent of the available data and the coverage of the relevant metabolic reactions by SoM prediction tools.

AUTHOR'S NOTE

The GLORY web service is available at the following address: https://acm.zbh.uni-hamburg.de/glory/.

AUTHOR CONTRIBUTIONS

CdBK and JK: conceptualization; CdBK, CS, and JK: methodology; CdBK, CS, MŠ, NK, and NJ: software development; CdBK: validation; JK and DS: resources; CdBK: data curation; all authors: writing—original draft preparation; CdBK: visualization; DS, NJ, and JK: supervision; JK: project administration; DS and JK: funding acquisition.

FUNDING

CS and JK are supported by the Deutsche Forschungsgemeinschaft (DFG, German Research Foundation)–project number KI 2085/1-1. DFG is a German research funding organization supporting research in science, engineering and the humanities. JK is also supported by the Bergen Research Foundation (BFS) [BFS2017TMT01]. BFS gives grants toward research and research supporting activities at the University of Bergen (UiB) and Haukeland University Hospital (HUS), and other Norwegian research institutions that cooperate with institutions in Bergen. The foundation also gives grants to support research at UiB and HUS at the interface between basic research and clinical research. MŠ and DS are supported by the Ministry of Education, Youth and Sports (MEYS)—project numbers MSMT No 20-SVV/2017, LM2015063 and RVO: 68378050-KAV-NPUI. MEYS is responsible for public administration in education, for developing educational, youth and sport policies and international cooperation in these fields. It is also the central administrative office responsible for research and development and one of the main public research coordinating and funding bodies of the Czech Republic.

ACKNOWLEDGMENTS

We thank Craig Knox, Michael Wilson, and David Wishart from the University of Alberta, AB, Canada and OMx Personal Health Analytics Inc., AB, Canada for sending us the structures of the metabolites in the DrugBank database prior to their being made freely available online.

SUPPLEMENTARY MATERIAL

Supplementary Tables | Reaction rules and additional evaluation results (DOCX).

Supplementary Data Sheet 1 | Test dataset containing SMILES for parent molecules and metabolites as well as publication references (CSV).

Supplementary Data Sheet 2 | Reference dataset containing SMILES (with stereochemistry information), InChI (without stereochemistry information), and DrugBank and MetXBioDB identifiers for parent molecules and metabolites (JSON).

REFERENCES

Bell-Parikh, L. C., and Guengerich, F. P. (1999). Kinetics of cytochrome P450 2E1-catalyzed oxidation of ethanol to acetic acid via acetaldehyde. *J. Biol. Chem.* 274, 23833–23840. doi: 10.1074/jbc.274.34.23833

Cruciani, G., Carosati, E., De Boeck, B., Ethirajulu, K., Mackie, C., Howe, T., et al. (2005). MetaSite: understanding metabolism in human cytochromes from the perspective of the chemist. *J. Med. Chem.* 48, 6970–6979. doi: 10.1021/jm050529c

Darvas, F. (1987). "Metabolexpert: an expert system for predicting metabolism of substances," in *QSAR in Environmental Toxicology - II*, ed K. L. E. Kaiser, (Dordrecht: Springer), 71–81.

Di, L. (2014). The role of drug metabolizing enzymes in clearance. *Expert Opin Drug Metabol. Toxicol.* 10, 379–393. doi: 10.1517/17425255.2014.876006

Djoumbou-Feunang, Y., Fiamoncini, J., Gil-de-la-Fuente, A., Greiner, R., Manach, C., and Wishart, D. S. (2019). BioTransformer: a comprehensive computational tool for small molecule metabolism prediction and metabolite identification. *J. Cheminform.* 11:2. doi: 10.1186/s13321-018-0324-5

Guengerich, F. P. (2001). Common and uncommon cytochrome P450 reactions related to metabolism and chemical toxicity. *Chem. Res. Toxicol.* 14, 611–650. doi: 10.1021/tx0002583

Judson, P. N. (2014). "Knowledge-based approaches for predicting the sites and products of metabolism," in *Drug Metabolism Prediction*, ed J. Kirchmair, Methods and Principles in Medicinal Chemistry (Weinheim: Wiley-VCH), 293–318.

Kirchmair, J., Göller, A. H., Lang, D., Kunze, J., Testa, B., and Wilson, I. D. (2015). Predicting drug metabolism: experiment and/or computation? *Nat. Rev. Drug Disc.* 14, 387–404. doi: 10.1038/nrd4581

Kirchmair, J., Williamson, M. J., Tyzack, J. D., Tan, L., Bond, P. J., Bender, A., et al. (2012). Computational prediction of metabolism: sites, products, S. A. R., P450 enzyme dynamics, and mechanisms. *J. Chem. Inform. Model.* 52, 617–48. doi: 10.1021/ci200542m

Klopman, G., Dimayuga, M., and Talafous, J. (1994). META. 1. a program for the evaluation of metabolic transformation of chemicals. *J. Chem. Inform. Comp. Sci.* 34, 1320–1325.

Kochev, N., Avramova, S., and Jeliazkova, N. (2018). Ambit-SMIRKS: a software module for reaction representation, reaction search and structure transformation. *J. Cheminform.* 10:42. doi: 10.1186/s13321-018-0295-6

Marchant, C. A., Briggs, K. A., and Long, A. (2008). *In silico* tools for sharing data and knowledge on toxicity and metabolism: Derek for Windows, Meteor, and Vitic. *Toxicol. Mechanisms Methods.* 18, 177–187. doi: 10.1080/15376510701857320

Mekenyan, O. G., Dimitrov, S. D., Pavlov, T. S., and Veith, G. D. (2004). A systematic approach to simulating metabolism in computational toxicology. I. the TIMES heuristic modelling framework. *Curr. Pharmaceutical Design.* 10, 1273–1293. doi: 10.2174/1381612043452596

Olsen, L., Montefiori, M., Tran, K. P., and Jørgensen, F. S. (2019). SMARTCyp 3.0: Enhanced cytochrome P450 site-of-metabolism prediction server. *Bioinformatics.* doi: 10.1093/bioinformatics/btz037. [Epub ahead of print].

Patlewicz, G., Jeliazkova, N., Safford, R., J., Worth, A., P., and Aleksiev, B. (2008). An evaluation of the implementation of the Cramer classification scheme in the Toxtree software. *SAR QSAR Environ. Res.* 19, 495–524. doi: 10.1080/10629360802083871

Ridder, L., and Wagener, M. (2008). SyGMa: combining expert knowledge and empirical scoring in the prediction of metabolites. *Chem. Med. Chem.* 3, 821–832. doi: 10.1002/cmdc.200700312

Rudik, A., Dmitriev, A., Lagunin, A., Filimonov, D., and Poroikov, V. (2015). SOMP: web server for *in silico* prediction of sites of metabolism for drug-like compounds. *Bioinformatics* 31, 2046–2048. doi: 10.1093/bioinformatics/btv087

Rudik, A. V., Bezhentsev, V. M., Dmitriev, A. V., Druzhilovskiy, D. S., Lagunin, A. A., Filimonov, D. A., et al. (2017). MetaTox: web application for predicting structure and toxicity of xenobiotics' metabolites. *J. Chem. Inform. Model.* 57, 638–642. doi: 10.1021/acs.jcim.6b00662

Rydberg, P., Gloriam, D. E., Zaretzki, J., Breneman, C., and Olsen, L. (2010). SMARTCyp: a 2D method for prediction of cytochrome p450-mediated drug metabolism. *ACS Med. Chem. Lett.* 1, 96–100. doi: 10.1021/ml100016x

Šícho, M., de Bruyn Kops, C., Stork, C., Svozil, D., and Kirchmair, J. (2017). FAME 2: simple and effective machine learning model of cytochrome P450 regioselectivity. *J. Chem. Inform. Model.* 57, 1832–1846. doi: 10.1021/acs.jcim.7b00250

Sing, T., Sander, O., Beerenwinkel, N., and Lengauer, T. (2005). ROCR: visualizing classifier performance in R. *Bioinformatics* 21, 3940–3941. doi: 10.1093/bioinformatics/bti623

Testa, B., Pedretti, A., and Vistoli, G. (2012). Reactions and enzymes in the metabolism of drugs and other xenobiotics. *Drug Disc. Today* 17, 549–560. doi: 10.1016/j.drudis.2012.01.017

Tian, S., Djoumbou-Feunang, Y., Greiner, R., and Wishart, D. S. (2018). CypReact: a software tool for *in silico* reactant prediction for human cytochrome P450 enzymes. *J. Chem. Inform. Model.* 58, 1282–1291. doi: 10.1021/acs.jcim.8b00035

Tyzack, J. D., Hunt, P. A., and Segall, M. D. (2016). Predicting regioselectivity and lability of cytochrome p450 metabolism using quantum mechanical simulations. *J. Chem. Inform. Model.* 56, 2180–2193. doi: 10.1021/acs.jcim.6b00233

Tyzack, J. D., and Kirchmair, J. (2018). Computational methods and tools to predict cytochrome P450 metabolism for drug discovery. *Chem. Biol. Drug Design* 93, 377–386. doi: 10.1111/cbdd.13445

Willighagen, E. L., Mayfield, J. W., Alvarsson, J., Berg, A., Carlsson, L., Jeliazkova, N., et al. (2017). The Chemistry Development Kit (CDK) v2.0: atom typing, depiction, molecular formulas, and substructure searching. *J. Cheminform.* 9:33. doi: 10.1186/s13321-017-0220-4

Wishart, D. S., Feunang, Y. D., Guo, A. C., Lo, E. J., Marcu, A., Grant, J. R., et al. (2018). DrugBank 5.0: a major update to the DrugBank database for 2018. *Nucleic Acids Res.* 46, D1074–D1082. doi: 10.1093/nar/gkx1037

Zaretzki, J., Matlock, M., and Swamidass, S. J. (2013). XenoSite: accurately predicting CYP-mediated sites of metabolism with neural networks. *J. Chem. Inform. Model.* 53, 3373–3383. doi: 10.1021/ci400518g

Permissions

All chapters in this book were first published by Frontiers; hereby published with permission under the Creative Commons Attribution License or equivalent. Every chapter published in this book has been scrutinized by our experts. Their significance has been extensively debated. The topics covered herein carry significant findings which will fuel the growth of the discipline. They may even be implemented as practical applications or may be referred to as a beginning point for another development.

The contributors of this book come from diverse backgrounds, making this book a truly international effort. This book will bring forth new frontiers with its revolutionizing research information and detailed analysis of the nascent developments around the world.

We would like to thank all the contributing authors for lending their expertise to make the book truly unique. They have played a crucial role in the development of this book. Without their invaluable contributions this book wouldn't have been possible. They have made vital efforts to compile up to date information on the varied aspects of this subject to make this book a valuable addition to the collection of many professionals and students.

This book was conceptualized with the vision of imparting up-to-date information and advanced data in this field. To ensure the same, a matchless editorial board was set up. Every individual on the board went through rigorous rounds of assessment to prove their worth. After which they invested a large part of their time researching and compiling the most relevant data for our readers.

The editorial board has been involved in producing this book since its inception. They have spent rigorous hours researching and exploring the diverse topics which have resulted in the successful publishing of this book. They have passed on their knowledge of decades through this book. To expedite this challenging task, the publisher supported the team at every step. A small team of assistant editors was also appointed to further simplify the editing procedure and attain best results for the readers.

Apart from the editorial board, the designing team has also invested a significant amount of their time in understanding the subject and creating the most relevant covers. They scrutinized every image to scout for the most suitable representation of the subject and create an appropriate cover for the book.

The publishing team has been an ardent support to the editorial, designing and production team. Their endless efforts to recruit the best for this project, has resulted in the accomplishment of this book. They are a veteran in the field of academics and their pool of knowledge is as vast as their experience in printing. Their expertise and guidance has proved useful at every step. Their uncompromising quality standards have made this book an exceptional effort. Their encouragement from time to time has been an inspiration for everyone.

The publisher and the editorial board hope that this book will prove to be a valuable piece of knowledge for researchers, students, practitioners and scholars across the globe.

List of Contributors

Yaxia Yuan
Beijing National Laboratory for Molecular Sciences, State Key Laboratory for Structural Chemistry of Unstable and Stable Species, College of Chemistry and Molecular Engineering, Peking University, Beijing, China

Jianfeng Pei
Center for Quantitative Biology, Academy for Advanced Interdisciplinary Studies, Peking University, Beijing, China

Luhua Lai
Beijing National Laboratory for Molecular Sciences, State Key Laboratory for Structural Chemistry of Unstable and Stable Species, College of Chemistry and Molecular Engineering, Peking University, Beijing, China
Center for Quantitative Biology, Academy for Advanced Interdisciplinary Studies, Peking University, Beijing, China
Center for Life Sciences, Academy for Advanced Interdisciplinary Studies, Peking University, Beijing, China

Giulio Rastelli and Luca Pinzi
Department of Life Sciences, University of Modena and Reggio Emilia, Modena, Italy

J. Jesús Naveja
PECEM, School of Medicine, Universidad Nacional Autónoma de México, Mexico City, Mexico
Department of Pharmacy, School of Chemistry, Universidad Nacional Autónoma de México, Mexico City, Mexico

José L. Medina-Franco
Department of Pharmacy, School of Chemistry, Universidad Nacional Autónoma de México, Mexico City, Mexico

Matic Pavlin, Angelo Spinello and Alessandra Magistrato
National Research Council – Institute of Materials (IOM) at International School for Advanced Studies (ISAS), Scuola Internazionale Superiore di Studi Avanzati (SISSA), Trieste, Italy

Luca Gelsomino, Ines Barone, Stefania Catalano and Sebastiano Andò
Department of Pharmacy, Health and Nutrition Sciences, Centro Sanitario, University of Calabria, Rende, Italy

Nuno G. Alves, Ana I. Mata and João P. Luís
Department of Chemistry, Coimbra Chemistry Centre, University of Coimbra, Coimbra, Portugal

Rui M. M. Brito and Carlos J. V. Simões
Department of Chemistry, Coimbra Chemistry Centre, University of Coimbra, Coimbra, Portugal
BSIM Therapeutics, Instituto Pedro Nunes, Coimbra, Portugal

Gaspar P. Pinto, Ondrej Vavra, Jan Stourac David Bednar and Jiri Damborsky
Loschmidt Laboratories, Department of Experimental Biology and RECETOX, Faculty of Science, Masaryk University, Brno, Czechia
International Centre for Clinical Research, St. Anne's University Hospital Brno, Brno, Czechia

Jiri Filipovic
Institute of Computer Science, Masaryk University, Brno, Czechia

Rafael A. A. Ferreira, Thiago S. Sampaio, Celso de O. Rezende Jr. and Luiz C. Dias
Instituto de Química, Universidade Estadual de Campinas, Campinas, Brazil

Adriano D. Andricopulo, Mariana L. de Souza, Ivani Pauli, Leonardo L. G. Ferreira, Luma G. Magalhães and Renata Krogh
Laboratório de Química Medicinal e Computacional, Centro de Pesquisa e Inovação em Biodiversidade e Fármacos, Instituto de Física de São Carlos, Universidade de São Paulo, São Carlos, Brazil

Rafaela S. Ferreira
Departamento de Bioquímica e Imunologia, Universidade Federal de Minas Gerais, Belo Horizonte, Brazil

Floriane Montanari, Bernhard Knasmüller, Stefan Kohlbacher, Christoph Hillisch, Christine Baierová, Melanie Grandits and Gerhard F. Ecker
Pharmacoinformatics Research Group, Department of Pharmaceutical Chemistry, University of Vienna, Vienna, Austria

Yifei Wu, Lei Lou and Zhong-Ru Xie
Computational Drug Discovery Laboratory, School of Electrical and Computer Engineering, College of Engineering, University of Georgia, Athens, GA, United States

Yanming Chen, Yafeng Tian, Ya Gao, Fengshou Wu, Xiulian Ju and Genyan Liu
Key Laboratory for Green Chemical Process of Ministry of Education, Hubei Key Laboratory of Novel Reactor and Green Chemical Technology, School of Chemical Engineering and Pharmacy, Wuhan Institute of Technology, Wuhan, China

Xiaogang Luo
Key Laboratory for Green Chemical Process of Ministry of Education, Hubei Key Laboratory of Novel Reactor and Green Chemical Technology, School of Chemical Engineering and Pharmacy, Wuhan Institute of Technology, Wuhan, China
School of Materials Science and Engineering, Zhengzhou University, Zhengzhou, China

Hajar Sirous
Bioinformatics Research Center, School of Pharmacy and Pharmaceutical Sciences, Isfahan University of Medical Sciences, Isfahan, Iran

Giulia Chemi, Sandra Gemma, Stefania Butini and Giuseppe Campiani
Department of Biotechnology, Chemistry and Pharmacy, Department of Excellence 2018-2022, University of Siena, Siena, Italy

Zeger Debyser and Frauke Christ
Molecular Medicine, K.U. Leuven and IRC KULAK, Leuven, Belgium

Afshin Fassihi and Lotfollah Saghaie
Department of Medicinal Chemistry, Faculty of Pharmacy, Isfahan University of Medical Sciences, Isfahan, Iran

Simone Brogi
Department of Pharmacy, University of Pisa, Pisa, Italy

Margherita Brindisi
Department of Pharmacy, Department of Excellence 2018-2022, University of Naples Federico II, Naples, Italy

Gurbet Tutumlu and Berna Dogan
Computational Biology and Molecular Simulations Laboratory, Department of Biophysics, School of Medicine, Bahcesehir University, Istanbul, Turkey

Serdar Durdagi
Computational Biology and Molecular Simulations Laboratory, Department of Biophysics, School of Medicine, Bahcesehir University, Istanbul, Turkey
Neuroscience Program, Health Sciences Institute, Bahcesehir University, Istanbul, Turkey

Muge Didem Orhan
Neuroscience Program, Health Sciences Institute, Bahcesehir University, Istanbul, Turkey
Neuroscience Laboratory, Health Sciences Institute, Bahcesehir University, Istanbul, Turkey

Timucin Avsar
Neuroscience Program, Health Sciences Institute, Bahcesehir University, Istanbul, Turkey
Department of Medical Biology, Bahcesehir University, School of Medicine, Istanbul, Turkey
Neuroscience Laboratory, Health Sciences Institute, Bahcesehir University, Istanbul, Turkey

Seyma Calis
Molecular Biology, Genetics and Biotechnology Graduate Program, Istanbul Technical University, Istanbul, Turkey
Neuroscience Laboratory, Health Sciences Institute, Bahcesehir University, Istanbul, Turkey

Xingping Quan, Xiaoying Hou, Xiaofeng Gong, Yao Wu, Yuqi Zhou, Jingwei Jiang, Shengtao Yuan and Li Sun
Jiangsu Key Laboratory of Drug Screening, China Pharmaceutical University, Nanjing, China

Hongzhi Du
School of Pharmacy, Hubei University of Chinese Medicine, Wuhan, China

Lei Shi and Jingjing Xu
Henan Key Laboratory of Organic Functional Molecules and Drug Innovation, School of Chemistry and Chemical Engineering, Henan Normal University, Xinxiang, China

Xiangyu Yang and Ligong Lu
Zhuhai Interventional Medical Center, Zhuhai Precision Medical Center, Zhuhai People's Hospital, Zhuhai Hospital Affiliated with Jinan University, Zhuhai, China

Benoît Baillif and David Rouquié
Bayer SAS, Bayer CropScience, Sophia Antipolis, France

Joerg Wichard
Department of Genetic Toxicology, Bayer AG, Berlin, Germany

Oscar Méndez-Lucio
Bayer SAS, Bayer CropScience, Sophia Antipolis, France
Department of Genetic Toxicology, Bayer AG, Berlin, Germany
Bloomoon, Villeurbanne, France

Christina de Bruyn Kops and Conrad Stork
Department of Computer Science, Center for Bioinformatics (ZBH), Faculty of Mathematics, Informatics and Natural Sciences, Universität Hamburg, Hamburg, Germany

Martin Šícho
Department of Computer Science, Center for Bioinformatics (ZBH), Faculty of Mathematics, Informatics and Natural Sciences, Universität Hamburg, Hamburg, Germany
National Infrastructure for Chemical Biology, Department of Informatics and Chemistry, Faculty of Chemical Technology, University of Chemistry and Technology Prague, Prague, Czechia

Daniel Svozil
National Infrastructure for Chemical Biology, Department of Informatics and Chemistry, Faculty of Chemical Technology, University of Chemistry and Technology Prague, Prague, Czechia

Nina Jeliazkova
Ideaconsult Ltd., Sofia, Bulgaria

Nikolay Kochev
Ideaconsult Ltd., Sofia, Bulgaria
Department of Analytical Chemistry and Computer Chemistry, University of Plovdiv, Plovdiv, Bulgaria

Johannes Kirchmair
Department of Computer Science, Center for Bioinformatics (ZBH), Faculty of Mathematics, Informatics and Natural Sciences, Universität Hamburg, Hamburg, Germany
Department of Chemistry, University of Bergen, Bergen, Norway
Computational Biology Unit (CBU), University of Bergen, Bergen, Norway

Index